Clinical Immunology

Clinical Immunology

Principles and Laboratory Diagnosis

Second Edition

Catherine Sheehan, MS, CLS(NCA), SI(ASCP)
Professor
Department of Medical Laboratory Science
College of Arts and Sciences
University of Massachusetts Dartmouth
North Dartmouth, MA

with 12 contributors

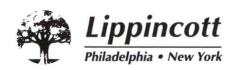
Lippincott
Philadelphia • New York

Acquisitions Editors: Kathleen P. Lyons; Lawrence McGrew
Editorial Assistant: Holly Collins
Senior Production Editor: Virginia Barishek
Production Service: P. M. Gordon Associates
Compositor: Circle Graphics
Color Separator: Chroma Graphics
Color Printer: Sheridan Press
Printer/Binder: Courier/Westford
Cover Designer: Larry Pezzato
Cover Printer: Lehigh Press

Second Edition

Cover photo credit (also Color Plates 19 and 20)—Sanofi Diagnostics Pasteur, Chaska, MN.

Library of Congress Cataloging-in-Publication Data

Clinical immunology: principles and laboratory diagnosis / Catherine Sheehan; with 12 contributors.—2nd ed.
    p.   cm.
    Includes bibliographical references and index.
    ISBN 0-397-55313-7
    1. Immunodiagnosis.   2. Clinical immunology.   I. Sheehan, Catherine.
    4. Immunologic Diseases.   QW 504 C6418 1997]
[DNLM: 1. Immune System. 2. Diagnosis, Laboratory. 3. Immunity
    RB46.5.C546   1997
616.07'56—dc21
DNLM/DLC
for Library of Congress   96-37572
                                                                                                                        CIP

Care has been taken to confirm the accuracy of the information presented and to describe generally accepted practices. However, the authors, editors, and publisher are not responsible for errors or omissions or for any consequences from application of the information in this book and make no warranty, express or implied, with respect to the contents of the publication.

The authors, editors and publisher have exerted every effort to ensure that drug selection and dosage set forth in this text are in accordance with current recommendations and practice at the time of publication. However, in view of ongoing research, changes in government regulations, and the constant flow of information relating to drug therapy and drug reactions, the reader is urged to check the package insert for each drug for any change in indications and dosage and for added warnings and precautions. This is particularly important when the recommended agent is a new or infrequently employed drug.

Some drugs and medical devices presented in this publication have Food and Drug Administration (FDA) clearance for limited use in restricted research settings. It is the responsibility of the health care provider to ascertain the FDA status of each drug or device planned for use in their clinical practice.

9 8 7 6 5 4 3 2 1

To my family and friends for their support and encouragement

Contributors

Ann C. Albers, PhD, MT(ASCP)
Chairman and Associate Professor
Department of Clinical Laboratory Sciences
School of Health and Rehabilitation Sciences
University of Pittsburgh
Pittsburgh, PA

Alice K. Chen, PhD, SC(ASCP)
Associate Professor
Department of Clinical Laboratory Sciences
School of Health and Rehabilitation Sciences
University of Pittsburgh
Pittsburgh, PA

Therese B. Datiles, MA, SI(ASCP)
Laboratory Supervisor
Diagnostic Immunology Laboratory
The Johns Hopkins Hospital
Baltimore, MD

Dorothy J. Fike, MS, MT(ASCP)SBB, CLS(NCA)
Associate Professor and Education Coordinator, Medical Technology
Department of Clinical Laboratory Sciences
Marshall University
Huntington, WV

Richard L. Humphrey, MD
Medical Director
Diagnostic Immunology Laboratory
The Johns Hopkins Hospital
Baltimore, MD

Anne E. Huot, PhD
Chairperson and Associate Professor
Department of Biomedical Technologies
University of Vermont
Burlington, VT

Karen James, PhD, MT(ASCP), Dipl. ABMLI
Consultant
Boone, NC

Ann Marie McNamara, ScD, MT(ASCP)
Director, Microbiology Division
U.S. Department of Agriculture
Food Safety and Inspection Service
Washington, DC

J. Patrick Reed, MS, MT(ASCP), SH(ASCP)
Associate Professor
Department of Biomedical Technologies
University of Vermont
Burlington, VT

Rosemarie Rumanek Romesburg, PhD, MT(ASCP)
Associate Professor
Department of Clinical Laboratory Sciences
School of Health and Rehabilitation Sciences
University of Pittsburgh
Pittsburgh, PA

Catherine Sheehan, MS, CLS(NCA), SI(ASCP)
Professor
Department of Medical Laboratory Science
College of Arts and Sciences
University of Massachusetts Dartmouth
North Dartmouth, MA

William C. Wagener, PhD, MT(ASCP)
Chairman and Associate Professor
Department of Clinical Laboratory Science
West Liberty State College
West Liberty, WV

Denise R. Zito, BS, MT(ASCP), SI(ASCP)
Operations Manager
Clinical Pathology Laboratories
University of Virginia Medical Center
Charlottesville, VA

Preface

The second edition of *Clinical Immunology: Principles and Laboratory Diagnosis* was developed for students in health-related programs and for practitioners who are interested in basic concepts of human immunology. More specifically, this book addresses the role of the clinical laboratory to provide information to diagnose and monitor disease. Although this book assumes little or no previous exposure to immunologic concepts, it does assume some understanding of related sciences, such as genetics, anatomy, physiology, microbiology, and chemistry. Experimental aspects of immunology, especially those from animal models, are minimized while immunologic principles of laboratory diagnosis of human disease are emphasized. This book is primarily intended for use by clinical laboratory science students in 2- or 4-year programs, in hospital- or campus-based programs, and in lecture or laboratory courses. This book may also be useful for clinical laboratorians who are cross-training between laboratory sections or for those returning to the laboratory workplace.

The second edition incorporates features to help the reader to understand the basic concepts and their application to human disease. These features include chapter outlines, instructional objectives, review questions, and case studies. Care has been taken to encourage easy readability. Color plates have been introduced to better show the cells, immunofluorescence, and electrophoresis. Illustrations have been revised or newly created to make visualizing and remembering relationships easier.

The text is divided into three sections. The first section is a discussion of reactions by the host in response to challenges. It addresses fundamental mechanisms of the immune system, such as antigen recognition, self versus non-self, beneficial specific and non-specific immune responses, tumor surveillance, and hypersensitivity. The second section is an in-depth discussion of antigens and antibodies and their interaction in serologic methods. Specific examples of commonly performed laboratory tests are presented following the general discussion about the method. The final section is a discussion of immunologic diseases in which measuring an immune product or reaction yields significant information for diagnosing and monitoring the disease.

Though immunology changes rapidly, all attempts have been made to ensure that the information presented is current. Equally important is the decision to include information that is widely accepted rather than speculative. The scope and depth of this book are based on two considerations. First, this book prepares the student for major national certification examinations, so the details related directly to laboratory practice must suffice for this goal. Secondly, this book is written to provide a foundation in immunology. This foundation should enable the reader to follow and understand immunology as it develops and unfolds in the future.

My sincere thanks to Jim Feeley for his expert preparation of the new and revised illustrations in the second edition. Also my appreciation to those at Lippincott–Raven Publishers, especially Andrew Allen and Holly Collins for working so cooperatively and patiently with me during the manuscript preparation. Finally, this book would not be possible if it were not for the dedication and hard work of the contributors.

Catherine Sheehan, MS, CLS(NCA), SI(ASCP)

Contents

PART I

Immunobiology

CHAPTER 1

Introduction to Immunology

Catherine Sheehan

WHAT IS IMMUNOLOGY?
ANTIGENS AND ANTIBODIES
SCOPE OF IMMUNOLOGY

Objectives

Upon completion of the chapter, the reader will be able to:

1. Define immunology, antigen, hapten, antibody, immunoglobulin, and immune complex
2. Compare and contrast innate and adaptive immunity
3. Given an example of immunity, classify it as innate or adaptive
4. Given an example of immunity, classify it as cellular or humoral
5. Classify an example of specific immune response as active, passive, or adoptive immunity

WHAT IS IMMUNOLOGY?

Immunology is the study of mechanisms that protect an individual from injury. The injury or challenge can result from exogenous microorganisms (e.g., bacteria, viruses, or fungi), exogenous chemicals (e.g., pollen, dander, or poison ivy), or endogenous cells (e.g., malignant or senescent cells). Collectively these mechanisms are the immune response and constitute a broad range of defense mechanisms, including inflammation, phagocytosis, antibody synthesis, and effector T lym-

phocytes. In addition to defense, the immune system monitors the cells of the host to detect and eliminate neoplastic cells and maintains homeostasis by removing normal dying cells.

The immune system is a complex, highly regulated set of processes that require the host to detect changes in host cells or undesirable exogenous cells. The goals of the immune response are to protect an individual from challenge and to restore homeostasis. These goals require the immune system to recognize offending challenges, to respond immediately or with some delay and then to repair the site. Some mechanisms primarily rely on cell-cell interactions, whereas others are mediated by humoral substances (soluble chemicals secreted by cells). Two types of immunity, innate and adaptive, have evolved and work together to provide human defense to diverse challenges. Figure 1-1 illustrates the sources of challenges and a model of host response.

Innate or nonspecific immune mechanisms are present from birth in all individuals, and once activated the same mechanism occurs regardless of which challenge is encountered or previous exposure. On the other hand, adaptive immunity is acquired or developed by an individual *only* after a specific challenge is encountered. The resulting adaptive immune products are effective only against the specific challenge. Also, immunologic memory in adaptive immunity provides greater efficiency should there be subsequent exposure to the same challenge.

Innate immunity is the first defense against exogenous challenging organisms. The mechanisms are nonspecific, that is, there is no discrimination between different challenges. Once the challenge is encountered, nonspecific immunity begins immediately. The physical

3

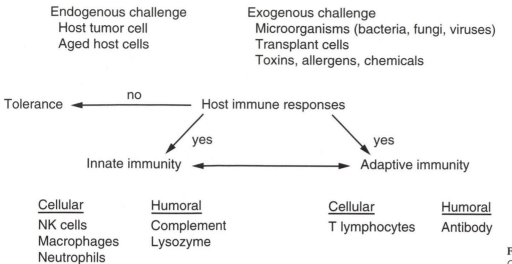

FIGURE 1-1
Overview of immune responses.

barrier of the skin and mucous membranes, for example, provides the first line of defense from invading organisms by preventing their entry into the host. Innate immunity also depends on the species, race or strain, and sex. For example, humans demonstrate natural resistance to dog distemper and viral feline leukemia, whereas dogs are resistant to anthrax, which can infect humans. Variation in susceptibility to some infectious diseases is related to race. African Americans and Native Americans are more susceptible to tuberculosis, while Caucasians are more susceptible to influenza and diphtheria.

Physiologic innate immunity reduces the likelihood of infection by providing an unfavorable environment for the infective organism: The acidity of the stomach destroys most ingested organisms, the tearing action of the eye flushes foreign material from the eye, the flow of urine prevents bacterial infection of the lower urinary tract, and the cilia and mucus of the respiratory tract remove particulate matter that enters from the air. Age and nutritional status also influence innate immunity. Children and the elderly are more susceptible to certain infections, such as *Escherichia coli* sepsis in the newborn and *Streptococcus pneumoniae* pneumonia in older people. Poor nutrition and alcohol may suppress the immune system.

Chemicals secreted by cells also contribute to innate immunity. Lysozyme, an enzyme found in secretions, disrupts the cell wall of bacteria and kills the organism. Skin secretions, such as lactic acid and saturated fatty acids, provide resistance to some bacteria and fungi. Mucoprotein in secretions prevents attachment of some viruses to cells, and thus prevents the virus from entering the cell. Interferon interrupts viral replication.

The two major physiologic processes in innate immunity are phagocytosis and inflammation. Phagocy-

tosis is the engulfment of particulate material by a cell. Neutrophils and macrophages are the most phagocytic cells of the immune system. The engulfed material is usually killed, digested, and thus eliminated, causing no further threat to the host. Inflammation is a series of events that promote changes in the vasculature, movement of cells to an affected area, cell responses to eliminate the challenge, and repair of tissue damage.

When innate immunity is insufficient to protect the individual from a challenge, adaptive or specific immune mechanisms are stimulated. These mechanisms are dormant until stimulated. An initial specific immune response requires time to activate cells and to synthesize immune products, such as antibody and cytokines. This is thus an acquired response. The adaptive immune response develops immune products that are specific for the challenge and immunologic memory that will result in a more intense and faster immune response on re-exposure to the challenge. The diversity of the specific immune response is shown by the ability of the system to synthesize multiple antibodies to one microorganism; to synthesize different antibody classes (such as IgG and IgM) against one microorganism; to synthesize antibodies against membrane components, intracellular products, and secreted products of cells; and to activate different cells to respond directly or to be mediated by cytokines.

The two major arms of effective specific immunity are humoral immunity and cell-mediated immunity. While historically these are quite distinct, current knowledge suggests that each time adaptive immunity is activated, both arms are activated. It becomes a matter of the degree to which each arm is activated.

Adaptive immunity may be classified based on the host's role in developing the adaptive specific immunity.

- Active immunity is generated when an immunocompetent host is exposed to the foreign challenge and the host's native immune cells respond by generating specific immune products.
- Passive immunity is bestowed to the host when preformed immune products are administered to the host.
- In adoptive immunity, immunocompetent cells are transplanted to an immunoincompetent host to restore the immune system.

Although the physiologic mechanisms are the same regardless of the type of adaptive immunity, it is the source of immune cells and products that determines if the adaptive response is active, passive, or adoptive. Table 1-1 is a summary of the types of immunities.

Active immunity requires the host's immune cells to interact with the stimulating challenge. The host will produce antibodies, sensitized lymphocytes, and cytokines. These immune products eliminate the stimulating agent and usually provide lifelong immunity. Active immunity requires competent host lymphocytes to generate immune products that are specific for the challenge. This process may take weeks to develop. Exposure to the stimulating agent may occur from natural infection or from immunization. Ideally, if an individual is infected with the live rubella virus or is immunized with the live attenuated rubella virus, the result should be the same—the stimulation of humoral and cellular adaptive mechanisms to protect the host from subsequent rubella virus infection. Often this protection is lifelong.

Passive immunity occurs when immune products, most often antibody preparations known as immune or gamma globulin, are administered to an individual. In this way, the antibody is immediately available to protect the individual. This is especially important when an individual is accidentally exposed to a challenge, such as hepatitis B virus. To prevent the morbidity and mortality associated with hepatitis B infection, immune globulin rich in hepatitis B antibodies is administered immediately and is able to prevent the hepatitis B virus from infecting the host. Thus the host receives protective antibody yet is not required to synthesize antibody.

TABLE 1-1
Types of Immunity

Innate (nonspecific)
Adaptive (specific)
    Active
    Passive
    Adoptive

The antibody will gradually be catabolized, thus providing only short-term protection.

Adoptive immunity is reserved for immunodeficient individuals or individuals rendered immunoincompetent. When immunocompetent cells or tissue are transplanted into an immunoincompetent individual, the cells or tissue can reconstitute the immune system. This allows the individual to actively respond to future challenges.

One way to evaluate specific humoral immune activation is by measuring the quantity of antibody secreted. B lymphocytes and plasma cells synthesize antibodies that specifically recognize and bind to a challenge. Antibody is especially effective in eliminating bacteria by enhancing phagocytosis.

Evidence of specific cell-mediated immune activation is evaluated by measuring the number and type of immune cells present in tissue and by measuring specific cytokines. T lymphocytes produce these cytokines and direct the cellular traffic and activation in response to aberrant host cells, transplanted cells, and foreign organisms. The cell-mediated response is especially effective in eliminating viruses, fungi, mycobacteria, tumor cells, and tissue grafts.

ANTIGENS AND ANTIBODIES

A general description of some terms in the context of immunology may be useful background. The term *challenge* has been used to signify any cell or substance that is capable of stimulating the nonspecific immune response, specific immune response, or both. In immunologic terminology, the challenge is an antigen. An antigen initiates immune mechanisms that result in immune products that can react with the antigen. In conventional thinking, antigens are exogenous, harmful substances that the body will try to eliminate. However, increasing attention is paid to endogenous self-antigens and their roles in tolerance and regulation.

Haptens are substances that react with products of the immune system but cannot initiate an immune response. Usually these are small molecules that fail to trigger a response.

The major immune product, antibody, is also known as immunoglobulin. Antibodies are protein molecules that are present in secretions and plasma. These proteins are bifunctional; one end of the molecule (Fab) is able to recognize and bind to the antigen, while the other end of the antibody (Fc) establishes the biologic properties of the antibody class. Thus differences in antibody class (IgG, IgM, IgA, IgE, and IgD) are set by the Fc portion of the antibody molecule. All antibodies of the same class share these properties, such as the ability to cross the placenta or to bind complement. Clinically, both the class and specificity of antibody are important.

When antigen binds to antibody, an immune or antigen-antibody complex is formed. Immune complexes vary in size based on the number of antigen and antibody molecules interacting. They may cause in vivo host damage (immune complex–mediated glomerulonephritis) or may be constructed in vitro to measure the concentration of an analyte by immunoassay.

SCOPE OF IMMUNOLOGY

Immunology is divided into 11 main areas of study, which will be addressed in the remaining chapters.[1] Allergy and hypersensitivity refer to deleterious effects of exaggerated immune responses that harm the host. Autoimmunity is the failure of the immune system to tolerate "self" or immune reactions directed against "self." Cancer immunology is the study of tumor antigens and the immunologic response to tumors. Cellular immunology investigates lymphocytes and lymphoid organs involved in the immune response. Immunochemistry studies immunoassays and antigen-antibody interactions. Immunogenetics is primarily concerned with the genetic control of immune responses, especially the major histocompatibility complex. Immunohematology is the study of blood groups, the genetic variation in blood cell antigens. Immunopathology is the study of organ damage by immune products or processes. Microbial immunology studies the antigens of bacteria, viruses, and other parasites and the development of vaccines. Molecular immunology analyzes the structure of antigens, antibodies, cytokines, and complement. Transplantation investigates tissue typing, graft rejection, and immunologic tolerance.

Review Questions

1. Which type of immunity does not require discrimination between different challenges?

   a. innate
   b. adaptive

2. Which form of immunity has memory?

   a. innate
   b. adaptive

3. Which cell most effectively eliminates transplanted cells?

   a. macrophage
   b. neutrophil
   c. T lymphocyte
   d. plasma cell

4. The hepatitis B virus vaccine was administered to a new hospital employee. Which type of immunity is expected to develop and provide long-term protection?

   a. active
   b. passive
   c. adoptive
   d. innate

5. Which form of immunity provides immediate yet short-lived protection?

   a. active
   b. passive
   c. adoptive
   d. cellular

6. A substance that induces an immune response is called a(n)

   a. antigen
   b. hapten
   c. antibody
   d. immune complex

7. The properties of an antibody class are defined by the

   a. size of the immune complex
   b. nature of the stimulating antigen
   c. Fab end of the molecule
   d. Fc end of the molecule

Reference

1. Nicholas R, Nicholas D: Immunology: An Information Profile, p 11. London, Mansell Publishing, 1985.

CHAPTER 2

Cells and Tissues of the Immune System

Dorothy J. Fike

CELLS OF THE IMMUNE SYSTEM
  Myeloid Cells
  Lymphocytes
  Accessory Cells
  Cytokines
ORGANS AND TISSUES OF THE IMMUNE SYSTEM
  Primary Lymphoid Organs
  Secondary Lymphoid Organs

Objectives

Upon completion of the chapter, the reader will be able to:

1. List the cells associated with the immune system
2. Discuss the function of each cell in the immune system
3. Compare and contrast between primary and secondary lymphoid organs
4. Discuss the functions of the lymphatic system and spleen
5. State the general organization found in the lymph node and spleen, and the predominant cells in each area
6. Trace the route of the lymphocyte circulation through a lymph node
7. For each cytokine discussed, state the predominant cell source and its primary function

CELLS OF THE IMMUNE SYSTEM

The diversity of cells of the immune system reflects the diversity of mechanisms of the specific and non-specific immune responses. Some cells originate from pluripotent stem cells in the bone marrow; others do not. Some cells travel throughout the body via the peripheral blood, whereas others are fixed in a tissue. Some cells require the presence of other cells or soluble mediators to be functional and others work independently. Immune system cells derived from pluripotent stem cells follow two cell lines: myeloid and lymphoid. Mature myeloid cells are monocytes, macrophages, and granulocytes; mature lymphoid cells are T cells, B cells, and large granular lymphocytes. Other cells to be discussed include antigen-presenting cells (dendritic cells and Langerhans cells) and mast cells.

Myeloid Cells

Myeloid cells are responsible for nonspecific immune responses. After leaving the bone marrow, these cells circulate in the peripheral blood and may enter tissue as needed.

MONOCYTES AND MACROPHAGES

Monocytes are approximately 4% to 10% of the nucleated cells in the blood. The monocyte has a diameter of 12 to 16 μm, a horseshoe-shaped nucleus, and cytoplasmic neutrophilic granules (Fig. 2-1; Color Plate 1). When monocytes migrate into tissue, the cell becomes larger, the granules are more prominent, and the cellular metabolism increases.[1] The monocyte is now a tissue macrophage. Macrophages have two important functions in the immune system: phagocytosis of particulate material and presentation of antigen to a T cell to initiate a specific immune response. The phagocytic process

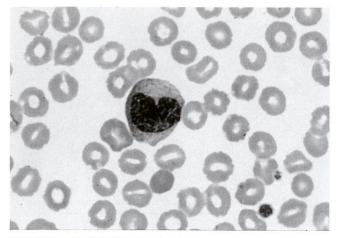

FIGURE 2-1 (COLOR PLATE 1)
Monocytes are found in the peripheral blood. When they migrate to the tissue, changes occur in their size and cytoplasm, and the cell is known as a macrophage. (From Lotspeich-Steininger CA, Steine-Martin EA, Koepke JA. Clinical hematology. Philadelphia, JB Lippincott, 1992.)

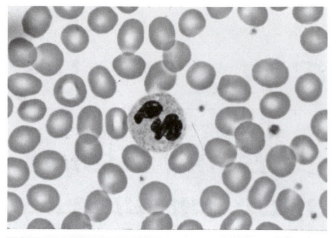

FIGURE 2-2 (COLOR PLATE 2)
The granules of the neutrophil are small. The nucleus of a mature neutrophil is segmented into three or more lobes. (From Lotspeich-Steininger CA, Steine-Martin EA, Koepke JA. Clinical hematology. Philadelphia, JB Lippincott, 1992.)

is nonspecific so that particles are ingested and eliminated without discrimination. Antigen presentation by macrophages begins the T-cell–dependent process to activate other T cells and B cells to eliminate the antigen via mechanisms of the specific immune response. Macrophages express surface receptors, including major histocompatibility complex (MHC) Class II molecules, complement receptors, and immunoglobulin (Fc) receptors on their surface, which aid in phagocytosis and antigen presentation.[2,3]

GRANULOCYTES

Granulocytes share a common lineage and have granules; cytoplasmic differences result in unique staining characteristics. Cells include neutrophils, eosinophils, and basophils. A mature cell has a diameter of 10 to 15 μm, contains a multilobed nucleus, has many cytoplasmic granules, and can migrate into surrounding tissues. Polymorphonuclear granulocytes have an important role in acute inflammation.

Neutrophils

Neutrophils, approximately 70% of the nucleated cells in the blood, contain cytoplasmic azurophilic granules (Fig. 2-2; Color Plate 2), which store enzymes such as hydrolase, myeloperoxidase, and muraminidase. These cells are very phagocytic and express complement (CD11b, CD35) and immunoglobulin (Fc, CD16) receptors on their cell surface.[1] CD (clusters of differentiation) is standardized nomenclature to describe antigenic expression by leukocytes that are identified by monoclonal antibody.

Eosinophils

Usually 2% to 5% of the circulating leukocytes are eosinophils. In allergic individuals this percentage may be increased. The cytoplasm of the eosinophil contains yellowish-red granules when stained with

Wright's stain. Eosinophils kill helminths by releasing the granular contents into the extracellular space. They also regulate the IgE-mediated response by releasing mediators (histaminase and aryl sulfatase), which inactivate the IgE-mediated allergic response (Fig. 2-3; Color Plate 3).[2,3]

Basophils

Basophils are myeloid cells with large, coarse granules that stain deep violet blue when stained with basophilic dyes. These granules contain histamine and other vasoactive amines. Unlike other granulocytic cells, the basophil expresses surface receptors for IgE only. When the IgE molecule crosslinks this surface receptor, the basophil releases the granular contents, which causes an allergic reaction to occur. Basophils are 0.5% to 1% of the circulating leukocytes (Fig. 2-4; Color Plate 4).[3]

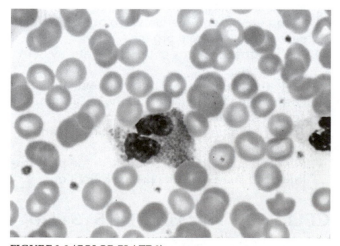

FIGURE 2-3 (COLOR PLATE 3)
The eosinophil is a granulocyte. Note that the granules of this cell are stained red and the nucleus is segmented into two lobes. (From Lotspeich-Steininger CA, Steine-Martin EA, Koepke JA. Clinical hematology. Philadelphia, JB Lippincott, 1992.)

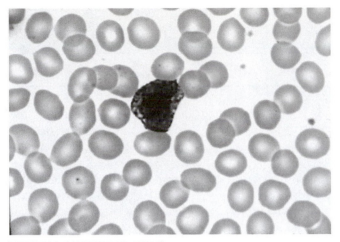

FIGURE 2-4 (COLOR PLATE 4)
The basophil is a granulocytic cell. The granules of this cell stain with basic dyes and are larger than the granules of neutrophils and eosinophils. The granules obscure the nucleus of the cells. (From Lotspeich-Steininger CA, Steine-Martin EA, Koepke JA. Clinical hematology. Philadelphia, JB Lippincott, 1992.)

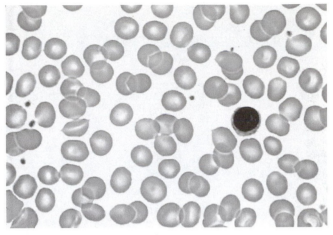

FIGURE 2-5 (COLOR PLATE 5)
Lymphocytes vary in size. A small lymphocyte that contains very little cytoplasm is shown. (From Lotspeich-Steininger CA, Steine-Martin EA, Koepke JA. Clinical hematology. Philadelphia, JB Lippincott, 1992.)

LYMPHOCYTES

Lymphocytes are produced in the bone marrow, are approximately 20% to 30% of peripheral blood leukocytes, and have a long life span. Lymphocytes may be classified according to size: Small lymphocytes have a diameter of 8 to 10 μm, with a high nuclear to cytoplasm (N/C) ratio. These small lymphocytes also lack cytoplasmic granules (Fig. 2-5; Color Plate 5). Small lymphocytes are divided into two different types, T and B lymphocytes, based on function. A third type, large granular lymphocytes (LGL), has a diameter of up to 16 μm, a smaller N/C ratio than small lymphocytes, and contains granules.

B Lymphocytes

B lymphocytes comprise approximately 5% to 15% of all circulating lymphocytes and express surface immunoglobulin (sIg) (Fig. 2-6). sIg is produced by the cell and serves as the receptor for a specific antigen. The surface immunoglobulin on the majority of cells in the peripheral blood is monomeric IgM and IgD. Some B cells also express immunoglobulins of another class. In mucosal-associated lymphoid tissue, the majority of the B cells express IgA on their membrane. Other surface markers include immunoglobulin Fc receptors (CD16), complement receptors (CD11b, CD35), and MHC Class II molecules. Monoclonal antibodies have identified other glycoproteins: CD19, CD20, and CD21 (Table 2-1 on p. 10).[1,3]

B-Lymphocyte Differentiation. B cells develop from committed lymphocytes under the influence of a special microenvironment. B lymphocytes differentiate in utero in the fetal liver, and later in the bone marrow. Bone marrow differentiation of B cells con-

tinues after birth. B-cell maturation occurs in two stages: antigen independent and antigen dependent (Fig. 2-7). Antigen-independent maturation begins when a stem B cell, which does not express immunoglobulin products, undergoes a series of cell divisions with immunoglobulin gene rearrangements to become a pre-B cell. The pre-B cell is a large lymphoblast that expresses IgM heavy chains in the cytoplasm (but not on the surface) and MHC Class II molecules and complement receptors (CD11b, CD35) on the surface. When the pre-B cell matures into the B cell, cytoplasmic μ heavy chains are no longer present but surface IgM and IgD are expressed.[1,3]

When a specific antigen is introduced to the B cell, further changes occur. There is cell activation, prolifer-

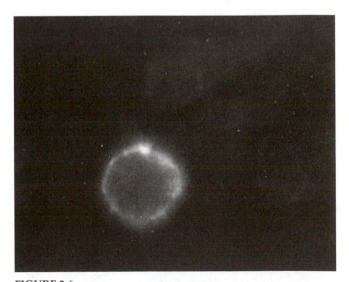

FIGURE 2-6
B cell stained to detect surface immunoglobulin. The majority of the membrane contains surface immunoglobulin.

TABLE 2-1
T- and B-Lymphocyte Markers

CD DESIGNATION	MOLECULAR WEIGHT	CELLULAR DISTRIBUTION	COMMENTS
CD1a	49 kDa	Thymocytes	
CD1b	45 kDa	Thymocytes	Also expressed on Langerhans cells
CD1c	43 kDa	Thymocytes	Also expressed on dendritic cells
CD2	50 kDa	All T cells, some NK cells	Associated with SRBC-receptor
CD3	19, 25 kDa	All T cells	Associated with T-cell antigen receptor
CD4	55 kDa	T_H cells	Receptor for MHC Class II molecule
CD8	32, 36 kDa	$T_{S/C}$ cells, some NK cells	Receptor for MHC Class I molecule
CD11b	165 kDa	NK cells, monocytes, granulocytes	Complement receptor 3 (CR3) alpha chain
CD16	50–65 kDa	NK cells, monocytes	Fc receptor
CD19	95 kDa	B cells	
CD20	35, 37 kDa	B cells	
CD21	140 kDa	Mature B cells	Complement receptor 2 (CR2) (C3d receptor)
CD35	160–260 kDa	B cells, some NK cells, monocytes, granulocytes	Complement receptor 1 (CR1)
CD56	135, 220 kDa	NK cells, some T cells	CAM associated

SRBC, sheep red blood cell; CAM, cell adhesion molecule

ation, and differentiation into plasma cells that synthesize and secrete specific immunoglobulins. The plasma cell expresses cytoplasmic immunoglobulin but does not express surface immunoglobulin, MHC Class II molecules, or CD19, CD20, and CD21 found on B lymphocytes (Fig. 2-8).[1,3]

T Lymphocytes

Most circulating lymphocytes (80%) are T cells that have two immunologic functions: effector and regulatory. Effector functions include cytolysis of virally infected cells, tumor targets, and lymphokine production. The regulatory function is accomplished by the ability

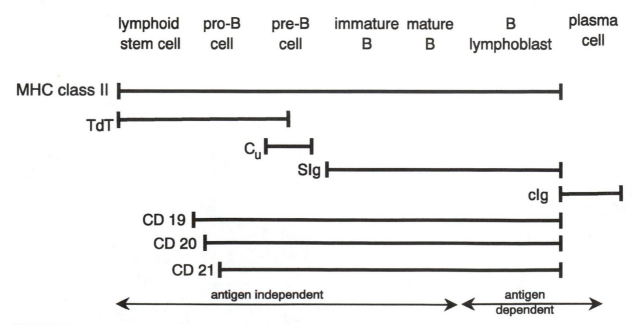

FIGURE 2-7
Stages of B-cell differentiation. Surface immunoglobulin appears during antigen-independent differentiation. Cytoplasmic immunoglobulin (CIg) appears when antigen is processed by the cell. Notice that surface Ig disappears when CIg appears.

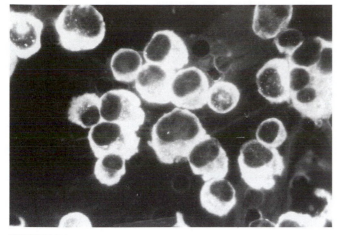

FIGURE 2-8
Plasma cells showing cytoplasmic immunoglobulin by direct immunofluorescence. Note the increase in cytoplasm compared with that in small lymphocytes.

of T cells to increase or suppress other lymphocytes and accessory cells. The classical T-cell surface marker, CD2, is the sheep red blood cell (SRBC) receptor. When T cells are incubated with SRBC, the SRBCs bind to T cells and form rosettes. In addition to CD2, all circulating T cells express CD3, which is associated with the T-cell antigen receptor complex. Two subsets of T cells express different CD markers and are functionally distinct. Helper T cells express the CD4 and suppressor T cells express the CD8.[1,3]

T-Lymphocyte Differentiation. The pre-T cells differentiate in the fetal liver or bone marrow. Pre-T cells migrate to the thymus, which provides the microenvironment for further T-cell maturation; lymphocytes in the thymus are also known as thymocytes (Fig. 2-9). The pre-T cell contains an enzyme, terminal deoxynucleotidyl transferase (TdT), in the nucleus, that is a marker for primitive T cells. Maturation in the cortex of the thymus results in CD2 and CD3 expression on the surface of the cell. As maturation progresses and while the cell is still in the cortex, CD4 and CD8 mole-

cules are coexpressed on the cell membrane. Thus, four CD molecules are located on the cell membrane: CD2, CD3, CD4, and CD8. When the immature T cell migrates into the thymus medulla, either the CD4 or CD8 molecule is lost. At this stage TdT is no longer produced by the T cell. Approximately 90% of the pre-T cells that migrate to the thymus die in the thymus and never become mature T cells. Cells with receptors that recognize self-antigens do not survive, while cells with receptors that recognize foreign antigens mature. Thus, one of the major outcomes of thymic differentiation is the ability to recognize self. This is important in cell interactions of the immune response.[2,4]

Large Granular Lymphocytes

A third population of lymphocytes described by its appearance in peripheral blood is the large granular lymphocytes (LGL). These cells are slightly larger than resting T or B cells, have cytoplasmic granules, and do not consistently express T- or B-cell markers. Some LGL are natural killer (NK) cells; others may be activated T lymphocytes. NK cells express CD2, CD16, and CD56. NK cells act to lyse virally infected cells, tumor cells, and allogeneic transplant cells without antibody, complement, MHC restriction, and generation of memory. NK cells also participate in antibody-dependent cell-mediated cytolysis (ADCC).[2]

ACCESSORY CELLS

Accessory cells contribute to an immune response by supporting, augmenting, or enabling physiologic mechanisms to occur. An important class of cells, the antigen-presenting cells (APCs) are necessary to initiate a specific immune response. In addition to macrophages, dendritic cells and Langerhans cells are essential for proper antigen presentation. Both express MHC Class II molecules and other markers (CD1a, CD1b, CD1c). The origin of these cells, the specificity for identifying these cells, and their longevity within a tissue site are unknown at this time. Langerhans cells are cells of the dermis and epidermis that play a critical

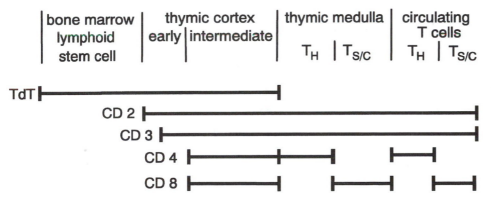

FIGURE 2-9
T-cell maturation occurs in both the bone marrow and thymus. When TdT appears in the cell, all of the T cells have the same surface markers. When TdT is no longer present, the T cells have differentiated into T_H and $T_{S/C}$ lymphocytes with different cell surface markers.

role in immune surveillance in the skin. Dendritic cells, so named because of their morphology, appear as cells with long, filamentous cytoplasmic projections in the lymphoid organs. Dendritic cells form an extensive web for trapping of antigen while allowing other cells to move and interact.[1,5]

The mast cell originates in the mesenchymal connective tissue. The IgE receptors on its surface allow crosslinking of IgE to release granular contents, causing an allergic reaction. This is the same allergic reaction mediated by basophils. The contents of the granules are the same in both cells, but mast cell granules are smaller and more plentiful. The mast cell membrane is less regular than that of a basophil.[1] Table 2-2 compares all cell types in the immune system.

CYTOKINES

Active research has led to a rapid increase in the number of known cytokines. Detecting blood levels of cytokines is useful for evaluating immune activation. The four major groups of cytokines are colony stimulating factors (CSF), interferons (IFN), tumor necrosis factors (TNF), and interleukins (IL). A partial list of cytokines is presented in Table 2-3.

Colony Stimulating Factors
Colony stimulating factors (CSF) cause the proliferation and differentiation of immature bone marrow cell. Granulocyte CSF (G-CSF) stimulates the growth of mature granulocytes while macrophage CSF (M-CSF) stimulates the growth of monocyte/macrophage colonies. Granulocyte-macrophage (GM-CSF) stimulates the formation of both mature granulocytes and monocyte/macrophage colonies.[3,6,7]

Interferons
Interferons are glycoproteins produced in response to viral infections, immune stimulation, or chemical stimulators. There are three types of interferon: interferon α (IFNα), produced by leukocytes; interferon β (IFNβ), produced by fibroblasts; and interferon γ (IFNγ), produced by T cells. IFNα and IFNβ are antiviral proteins that inhibit viral replication, increase the expression of MHC Class I molecules on virally infected cells, and activate NK cells. IFNα and IFNβ inhibit viral replication by interfering with viral RNA and ultimately protein production. Enhanced expression of MHC Class I molecules on virally infected cells increases the ability to present viral antigen associated with MHC Class I molecules to cytotoxic T cells. Cytotoxic T cells and activated NK cells can kill the virally infected cell.[8,9]

In addition to its antiviral effects, IFNγ regulates the specific immune response. The most important function of IFNγ is to activate macrophages and to increase the expression of MHC Class I and Class II molecules on activated macrophages and other cells. NK cells are activated, and activated B cells are stimulated to secrete antibody.[8,9]

TABLE 2-2
Cells Involved in the Immune Response

CELLS	FUNCTION	CELL SURFACE MOLECULES
Monocyte/macrophage	Phagocytosis/APC	MHC Class II, CR, Fc receptor
GRANULOCYTES		
Neutrophils	Phagocytosis Inflammation	Fc receptor, CD11b, CD35
Eosinophils	Allergies Helminth destruction	
Basophils	Allergic reactions	IgE receptors
LYMPHOCYTES		
T cells	Cellular immunity helper/cytotoxic or suppressor functions	MHC Class II (activated) CD2, CD3, and CD4 CD2, CD3, and CD8
B cells	Antibody formation	sIg, Fc receptor, MHC Class II, CR
Large granular	Natural killing	CD2, CD16
OTHER		
Mast cells	Allergic reactions	IgE receptors
Langerhans cells	APC in skin	MHC Class II, CD1
Dendritic cells	APC in lymphoid tissue	MHC Class II, CD1

APC, antigen-presenting cells; CR, complement receptor

TABLE 2-3
Some Cytokines Produced by Cells

CYTOKINE	PRODUCED BY	FUNCTION
IL-1	Monocytes, dendritic cells, fibroblasts	Immunoregulation, inflammation, fever
IL-2	T cells, NK cells	Proliferation, activation of T and B cells, macrophage production of TNF and interferon α
IL-3	T cells	Colony stimulating factor
IL-4	T cells	Proliferation and differentiation of T and B cells
IL-5	T cells	Differentiation of B cells and eosinophils
IL-6	Macrophages, T cells	Differentiation, acute phase protein synthesis
TNFα	Macrophages, lymphocytes	Inflammation, kills cells, production of adhesion molecules
TNFβ	Macrophages, lymphocytes	Same as TNFα
IFNα	Leukocytes	Antiviral
IFNβ	Fibroblasts	Antiviral
IFNγ	T cells, NK cells	Immunoregulation, antiviral
GM-CSF	Macrophage	Proliferation of granulocyte and monocyte colonies
G-CSF	Macrophage, fibroblasts	Proliferation of granulocyte colonies
M-CSF	Fibroblasts, activated T and B cells	Proliferation of monocyte colonies

Tumor Necrosis Factors

There are two tumor necrosis factors, α and β. TNFα is produced by macrophages, monocytes, lymphocytes, and NK cells in response to bacterial lipopolysaccharides, viruses, tumor cells, bacterial toxins, a complement component (C5a), and bacterial, fungal, and parasitic toxins. TNFα can kill some human tumor cell lines and helps to regulate the immune response by increasing the production of B and T cells. There is a suppressor effect on other hematologic cell lines. TFNα suppresses hematologic progenitors of myeloid and erythrocyte cell lines but does increase the rate of differentiation of the existing progenitors present. The end result may be a decrease in red cell production leading to anemia, because few erythrocyte precursor cells are available. TNFβ, previously known as lymphotoxin, is produced by CD4+ and CD8+ cells after exposure to antigen and is directly cytotoxic for selected cells.[8–10]

Interleukins

The fourth group of cytokines are the interleukins (IL), which are primarily produced by leukocytes and act on leukocytes and other cells.

Interleukin 1. Interleukin 1 (IL-1) is produced mainly by macrophages and fibroblasts. IL-1 acts as an initiation molecule for immunologic and inflammatory responses. IL-1 activates T cells and causes the T cells to release other lymphokines. IL-1 also supports B-cell proliferation. IL-1 acts in the differentiation of T and B cells, and also acts on the bone marrow to produce CSFs. IL-1 activates and increases the number of T and B cells and activates NK cells. IL-1 also activates the vascular endothelium, induces fever, increases the synthesis of acute phase proteins by the liver, and induces the growth and differentiation of hematopoietic precursors. Activated cells produce and release other cytokines and mediators of inflammation to increase the specific immune response.[8,9,11]

Interleukin 2. IL-2, a glycoprotein, is produced by CD4+ lymphocytes in response to an appropriate stimulus. IL-2 causes the proliferation of activated T and B cells, and increased production of NK cells by the bone marrow. Also, T cells are induced to express IL-2 receptors for the IL-2, B cells are stimulated to produce more antibody, and NK cells are activated.[8,9,12]

Interleukin 3. IL-3 is a glycoprotein also produced by activated T cells and a growth factor for many hematopoietic precursors. There is an increase in the number of mast cells in the skin, spleen, and liver with IL-3.[8,9]

Interleukin 4. Another glycoprotein, IL-4, is produced by activated T cells, and increased production occurs in the presence of IL-2 or IL-4. The in vivo effects of IL-4 are unknown, although there is indirect evidence that IgE levels are increased. In vitro, the effects of IL-4 include proliferation of T cells, B cells, and NK cells, and suppression of T-cell production of IFNγ, TNFα, and TNFβ.[8,9,13]

Interleukin 5. IL-5 is a produced by activated T cells and stimulates B cells to produce antibody. In mice, IL-5 increases the number of eosinophils and IgE antibody concentrations.[8]

Interleukin 6. IL-6 is produced by activated T and B cells as well as monocytes and fibroblasts. The half-life of IL-6 is approximately 1 hour. IL-6 may play a major role in host defense systems by regulating hematopoiesis, acute phase protein production in hepatocyte responses, and antibody production.[8,14]

Interleukins 10 and 12. IL-10 inhibits IFNγ production, antigen presentation, and macrophage production of IL-1. IL-12 acts in a manner opposite that of IL-10. It activates macrophage and NK cells and increases IFNγ production.[8]

ORGANS AND TISSUES OF THE IMMUNE SYSTEM

The lymphoid tissue must be organized so that immune cells can develop and there is adequate opportunity for antigen to interact with cells of the immune system and subsequent immune cell interactions. The blood or lymphatic fluid passes through the reticula, a loose network of fibers to which phagocytes adhere. This system acts as a filter to trap antigens and is known as the *reticuloendothelial system*. It is present in all secondary lymphoid organs (spleen and lymph nodes), bone marrow, liver, and lungs.

Lymphoid organs are divided into two categories based on their general function. Primary lymphoid organs are central and are the site of antigen-independent differentiation of lymphocytes. The bone marrow, fetal liver, and thymus comprise the primary lymphoid organs. Cells are protected from antigen, mature, are released to the circulation, and migrate to the secondary lymphoid organs. The secondary lymphoid organs and tissues are peripheral and are the sites where antigen-dependent activation and differentiation occur.[1,3,5] The spleen, lymph nodes, and mucosal-associated lymphoid tissue (MALT) are all secondary lymphoid organs. The spleen and lymph nodes are encapsulated organs, while MALT is an aggregation of lymphoid cells lining the gut, lungs, and urinary tract.[1,5] Secondary lymphoid organs are located throughout the body and trap antigens, providing a network for lymphocyte-antigen interactions and the release of immune response products.[1,5]

Primary Lymphoid Organs

BONE MARROW

The bone marrow is the site of blood cell production in late fetal and adult life, similar to the fetal liver in early fetal life. The pluripotent stem cell can be committed to the lymphocyte, erythrocyte, megakaryocyte, or myelomonocyte cell lines. In terms of the immune system, the bone marrow is the site where lymphocytes develop into B cells. The bone marrow may also serve as a secondary lymphoid organ, which is supported by the presence of T cells and plasma in the bone marrow.[1,3,5]

THYMUS

The thymus gland develops from the third and fourth embryonic pharyngeal pouches. In fetal life, the thymus begins as an outpouching of the endodermal epithelium. The fetal lymphocytes that have been produced in either the liver or spleen migrate to these outpouches. The thymus, a bilobed gland that is located in the anterior mediastinum, reaches its maximum size in puberty. Subsequently, the thymus gland begins to atrophy, with fatty tissue replacing thymic tissue, leading to a loss of function. This process is known as *thymic involution*. Atrophy of the thymus gland can be accelerated by corticosteroids. If the adrenal glands produce an increased amount of corticosteroids or if the person is on corticosteroid therapy, atrophy increases. This is known as *stress involution* because corticosteroid levels increase in stress and disease.[15]

Structurally, the thymus is organized into lobules separated by connective tissue septa (Fig. 2-10). Microscopically, each lobule is divided into the outer cortex and the inner medulla. The pre-T lymphocytes migrate from the bone marrow, enter the cortex, and then move to the inner medulla. T-cell maturation occurs in both the cortex and the medulla. The T cells in the outer cortex are immature and divide frequently. Mature T cells are found in the inner medulla. These T cells migrate to the circulatory and lymphatic systems. The network of epithelial and interdigitating cells found in the thymus is thought to be important in self versus non-self recognition. Hassall's corpuscles are also found in the thymic medulla, although their function is not well understood.[1,3,5]

Besides the differentiation of T cells, the thymus also produces some soluble mediators that play an important role in the maintenance of cell-mediated

thymus

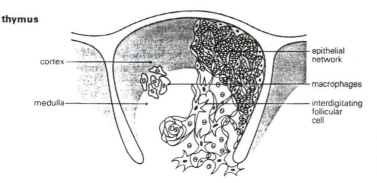

immunity by controlling the process and rate of T-cell development. These mediators act on the T cells at different stages of development. Thymosin, with a molecular weight of 31 to 52.5 kDa, is one of the best characterized thymic hormones. If thymosin is injected into a mouse without a thymus, T-cell function is restored. A second thymic hormone, thymopoietin (molecular weight 55 kDa), also induces T-cell maturation. Serum thymic factor (molecular weight 847 kDa) causes expression of some CD markers. The majority of the thymic factors are produced by the thymic epithelial cells, but macrophages found in the thymus also produce a mitogenic factor that aids in the development of T cells.[15]

Secondary Lymphoid Organs

The specific or antigen-dependent immune response begins in the secondary lymphoid organs. All secondary lymphoid organs have several common structural characteristics. Each has a specialized port of entry, discrete areas to which T and B lymphocytes migrate, and an elaborate architecture that maximizes the trapping of antigens and lymphocyte-antigen interactions.[3,5,16]

The specific migration of T and B lymphocytes has been demonstrated in animal experiments. If the bursa of Fabricius (the site where cells becomes committed to the B-cell lineage) is removed from a bird, no lymphoid follicles develop in the cortex of the lymph node but the diffuse paracortex of the node is normal. Conversely, if the thymus is removed, lymphocytes are depleted in the diffuse paracortex, but the follicles have normal cellularity. These experiments demonstrate the functional duality of the structural organization in secondary lymphoid organs.

LYMPH NODE

The typical lymph node is an encapsulated, round or bean-shaped organ, 1 to 25 mm in diameter. Subcapsular sinuses surround the lymphoid tissue. The lymphoid tissue is organized into an outer cortex and inner medulla (Fig. 2-11). The cortex is composed of the follicles, to which primarily B cells migrate, and the dif-

fuse paracortex, to which the T cells migrate. Follicles found in the lymph node are of two types: primary and secondary. The primary follicle is an aggregate of small B lymphocytes in the dendritic meshwork. Following antigenic stimulation, a primary follicle develops into a secondary follicle. The secondary follicle has a germinal center surrounded by a mantle zone. The germinal center contains small and large lymphocytes, blast cells, macrophages, and dendritic cells. The mantle zone has small lymphocytes. The diffuse paracortex is a mixture of cells, predominantly small T lymphocytes with antigen-presenting cells (macrophages and interdigitating cells). The inner medulla has an extensive sinus and cords that contain plasma cells and large lymphocytes.[5,16]

Lymph nodes are located at the junctions of lymphatic vessels throughout the body. These vessels and lymph nodes form a network that drains and filters the extravasated fluid (lymph) from the extracellular spaces of the tissues. This fluid enters the vessels by osmotic pressure and muscular contractions. The fluid then en-

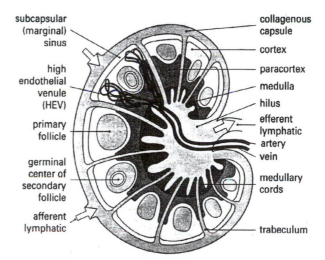

ters the subcapsular sinuses of a lymph node through the afferent lymphatic vessels. When in the lymph node, the fluid travels through a series of sinusoids located throughout the node. The fluid leaves the lymph node by the efferent lymphatic vessels, and eventually the lymph enters the venous system by the thoracic duct.[5,16]

Antigens that enter tissue spaces are carried into a regional lymph node by the lymphatic circulation. The majority of the antigens are trapped in the lymph node and phagocytosed by macrophages. Antigens are degraded and presented to the lymphocytes as they pass through the node. Lymphocytes enter the lymph node from the arterial blood stream that supplies the lymph node. The T and B cells adhere to the endothelial cells of the postcapillary venules (also known as the high endothelial venule) and cross these walls to the diffuse paracortical area. Although both types of lymphocytes migrate to the paracortical area, only T cells remain in that area and B cells migrate further to the follicles. The lymphocytes leave the lymph node after entering the efferent lymphatic vessel (see Fig. 2-11).[5,16]

SPLEEN

The largest lymphoid organ, the spleen, is specialized for filtering blood. The spleen is located beneath the diaphragm in the left upper quadrant behind the stomach. The spleen is organized into red pulp and white pulp. The red pulp is mainly red blood cells and functions to destroy old or abnormal cells. The white pulp is composed of lymphoid tissue surrounding the central arterioles and has a structure similar to lymph node. The tissue immediately surrounding the central arteriole is the T-cell area, adjacent to which is the B-cell follicle area. Both primary and secondary follicles are found in the spleen. The periarteriolar lymphoid sheath is surrounded by the marginal zone, which contains blood vessels, macrophages, and lymphocytes (Fig. 2-12).[5,16]

The lymphocytes enter and leave the white pulp through capillary branches of the central arteriole in the marginal zone. As with the lymph nodes, both T and B lymphocytes enter the diffuse area and then the B cells migrate to the follicles. When presented with antigen from an antigen-presenting cell, the lymphocytes are retained in the spleen while mounting an immune response. If no antigen is present, unstimulated cells may freely circulate from the marginal zone of the white pulp. Some lymphocytes as well as plasma cells may enter the red pulp and venous circulation.[5,16]

MUCOSAL-ASSOCIATED LYMPHOID TISSUES

The noncapsulated lymphoid cell aggregates known as the mucosal-associated lymphoid tissues (MALT) are located in the submucosal areas along the gastroin-

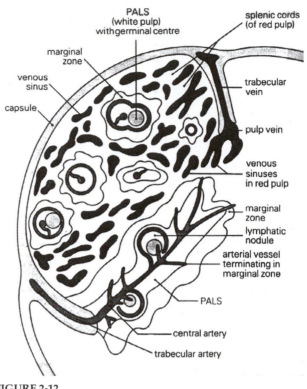

FIGURE 2-12
Structure of a spleen nodule. The spleen is composed of both red and white pulp, with the red pulp surrounding areas of the white pulp. The white pulp contains primary follicles and germinal centers as in the lymph node. (From Roitt IM, Brostoff J, Male DK. Immunology, 4th ed. London, Mosby, 1996.)

testinal, respiratory, and urogenital tracts. These tracts interface with the external environment, providing an important early immune response. MALT may be organized into follicles containing germinal centers, as in other secondary lymphoid organs. The lamina propria of the intestinal wall usually contains diffuse lymphoid cells. The Peyer's patches, located in the ileum, often contain follicles and germinal centers.[5,16]

LYMPHOID CIRCULATION

After release from the primary lymphoid organs, the mature lymphocytes migrate from one secondary lymphoid organ to another, using both the circulatory and lymphatic channels. Figure 2-13 is a schematic diagram of the lymphocyte circulation. After migrating through their respective areas of the lymph node, the T and B cells leave the node through the efferent lymphatics and the lymphatics drain into the blood stream from the thoracic duct, which returns the T and B cells to the peripheral blood. The spleen has a different migratory pattern. The lymphocytes leave the peripheral blood from the capillaries in the marginal zone. The lymphocytes migrate from the white pulp of the spleen by way of the sinusoid, which goes to the splenic vein.

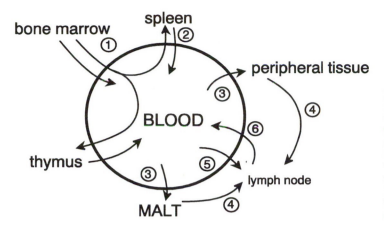

FIGURE 2-13
(**1**) Lymphoblasts travel via the blood to the spleen and thymus. After maturation, the lymphocytes are released into the blood. (**2**) Mature lymphocytes can enter and leave the spleen as needed. (**3**) Mature lymphocytes can enter the mucosal-associated lymphoid tissue (MALT) and peripheral tissue. (**4**) Lymphocytes leave the MALT and peripheral tissue via the lymphatics. (**5**) Lymphocytes enter a lymph node by passing through specialized cells lining the postcapillary venule. (**6**) Lymphocytes leave the lymph node in the lymph, and then re-enter the blood at the thoracic duct.

Under normal circumstances, there is a continuous flow of lymphocytes between the circulatory and lymphoid systems. When there is antigenic stimulation, the specific lymphocytes are preferentially retained in the lymphoid organ, which drains the area of the antigen entrance. This sequestration of antigen-specific lymphocytes allows the recognition of the antigen and a specific response to that antigen. The constant movement of lymphocytes between the circulatory and lymphatic systems allows for prompt recognition of the invading antigen.[16]

Review Questions

1. Antibody production is most likely to take place in the

   a. red pulp of the spleen
   b. bone marrow
   c. site of inflammation
   d. blood
   e. lymph nodes

2. Match the function with the cell type.

Cell	Function
_____ a. T lymphocyte	1. parasitic infections
_____ b. B lymphocyte	2. cellular immunity
_____ c. eosinophil	3. phagocytosis
_____ d. neutrophil	4. antibody production
_____ e. macrophage	5. antigen presentation

3. The function of interferon is to aid in

   a. antibody formation
   b. resistance to viral infections
   c. antigen presentation
   d. phagocytosis
   e. fever production

4. Match the function with the cytokine.

Cytokine	Function
_____ a. IL-1	1. activates NK cells
_____ b. G-CSF	2. growth factor for T and B cells
_____ c. IFNγ	3. inhibits macrophage
_____ d. TNFα	4. stimulates granulocyte production
_____ e. IL-10	5. kills human tumor cells

5. Lymphocytes leave the blood stream and enter a lymph node by

   a. crossing the endothelium of the postcapillary venule
   b. passing through the thoracic duct
   c. adhering to the afferent lymphatic vessels
   d. forming immune complexes

References

1. Lydyard P, Grossi C: Cells involved in the immune response. In Roitt I, Brostoff J, Male D (eds): Immunology, 4th ed, p 2.1. London, Mosby, 1996
2. Reinherz EL, Schlossman S: The differentiation and function of human T lymphocytes. Cell 19:821, 1981

3. Nelson DA, Davey FR: Hematopoiesis. In Henry JB (ed): Clinical Diagnosis and Management by Laboratory Methods, 18th ed, p 605. Philadelphia, WB Saunders, 1991

4. Osmond DG: The ontogeny and organization of the lymphoid system. J Invest Dermatol 85 (Suppl):2s, 1985

5. Abbas AK, Lichtman AH, Pober JS: Cellular and Molecular Immunology, 2nd ed, p 14. Philadelphia, WB Saunders, 1994

6. Souza LM: Granulocyte stimulating factor. In Aggarwal BB, Gutterman JU (eds): Human Cytokines: Handbook for Basic and Clinical Research, p 221. Boston, Blackwell Scientific, 1992

7. Crozier PS, Garnick MB, Clark SC: Granulocyte-macrophage colony stimulating factor. In Aggarwal BB, Gutterman JU (eds): Human Cytokines: Handbook for Basic and Clinical Research, p 238. Boston, Blackwell Scientific Publications, 1992

8. Feldman M: Cell cooperation in the antibody response. In Roitt I, Brostoff J, Male D (eds): Immunology, 4th ed, p 8.1. London: Mosby, 1996

9. Abbas AK, Lichtman AH, Pober JS: Cellular and Molecular Immunology, 2nd ed, p 239. Philadelphia, WB Saunders, 1994

10. Aggarwal BB: Tumor necrosis factor. In Aggarwal BB, Gutterman JU (eds): Human Cytokines: Handbook for Basic and Clinical Research, p 270. Boston, Blackwell Scientific, 1992

11. Dower SK: Interleukin-1. In Aggarwal BB, Gutterman JU (eds): Human Cytokines: Handbook for Basic and Clinical Research, p 46. Boston, Blackwell Scientific, 1992

12. Lotze MT: Interleukin-2. In Aggarwal BB, Gutterman JU (eds): Human Cytokines: Handbook for Basic and Clinical Research, p 81. Boston, Blackwell Scientific, 1992

13. de Vries JEL: Interleukin-4. In Aggarwal BB, Gutterman JU (eds): Human Cytokines: Handbook for Basic and Clinical Research, p 113. Boston, Blackwell Scientific, 1992

14. Taga T, Yokota T: Interleukin-6. In Aggarwal BB, Gutterman JU (eds): Human Cytokines: Handbook for Basic and Clinical Research, p 143. Boston, Blackwell Scientific, 1992

15. Weiss L. The thymus. In Histology: Cell and Tissue Biology, 5th ed, p 510. New York, Elsevier, 1983

16. Lydyard P, Grossi C. The lymphoid system. In Roitt I, Brostoff J, Male D (eds): Immunology, 4th ed, p 3.1. London: Mosby, 1996

CHAPTER 3

Mechanisms of the Specific Immune Response

Anne E. Huot

Objectives

Upon completion of this chapter, the reader will be able to:

1. Define specificity and immunological memory
2. Describe the steps involved in B-cell and T-cell antigen recognition
3. List the characteristics that differentiate T-dependent and T-independent antigens
4. Explain the activation of T_H, T_C, and B cells
5. Describe the mechanisms involved in the elimination of antigen by T_C, natural killer cells, antibodies, and macrophages

OVERVIEW

Specific immune responses are traditionally classified as humoral or cell-mediated. The humoral immune response involves antibody production by the B lymphocytes with or without the aid of T lymphocytes, whereas the cell-mediated immune response involves cell-cell communication, mainly mediated by T lymphocytes and their products. The division of humoral and cell-mediated immune responses is not absolute, and the occurrence of one type of response in the complete absence of the other is extremely rare. However, certain antigens may tend to elicit a predominantly antibody response with a minimal cell-mediated response, or vice versa. An elaborate cascade of cellular interaction is required for a specific T-cell–mediated immune response to occur. The steps involved include: antigen processing, antigen presentation, lymphocyte activation, release of cytokines, and activation of effector cells.

Lymphocytes belong to two distinct lineages, T and B. T cells are educated in the thymus, whereas B cells are educated in the bone marrow in humans. T cells can be divided into subsets based on their surface glycoproteins, CD4 and CD8. CD4-positive cells are generally referred to as T-helper (T_H) cells and can be divided into subsets (T_H1, T_H2) based on the cytokines that they secrete. CD8-positive cells are either T cytotoxic lymphocytes (T_C) or T suppressor (T_S) cells. B lymphocytes are capable of differentiating into antibody-producing plasma cells. T_H and T_S cells regulate the cell-mediated immune response, whereas B lymphocytes and T_C lymphocytes carry out effector functions.

Specificity and memory are important concepts in specific immune responses because they represent a major difference between these responses and those of the innate immune system. Irrespective of whether the specific response is humoral or cell-mediated, the response is induced by a specific antigen, and the effector mechanisms activated are aimed at that specific antigen. For example, B cells activated by an antigen differentiate into plasma cells, which produce antibody that specifically binds to that antigen and in so doing aids in the elimination of that antigen.

Memory is a feature of specific immune responses that involve T_H cells. When appropriately stimulated, the T_H cell secretes cytokines, which induce activated B and T cells to become memory cells. The purpose of memory cells is, as the name implies, to quickly produce their effector molecules and carry out their effector functions, when the specific antigen that elicited the primary response is encountered, resulting in rapid elimination of the antigen.

ANTIGEN RECOGNITION

Antigen Processing

T and B cells recognize different forms of antigens. B cells are capable of binding to antigens in their native form. The antigens are generally polysaccharide or protein in nature, and the portion of the antigen that binds to the B-cell antigen receptor is referred to as a *conformational epitope*. T cells recognize only protein antigen that has been processed by antigen-presenting cells (APCs). The portion of the processed antigens that binds to the T-cell antigen receptor is referred to as a *linear epitope*. Further, the binding of a T cell to an APC is major histocompatibility complex (MHC) restricted. T_H cells are MHC Class II restricted, and $T_{S/C}$ cells are MHC Class I restricted.[1] Only a limited number of APCs are capable of interacting with T_H cells, including macrophages, dendritic cells, interdigitating cells, Langerhans cells, and B lymphocytes. The common characteristic of these APCs is that they are rich in surface MHC Class II molecules.[2,3] All nucleated cells express MHC Class I proteins on their surface and therefore are capable of interacting with T_C cells.

The processing of antigen for presentation to CD4- and CD8-positive cells is different.[4] For CD4-positive cells, antigen external to the cell is taken up by an APC and broken down into peptide fragments. The peptide fragments are then packaged with MHC Class II molecules, and the peptide/MHC complex is exported to the surface of the APC for presentation to the T_H cell. For CD8-positive cells, antigen, which is endogenous to the cell, is broken down into peptide fragments and complexed to MHC Class I molecules, and then the peptide/MHC complex is exported to the cell for presentation to T_C cells. This type of antigen processing is common in cells that are infected with a virus. As the virus replicates, viral protein generated inside the cell can be broken down and processed in this fashion. For both types of antigen presentation, processing of the protein antigen requires time and metabolism.

Antigen Receptors

B CELL

The B-cell antigen receptor is surface immunoglobulin. The immunoglobulin is composed of two identical heavy chains and two identical light chains joined together by interchain disulfide bonds and embedded into the membrane of the B cell (Fig. 3-1). The heavy and light chains have constant and variable regions. The variable regions of the heavy and light chain come together to form an antigen binding pocket. Therefore, each surface immunoglobulin has two identical antigen binding pockets that bind to the conformational epitopes of antigens in their native form.[5] Each clone of B cell puts only one specificity of immunoglobulin on its surface.

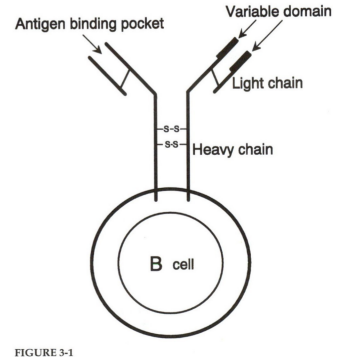

FIGURE 3-1
B-cell antigen receptor.

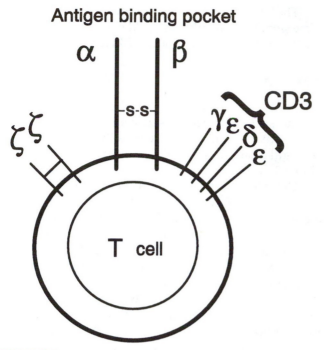

Antigen binding pocket

FIGURE 3-2
T-cell antigen receptor.

T CELL

The T-cell receptor (TCR) is a complex consisting of the peptide/MHC binding pocket and a glycoprotein, CD3. CD3 is a five-subunit molecule that transmits the signal into the cell to which the TCR has bound its MHC/peptide complex. This, in turn, leads to the activation of signal transduction pathways that activate the cell. The TCR belongs to the immunoglobulin super gene family in that it shares structural and sequence homology to the immunoglobulin. Like the immunoglobulin, each clone of T cells expresses a unique receptor. The majority of T cells have a TCR composed of an alpha and a beta polypeptide chain. Approximately 1% are composed of a gamma and a delta polypeptide chain. The function of gamma/delta T cells remains unclear. A schematic representation of a T-cell antigen receptor complex is depicted in Figure 3-2. The distal regions of the polypeptide chains form the antigen binding pocket, which recognizes the processed antigen in its linear form.[6]

Types of Antigens

As discussed previously, the antibody response to the majority of antigens requires T_H cells. These antigens are known as T-dependent antigens. They tend to be highly complex structures that are protein in nature. There are, however, a small number of substances that are capable of activating B cells without T-cell help;

these are known as T-independent antigens. In general, T-independent antigens are large molecules with repeating epitopes that elicit mainly IgM responses; the primary and secondary responses are indistinguishable, and immunologic memory and antibody affinity maturation do not occur.[7]

EFFECTOR MECHANISMS

T Cells

T_H-CELL ACTIVATION

Upon stimulation with antigen-charged APCs, the T_H cells undergo an activation process known as blast transformation. A series of cellular events occurs during this process. The noticeable changes in the cell morphology are increased cell size and the appearance of prominent nucleoli. At the molecular level the cell increases its mRNA and DNA synthesis, which leads to cell division and cell differentiation. Thus, the number of functional T_H cells increases. Direct contact between T_H cell and antigen-charged APC is necessary for T-cell activation.[7] Not only must the T_H cell recognize the antigen, but it must also recognize the MHC Class II molecules presented on the APC surface. This recognition is accomplished by the TCR on the surface of the T_H cell (Fig. 3-3). Such a dual recognition of antigen and MHC

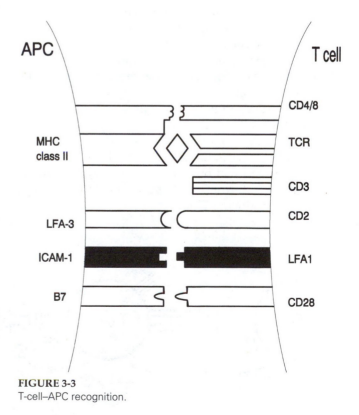

FIGURE 3-3
T-cell–APC recognition.

Class II molecule is possible only when the two inter-acting cells are from the same host or genetically simi-lar individuals. This phenomenon is known as MHC re-striction. Thus, the T_H cell–APC interaction is MHC Class II restricted.[3]

The TCR is a complex molecule with two distinct binding portions, one that recognizes the host MHC molecules and another that recognizes processed pep-tides presented in the cleft of the MHC on the surface of the APC. A number of other proteins on the surface of the T lymphocyte and the APC bind to each other in order to hold the T lymphocyte and APC together for a time sufficient for the transmission of intracellular sig-nals that activate the cell. One of these molecules is the CD4 protein that binds to MHC II proteins. Other pro-teins involved in cell-cell binding include the intracel-lular adhesion molecules (ICAM), leukocyte function antigens (LFA), CD2, CD28, and B7. The APC expresses ICAM-1, LFA-3, and B7. The T_H cell expresses LFA-1, which binds ICAM-1, CD2, which binds LFA-3, and CD28, which binds B7. Possible mechanisms of T_H cell–APC interaction are schematically represented in Figure 3-3.[3,7]

T-cell activation requires both soluble mediators and direct cell contact. The well-characterized soluble mediators are interleukin-1 (IL-1) and interleukin-2 (IL-2). IL-1 is a cytokine synthesized by various cell sources, including macrophages. IL-2 is a cytokine pro-duced by antigen-sensitized T cells. T-cell activation is a multistep process:

1. A T_H cell recognizes the antigen in conjunction with an MHC Class II molecule on the APC surface.
2. During the cell contact, the APC may receive a sig-nal or signals from the T_H cell and releases IL-1.
3. IL-1 promotes IL-2 receptor expression or IL-2 syn-thesis by T cells. Only T cells that are already sensi-tized by the antigen can respond to IL-1.
4. An effector T cell that is sensitized by the antigen and stimulated by IL-1 expresses IL-2 receptors.
5. In the presence of IL-2, the effector T cell undergoes blast transformation, cell division, and differentia-tion. The effector T cells may be cytotoxic or cy-tokine-producing T cells.

Therefore, activation of an effector T cell requires three signals: antigenic stimulation, IL-1, and IL-2. Fig-ure 3-4 outlines the sequence of T-cell activation.[1,8]

CYTOKINES

Cytokines are protein molecules that essentially trans-mit messages between cells. Recent experimental data suggest that the primary biologic activities of cytokines are regulation of cell growth and cellular differentiation (Table 3-1).

Cytokines primarily produced by activated T cells include IL-2, a T-cell growth factor that induces prolif-eration of antigen-activated T cells and enhances nat-ural killer (NK) cell cytolytic activities. Activated T cells also produce B-cell growth factors: interleukin-4 (IL-4, also known as B-cell growth factor 1), which stimulates proliferation of antigen-activated B cells, and inter-leukin-6 (IL-6, also known as B-cell growth factor 2), which induces differentiation of proliferating B cells into antibody-secreting plasma cells. Macrophage mi-gration inhibition factor (MIF) and macrophage acti-vating factor (MAF) are activated T-cell products that regulate macrophage functions described in a subse-quent section. Interferon gamma is also a T-cell cy-tokine that is known to have biologic functions, includ-ing enhancement of NK cells' cytolytic activities, activation of macrophages, and enhancement of MHC protein expression on cell surfaces.[9]

Two well-characterized cytokines produced by macrophages are IL-1 and tumor necrosis factor (TNF). IL-1 stimulates IL-2 receptor expression and IL-2 syn-thesis by antigen-activated T cells. Tumor necrosis fac-tor has direct cytolytic activity against tumor cells.[10]

CYTOKINE-MEDIATED CELL-CELL COMMUNICATION

The nature of the communication between the interact-ing T_H cell and APC is not completely elucidated. Dur-ing the antigen-presenting process, the APC also re-leases IL-1, which, in conjunction with binding of the MHC II-peptide complex to the TCR, results in the syn-thesis of both IL-2 and IL-2 receptors by the T_H cell. The

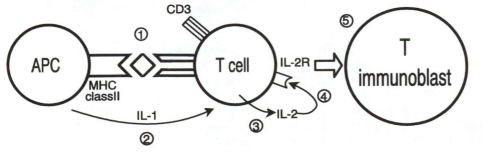

FIGURE 3-4
T-cell activation.

TABLE 3-1
Cytokines

CYTOKINES	IMMUNOBIOLOGIC ACTIVITIES
REGULATES OTHER LYMPHOCYTES	
IL-1	Stimulates antigen-activated T cells to express IL-2 receptors or to produce IL-2
IL-2	Stimulates antigen-activated T-cell proliferation
IL-4 (B-cell growth factor 1)	Stimulates antigen-activated B-cell proliferation
IL-6 (B-cell growth factor 2)	Induces proliferating B-cell differentiation into a plasma cell
IL-10	Augments IgM and IgG production, suppresses cytokine production by T_H1 cells
REGULATES HEMATOPOIESIS	
IL-3	Supports hematopoietic stem cell growth
Granulocyte-monocyte colony stimulating factor	Stimulates the growth of hematopoietic cells that are committed to granulocyte or monocyte lineage
REGULATES OTHER EFFECTOR CELLS	
MIF	Inhibits macrophage migration
MAF	Activates macrophages
Interferon γ	Enhances NK cells' cytotoxicity, activates macrophages, antiviral activity
DIRECT TOXICITY TO TARGETS	
TNF (α and β)	Causes tumor cell death

IL-2 serves as an autocrine growth factor for the T_H cell, causing the proliferation of the activated T_H-cell clone. Once fully activated, the T_H cell secretes other cytokines, which in turn communicate with effector cells involved in the response. The type of cytokine secreted is determined by the T_H-cell subset. T_H1 cells secrete interferon-gamma and IL-2, which promote inflammation and further activation of macrophages, T_C cells, and natural killer cells. T_H2 cells secrete IL-4, IL-6, and IL-10, which promote B-cell activation, proliferation, and differentiation into antibody-producing plasma cells. Other proliferation and differentiation factors are also produced by the activated T_H cells. Thus, the activation of a few T_H cells results in an amplification process whereby large numbers of identical cells are produced, which in turn regulate the activation of the inflammation process and B-cell and T_C-cell activation. Therefore, the immune system is made efficient by this amplification process, which is mediated by signal transduction (Fig. 3-5).[11]

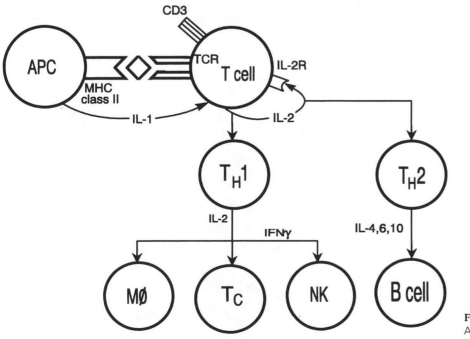

FIGURE 3-5
Amplification of the immune response.

CELL-MEDIATED IMMUNITY

The cell-mediated immune response is mediated primarily by T_H lymphocytes. The T_C cells and cytokines are important effectors of cell-mediated immune responses. Whereas the former destroy targets by direct cell contact, the latter recruit and activate other cells, such as macrophages, amplifying the response. In addition, cytokines may be directly toxic to the target cells (Table 3-1). Macrophages play dual roles in a cell-mediated immune response. They present antigen to the T cells during the induction phase and become activated in response to cytokines during the effector phase. There is yet another group of lymphocytes, known as natural killer (NK) cells, that is able to destroy targets without previous antigen sensitization. Finally, an effector mechanism that involves antibodies and cells for target destruction is known as antibody-dependent cell-mediated cytolysis (ADCC).

T_C-CELL ACTIVITY

T_C cells are capable of destroying target cells without involving antibody. Direct cell contact is required for target cell killing. This cell contact is achieved by the T-cell receptor, which binds to the target peptide/MHC Class I complex on the target cell surface. Upon contact, the T_C cell releases toxic molecules, which kill the target cell. A T_C can go through many cycles of target cell destruction; after killing one target cell, the T_C can attach to another target cell and repeat the killing activity. In order for a T_C cell to become fully activated and to be capable of destroying target cells, it must receive cytokine signals from activated T_H cells (Fig. 3-6). IL-2 is a cytokine released by the T_H cells that activates the T_C cell. Thus, activation of T_C cells is mediated by T_H cells. The main function of T_C is to eliminate virally infected

host cells. These T_C are CD8-positive cells with MHC Class I restriction.[1]

B Cells

B-CELL ACTIVATION

Antigens capable of eliciting an immune response are macromolecular structures with many epitopes, both conformational and linear. On any given macromolecular structure, there are some epitopes recognized by B cells and others by T cells. Historically, these epitopes are referred to as haptens and carriers, respectively. In this sense, the hapten is defined as a substance of low molecular weight that is not capable of eliciting an immune response unless it is bound to a larger macromolecular structure referred to as the carrier.

The activation of a B cell that ultimately results in antibody production requires binding of the immunoglobulin receptor to the antigen. Binding alone is not sufficient for full activation to occur. Cytokines such as IL-2, IL-4, IL-6, and IL-10 are required for B-cell proliferation and subsequent differentiation into plasma cells. These cytokines are provided by macrophages in a T-independent response and T_H cells in a T-dependent response. One may envision that macromolecular structures that activate the immune response have many epitopes on the larger carrier surface. Thus, in any given immune response, several clones of lymphocytes can be activated by different epitopes on the surface of a macromolecular carrier. This is referred to as a polyclonal response.

ANTIBODY DIVERSITY

The immune system is capable of synthesizing different antibody molecules that collectively recognize an unlimited number of antigens. Yet, the cells that produce

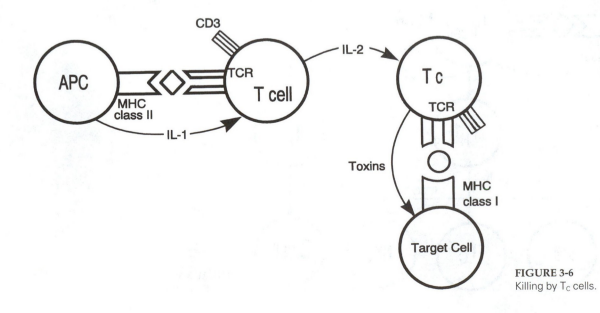

FIGURE 3-6
Killing by T_C cells.

antibodies, the B cells, are limited in number. The ability of the B cell to create such antibody diversity has fascinated immunologists throughout history because it is known that the B-cell antigen receptor is an immunoglobulin and that each clone of B cells makes only one specificity of immunoglobulin with respect to antigen binding character.[12]

In 1930 the instructionist theory was proposed, which stated that an antigen could serve as a template to which complementary antibody molecules were synthesized. This theory was ruled out when it was realized that the three-dimensional structure of an antibody molecule is determined by its amino acid sequence. The germline theory was formulated in 1960. It hypothesizes that antibody genes arise during vertebrate evolution by gene duplication, mutation, and selection. Thus, each individual is endowed with a complete antibody gene repertoire at conception, and antibody production merely requires antigen stimulus. On the contrary, the somatic mutation theory states that diversified antibody genes arise from a relatively small number of germline genes by mutation or recombination of the genes during development.

An understanding of structure and gene rearrangements of the antibody gene families offers good insight to the mechanism for generating antibody diversity. Antibody genes are located on three separate chromosomes: Heavy chain genes are located on chromosome 14, λ light chain genes are located on chromosome 22, and κ light chain genes are located on chromosome 2. The variable region of a heavy chain (V_H) is encoded by three genes, which are transcribed into three polypeptide segments: V_H, D, and J_H. The variable region of a light chain (V_L) is encoded by two separate genes that are transcribed into two polypeptide segments: V_L and J_L. These are known as *variable-segment genes* (V genes) of heavy and light chains.

There are many different genes for each variable-segment gene. For example, there are about 100 different genes that encode for V_H segment, four for D segment, and six for J_H. Each antibody molecule requires only one of each of these pieces in order to create a gene that will give rise to the variable region polypeptide component of the heavy chain. Thus, a B cell is provided with an enormous gene library from which it selects the appropriate combination of V genes for V_H and V_L chain synthesis (Fig. 3-7). This process of V-gene recombination occurs early in B-cell development, allowing the emergence of diversified B-cell populations that collectively recognize an unlimited number of antigens. Thus, the ability of an individual to produce a particular antibody is predetermined by gene rearrangements in the immature B cell. This rearrangement happens in the absence of any antigenic stimulation. Additional diversification comes from imprecision in joining the recombining gene pieces. This phenomenon is known as *junctional diversity*. Furthermore, the high mutational rate of V genes also contributes to antibody diversity. In conclusion, the immune system is capable of responding to an unlimited number of antigens with exquisite specificity. Such a diversified response is made possible through

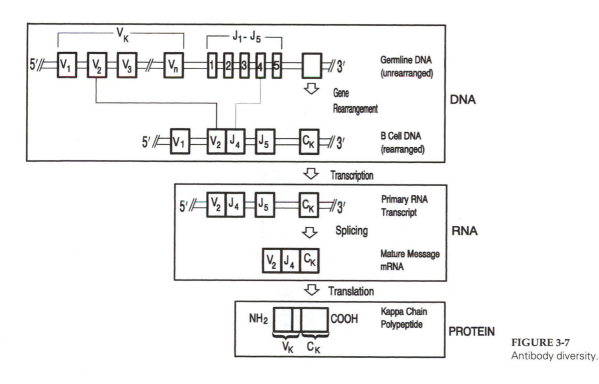

FIGURE 3-7
Antibody diversity.

gene recombination, junctional diversity, and V-gene mutation.[13–15]

When a B cell begins the maturation process, it must synthesize and put on its surface an immunoglobulin receptor. Each clone of B cells expresses a unique receptor. This receptor is generated by combining different gene pieces such that the combination yields a functional protein. Initially, the heavy chain variable region gene pieces are rearranged. If the first allele is successful, the second is prevented from rearranging (allelic exclusion). If the first is unsuccessful, the second is attempted. If the second is successful, the variable light chain genes are rearranged (also governed by allelic exclusion). If the second is not successful, the cell dies. Through this process of combinatorial and junctional gene rearrangement, enough antibody idiotypes are generated to cover the diversity of possible antigens that will be encountered. Once the gene pieces have been rearranged, this is a permanent change and the B cell will never change its idiotype (except for affinity maturation). The gene pieces making up the idiotype are spliced together, transcribed into nuclear RNA, spliced into messenger RNA, and translated into immunoglobulin protein. The constant regions of the heavy chain switch throughout the life of a B cell in response to cytokines made by T$_H$ cells. The class of antibody family determines the effector functions of which the antibody is capable. For example, only certain antibody families are capable of fixing complement.

ANTIBODY PRODUCTION

Primary and Secondary Antibody Response

The quality, magnitude, and tempo of an antibody response depend greatly on the host's experience with the antigen. A primary response is elicited when the antigen is introduced to an animal for the first time. During a primary response, a latent phase occurs in which there is no detectable circulating antibody. The length of the latent phase is usually between 5 and 7 days; however, it may vary, depending on the individual and the antigen. The latent phase is followed by a gradual rise, plateau, and final decline of the antibody titer. The final decline in the antibody titer is due to several factors, including the cessation of antibody production, clearance of antibody in the form of immune complexes, and catabolism of the antibody. The first immunoglobulin class to appear in a primary antibody response is IgM, which is followed by the production of IgG. Introduction of the same antigen for the second time evokes a secondary antibody response that differs from the primary response in many aspects (Fig. 3-8).[16]

1. The latent phase is shorter.
2. The circulating antibody reaches higher titer.
3. IgG is the predominant immunoglobulin produced.
4. The antibody response tends to persist for a longer time period.

Thus, the secondary response is "faster" and "bigger" than the primary response. It is also called an anamnestic response because the immune system seems to remember the previous antigenic exposure. Presumably, both memory T and B cells are generated during the primary response. Further, during secondary responses new primary responses are initiated in response to other epitopes on the macromolecular structure. Thus, some IgM is produced during a secondary response, but this production represents a primary response to new epitopes on the antigen.

Affinity Maturation

Antibodies produced during the secondary response have a higher affinity for the antigen than those produced during the primary response. This phenomenon is known as *affinity maturation*. Most likely, affinity maturation involves the selective activation of B cells that have high affinity receptors (i.e., surface immunoglobulin with high affinity for the antigen). This is supported by both the biology of B cells and experimental observations. It is likely that these B cells with high-affinity receptors are memory B cells made during the previous immune response to a particular epitope. The genes that code for the immunoglobulin receptor on these memory B cells undergo somatic mutations in the hypervariable regions of the antigen binding pocket, which results in a receptor with increased affinity for the epitope. However, the overall idiotype of the antibody remains unchanged.[17]

Both the surface immunoglobulin of a B cell and the immunoglobulin secreted by the same B cell are coded

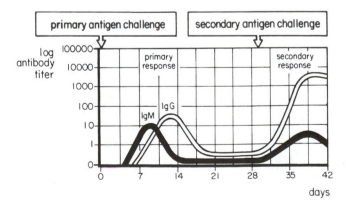

FIGURE 3-8
Primary and secondary antibody response. (From Roitt IM, Brostoff J, Male DK: Immunology. London, Gower Medical Publishing, 1985.)

by the same set of genes, which remain unchanged throughout the cell's life span. Consequently, the surface immunoglobulin of a B cell and the immunoglobulin secreted by a plasma cell have identical antigen specificity and affinity. A high antigen dose generally elicits antibodies that have low affinity for the antigen. In antigen excess, both B cells with high and those with low affinity have the opportunity to interact with the antigen to become activated. On the contrary, at a low antigen dose the B cells compete for the antigens, and only those B cells with high affinity will succeed in binding to the antigen, becoming activated, and producing high-affinity antibodies.[7,18] This correlates with the concept of T-dependent and T-independent antigens in that T-independent antigens are high-dose antigens that fail to elicit a memory response whereas T-dependent antigens tend to be in low dose and do elicit a memory response and therefore affinity maturation of the immunoglobulin receptor. Further, this is useful in that memory B and T cells take up residence in local secondary lymphatic tissue and are capable of high-efficiency antigen processing, which in turns leads to a quick and heightened immunoglobulin response.

T- and B-Cell Interactions

In a secondary immune response, T and B cells interact in a linked fashion, during which the B cell is the APC for the T_H cell. Because B cells have highly specific antigen receptors (immunoglobulins) on their surface, they are much more efficient APCs than macrophages. Thus, a small amount of antigen can be efficiently processed by a B cell. This is particularly important in secondary immune responses, where the goal is to generate large quantities of antibody quickly. In these responses, the B cell acts as the antigen-presenting cell. The B cell binds to the hapten portion of a macromolecular structure, internalizes the structure, and processes and presents peptide portions of the carrier molecule in association with MHC Class II proteins to the T_H cell. The T_H cell, in turn, secretes cytokines, which further activate the cell. These linked interactions result in heightened amplification of the proliferation and differentiation of the activated T and B cells. Thus, the production of antibody is increased and maintained for an extended period of time (Fig. 3-9). The direct T- and B-cell contact appears to enhance the communication between two interacting cells.[3,19]

Communication between interacting T and B cells is mediated by soluble cytokines released by the T cells. This is proven by cell culture experiments. In vitro antibody production is not inhibited when T and B cells are separated by a membrane; the membrane prevents cell contact yet allows antigen and soluble factors to diffuse freely (Fig. 3-10).[7] Two B-cell growth factors have been reported. B-cell growth factor 1 (also known as

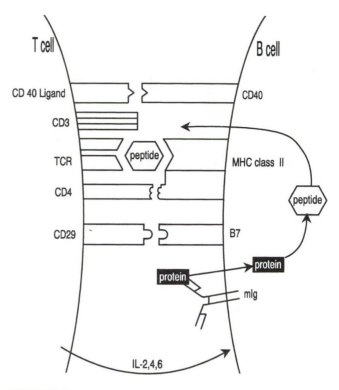

FIGURE 3-9
T- and B-cell interactions.

IL-4) stimulates proliferation of antigen-activated B cells, and B-cell growth factor 2 (also known as IL-6) induces differentiation of proliferating B cells.[9,20–23]

Other Cells

MACROPHAGES

Macrophages are important inflammatory cells whose functions are often modulated by cytokines. For example, macrophage MIF inhibits the migration of macrophages so that they are retained at the site of antigen response. Furthermore, their microbicidal and tumoricidal activities are greatly enhanced by yet another ac-

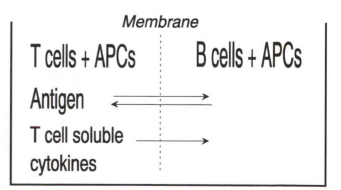

FIGURE 3-10
Soluble mediators of T- and B-cell interactions.

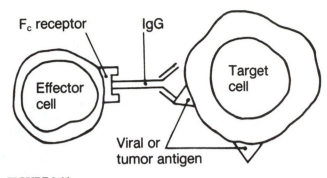

FIGURE 3-11
Antibody-dependent cell-mediated cytolysis.

tivated T-cell product, MAF. However, the biologic activities of macrophages are not antigen specific. Cytokines produced by the T cells sensitized to one antigen may activate macrophages that will destroy the sensitizing antigens as well as other unrelated targets. Therefore, the process of cytokine production is antigen specific, whereas the biologic activity of cytokine-activated macrophages is not antigen specific.[1]

NATURAL KILLER CELLS

A group of large lymphocytes with cytoplasmic granules is capable of killing virally infected cells or neoplastic cells without previous antigen sensitization. These are known as natural killer (NK) cells. NK cells do not express T- or B-cell markers; however, they consistently express Fc receptors on their cell surface. Their cellular activities are modulated by cytokines. For example, IL-2 stimulates their proliferative activities, and interferon gamma enhances their cytolytic activities.[1,24,25] Although experimental evidence demonstrates that NK cells are antigen specific and discriminate self from non-self, the receptor that binds to the antigen and the self–non-self education process have yet to be elucidated.

ANTIBODY-DEPENDENT CELL-MEDIATED CYTOLYSIS

Effector cells with cytolytic activity and Fc receptors are able to lyse antibody-coated target cells (Fig. 3-11). This phenomenon is known as antibody-dependent cell-mediated cytolysis (ADCC). Direct effector–target cell contact is required for target cell lysis, and it probably involves the cytolytic mediator released by the effector cell. The antibody involved is usually IgG, which is directed against viral or tumor antigens on the target cell surface. Therefore, the antigen specificity in this cytolytic activity resides in the antibody molecule. The effector cells are poorly defined. NK cells probably play an important role; however, all Fc receptor–positive cells, including macrophages, monocytes, and neutrophils, have the potential to be effector cells.[1]

REGULATORY MECHANISMS

Regulatory Effect of Antibody

Antibody can have a negative feedback effect on its own production. Two possible mechanisms are suggested by which the antibody suppresses its further synthesis. Circulating antibodies and the B cell may compete for antigen binding. Thus, as the serum antibody titer increases, antigen is bound by the antibody and less antigen is available for the activation of B cells with the same antigen specificity. Circulating antibodies may also bind to the B-cell surface by way of Fc receptors. Crosslinking between B-cell surface Fc receptor and surface immunoglobulin may occur when a multivalent antigen binds to the surface immunoglobulin and antibody that has been passively adsorbed by the Fc receptor. Such a crosslinkage of B-cell surface receptors will lead to B-cell inactivation, thus decreasing antibody synthesis (Fig. 3-12).[7]

Regulatory Effect of Anti-Idiotype Antibody

The antigen binding sites of an immunoglobulin molecule are known as the idiotypes. Because each B-cell clone produces immunoglobulin of a single antigen binding character, each molecule can be categorized according to its idiotypes. The antigen binding site of an immunoglobulin is immunogenic and is therefore capable of eliciting an immune response. The antibody produced against the idiotype portion of an another antibody is called anti-idiotypic antibody. During the course of an immune response, anti-idiotypic antibodies are made by the host to regulate the response. This is accomplished via both removal of circulating antibody and binding of the anti-idiotype antibodies to the target idiotype on the B-cell surface immunoglobulin, leading to the B-cell inactivation.[7]

Jerne proposed this theory of idiotypic network based on the observations made by two independent groups, Kunkle et al. and Oudin and Michel.[26] The theory postulates that the immune system consists of a net-

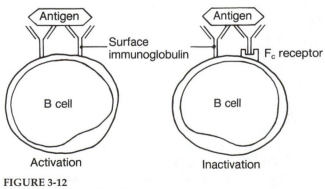

FIGURE 3-12
B-cell activation and inhibition.

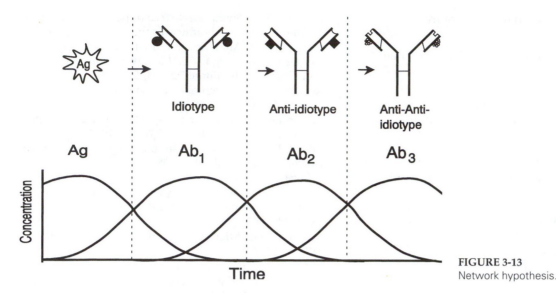

FIGURE 3-13
Network hypothesis.

work of idiotypes (Fig. 3-13). Antibodies generated in response to an antigen constitute the first wave of antibody response. The second wave of antibody response is initiated by the idiotypes of the first-wave antibodies. The second-wave antibodies are known as anti-idiotypic antibodies and express idiotypes that generate a third wave of antibody response (anti–anti-idiotypic antibody). In theory, the preceding idiotype–anti-idiotype response can continue indefinitely; however, the circuit is ended when one of the antibody's idiotypes resembles that of an earlier antibody's idiotypes.[27,28]

Regulatory Effect of Suppressor T Cells

Whereas T_H cells promote B-cell activation, T_S cells downregulate B-cell activity. T_S activity has been demonstrated in cell transfer experiments. In these experiments an animal is made tolerant to a specific antigen and the cells and plasma are collected. Naive animals are then given either the cells or the plasma from the tolerized animals and then are challenged with the antigen. The animals receiving the cells do not produce antibody in response to the antigen.[7] The mechanisms by which T_S cells work is at present unclear.[29]

Regulation of T Cells

In principle, T and B cells should share similar regulatory mechanisms. The search for T-cell idiotypes has proved to be rewarding: The existence of an idiotype profile of the variable regions of T-cell antigen receptor is well documented. Thus, the potential for the T cells to be regulated by way of the idiotypic network exists.[30,31] The idiotypic network of T-cell antigen receptor is likely to be more complex than the antibody idiotypic network because two types of regulatory T cells, in-

ducer and suppressor T cells, exist. Undoubtedly, T suppressor cells are also likely to play a role in the regulation of the T-cell–mediated immune responses.

Review Questions

1. Which of the following pairs of genes are found on the same chromosome?

   a. V gene for lambda and C gene for kappa
   b. C gene for gamma and C gene for kappa
   c. V gene for lambda and V gene for heavy chain
   d. C gene for gamma and D gene for heavy chain

2. Which of the following glycoproteins is composed of five polypeptides found closely associated with the T-cell receptor and is responsible for transducing the signal that antigen and TCR have interacted?

   a. CD4
   b. CD3
   c. CD2
   d. CD8

3. Interferon gamma

   a. enhances expression of MHC proteins.
   b. is mainly made by macrophages.
   c. is made by T_H2 cells.
   d. is an autocrine growth factor for T cells.

4. Which of the following is true regarding cell surface adhesion molecules?

   a. LFA-1 binds ICAM-1.
   b. Blocking LFA-1 has no effect on natural killer cell activity.
   c. LFA-3 binds ICAM-1.
   d. Blocking LFA-3 has no effect on cell-mediated immunity.

5. A difference between innate and acquired immunity is

   a. innate responses are enhanced by subsequent exposures
   b. memory is a feature of acquired immunity
   c. inflammation is part of acquired immunity
   d. innate immunity is controlled by immune response genes

6. Effector molecules are produced in response to specific epitopes. Which of the following statements is true?

   a. CD8 cells secrete porins.
   b. B cells secrete antibody.
   c. CD4 cells are involved in direct cell-cell killing.
   d. CD4 cells are involved in T-independent pathways.

7. Which of the following is true?

   a. Antigen recognition by B cells is MHC restricted.
   b. T cells bind soluble antigen.
   c. The B-cell antigen receptor has preprogrammed specificity.
   d. IL-1 is an autocrine growth factor for T cells.

8. IL-2 is produced mainly by

   a. B cells
   b. T cells
   c. macrophages
   d. plasma cells

9. Suppressor cells are likely to have the following characteristics

   a. IgD on their surface
   b. CD2 on their surface
   c. the ability to mature into plasma cells
   d. the presence of MHC Class II proteins on their surface

10. During its lifetime a B lymphocyte may switch its

   a. immunoglobulin light-chain isotype
   b. immunoglobulin heavy-chain isotype
   c. constant region of the immunoglobulin light chain
   d. immunoglobulin idiotype

References

1. Roitt I, Brostoff J, Male D: Immunology, p 11.1. London, Gower Medical Publishing, 1985
2. Thiele DI, Lipsky PE: The accessory function of phagocytic cells in human T-cell and B-cell responses. J Immunol 129:1033, 1982
3. Schwartz RH: T-lymphocyte recognition of antigen in association with gene products of the major histocompatibility complex. Annu Rev Immunol 3:237, 1985
4. Neejles JJ, Momburg F: Cell biology of antigen presentation. Curr Opin Immunol 5:27–34, 1993
5. Reth M: Antigen receptors on B lymphocytes. Annu Rev Immunol 10:97–121, 1992
6. Leiden JM: Transcriptional regulation of T-cell receptor genes. Annu Rev Immunol 11:539–570, 1993
7. Roitt I, Brostoff J, Male D: Immunology, p 8.1. London, Gower Medical Publishing, 1985
8. Schwab R, Crow MK, Russo C, Weksler HE: Requirements for T-cell activations by OK3 monoclonal antibody: Role of T3 molecules and interleukin-1. J Immunol 135:1714, 1985
9. Dinarello CA, Mier JW: Lymphokines. N Engl J Med 317:940, 1987
10. Le J, Vilcek J: Tumor necrosis factor and interleukin-1: Cytokines with multiple overlapping biological activities. Lab Invest 36:234, 1987
11. Biron CA: Cytokines in the generation of immune responses to, and resolution of, virus infection. Curr Opin Immunol 6:530–538, 1994
12. Jongstra J, Misener V: Developmental maturation of the B-cell antigen receptor. Immunol Rev 132:107–123, 1993
13. Roitt I, Brostoff J, Male D: Immunology, p 8.1. London, Gower Medical Publishing, 1985
14. Yancopoulus GD, Alt FW: Regulation of the assembly and expression of variable-region genes. Annu Rev Immunol 4:339, 1986
15. Griffiths GM, Berek C, Kaartinen M, et al: Somatic mutations of immune response to 2-phenyl oxazolone. Nature 312:271, 1984
16. Lu YJ, Kassir R, Kelsoe G: Studies of specific B cell activation in primary and secondary responses to T cell dependent and T cell independent antigens. J Exp Med 173:1165–1175, 1991
17. Neuberger MS, Milstein C: Somatic hypermutation. Curr Opin Immunol 7:248–254, 1995
18. Hood LE, Weissman IL, Wood WB, et al: The immune response: Affinity maturation and immunologic memory. In: Immunology, 2nd ed, p 287. Menlo Park, CA, Benjamin/Cummings, 1984
19. Mehta SR, Sandler RS, Ford RJ, et al: Cellular interaction between B and T lymphocytes: Enhanced release of B cell growth factor. Lymphokine Res 5:49, 1986
20. Howaed M, Paul WE: Interleukins for B lymphocytes. Lymphokine Res 1:1, 1982
21. Maizel AI, Sahasrabuddhe C, Mehta S, et al: Characterization of B-cell growth factor. Lymphokine Res 1:9, 1982
22. Sharma S, Mehta S, Morgan J, Maizel A: Molecular cloning and expression of a B-cell growth factor gene in *Escherichia coli*. Science 235:1489, 1987
23. Yokoda T, Otsuka T, Mosmann T, et al: Isolation and characterization of a human interleukin cDNA clone, homologous to mouse B-cell stimulatory factor 1, that expresses B-cell and T-cell stimulating activities. Proc Natl Acad Sci USA 83:5894, 1986
24. Lazarus AH, Baines MG: Studies on the mechanism of specificity of human natural killer cells for tumor cells: Correlation between target cell transferin receptor ex-

pression and competitive activity. Cell Immunol 96:255, 1985

25. MacDougall SL, Shustik C, Sullivan AK: Target cell specificity of human natural killer cells. Cell Immunol 103:352, 1986

26. Jerne NK: Idiotypic network and other preconceived ideas. Immunol Rev 79:5, 1984

27. Burdette S, Schwartz RS: Idiotypes and idiotypic networks. N Engl J Med 317:219, 1987

28. Rajewsky K, Takemori T: Genetics, expression, and function of idiotypes. Annu Rev Immunol 1:569, 1983

29. Murphy DB: T cell mediated immunosuppression. Curr Opin Immunol 5:411–417, 1993

30. Geha RS: Idiotypic determination on human T cells and modulation of human T cell receptors by anti-idiotypic antibodies. J Immunol 133:1846, 1984

31. Sim GK, Mackneil A, Augustin AA: T helper receptors; idiotypes and repertoire. Immunol Rev 90:49, 1986

CHAPTER 4

Mechanisms of the Nonspecific Immune Response

Karen James

Objectives

Upon completion of the chapter, the reader will be able to:

1. Define the cells involved in the nonspecific immune response
2. Describe the functions of polymorphonuclear leukocytes, eosinophils, basophils and other mediator cells, and mononuclear phagocytes
3. Recall the abnormalities or disease states that result from abnormalities in polymorphonuclear leukocyte function
4. Define the 14 complement components
5. Describe the functions of each of the complement components, whether each is involved in the classical and/or alternative pathway, and the activity unit of each (recognition, activation, membrane attack)
6. Define the complement component control proteins
7. Describe how the complement control proteins exhibit their function
8. Recall the disease states that result from abnormalities in complement components or control proteins of the complement sequence
9. Define the acute phase proteins
10. Describe the phases or events that constitute inflammation

CELLULAR MECHANISMS OF THE NONSPECIFIC IMMUNE RESPONSE

Barrier Epithelial Cells

The body's first line of defense is an intact barrier of epithelial cells. This includes the skin and mucous membrane linings of the respiratory, urinary, and gastrointestinal tracts. The skin is the largest single organ of the body, with one of its chief functions being protection from the external environment.[1] The layers of the skin are essentially continuous with the mucous membranes of the digestive, respiratory, and genitourinary tracts. When epithelial structures are damaged (e.g., cuts or punctures) or destroyed (severe burns), the protective effect of the epithelial barrier is destroyed and the danger of an infectious process is significantly increased. Most infections enter the body through the mucous membranes, which are protected not only by epithelial barrier cells, but also by biochemical defense mechanisms in the secretions (e.g., lysozyme, stomach acid, secretory immunoglobulins).

Polymorphonuclear Neutrophils

Polymorphonuclear neutrophils (PMNs) comprise the largest population of leukocytes in the peripheral blood. The mature PMN is primarily a phagocytic cell with distinct granules.[2] The granules contain acid hydrolases, microbicidal proteins (e.g., myeloperoxidase, lysozyme), proteases, and other proteins (e.g., lactoferrin). Each of these biochemical components performs either a bactericidal function or serves to degrade the organic materials that remain after bacteria are killed.[3]

PMNs are involved in the nonspecific immune response through a series of steps: (1) adhesion or attachment to the damaged epithelium, (2) locomotion or amoeboid movement, (3) diapedesis or emigration through the wall of the blood vessel into the tissues, (4) chemotaxis or directed movement toward the particles to be engulfed, (5) phagocytosis or ingestion of the bacteria, (6) increased metabolism through glycolysis, (7) degranulation, and (8) digestion of the foreign material.[4,5]

The specific adhesion of cells to each other or to an extracellular matrix is a fundamental mechanism of cell migration, recognition, inflammation, and immune reactions. The group of proteins named integrins have specific adhesion functions.[6] One important mechanism of integrin function is the activation of these molecules to rapidly change from a low-adherence state to a high-adherence state because of a controllable conformational change. This controllable adhesiveness provides for the tight adherence of circulating leukocytes to vascular endothelium, followed by intermediate adhesion during transendothelial migration and de-adhesion (release of adherence) at extravasation (release from the capillary into the surrounding tissue).[6]

Locomotion of PMNs is similar to the movements of amebae.[5] PMNs can crawl about on the surfaces of blood vessel walls, changing direction every 20 μm or so by sending out pseudopods from a different part of the cell surface. In the absence of specific stimuli, this locomotion is not in a straight line and is not directed toward anything in particular. For diapedesis to occur, locomotion is necessary, as is adherence to the walls of the capillaries.

Diapedesis, or emigration through the wall of the blood vessel, occurs following adherence to the endothelium (Fig. 4-1). The PMN inserts pseudopods between the endothelial cell junctions, disrupting the basement membrane at that location so that the PMN can "squeeze" itself out of the blood vessel into the surrounding tissue spaces.

Chemotaxis is the directed movement of phagocytic cells either toward or away from substances or particles in the environment. Directed migration of PMNs is mediated primarily by fluid-phase components of the complement system, particularly C5a, which is discussed later in this chapter. Other factors that are known to be chemotactic include certain products of the coagulation or fibrinolytic pathways and certain bacterial products.[2]

Phagocytosis has been studied for over 75 years. The external cell wall of the PMN seems to adhere to and completely surround the offending bacterium or other particle, encapsulating the foreign substance with a layer of inside-out membrane called a phagosome (Fig. 4-2). Opsonins such as C3b and IgG clearly increase the rate and quantity of particle uptake. Opsonins have been described as the "butter on the bread" that makes the particle more "appetizing" to the phago-

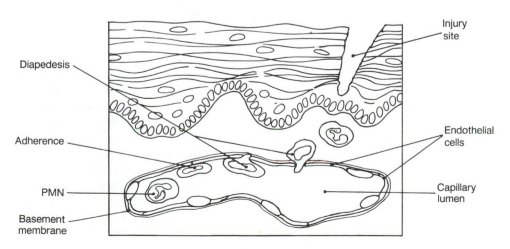

FIGURE 4-1
Adherence and diapedesis of PMNs.

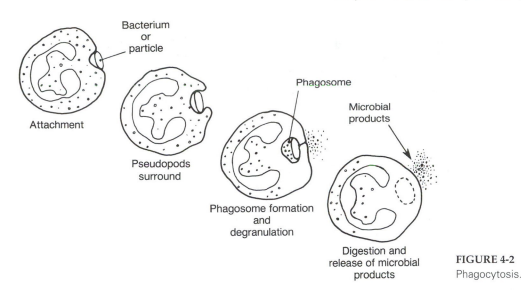

FIGURE 4-2
Phagocytosis.

cytic cell. C3b and immune complexes bind to specific Fcγ receptors (FcRI, FcRII, FcRIII), C3b receptors (CRI or CRII), IgA receptors, or IgE receptors.[7]

During phagocytosis, the metabolism of leukocytes changes rather dramatically. O_2 and glucose are consumed, primarily through the hexose monophosphate shunt. H_2O_2 is produced in the respiratory burst that occurs as the phagocytosed particle is digested.

Degranulation of granulocytes involves the fusion of intracellular granules with the plasma membrane of the PMN. The contents of the granules are then released either into the phagosome or into the accumulated fluid outside of the cell.[3,5] As is discussed in the section on inflammation, much of the tissue damage associated with injury can be attributed to the release of the contents of the granules during degranulation of PMNs. Digestion occurs following the degranulation step. When the granules are fused with the vacuole containing the phagocytosed particle, the particle is exposed to the lytic action of the enzymes. The mechanism by which many types of bacteria are killed following ingestion by phagocytes requires H_2O_2 and the enzyme myeloperoxidase (MPO).

Dysfunctions of Polymorphonuclear Neutrophils

Diseases associated with dysfunctions of PMNs include chronic granulomatous disease (CGD), glucose-6-phosphate dehydrogenase (G6PD) deficiency, myeloperoxidase (MPO) deficiency, and Chediak-Higashi (CH) syndrome.[8] CGD is a heterogeneous group of disorders characterized by molecular defects in the NADPH-oxidase enzyme system that result in abnormalities of neutrophil function. Molecular biology techniques have facilitated identifying several genetic abnormalities that result in CGD.[9] The majority (67%) of CGD patients have an X-linked defect of the β subunit of flavocytochrome b. (Flavocytochrome b is a small heme protein, present in the endoplasmic reticulum, involved in the electron transport pathway). The remaining one third of CGD patients exhibit autosomal recessive patterns of inheritance at three different chromosome locations. CGD is characterized by infections, predominantly at epithelial surfaces with environmental contact (skin, mucous membranes, lung, and gut). Failure to thrive is an associated response to the chronic infections in children. The bacteria responsible for the majority of infections include *Staphylococcus aureus* and enteric Gram-negative rods, such as *Salmonella, Klebsiella, Aerobacter, Pseudomonas*, and *Serratia. Aspergillus* species of fungi are also frequently implicated.

The laboratory test most useful in the diagnosis of CGD is the nitroblue tetrazolium (NBT) test. NBT is a yellow, water-soluble compound that turns blue upon reduction. The dye is ingested in the presence of latex particles. When H_2O_2 is produced along with other events associated with the respiratory burst, the dye is reduced by normal PMNs; blue granules can be seen morphologically or the NBT can be extracted and the reaction read at A_{580} to measure NBT reduction as a ratio to ingestion.[10] The normal ratio is ≥2.5. In the absence of bacteria, the CGD PMN cannot produce H_2O_2, so the dye remains yellow, with a resulting NBT reduction/ingestion ratio ≤1.5. Females with a ratio between 1.5 and 2.5 have a subpopulation of PMNs that do not reduce NBT and are carriers of the X-linked disease, exhibiting a mixed population of NBT-positive and NBT-negative cells.[11] Carrier states for the autosomal types of CGD do not show such aberrations; their detection requires genetic analysis.

Theoretically, CGD could be cured by allogeneic stem cell transplantation, but the risks outweigh the potential benefits. An alternative strategy would be gene therapy, delivering the genetic material in vitro or in vivo by retroviral vectors to hematopoietic progenitors derived from the patients.[9]

G6PD deficiency is an X-linked recessive disorder resulting in a defective enzyme rather than an absence of enzyme. Several hundred variants of the enzyme have been described, only a few of which lead to severe hemolysis in the absence of defined oxidative stress. The form of G6PD deficiency seen in African Americans does not result in hemolysis unless stimulated by a drug (e.g., quinine) or rarely by a febrile illness or diabetic ketoacidosis.[11] The G6PD enzyme is the first in the hexose monophosphate shunt pathway. Only in recent years has it been recognized that these patients also have a defect in leukocyte function.[8] Although G6PD deficiency is inherited in an X-linked manner, leukocyte function in both males and females can be affected. The susceptibility to organisms is similar to that of CGD patients, but the onset of the disease is usually later in life and associated with anemia. Laboratory diagnosis is by the NBT test and by detection of the G6PD deficiency.

MPO deficiency and CH syndrome are relatively rare disorders.[8] Functional and immunochemical absence of the enzyme MPO from granules of neutrophils and monocytes, but not from eosinophils, is inherited as an autosomal recessive trait.[11] MPO potentiates the microbicidal effectiveness of H_2O_2 in the phagosome, which is necessary for killing certain organisms, particularly *Candida* species and staphylococcal species. MPO deficiency can be diagnosed in the laboratory by peroxidase-staining peripheral blood leukocytes.

CH syndrome is a rare, genetically determined disease manifested clinically by abnormal leukocyte granulation, defective pigmentation, and increased susceptibility to infections.[12] Morphologically, CH is characterized by giant cytoplasmic granular inclusions in PMNs and platelets that are discernible by light microscopy. The metabolic and biochemical pathways associated with other enzyme deficiencies appear to be normal, but the PMNs of these patients have abnormal intracellular killing of organisms, which include streptococcal and pneumococcal species as well as those listed earlier for MPO deficiency. CH syndrome patients have also been shown to have defective natural killer (NK) cells,[12] a defect that can be partially reversed in vitro by substances known to increase cyclic GMP or decrease cyclic AMP. Such substances have normalized both bacterial killing and NK response.[12,13] The laboratory diagnosis of CH syndrome can be made by light microscopic examination of PMNs and platelets.

Eosinophils

The eosinophilic granulocytes constitute less than 3% of the circulating leukocytes in the blood of normal humans. Eosinophils arise from a common progenitor cell with PMNs but are much less efficient at phagocytosis. The granules of eosinophils do not contain lysozyme but are rich in acid phosphatase and peroxidase activity.[14] Although the role of eosinophils is not known, two roles have been postulated: Ingestion of immune complexes and limiting inflammatory reactions by antagonizing the effects of mediators (discussed later). Eosinophil granules also have a unique protein called eosinophilic basic protein, which has been found to be toxic to certain parasites, the clearance of which is also attributed to eosinophils.[14] Eosinophilia (>10% of leukocytes in peripheral blood) is associated with allergic reactions as well as parasitic infections.

Mediator Cells

Cells that participate in immunologic reactions by release of biochemical substances (mediators) include mast cells, basophils, and platelets.[14] The biologic activities of these mediators include increased vascular permeability, smooth muscle contraction, and augmentation of the inflammatory response (Fig. 4-3). Blood platelets contain serotonin and lysosomal enzymes that are released from the granules during platelet aggregation. Serotonin apparently does not have a pharmacologic role in humans, but lysosomal enzymes participate in digestion of foreign materials.

Skin and the gastrointestinal tract are particularly rich in mast cells. Granules containing the potent mediators are released from mast cells upon injury to these

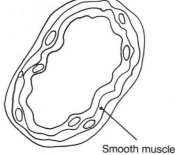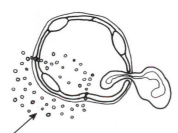

Smooth muscle
contraction

Increased
vascular
permeability

FIGURE 4-3
Biologic activities of mediator substances.

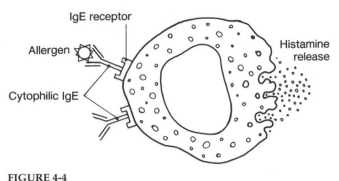

FIGURE 4-4
Basophil/mast cell histamine release.

tissues.[15] The biochemical components of these granules include heparin, histamine, tumor necrosis factor (TNFα), superoxide dismutase, peroxidase, and acid hydrolases. Immunologic reactions involving IgE that binds to high affinity Fc receptors for IgE (FcεRI) on the surface of mast cells and basophils can trigger degranulation and release of the mediators into the circulation (Fig. 4-4). Mast cells can be stimulated to degranulate by nonimmunologic mechanisms (e.g., infections of the skin or mucous membranes, surgical incisions, heat, pressure, and certain other agents).

Basophils make up 0.5% to 2% of circulating leukocytes. At one time it was thought that basophils were circulating mast cells (or that mast cells were stationary basophils), but further study has shown these two cell types differ in the structure and content of their granules. Basophilic granules contain primarily histamine and a group of sulfidopeptide leukotrienes, LTC$_4$, LTD$_4$, and LTE$_4$ (formerly called slow-reacting substance of anaphylaxis [SRS-A]), which are potent spasmogenic agents causing constriction of smooth muscle.[16]*

Like mast cells, basophils respond to IgE-containing immune complexes that bind to the IgE receptors on the basophils to stimulate degranulation. The primary function of the basophil appears to be to amplify the reaction that starts with the mast cells at the site of entry of the antigen. For example, initial evidence of sensitivity to the antigenic substances from penicillin might be a skin rash, but a severe allergic reaction to penicillin can result in disseminated effects from the histamine released from basophils within the circulation. Rare cases of basophil leukemia have been reported, but no specific diseases have been associated with a general basophilia.

*LTC$_4$ *5S-hydroxy-6R-S-glutathionyl-7,9-trans-11,14-cis-eicosatetraenoic acid (leukotriene C$_4$).*
LTD$_4$ is LTC$_4$ cleaved by gamma glutamyl transpeptidase to 5S-hydroxy-6R-S-cysteinylglycyl-7,9-trans-11,14-cis-eicosatetraenoic acid (leukotriene D$_4$).
LTE$_4$ is LTD$_4$ cleaved by a dipeptidase to 5S-hydroxy-6R-S-cysteinyl-7,9-trans-11,14-cis-eicosatetraenoic acid (leukotriene E$_4$).

Mononuclear Phagocyte System

The term *reticulendothelial system* (RES) was introduced by Aschoff in 1924 to designate all actively phagocytic cells.[5] The current definition of the RES is limited to mononuclear phagocytic cells and has been renamed the *mononuclear phagocyte system* (MPS). Mononuclear phagocytes include tissue macrophages located primarily in the reticular connective tissue framework of the spleen, liver, and lymphoid tissues and their immature circulating form as blood monocytes.[2] Debris removed by the MPS include old or injured red cells, white cells and platelets, bacteria, antigen-antibody complexes, and degenerated or damaged cell membranes.[17] The Kupffer cells of the liver are the most actively phagocytic cells in the MPS. Other histiocytes (tissue macrophages) actively involved in phagocytosis include alveolar (pulmonary) macrophages, splenic macrophages, and macrophages of the lymph nodes, peritoneum, and other areas (Fig. 4-5). At times when the MPS is actively involved in eliminating debris from circulation, organs that are rich in tissue macrophages become involved, resulting in lymphadenopathy (enlarged lymph nodes), splenomegaly (enlarged spleen), or hepatomegaly (enlarged liver). It is the intent of the body's defense mechanisms that these secondary barriers stop the spread of infection, but in some cases even the MPS becomes overwhelmed.

Mechanisms of phagocytosis that were described earlier for PMNs also occur with monocytes and macrophages. Circulating PMNs, however, are end-stage cells (i.e., after phagocytosis and degranulation, these cells die). Macrophages, conversely, appear to be stimulated by the processes involved with phagocytosis, become secretory cells, synthesize acute phase proteins, and may even proliferate locally within the tissues.[2]

Mononuclear phagocytes respond to the same chemotactic factors that attract PMNs (e.g., the C5a

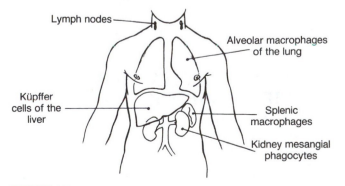

FIGURE 4-5
Organs and cells of the MPS.

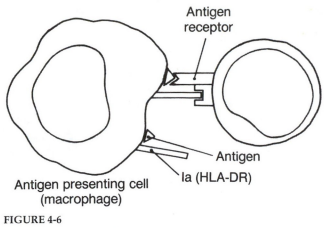

FIGURE 4-6
HLA-DR(Ia)+ monocyte-bound antigen.

peptide of complement). The primary chemotactic materials to which macrophages respond are soluble factors (cytokines) released from T lymphocytes, which are discussed in more detail in a later chapter. Peripheral blood monocytes are much less efficient at phagocytosis and killing bacteria than are PMNs. Macrophages use predominantly the oxygen-dependent metabolic pathways to provide energy for the cell.

Mononuclear phagocytes are less efficient than PMNs at killing bacteria, and the mechanisms of killing are not as well understood. When macrophages are stimulated by phagocytic events, they become secretory cells that produce and secrete a wide variety of biologically active factors that influence the activities of lymphocytes.[2] One factor, interleukin-1 (IL-1), has specificity for activating T cells, but most of the factors secreted by macrophages nonspecifically suppress the activities of lymphocytes. These include interferon, prostaglandins, complement components, and certain other acute phase proteins.

Antigen presentation is another very important function of a subset of macrophages with major histocompatibility complex (MHC) antigens on their surface.[18] Macrophages process antigen by phagocytosis, partial degradation of foreign antigen into discrete antigenic fragments (peptides), and displaying those peptides in association with MHC molecules providing an effective antigenic stimulus for T lymphocytes (Fig. 4-6).

HUMORAL MECHANISMS OF THE NONSPECIFIC IMMUNE RESPONSE

Complement

The complement system consists of 14 components that are involved in two separate pathways of activation. The five proteins that are unique to the classical pathway include the trimolecular complex of C1 (C1q, C1r, C1s), C4, and C2. Three proteins are unique to the alternative pathway, including Factor B, Factor D, and P (properdin). Six components that participate in both the classical and alternative pathways include C3, C5, C6, C7, C8, and C9. These components were named in the order in which they were described; consequently, the sequence of activation is not in numerical order. Although complement activation is complex, the components interact in a specific cascading sequence. Both pathways can be divided into three units (recognition, activation, and membrane attack), which simplifies the study of complement.[19]

CLASSICAL PATHWAY

Recognition Unit

The C1q molecule consists of a collagenous region with six globular head groups. This component appears to be like a flower pot with six flowers. When a specific antibody interacts with its corresponding antigen, binding sites for the globular head groups of C1q are exposed on the Fc region of the antibody molecule (Fig. 4-7). At least two molecules of IgG or C-reactive protein (CRP) or one molecule of IgM are required for the binding of C1q.[20] When circulating in plasma, the collagen portion of C1q is surrounded by two molecules of C1r and two molecules of C1s. When C1q binds to the Fc region of IgG or IgM, or the equivalent region of CRP, a conformational change occurs in C1q. This change in C1q causes the proenzyme C1r to become the enzymatically active C1r. The substrate for the enzyme C1r is C1s, which is then cleaved to become the serine esterase C1s.

Activation Unit

The active enzyme of C1s cleaves two proteins, C4 (into C4a and C4b) and C2 (into C2a and C2b), in a magnesium-dependent reaction. C4b and C2a combine to form an active enzyme C4b2a, which is the classical pathway C3 convertase (Fig. 4-8). C4a and C2b are byproducts of the process of activation of the classical pathway. The enzymatically active C4b2a complex can cleave many molecules of C3 into C3a and C3b. The C3b can then either form a covalent bond with the antigen or with bystander surfaces (e.g., erythrocytes) in immune adherence (discussed later) or can bind to C4b2a to form C4b2a3b, an enzyme with specificity for C5. The final enzymatic step of the classical complement pathway is the cleavage of C5 into C5a and C5b by the C5 convertase, C4b2a3b. At this point, the classical pathway and the alternative pathway converge, with both pathways using the same membrane attack unit.

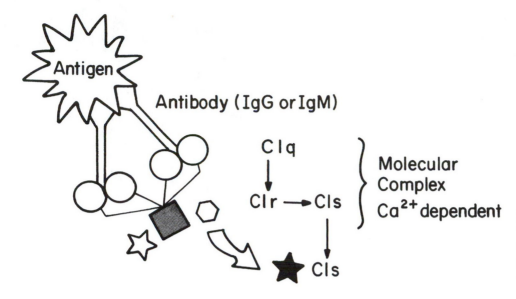

FIGURE 4-7
The classical pathway recognition unit. (From James K. Complement: Activation, consequences, and control. Am J Med Technol 48:735, 1982.)

Membrane Attack Unit

C5b binds to one molecule of C6 to form a stable bimolecular complex, C5b6. If C7 is present, a trimolecular complex, C5b67, is formed. C5b67 binds hydrophobically to a membrane (Fig. 4-9). Once C5b67 is bound, C8 can attach to form a functional transmembrane channel. Up to six molecules of C9 can surround the puncture site, which effectively prevents the channel

from being resealed. C9 is not essential for the lytic event, but it does accelerate lysis.

ALTERNATIVE PATHWAY

Recognition Unit

Efficient activation of the alternative pathway is dependent upon the availability of an activating surface. Sub-

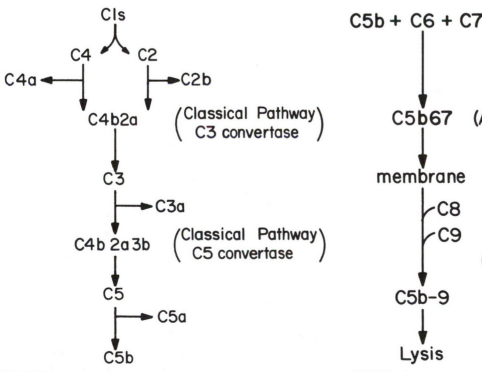

FIGURE 4-8
The classical pathway activation unit. (From James K. Complement: Activation, consequences, and control. Am J Med Technol 48:735, 1982.)

FIGURE 4-9
The membrane attack unit, common to both pathways. (From James K. Complement: Activation, consequences, and control. Am J Med Technol 48:735, 1982.)

stances known to provide an activation surface are bacterial cell walls, bacterial lipopolysaccharide, fungal cell walls, some virus-infected cells, and rabbit erythrocytes.[21] The "activating surface" protects spontaneously hydrolyzed C3 (non-enzymatically cleaved into C3a and C3b) from being inactivated by the control proteins.[22] Hydrolyzed C3 becomes C3b-like (Fig. 4-10). In the presence of Factor D and magnesium, this C3b-like molecule can cleave Factor B into Ba and Bb. Ba becomes a byproduct, while Bb binds to C3b to form an alternative pathway C3 convertase, C3bBb. By itself, C3bBb is a very unstable molecule and would be quickly inactivated by control proteins unless it is bound to an activating surface such as those listed previously.

Activation Unit

When protected by an activating surface and stabilized by P (properdin), the C3bBbP enzymatic complex can cleave additional molecules of C3. If a second C3b molecule is inserted into the C3 convertase to become C3bBb3bP, this becomes a C5 convertase, which can cleave C5 into C5a and C5b (Fig. 4-11).

Membrane Attack Unit

The membrane attack unit for the alternative pathway begins with C5b and progresses through C6, C7, C8, and C9 in exactly the same sequence as it does for the classical pathway.

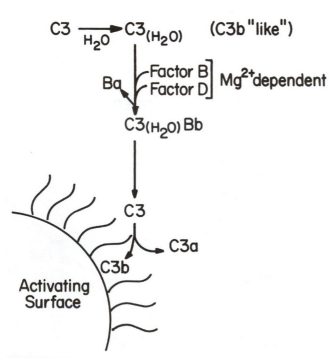

FIGURE 4-10

The alternative-pathway recognition unit. (From James K. Complement: Activation, consequences, and control. Am J Med Technol 48:735, 1982.)

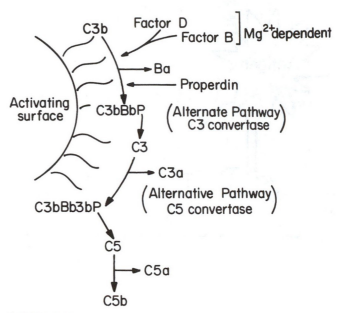

FIGURE 4-11

The alternative-pathway activation unit. (From James K. Complement: Activation, consequences, and control. Am J Med Technol 48:735, 1982.)

BIOLOGIC CONSEQUENCES OF COMPLEMENT ACTIVATION

Amplification

C3b can be generated either by the classical pathway C3 convertase (C4b2a) or by the alternative pathway C3 convertase (C3bBbP). This provides a feedback loop that uses the alternative pathway components (B, D, and P) in both pathways to amplify the activation of the C3 through C9 components of activation and membrane attack (Fig. 4-12).

Anaphylatoxins

The cleavage of C4, C3, and C5 results in the release of the biologically active peptides C4a, C3a, and C5a (Fig. 4-13). These anaphylatoxins mediate inflammation by inducing the release of histamine from basophils and mast cells, by causing smooth muscle to contract, and by increasing vascular permeability.[23]

Immune Adherence

Immune adherence is the covalent bonding between the cleaved form of C3 (C3b) and nearby soluble immune complexes or surfaces of particles (Fig. 4-14). The portion of C3b that does not adhere is exposed and available for binding to the receptor for C3b (CRI) on human erythrocytes, B lymphocytes, monocytes, glomerular epithelial cells, or mast cells. B lymphocytes and macrophages also have receptors for C3d (CRII), which is formed by cleaving C3b into C3c and C3d. One biologic purpose for immune adherence would be to facilitate removal of soluble immune complexes. Immune

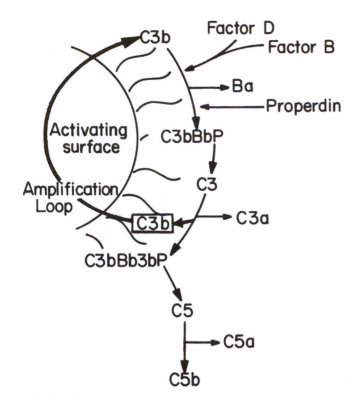

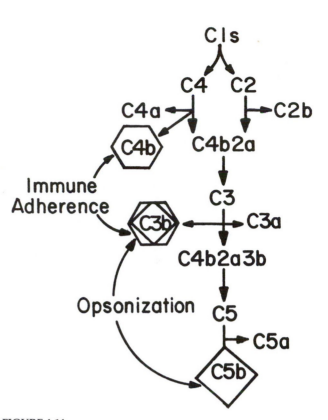

FIGURE 4-12

The amplification loop of the alternative pathway. (From James K. Complement: Activation, consequences, and control. Am J Med Technol 48:735, 1982.)

FIGURE 4-14

Immune adherence, mediated by C3b and C4b. Opsonization, mediated by C3b and C5b. (From James K. Complement: Activation, consequences, and control. Am J Med Technol 48:735, 1982.)

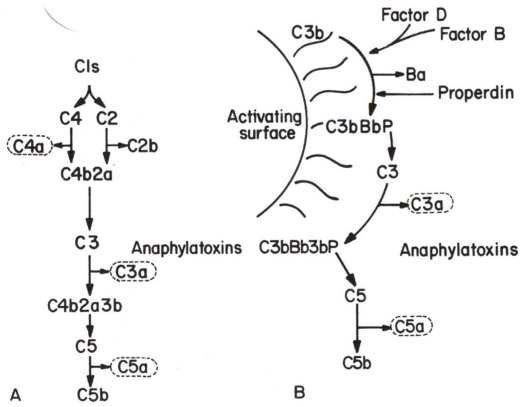

FIGURE 4-13

The anaphylatoxins are biologically active cleavage products resulting from the cleavage of C4, C3, and C5. (From James K. Complement: Activation, consequences, and control. Am J Med Technol 48:735, 1982.)

adherence provides a mechanism for the soluble complexes to bind to erythrocytes, facilitating removal of the complexes by the MPS.

Opsonization

Immune adherence is the covalent binding of C3b to a surface; however, if C3b and IgG are present on that surface, phagocytosis by PMNs or monocytes is enhanced. The C3b receptors on these cells bind to the exposed C3b on the surface of the particle. The membrane of the phagocytic cell surrounds the opsonized particle, much like the two sides of a zipper fusing together. When the particle is completely surrounded, the cell membrane fuses together, thereby engulfing or phagocytosing the particle (see Fig. 4-2).

Chemotaxis

The byproduct resulting from the cleavage of C5 by either the classical or alternative pathway C5 convertase is C5a (Fig. 4-15). C5a is a potent chemotactic factor as well as an anaphylatoxin. C5a induces the directed migration of neutrophils and monocytes into the area of inflammation.[23]

Kinin Activation

The fragment of C2 (C2b) released during cleavage by C1s interacts with plasmin to produce kinin-like activity (Fig. 4-16). The biologic activity of C2b results in smooth muscle contraction, mucous gland secretion, increased vascular permeability, and pain.[24]

Lysis

In the laboratory, the activity of complement is studied by measuring the degree of lysis that occurs in sheep red blood cells. Lysis, however, plays a relatively minor biologic role. One example of lysis as the biologic consequence of complement activation is an antibody-mediated transfusion reaction. The lytic function of complement also appears to be necessary for host defense against *Neisseria*, which is discussed later in this chapter.

DEFICIENCIES OF COMPLEMENT COMPONENTS

It is important to distinguish consumption of complement from complement deficiencies. The most common causes of complement *consumption* are infections and collagen vascular diseases. The clinical immunology laboratory generally quantitates the C3 and C4 proteins to detect complement consumption to monitor disease activity. Because C4 (10 to 20 mg/mL) is found in a much lower concentration than C3 (80 to 120 mg/mL), C4 is more sensitive than C3 in detecting classical pathway complement consumption that occurs in an im-

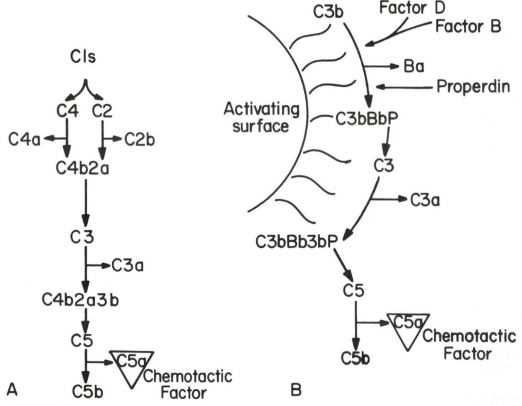

FIGURE 4-15
Chemotactic attraction of phagocytic cells, mediated by C5a. (From James K. Complement: Activation, consequences, and control. Am J Med Technol 48:735, 1982.)

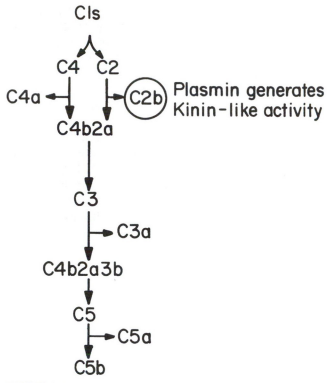

Plasmin generates
Kinin-like activity

FIGURE 4-16
Kinin-like activity, mediated by a fragment of activated C2. (From James K. Complement: Activation, consequences, and control. Am J Med Technol 48:735, 1982.)

mune-complex–mediated diseases such as systemic lupus erythematosus (SLE) or certain forms of vasculitis. C3 is an acute phase reactant, so the level elevates during inflammation, thereby sometimes masking the consumption of C3. Decreased C4 and normal C3 levels would indicate mild classical pathway complement activation with detectable consumption of C4 and probable consumption of C3 that has been compensated for by the acute phase response. A quantitative decrease in both C4 and C3 would be consistent with significant immune complex–mediated activation of the classical pathway. Because the alternative complement pathway bypasses C1, C4, and C2, decreased C3 and normal C4 levels would be found during activation of the alternative complement pathway, where C3 is consumed. Certain bacterial infections and glomerulonephritis can cause activation of the alternative pathway.

Functional complement activity is measured using a hemolytic assay, CH50 (or CH100) to determine the integrity of the entire classical complement pathway. Alternative pathway functional activity can be measured using rabbit erythrocytes instead of sensitized (antibody-coated) sheep erythrocytes in the CH50 assay. The primary use of the functional assays would be to screen for hereditary or acquired complement deficiencies that result in the absence of or markedly diminished lytic function.

Hereditary deficiencies reported for most of the complement components are summarized in Table 4-1.[25] The complement components are inherited as autosomal codominants, with each of two genes contributing 50% of normal protein levels. Consequently, a normal human with two functioning production genes will have 100% of the normal level of each complement component. A heterozygotic deficient patient (with one defective gene and one normal gene) will have 50% of the normal level of the protein. A homozygous deficient patient (with two defective or deficient genes) will have 0% to 10% of the normal level of the protein both quantitatively and functionally. The heterozygous state is usually not associated with any disease process unless the patient is compromised by some other medical problem.

Patients with homozygous deficiencies of complement proteins have an increased incidence of collagen vascular diseases.[25] Deficiencies of the early complement proteins of the classical pathway (C1, C4, C2) have a significantly higher incidence of lupus-like disease; 50% of C2-deficient patients develop SLE or related illnesses.[26]

C2 deficiency is the most common hereditary complement component deficiency, occurring in 1 in 10^5 individuals.[25] The gene for Factor B appears to be closely associated with the gene for C2, because C2-deficient patients have been reported to have decreased levels of Factor B. Patients with C3 deficiency have an inability to opsonize antigens, have recurrent pyogenic infections, and exhibit a clinical picture that is similar to X-linked agammaglobulinemia. C3 deficiency is a rare occurrence as an autosomal recessive inherited disease. Other complement component deficiencies are very rare.

The most common deficiency of a soluble serum complement control protein is C1INH deficiency. Deficiencies of C3 control proteins have been reported, all of which result in markedly decreased levels of C3 caused by activation or consumption of C3. Deficiency of the integral membrane complement proteins decay accelerating factor (DAF) and membrane inhibitor of

TABLE 4-1
Deficiencies of Complement Components

DEFICIENT COMPONENT	DISEASE ASSOCIATION
C1 (q, r, or s)	Lupus-like disease
C4	Lupus-like disease
C2	Lupus-like disease
C3	Overwhelming infection
C5, C6, C7	*Neisseria* infections
C9	No known disease association
C1INH	Angioedema
H or I	Recurrent bacterial infections

reactive lysis (MIRL) result in paroxsymal nocturnal hemoglobinuria (PNH).[26]

Deficiencies of the complement components involved in the membrane attack complex (C5, C6, C7) have a high incidence of infections, particularly with *Neisseria* organisms. These patients have recurrent gonococcal or meningococcal infections, organisms that require complement-dependent lysis to be destroyed. C9 deficiencies do not appear to be associated with any particular disease state.

CONTROL MECHANISMS

If any or all of the biologic consequences of complement activation were to go uncontrolled, the effects of even minor inflammatory processes involving activation of either complement pathway would be potentially devastating. The body, however, does not leave a reaction uncontrolled. The first means of control is the extreme lability of activated complement components. If an activated enzyme does not combine with its substrate within milliseconds, the activity is lost or markedly decayed.[21] "Innocent bystander" cells in the vicinity of activated complement would be rapidly destroyed if the activated components were not so highly labile. Additionally, soluble serum proteins and integral membrane proteins serve as inhibitors or inactivators of specific reactions or products involved in the complement cascade. Other serum proteins that modulate complement activity will also be described.

Soluble Serum Inhibitory Proteins
C1 Inhibitor (C1INH). C1INH forms an irreversible complex with both C1r and C1s (Fig. 4-17) that blocks their enzymatic activities and dissociates them from C1q.[27] The hereditary or acquired deficiency of this protein results in uncontrolled activation of the classical pathway. Control proteins that exercise their activity at the level of C3 or later are still functioning, retarding the amplification loop and other biologic consequences of C3–C9 activation. C1s, in the absence of C1INH, continues to cleave C4 and C2 unchecked, resulting in release of C2b kinin-like activity and C4a anaphylatoxin activity.

The disease process associated with C1INH deficiency is angioedema (*angio* denoting relationship to blood vessels and *edema* indicating the presence of extraordinary amounts of fluid in the tissue spaces). C2b and C4a can both stimulate smooth muscle to contract and cause increased vascular permeability, which allows the fluid part of the blood to leak out into the extravascular spaces, causing edema. The hereditary form of the disease, hereditary angioedema (HAE), is transmitted as an autosomal dominant trait and occurs in approximately 1 in 10^6 individuals.[28] The C2b also causes excess mucous membrane secretions, reflected in HAE when the episodes involve the respiratory tract (which can be life threatening) and by the intense gastrointestinal pain. Acquired forms of angioedema are much rarer and are usually associated with lymphoproliferative diseases.[29] Both forms of the disease are treated with an anabolic steroid, danazol, which appears to stimulate the liver to produce C1INH as well as other proteins. The most effective screening test for C1INH is a serum C4 level, because C4 is decreased due to activation of C4 and C2. (C2 is not generally measured in the laboratory because normal levels are not of sufficient quantity to be detected by precipitation or nephelometric techniques used to detect C3 and C4.) The protein C1INH can be quantitatively analyzed by radial immunodiffusion or nephelometry, or can be qualitatively evaluated by a modification of the total hemolytic complement assay. A small but significant percentage (15%) of individuals with HAE have normal levels of nonfunctional protein. In those cases, the level of C1INH would be normal to elevated, but the qualitative or functional assay shows deficiency in activity.

β1H (H) and C3b Inactivator (I). The most important biologic consequence of complement activation is the feedback loop amplification mediated by C3b. Proteins H and I serve to tightly control the enzymes that cleave C3 and C5 (Fig. 4-18). I inactivates C3b and C4b, whereas H accelerates the decay of the alternative pathway C3 convertase by dissociating Bb from the enzyme.[30] H and I are both involved in cleaving C3b into its hemolytically inactive form, C3bi, which is further cleaved into C3c and C3d. Fluid-phase C3b is rapidly inactivated by H and I. Consequently, activation of the alternative pathway is dependent upon the presence of a protective (activating) surface, which shelters C3b from these two control proteins.

In patients with deficiencies of I or H, a very low serum C3 is found because of the uncontrolled formation of the alternative-pathway C3 convertase, which results in a rapid catabolism of C3 and Factor B.[21,30]

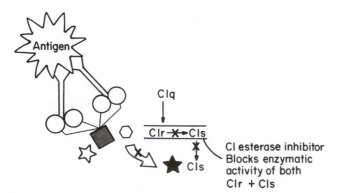

FIGURE 4-17
C1INH controls activation by blocking the enzymatic activity of C1r and C1s. (From James K. Complement: Activation, consequences, and control. Am J Med Technol 48:735, 1982.)

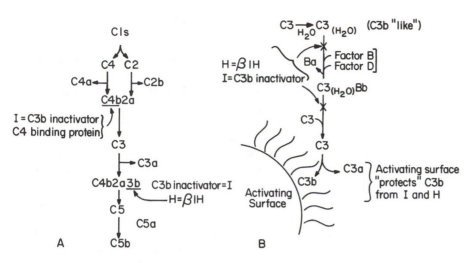

FIGURE 4-18

H and I control the amplification loop by dissociating Bb from the C3 convertase, thus inactivating C3b. (From James K. Complement: Activation, consequences, and control. Am J Med Technol 48:735, 1982.)

These patients are subject to recurrent bacterial infections because of poor opsonization and chemotaxis. A serum C3 level would effectively screen for the deficiencies of H and I control proteins. C3b inactivator (I) can also cleave and inactivate C4 but requires an accessory protein, C4 binding protein (Fig. 4-18).

Anaphylatoxin Inactivator. Carboxypeptidase controls the effects of C4a, C3a, and C5a by removing a single amino acid, a carboxy-terminal arginine.[23] Cleavage of this amino acid destroys the anaphylatoxin activity of these peptides (Fig. 4-19) but leaves the chemotactic effect of C5a remaining.

Membrane Attack Complex (MAC) Inhibitors. S protein (vitronectin) binds to C5b-7 complex and prevents membrane insertion of the MAC. SP-40 interacts with C5b-9 to modulate MAC formation.[26]

Integral Membrane Inhibitory Proteins[26]

Complement Receptor Type 1 (CRI, CD35). CRI are found on all peripheral blood cells except platelets and most T lymphocytes, and are also found on the epithelial cells of the kidney glomerulus. CRI binds C3b and C4b complement activation products, thus inhibiting the amplification loop. CRI on erythrocytes are responsible for binding circulating immune complexes and/or microorganisms that have activated complement and transporting them to the liver or spleen for clearance. CRI has decay accelerating activity for the classical and alternative pathway C3 convertases. CRI also acts as a cofactor for Protein I–mediated cleavage of C3b and C4b.

Complement Receptor Type 2 (CRII, CD21). CRII is the Epstein-Barr virus receptor and is found on mature B lymphocytes, follicular dendritic cells, and probably on epithelial cells. CRII binds C3d. In addition to regulating complement activation, CRII helps mediate B-cell growth and differentiation.

Complement Receptor Type 3 (CDIII, CD11b/18). CRIII binds C3bi, which is C3b that has been inactivated by cleavage by proteases. Interaction with this receptor is the primary triggering mechanism for phagocytosis of coated particles. CRIII also binds carbohydrates with a lectin-binding capacity.

Anaphylatoxin Receptors. Membrane receptors for C3a and C4a are found on mast cells, basophils, lymphocytes, and smooth muscle cells. Receptors for C5a are found on granulocytes, monocytes, mast cells, and basophils. C5a receptors are particularly abundant on

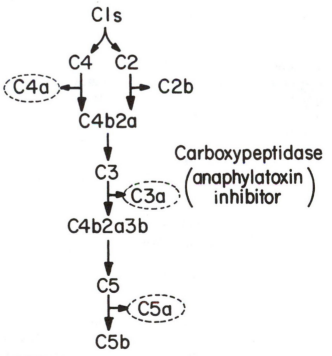

FIGURE 4-19

Carboxypeptidase inactivates anaphylatoxins. (From James K. Complement: Activation, consequences, and control. Am J Med Technol 48:735, 1982.)

neutrophils, where they affect the chemotactic function as well as stimulating the release of granule contents in response to the anaphylatoxin activities of C5a.

Decay Accelerating Factor (DAF). DAF is found on most peripheral blood cells (except NK cells, bone marrow mononuclear cells, erythroid progenitors, and epithelial and endothelial cells).[31] Soluble DAF is found in body fluids, including plasma and urine. DAF binds C4b2b and C3bBb to accelerate dissociation of these classical and alternative pathway C3 convertases.

Membrane Cofactor Protein (MCP, CD46). MCP is found on most peripheral blood cells (except erythrocytes, endothelial and epithelial cells, and fibroblasts). MCP binds C3b and C4b, and functions as a cofactor to Protein I–mediated cleavage of C3b and C4b.

Homologous Restriction Factor (HRF). HRF is found on erythrocytes, lymphocytes, monocytes, neutrophils, and platelets. MCP binds to fluid-phase C8 and C9, blocking their binding to the MAC of autologous cells. The action of this membrane protein is restricted to C8 and C9 of the same species. This blocking function prevents the lysis of bystander cells (reactive lysis).

Membrane Inhibitor of Reactive Lysis (MIRL, CD59). MIRL is found on erythrocytes, lymphocytes, monocytes, neutrophils, platelets, and endothelial and epithelial cells. MIRL binds to C7 and C8, preventing MAC formation. The action of MIRL is species specific and inhibits the lysis of bystander cells (reactive lysis).

Complement Enhancing Proteins

Properdin (P). Properdin is an enhancer. While not required for the activation sequence of the alternative pathway, P stabilizes the C3 and C5 convertases to prolong their activity.

C3 Nephritic Factor (NF). NF is a pathologic enhancing protein. NF is an IgG antibody with specificity for the alternative pathway C3 convertase.[32] NF binds to the C3 convertase and thus prevents inactivation by the control proteins H and I. When NF is present, C3 activation proceeds uncontrolled, thereby markedly depleting C3.

Patients with C3NF present with recurrent bacterial infections and frequently also have partial lipodystrophy, which is a disturbance in fat metabolism that leaves people emaciated.[21] Serum C3 levels are markedly depleted, while C4 levels are normal. To distinguish C3NF from alternative pathway activation or deficiency of H or I, Factor B levels are helpful. Factor B levels are normal in C3NF but decreased in alternative pathway activation, H deficiency, or I deficiency.

SYNTHESIS OF COMPLEMENT COMPONENTS

Most complement components are synthesized in the liver, with the exception of C1, which is synthesized in the epithelial cells of the intestine.[33] Limited quantities of most complement components, including C1q, can be synthesized by activated macrophages/monocytes. Synthesis by these mononuclear phagocytes takes place at the site of inflammation, providing for a microenvironment that perpetuates the inflammatory process.

The level of C1q parallels the relative levels of the immunoglobulins, i.e., C1q is low in hypogammaglobulinemia, while in hypergammaglobulinemia, C1q is present in high levels. Several of the other complement components (especially C3 and Factor B) are acute phase reactants, i.e., elevate in response to inflammation. For that reason, the levels of these proteins should be interpreted in light of other measurements of inflammation, such as erythrocyte sedimentation rate or C-reactive protein.[34] Levels that are in the "normal range" may reflect activation or depletion if the patient is in the acute phase.

SUMMARY

The activation of complement provides the humoral (fluid-phase) effector mechanism most responsible for immune-mediated injury. The classical pathway is activated by an antigen-antibody reaction. The binding of C1q initiates the sequential activation of the eleven proteins. The classical pathway has a calcium-dependent step (C1q, C1r, C1s) and a magnesium-dependent reaction, the enzymatic action of C1s on C4 and C2.

The alternative pathway appears to be spontaneously activated, but the perpetuation of that activation is dependent upon the availability of an activating (or protective) surface that interferes with the inactivation of C3b by control proteins. The alternative pathway has a magnesium-dependent step, the binding of B to C3b to form the C3 convertase. Once initiated, the alternative pathway activation results in the sequential activation of nine proteins, six of which are common to both pathways.

The activation of complement results in a variety of biologic consequences that can cause injury to the host. The potential destructiveness of the effects of complement activation is modulated by a series of control proteins. Detection of complement component consumption is the primary reason for quantitating C3 and C4 in the clinical laboratory. Measurement of the functional integrity of either the classical or alternative pathway can be accomplished using hemolytic assays that are most useful for detecting hereditary deficiencies of complement components.

Deficiencies of complement component or control proteins are not as uncommon as once thought. Patients with homozygous deficiencies appear to have an increased incidence of collagen vascular diseases. Deficiencies in C3 or control proteins that regulate C3 result in life-threatening diseases, such as fulminant or recurrent bacterial infections. Patients with deficiencies in complement components involved in the MAC have a high incidence of infections with neisserial organisms that appear to require complement-induced lysis of the organisms.[35]

Acute Phase Response

When the body is injured, among the many ways it responds is by increasing the hepatic synthesis of a number of plasma proteins. This increased synthesis results in an increase in the concentration of these proteins in the plasma and at the site of injury. Experimental evidence indicates that these acute phase proteins play a major role in wound healing.[36]

From a teleological (adapting to the environment) perspective, the systemic acute phase response helps to ensure survival during the period immediately following injury. The systemic response must help to achieve the same goals as the localized inflammatory response, that is, to contain or destroy infectious agents, to remove damaged tissue, and to repair the affected organ.[37] Studies of the acute phase response have involved infections, surgical wounds or other traumas with definite onsets, burns, and myocardial infarctions. Certain of the acute phase proteins are elevated in pregnancy and neoplasia (malignancies).

One of the first acute phase responses recognized was fever, which may occur following many types of inflammatory stimuli, including noninfectious states. Fever reflects the effects of endogenous pyrogens (IL-1), which elevate the set point of the hypothalmic center for body temperature.[37] Another long recognized but variable, acute phase response is an increase in the granulocyte count in the blood. This initially reflects release from the storage pool and later reflects increased production by the bone marrow. The best studied acute phase proteins differ markedly in the magnitude of their rise after the onset of injury. They may be classified into three groups based on the degree of elevation during the acute phase response (Table 4-2).

C-REACTIVE PROTEIN (CRP)

The discovery of C-reactive protein in 1930 focused attention on the acute phase response and the role of the proteins produced as a result of an injury to the body. CRP was recognized because of its ability to precipitate with the C-polysaccharide extract of pneumococcus.[38] CRP is normally present in nanogram (ng/mL) quantities, but may increase dramatically to hundreds of micrograms per milliliter (μg/mL) within 3 days following tissue injury. This represents a 100- to 1000-fold increase within hours of tissue damage. Although CRP was recognized as being distinct from antibody, many parallels between the two molecules are evident. Two of the most striking examples of the similarity between CRP and immunoglobulins include the initiation of the complement cascade through C1 activation by complexed CRP in a manner analogous to antibody-antigen complexes, and the ability of CRP to bind to red cells coated with C-polysaccharide for ingestion by phagocytic cells.[39]

The functional similarities between CRP and antibody are striking, but CRP is produced by liver hepatocytes, unlike antibody, which is synthesized by lymphoid tissue and plasma cells. Additionally, there is little physical or biochemical resemblance between CRP and antibody. The binding of CRP to C-polysaccharide or other phosphocholine-containing com-

---

TABLE 4-2
Acute Phase Proteins Listed by Relative Change

CONCENTRATION USUALLY INCREASES ABOUT 50%

α2-Macroglobulin

Ceruloplasmin

C3 (and other complement components)

CONCENTRATION USUALLY INCREASES TWOFOLD TO FOURFOLD

α_1-Antitrypsin

Fibrinogen

Haptoglobin

CONCENTRATION USUALLY INCREASES SEVERAL HUNDRED TIMES

C-reactive protein (CRP)

CONCENTRATION USUALLY DECREASES

Albumin

pounds is calcium dependent. Approximately one phosphate is bound per CRP subunit (of which there are five), requiring two calcium ions per CRP subunit.

CRP may be considered to be a primitive form of an antibody molecule with specificity for components found in cell membranes of microorganisms, such as bacteria and fungi, as well as for damaged membranes of cells from normal humans. When complexed to a binding specificity, CRP can activate complement, which may enhance opsonization and clearance of the microorganisms *prior* to the production of specific IgM or IgG. Complexed CRP can bind to NK cells and to monocytes and may serve to activate these cells to be tumoricidal.[40,41] CRP is produced very early in the inflammatory response and may also play a role in tumor surveillance prior to the production of antibody or the activation of specific cytotoxic T cells.

HAPTOGLOBIN

The principal biologic function of haptoglobin is to bind to and remove free hemoglobin released by intravascular hemolysis. Haptoglobin irreversibly binds to free hemoglobin, forming a complex that is rapidly cleared by hepatocytes.[42] Following injury, haptoglobin increases two- to fourfold and is frequently found in inflammatory exudates. The rise in plasma haptoglobin in response to inflammation is caused by the de novo synthesis of the protein by the liver and does not involve the release of previously formed haptoglobin from other sites.[42]

Low haptoglobin levels are always clinically significant after the first year of life. In some cases, the cause may be decreased synthesis due to liver disease, but in the majority of patients the cause is intravascular hemolysis and rapid clearance of the haptoglobin-hemoglobin complex. No quantitative correlation is possible between the plasma haptoglobin content and the severity of hemolysis because relatively minor hemolytic events have the potential of markedly depleting the haptoglobin in the absence of an inflammatory response. Because haptoglobin increases during infections or inflammation, a "normal" haptoglobin level may not rule out the diagnosis of intravascular hemolysis if the patient is in the acute phase. In such situations, the haptoglobin level should be interpreted in light of the levels of another acute phase protein, for example, CRP.[34]

FIBRINOGEN

Fibrinogen accumulates at the site of injury for the first or second week after a surgical incision. In the presence of enzymes released from PMNs and platelets, fibrin is formed.[36] Fibrin increases the tensile strength of the wound and stimulates fibroblast proliferation and growth. Fibrinogen synthesis, but not haptoglobin synthesis by hepatocytes, can be stimulated by fibrinogen or fibrin degradation products (FDP), suggesting a feedback amplification loop.[43] The macrophage is necessary in this loop, because FDP does not directly stimulate hepatocyte synthesis of fibrinogen, but FDP does promote the production of IL-1 by peripheral blood monocytes or Kupffer cells.

α-1 ANTITRYPSIN

α-1 Antitrypsin is one of a family of serine protease inhibitors in human plasma. Although named *antitrypsin*, the physiologic targets are the proteases (e.g., elastase) released from leukocytes rather than trypsin.[44] Elastase is an endogenous enzyme capable of degrading elastin and collagen. In chronic pulmonary inflammation, lung tissue is damaged because of the activities of these leukocyte proteases released during phagocytosis and digestion of microorganisms and other debris. Once bound to α-1 antitrypsin, the activity of the proteases is completely inhibited, being later removed and catabolized. α-1 Antitrypsin is synthesized by the liver, where synthesis can increase fourfold when stimulated by an inflammatory process. In contrast to complexes of proteases with α-2 macroglobulin, α-1 antitrypsin–protease complexes are not taken up by macrophages.[36]

A loss of lung elasticity is a normal feature of aging, but this loss can be accelerated and cause premature emphysema in either the smoker or the patient with homozygous α-1 antitrypsin deficiency. When the two were combined (smoking and α-1 antitrypsin deficiency), emphysema onset was as early as age 30 years, with death by the age of 50. Air pollution and/or respiratory infections are also detrimental to the α-1 antitrypsin–deficient patient.

α-1 Antitrypsin deficiency is also associated with liver disease.[44] Homozygous deficient infants may develop neonatal cholestasis, which can progress to cirrhosis as children. Adults who are homozygous invariably show histologic evidence of liver damage, with about 20% of these individuals developing cirrhosis.

Heterozygous individuals are at more risk than normal individuals for developing liver disease, connective tissue disease (e.g., rheumatoid arthritis), inflammatory eye disease, and glomerulonephritis.[45] α-1 Antitrypsin has a role in several mediator pathways involved in the inflammatory response. Consequently, in the absence of this protein these proteases attack the tissue surrounding the inflammatory process and cause damage that may lead to a chronic inflammatory process.

CERULOPLASMIN

Ceruloplasmin is a glycoprotein that is the principal copper-transporting protein in human plasma.[36] Eighty to 95% of the total circulating copper is bound to ceruloplasmin, the rest being bound more loosely to albumin and amino acids. Ceruloplasmin appears to be the primary copper transport protein for transferring copper to cytochrome C oxidase, vital to aerobic energy production, which, along with glycolysis, increases during wound healing.[46] Ceruloplasmin and the copper it carries are essential to collagen formation and the extracellular crosslinking and maturation of collagen and elastin.[36] Ceruloplasmin and the copper it contains may also serve to protect the matrix of healing tissue against superoxide ions, generated by phagocytes in the course of clearing tissue debris or microorganisms.

An absence or marked depletion of ceruloplasmin is associated with a degenerative process named Wilson's disease, which is an autosomal recessive trait and a relatively rare disease.[47] There is a gastrointestinal absorption defect that allows copper to be taken up in excessive amounts. In the absence of ceruloplasmin, copper is massively increased in the tissues. The disease is also characterized by massive renal tubular reabsorption defects, which result in excessive urinary excretion of proteins, glucose, and other elements. (Wilson's disease is one of many inherited or acquired conditions caused by deposition of abnormal metabolic products that results in proximal tubular abnormalities. Collectively, these renal manifestations are referred to as Fanconi syndrome.)

α-2 MACROGLOBULIN

α-2 Macroglobulin is one of two principal protease inhibitors in human plasma, the other being α-1 antitrypsin. Proteolytic enzymes released from damaged tissues as well as from phagocytic cells have their activity inhibited partially by being bound by α-2 macroglobulin. These complexes of proteases and α-2 macroglobulin are rapidly phagocytosed by macrophages and fibroblasts.[48] α-2 Macroglobulin appears to be a backup protein, i.e., a scavenger protease inhibitor that acts to take up any excess molecules that cannot be handled by

the intended inhibitor. In that role, it functions in hemostasis, coagulation, fibrinolysis, and complement pathways.[49] No diseases have been associated with a deficiency in α-2 macroglobulin, so deficiency of this protein may be incompatible with life.

Inflammation

The preceding sections provide a foundation of knowledge about each of the specific systems (cellular and humoral) involved in the inflammatory process. Celcius of Rome first described the famous "four cardinal signs" of inflammation: redness, swelling, heat, and pain.[50,51] Loss of function was later recognized as another sign of inflammation. Inflammation appears to represent an orderly sequence of coordinated events designed to protect the host from a foreign invader, minimizing damage to the host tissue. In addition to killing off the adversary, the inflammatory process is intended also to eliminate the debris and to repair the damaged tissues. The localized inflammatory reaction can be divided into four stages: (1) increased vascular permeability, (2) emigration of neutrophils, (3) emigration of mononuclear cells, and (4) cellular proliferation.

VASCULAR PERMEABILITY

The vascular phase of the inflammatory response primarily involves the microcirculation, that is, the capillaries, the arterioles, and the venules. Following injury, the first phase is hyperemia (a rush of blood into the affected area), initially confined to the vicinity of the site of the injury (Fig. 4-20). This is facilitated by the localized dilatation (dilated or stretched beyond normal dimensions) of capillaries and venules resulting from the chemical mediators released as a direct result of the injury (e.g., histamine released from mast cells in skin that has been punctured).

After the hyperemia phase, transudation begins. Transudation is the passage of serum or other body flu-

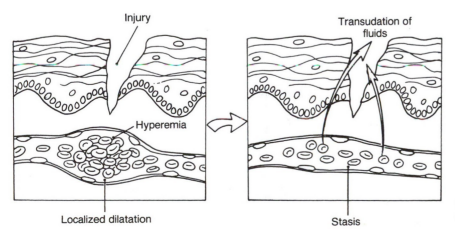

FIGURE 4-20

Vascular phase of inflammation.

ids through a membrane. A transudate, in contrast to an exudate, is characterized by a low protein content and few cells. Transudation is brought about by chemical mediators such as histamine and kinins, which increase vascular permeability by causing the endothelial cells' smooth muscle to contract. As the endothelial cells contract, adjacent cells separate from one another, creating gaps where fluids and even diapedetic PMNs can escape through the basement membrane and move into the tissues. If fibrinogen is extravasated into the tissues, the clotting mechanism is activated and fibrin forms from fibrinogen—the body's effort to "plug the leak."

As transudation proceeds, the blood flow in the dilated capillaries and venules slows. In severe injury, the blood flow may cease completely (stasis), which is caused by hemoconcentration when the fluids are lost by transudation. During stasis, the red blood cells, which normally repel each other, clump into tight stacks. Stasis (in contrast to thrombosis) is completely reversible; that is, when blood flow is restored, the red cell aggregates break up and normalcy resumes. Depending on the type and severity of the inflammation, microthrombus formation and platelet aggregation may also occur and may not be reversible.

EMIGRATION OF NEUTROPHILS

Shortly after the initial injury, the endothelial cells become "sticky" and circulating PMNs begin to adhere to the endothelium. Initially, the numbers of cells involved are small and the adherence seems transitory, but soon the endothelial surface becomes completely "pavemented" by leukocytes. PMNs are the most conspicuous, but eosinophils and basophils, platelets, and even erythrocytes do participate.

Following pavementing, the leukocytes exhibit amoeboid movement and actively migrate through the wall of the blood vessel by a process called diapedesis (see Fig. 4-1). Erythrocytes that appear in the tissues apparently have been passively forced through the gaps in damaged epithelium. It is the hemoglobin breakdown products that result in the purple, then green, and finally yellow color of a bruise. Bruise spots can occur following the most minor of injuries and are probably explainable by extravasating red blood cells rather than actual blood vessel damage and spilling of blood into the tissues.

The emigration of significant numbers of neutrophils into the area of inflammation is dependent upon chemotactic factors. If immune complexes are involved in initiating the inflammation, the chemotactic factors released during complement activation (C5a) will attract PMNs. Neutrophil granules themselves, when released from the PMNs arriving first on the scene, are chemotactic for other PMNs. Certain bacterial products are also chemotactic for neutrophils. The intensity and duration of the neutrophil emigration may last 24 to 48 hours and is proportional to the amount of chemotactic factor present in the inflamed area.

Neutrophils participate in the inflammatory process in many ways. They are actively phagocytic for microorganisms and other foreign material. Their lysosomes contain a number of biologically active macromolecules. The active aerobic glycolysis of PMNs is responsible for the formation of large amounts of the lactic acid (causing pain) found in inflamed tissues. When the amount of foreign material attracts a large number of neutrophils, it also stimulates the accumulation of fibroblasts and the proliferation and synthesis of collagen, and may result in the formation of a walled-off abscess, which may require drainage before healing can occur.[50]

EMIGRATION OF MONONUCLEAR CELLS

The third stage of the inflammatory response is the emigration of mononuclear cells in the affected area. This begins about 4 hours after the initial stimulus and may reach a peak (during a defined and single injury) at 16 to 24 hours. A few mononuclear cells may be found along with the PMNs early in the cellular phase of the response. These few monocytes either are directly stimulated by phagocytosis of the debris or are indirectly stimulated by products of PMN phagocytosis and degranulation to produce cytokines, for example, interleukin-1 (IL-1).[52] IL-1 is also released from neutrophils, epithelial cells, fibroblasts, and many other cell types. IL-1 (originally called endogenous pyrogen) is associated with many of the manifestations of inflammatory reactions, such as fever, elevation of acute phase proteins, and infiltration of inflammatory sites by leukocytes. Thus, another feedback amplification loop has begun. IL-1 attracts and activates other monocytes/macrophages as well as lymphocytes into the area of inflammation.[53] IL-1 can stimulate (or activate) T lymphocytes to produce IL-2, which in turn enhances the proliferation of T lymphocytes (Fig. 4-21).

CELLULAR PROLIFERATION AND REPAIR

Resolution and repair are the final stages of the inflammatory process.[50] Fibroblast proliferation begins within 18 hours and peaks by 48 to 72 hours. During proliferation, fibroblasts produce acidic mucopolysaccharides to neutralize the effects of some of the chemical mediators that are still being released by damaged mast cells and basophils. The end stage of inflammation may result in complete repair and restoration of function of the affected area. Alternatively, an injury may lead to the formation of an abscess with at least some loss of function. Another end stage of inflammation may be the formation of a granuloma, a tightly packed pocket of inflammatory cells that dies and degenerates from the center out, resulting

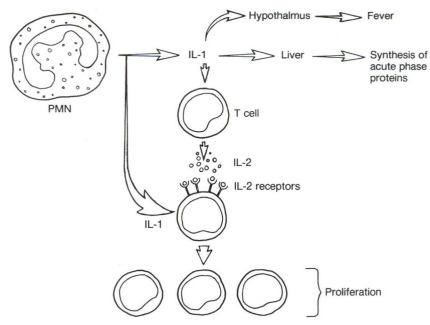

FIGURE 4-21
Soluble factors influencing the inflammatory response.

in necrosis. Granuloma formation is a typical end-stage result of delayed hypersensitivity of cell-mediated immunity and is further described in a later chapter.

Review Questions

1. Which of the following cell types are responsible for the majority of the effects of inflammation?

   a. basophils
   b. polymorphonuclear neutrophils
   c. eosinophils
   d. macrophages

2. Which mediator cells respond to IgE-containing immune complexes?

   a. basophils
   b. polymorphonuclear neutrophils
   c. eosinophils
   d. macrophages

3. Which of the following cell types is primarily responsible for antigen processing?

   a. basophils
   b. polymorphonuclear neutrophils
   c. eosinophils
   d. macrophages

4. Which complement components are associated only with classical pathway activation?

   a. C1q, C1r, C1s
   b. C3
   c. C5, C6, C7
   d. C8 and C9

5. Which complement component is associated with the amplification loop?

   a. C1q
   b. C3
   c. C4
   d. C5

6. The measurement of which complement component is an effective screening test for C1INH deficiency?

   a. C1q
   b. C3
   c. C4
   d. C5

7. The deficiency of which complement control protein is associated with paroxysmal nocturnal hemoglobinuria (PNH)?

   a. C3b inactivator (I)
   b. complement receptor 3 (CRIII)
   c. membrane cofactor protein (MCP)
   d. decay accelerating factor (DAF)

8. Which acute phase protein is associated with cirrhosis in children?

   a. C-reactive protein
   b. haptoglobin
   c. α-1 antitrypsin
   d. α-2 macroglobulin

References

1. Mescon H, Grots IA: The skin. In Robbins SL (ed): Pathologic Basis of Disease, p 1374. Philadelphia, WB Saunders, 1974

2. Parslow TG: The phagocytes: Neutrophils and macrophages. In Stites DP, Terr AI, Parslow TG (eds): Basic & Clinical Immunology, pp 9–20. Los Altos, CA, Lange Medical, 1994

3. Gallin JI: Inflammation. In Paul WE (ed): Fundamental Immunology, p 1026. New York, Raven Press, 1993

4. Cooper EL: Granulocytes and mast cells. In General Immunology, p 92, New York, Pergamon Press, 1982

5. Park BH, Good RA: Phagocytosis and host resistance. In Principles of Modern Immunobiology, p 159, Philadelphia, Lea & Febiger, 1974

6. Imhof BA, Dunon D: Leukocyte migration and adhesion. Adv Immunol 58:345–416, 1995

7. Greenberg S, Silverstein SC: Phagocytosis. In Paul WE (ed): Fundamental Immunology, p 941–949. New York, Raven Press, 1993

8. Ammann AJ: Phagocytic dysfunction diseases. In Stites DP, Terr AI, Parslow TG (eds): Basic & Clinical Immunology, pp 303–308. Los Altos, CA, Lange Medical, 1994

9. Thrasher AJ, Keep NH, Wientjes F, Segal AW. Chronic granulomatous disease. Biochim Biophys Acta 1227:1, 1994

10. Stites DP: Clinical laboratory methods for detection of cellular immunity. In Stites DP, Terr AI, Parslow TG (eds): Basic & Clinical Immunology, pp 212–214. Los Altos, CA, Lange Medical, 1994

11. Boxer LA, Stossel TP: Neutrophil disorders—qualitative abnormalities of neutrophils. In Williams WJ, Beutler E, Erslev AJ, et al (eds): Hematology, p 809. New York, McGraw-Hill, 1983

12. Roder JC, Haliotis T, Klein M, et al: A new immunodeficiency disorder in humans involving NK cells. Nature 284:553, 1980

13. Hayward A: Immunodeficiency. In Lachmann PJ, Peters DK (eds): Clinical Aspects of Immunology, p 1691. Oxford, Blackwell Scientific, 1982

14. Bellanti JA, Kadlec JV: General immunobiology. In Bellanti JA (ed): Immunology III, p 16. Philadelphia, WB Saunders, 1985

15. Terr AI: Inflammation. In Paul WE (ed): Fundamental Immunology, pp 139–141. New York, Raven Press, 1993

16. Lee TH, Austen F: Arachidonic acid metabolism by the 5-lipogenase pathway, and the effects of alternative dietary fatty acids. Adv Immunol 39:145, 1986

17. Robbins SL: Inflammation and repair. In Robbins SL (ed): Pathologic Basis of Disease, p 55. Philadelphia, WB Saunders, 1974

18. Berzofsky JA, Berkower IJ: Immunogenicity and antigen structure. In Paul WE (ed): Fundamental Immunology, pp 256–270. New York, Raven Press, 1993

19. James K: Complement: Activation, consequences, and control. Am J Med Technol 48:735, 1985

20. Gewurz H, Lint TF: Alternative modes and pathways of complement activation. In Day NK, Good RA (eds): Comprehensive Immunology, Vol 2, Biological Amplification Systems in Immunology, p 17. New York, Plenum Press, 1977

21. Lint TF, Gewurz H: Testing for complement defects. Clin Immunol Allergy 1:561, 1981

22. Pangburn MK, Schreiber RD, Muller-Eberhard HJ: Formation of the initial C3 convertase of the alternative complement pathway: Acquistion of the C3b-like activities of spontaneous hydrolysis of the putative thioester in native C3. J Exp Med 154:856, 1981

23. Hugli TE, Muller-Eberhard HJ: Anaphylatoxins: C3a and C5a. Adv Immunol 26:1, 1978

24. Donaldson VH, Rosen FS, Bing DH: Role of the second component of complement (C2) and plasmin in kinin release in hereditary angioneurotic edema (H.A.N.E.) plasma. Trans Assoc Am Physicians 90:174, 1977

25. Agnello V: Complement deficiency states. Medicine (Baltimore) 57:1, 1978

26. Liszewski MK, Atkinson JP: The complement system. In Paul WE (ed): Fundamental Immunology, p 917. New York, Raven Press, 1993

27. Ziccardi RJ, Cooper NR: Active disassembly of the first component, C1, by C1 inactivator. J Immunol 123:788, 1979

28. Frank MM, Gelfand JA, Atkinson JP: Hereditary angioedema: The clinical syndrome and its management. Ann Intern Med 84:580, 1976

29. Luskin AT, Tobin MC: Alterations of complement components in disease. Am J Med Technol 48:749, 1982

30. Pangburn MK, Muller-Eberhard HJ: Relation of a putative thioester bond in C3 to activation of the alternative pathway and the binding of C3 to biological targets of complement. J Exp Med 152:1102, 1980

31. Nicholson-Weller A, March JP, Rosen CE, Spicer DB, Austen KF. Surface membrane expression by human blood leukocytes and platelets of decay-accelerating factor, a regulatory protein of the complement system. Blood 65:1237, 1985

32. Davis AE, Ziegler JB, et al: Heterogeneity of nephritic factor and its identification as an immunoglobulin. Proc Natl Acad Sci USA 74:3980, 1977

33. Colten HR: Biosynthesis of complement. Adv Immunol 22:67, 1976

34. Witte DA: Laboratory tests to confirm or exclude iron deficiency. Lab Med 16:671, 1985

35. Nicholson A, Lepow IH: Host defense against *Neisseria meningitidis* requires a complement-dependent bactericidal activity. Science 205:298, 1979

36. Powanda MC, Moyer ED: Plasma proteins and wound healing. Surg Gynecol Obstet 153:749, 1981

37. Kushner I: The phenomenon of the acute phase response. In Kushner I, Volanakis JE, Gewurz H (eds): C-reactive protein and the plasma protein response to tissue injury. Ann NY Acad Sci 389:39, 1982

38. Tillett W, Francis T: Serological reactions in pneumonia with nonprotein somatic fraction of pneumococcus. J Exp Med 52:561, 1930

39. James KK: Studies of the interaction of C-reactive protein with mononuclear leukocytes, p 1. Thesis, 1980

40. James K, Baum L, Adamowski C, et al: C-reactive protein antigenicity on the surface of human lymphocytes. J Immunol 131:2930, 1983

41. Deodhar SD, James K, Chiang T, et al: Inhibition of lung metastases in mice bearing a malignant fibrosarcoma by treatment with liposomes containing human C-reactive protein. Cancer Res 42:5084, 1982

42. Javid J: Human haptoglobin. Curr Top Hematol 1:151, 1978

43. Fuller GM, Ritchie DG: A regulatory pathway for fibrinogen biosynthesis involving an indirect feedback loop. In

Kushner I, Volanakis JE, Gewurz H (eds): C-reactive protein and the plasma protein response to tissue injury. Ann NY Acad Sci 389:308, 1982

44. Carrell RW: Alpha-1 antitrypsin: Molecular pathology, leukocytes, and tissue damage. J Clin Invest 78:1427, 1986
45. Breit SN, Wakefield D, Robinson JP, et al: The role of alpha-1 antitrypsin deficiency in the pathogenesis of immune disorders. Clin Immunol Immunopathol 35:363, 1985
46. Goldstein IM, Kaplan HB, Edelson HS, et al: Ceruloplasmin: An acute phase reactant that scavenges oxygen-derived free radicals. In Kushner I, Volanakis JE, Gewurz H (eds): C-reactive protein and the plasma protein response to tissue injury. Ann NY Acad Sci 389:368, 1982
47. Foley JM: The nervous system: Degenerative diseases. In Robbins SL (ed): Pathologic Basis of Disease, p 1539. Philadelphia, WB Saunders, 1974
48. Van Leuven F, Cassiman JJ, Van-den Berghe H: Uptake and degradation of alpha-2 macroglobulin protease complexes in human cells in culture. Exp Cell Res 117:273, 1978
49. Roberts RC: Protease inhibitors of human plasma: Alpha-2 macroglobulin. J Med 16:149, 1985
50. Bach FH, Good RA: Inflammation. In Bach FH (ed): Clinical Immunobiology, p 139. New York, Academic Press, 1980
51. Gallin JI: Inflammation. In Paul WE (ed): Fundamental Immunology, pp 1015–1032. New York, Raven Press, 1993
52. Oppenheim JJ, Ruscetti FW, Faltynek CV: Cytokines. In Stites DP, Terr AI, Parslow TG (eds): Basic & Clinical Immunology, pp 107–110. Los Altos, CA, Lange Medical, 1994
53. James K: Cellular and humoral mediators of inflammation. In McClatchey KD (ed): Clinical Laboratory Medicine, pp 1543–1567. Baltimore, MD, Williams & Wilkins, 1994

CHAPTER 5

Major Histocompatibility Complex

Catherine Sheehan

Objectives

Upon completion of the chapter, the reader should be able to:

1. Define heterodimer, MHC, HLA, gene, allele, gene product, polymorphism, haplotype, genotype, linkage disequilibrium, and relative risk
2. Compare and contrast the MHC Class I, II, and III products with respect to structure, cellular or humoral distribution, function, and method of detection
3. Given an HLA designation, identify the specificity
4. Explain the principles of complement-mediated cytotoxicity, one-way mixed-lymphocyte culture, and the primed lymphocyte test
5. Given the HLA phenotypes of parents and offspring, determine the genotype and haplotype of each
6. Given the HLA phenotypes of an alleged father, mother, and offspring, determine if the alleged father is excluded as the biologic father, if possible
7. Describe how relative risk can be related to a disease

The major histocompatibility complex (MHC) is a group of genes that produce cell surface markers that are important in transplantation, immune regulation, and immune responsiveness. These cell surface markers are used to distinguish self from non-self. This distinction allows an appropriate response to non-self antigens while preventing an immune response to self antigens. The importance of the MHC is underscored by the fact that all mammalian species studied thus far have an MHC.

For centuries, people observed that tissue transplanted from one individual to another rarely survived. Apparently genetic differences between individuals were recognized, and an immune response was mounted to reject the transplanted tissue. In the 1950s it was observed that sera from multiply transfused patients contained leukoagglutinins that could clump leukocytes.[1,2] Later it was shown that leukoagglutinins were actually antibodies to leukocytes when characterized from the sera of multiparous women.[3,4] Because antibodies were able to agglutinate leukocytes, the antigens were called human leukocyte antigens (HLA). Since 1968, the HLA Nomenclature Committee of the World Health Organization has met periodically to evaluate serologic data, to standardize the HLA specificities, and to set the nomenclature.[5] HLA antigens are now known to be products of the major histocompatibility complex and are the major barrier to tissue transplantation.

MHC PRODUCTS

The MHC is located on the short arm of chromosome 6, as shown in Figure 5-1.[6,7] The MHC encodes for polypeptides included in three classes of products: Class I products are the classical HLA-A, -B, and -C. Other Class I products—HLA-E, -F, -G, -H, and -J—have been described. These are considered nonclassical because the product is structurally or functionally dissimilar from those of the classical HLA-A, -B, and -C. Class II products are HLA-D, -DR, -DQ, and -DP. Class III products are C2, C4, and Factor B. Classes I and II are the cell surface markers, whereas Class III products are soluble complement components.

Structure

All classical Class I products are composed of two polypeptides: the α heavy chain, which is encoded in the MHC, and the invariant (nonpolymorphic) light chain, β_2 microglobulin, which is encoded on another chromosome. The heavy chain is a single glycoprotein chain composed of 338 amino acids with a molecular weight of 44 kDa. This integral protein has an extracellular section (281 amino acids), a transmembrane section (25 amino acids), and an intracellular tail (30 amino

acids) (Fig. 5-2). The extracellular section is divided into three domains, each with approximately 90 amino acids. $\alpha1$ and $\alpha2$ are highly polymorphic and account for the specificity of the chain. β_2 Microglobulin is loosely associated with all classical Class I heavy chains.

Class II products are transmembrane heterodimers. Both chains are encoded in the MHC. One chain is designated α and ranges from 33 to 35 kDa, while the second chain is β and is slightly smaller (26 to 28 kDa). As shown in Figure 5-3, each chain has two extracellular domains, a transmembrane section and an intracellular tail. The specificity is in the outermost domains $\alpha1$ and $\beta1$. During synthesis, these chains are joined together by another intracellular protein until the Class II heterodimer is incorporated into the cell membrane. This assures that the α and β chains function together on the cell surface.[8]

There are 36 genes in the Class III region. Products include complement peptides (C4A, C4B, C2, Factor B), enzymes (steroid 21-hydroxylase α and β), tumor necrosis factor α and β, and heat shock proteins (HSP70-1 and HSP70-2).

Distribution and Function

Class I products are found on nearly all nucleated cells, although the level of expression may vary. Only remnants remain on the surface of red blood cells and are referred to as Bg antigens. A Class I product is necessary to present a peptide antigen to cytotoxic T cells (T_c), as shown in Figure 5-4A. The antigen receptor on the T_c recognizes the peptide antigen, while CD8 on the T_c simultaneously recognizes the Class I product. It is postulated that these peptide antigens are generally from intracellular constituents.[9] T_c eliminates transplanted cells, virally infected cells, and tumor cells.

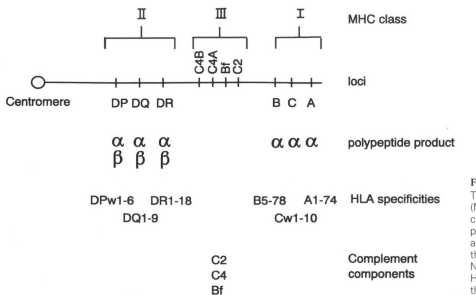

FIGURE 5-1
The major histocompability complex (MHC) is located on the short arm of chromosome 6. Class I and II loci code for peptides that are part of the HLA antigens. Class III loci code for peptides that are part of complement components. Note that the numbering of HLA-A and HLA-B specificities is continuous between the two designations.

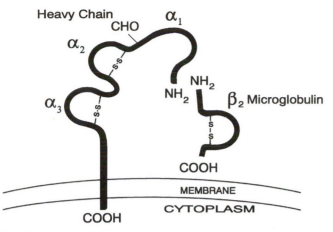

FIGURE 5-2
For Class I antigens the α chain is closely associated with β₂ microglobulin.

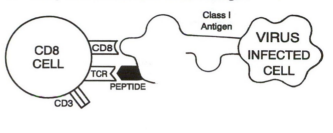

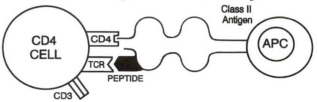

FIGURE 5-4
The MHC regulates the immune response. (**A**) The cytotoxic T cell (CD8) recognizes a peptide in association with a Class I molecule found on the virally infected cell. (**B**) The helper T cell (CD4) recognizes a peptide in association with a Class II molecule on the antigen-presenting cell (APC).

Class II products are found on selected immuno-competent cells, including monocytes, macrophages, B lymphocytes, activated T lymphocytes, dendritic cells, Langerhans cells, and some epithelial cells. Often the level of expression is increased by cytokine stimulation. A Class II product is necessary to present a peptide antigen to helper T (T_H) cells, as shown in Figure 5-4B. The antigen receptor on the T_H cell recognizes the peptide antigen, while the CD4 on the T_H cells simultaneously recognizes the Class II product. It is postulated that these peptide antigens are generally from endocytosed constituents.[9] T_H cells induce antibody synthesis and promote cell-mediated immunity.

Class III products are soluble proteins and are not associated with cell surfaces. C4 and C2 are necessary to generate the classical pathway C3 convertase, while Factor B is necessary to generate the alternative pathway C3 convertase.

Nomenclature

The loci of the MHC are highly polymorphic. Polymorphism occurs when more than one allele exists for a single locus. This can be thought of as inherited gene variants. The MHC Class I and Class II loci are the most polymorphic loci known in humans. Class III loci are less polymorphic than those of Class I and Class II.

The WHO Nomenclature Committee for factors of the HLA system met in 1991 to update the Class I and Class II specificities. A complete listing of HLA specificities is found in Table 5-1.[7] At each HLA locus, an allele codes for a specific peptide chain. The HLA product expressed by a cell is known as the HLA antigen specificity. The specificities are designated by the letter designation of A, B, C, Dw, DR, DQ, or DP, which is followed by a number. This number is assigned to the specificity based on its identification by traditional serologic and cellular methods. Using HLA-A2 as an example, the locus is A and the allele is 2.

Variation in the amino acid sequence of a single HLA specificity was detected. For example, HLA-B3901

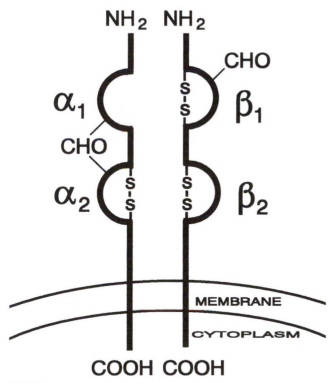

FIGURE 5-3
The Class II antigens are heterodimers, composed of an α chain and β chain in close proximity.

TABLE 5-1
HLA Specificities[7]

A	B	C	D	DR	DQ	DP
A1	B5	Cw1	Dw1	DR1	DQ1	DPw1
A2	B7	Cw2	Dw2	DR103	DQ2	DPw2
A203	B703	Cw3	Dw3	DR2	DQ3	DPw3
A210	B8	Cw4	Dw4	DR3	DQ4	DPw4
A3	B12	Cw5	Dw5	DR4	DQ5(1)	DPw5
A9	B13	Cw6	Dw6	DR5	DQ6(1)	DPw6
A10	B14	Cw7	Dw7	DR6	DQ7(3)	
A11	B15	Cw8	Dw8	DR7	DQ8(3)	
A19	B16	Cw9(w3)	Dw9	DR8	DQ9(3)	
A23(9)	B17	Cw10(w3)	Dw10	DR9		
A24(9)	B18		Dw11(w7)	DR10		
A2403	B21		Dw12	DR11(5)		
A25(10)	B22		Dw13	DR12(5)		
A26(10)	B27		Dw14	DR13(6)		
A28	B35		Dw15	DR14(6)		
A29(19)	B37		Dw16	DR1403		
A30(19)	B38(16)		Dw17(w7)	DR1404		
A31(19)	B39(16)		Dw18(w6)	DR15(2)		
A32(19)	B3901		Dw19(w6)	DR16(2)		
A33(19)	B3902		Dw20	DR17(3)		
A34(10)	B40		Dw21	DR18(3)		
A36	B4005		Dw22			
A43	B41		Dw23	DR51		
A66(10)	B42					
A68(28)	B44(12)		Dw24	DR52		
A69(28)	B45(12)		Dw25			
A74(19)	B46		Dw26	DR53		
	B47					
	B48					
	B49(21)					
	B50(21)					
	B51(5)					
	B5102					
	B5103					
	B52(5)					
	B53					
	B54(22)					
	B55(22)					
	B56(22)					
	B57(17)					
	B58(17)					
	B59					
	B60(40)					
	B61(40)					
	B62(15)					
	B63(15)					
	B64(14)					
	B65(14)					
	B67					
	B70					
	B71(70)					
	B72(70)					
	B73					
	B75(15)					
	B76(15)					
	B77(15)					
	B7801					
	Bw4					
	Bw6					

and HLA-B3902 are recognized serologically by the same antibody but differ in their amino acid sequence. Differences in amino acid sequence are indicated by the last two numbers added to the specificity designation.

More recently, molecular methods have been used to directly investigate HLA genes rather than the gene products. The polymerase chain reaction and restriction fragment length polymorphism analysis evaluate the nucleotide sequence. Multiple forms of a single specificity have been discovered. Thus the nomenclature has been modified to more definitively describe the alleles. For example, the two gene variants of the HLA-A29 specificity are known as A*2901 and A*2902.

The "w" designation is now used in three situations: (1) to distinguish Bw4 and Bw6 as epitopes rather than alleles, (2) to distinguish HLA-C specificities from complement components, and (3) to identify that HLA-D specificities are defined by the mixed lymphocyte reaction and that HLA-DP specificities are defined by primed lymphocyte testing.

In some cases what was originally thought to be one HLA specificity when recognized serologically was also found on other HLA specificities. Thus an epitope was shared by more than one conventionally detected HLA antigen. For example, an epitope of the original broad specificity of B12 is also on B44 and B45. These antigens are known as "splits." The original broad specificity is listed in parentheses in Table 5-1.

HLA DETECTION

Depending on the HLA antigen to be detected, either a serologic or cell-mediated assay is needed. All serologic assays use antibody to recognize the specificity of the HLA antigen. HLA-A, -B, -C, -DR, and -DQ are detected serologically by complement-mediated cytotoxicity.[10] In this assay patient lymphocytes are added to reagent antibody, which is in the microtitration well. After incubation, rabbit complement is added. Cytolysis can be observed by adding a supravital stain or viewing with phase contrast microscopy. When the reagent antibody recognizes an HLA antigen on the patient cell, it binds and then activates rabbit complement. The resulting cytolysis is detected when the supravital stain enters the dead cells. HLA-A, -B, and -C are most often detected using purified peripheral blood mononuclear cells, which are predominantly T lymphocytes. HLA-DR and -DQ require a B-lymphocyte–enriched cell preparation because these MHC Class II molecules are not expressed on resting peripheral blood T cells.

Cell-mediated assays require viable lymphocytes to recognize and react to an HLA specificity. HLA-Dw and -DPw are detected by cellular reactions. The one-way mixed-lymphocyte culture (MLC) is used to type

HLA-Dw. In the MLC, homozygous typing cells (HTC) that express a single HLA-D specificity are the reagent used to stimulate the patient lymphocytes. When the patient lymphocytes recognize that the HLA-Dw on the HTC is different than its own, the patient lymphocytes will respond and become transformed. The transformed lymphocytes will incorporate radiolabeled thymidine into its DNA. When a high level of radiolabel is taken up by the activated cells, it indicates that the patient lymphocytes do not express the same HLA-D as that on the HTC. The HLA-Dw phenotype may be a composite of HLA-DR, -DQ, and -DP specificities and may not be a unique product.

HLA-DPw is detected using a primed lymphocyte test. Cells matched for other HLA antigens are allowed to react in a mixed lymphocyte reaction with stimulator cells. These primed cells are then incubated with irradiated unknown cells in a second MLR to determine if the unknown cells will cause a response.[11] Refer to Chapter 17 for more information about cellular assays.

INHERITANCE OF HLA

The MHC loci encompass approximately 3500 kilobases. Thus the numerous loci are considered to be closely linked and are usually inherited as a unit on a single chromosome. The combination of HLA alleles inherited as a package is the haplotype. Recombination during meiosis is infrequent so that one haplotype is inherited without alteration from the father and one from the mother to the offspring. Two haplotypes constitute a genotype. The expression of HLA products is codominant. As shown in Figure 5-5, the frequency of inheriting each haplotype (designated as a, b, c, or d) from each parent is equal. Note that each offspring is 50% matched to each parent; this means that 100% of the time one haplotype is identical. Between siblings there is a 25% chance that the siblings will share no haplotype, a 50% chance of sharing one haplotype, and a 25% chance of sharing both haplotypes. When both haplotypes are shared, the HLA match is the best.

Lymphocytes can be tested to determine which HLA antigens are expressed to identify the phenotype. From the phenotype of parents and siblings, it is possible to determine the genotype and haplotype of individuals. In Table 5-2, the results of HLA-A and HLA-B typing within a family are presented. It is assumed that the mother is the true mother and the father is the true father. Remember that other HLA products could also be typed and that only two are shown here as an example. The laboratory detected A1, A2, B7, and B27 on the paternal cells. Thus the phenotype is A1, A2 and B7, B27. Possible genotypes are A1, B7/A2, B27 or A1,

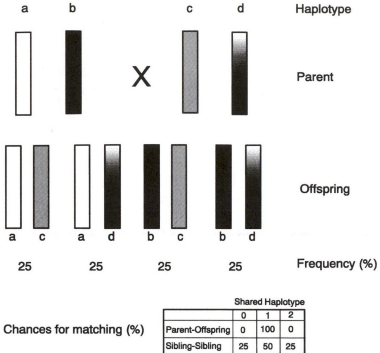

FIGURE 5-5
Inheritance of haplotypes.

B27/A2, B7. One half of the genotype would be inherited as a haplotype by the offspring. Thus, by examining the offspring phenotype, the paternal haplotype and genotype can be established. Looking at the phenotype of offspring 1, it can be seen that A1 and B7 must have been inherited from the father and therefore must have been on the same chromosome. Thus the paternal genotype is A1, B7/A2, B27. Note that in offspring 2, only one A specificity was detected; this is known as a blank. This could mean that two copies of the same allele were inherited (as was proven in this case); an alternative explanation is that the specificity was not detectable by the antiserum panel used.

Sometimes the inheritance pattern in a family may not exhibit the expected haplotypes. This may be due to chiasmata (or crossing over) of a segment of one chromosome to the sister chromosome during cell division (either mitosis or meiosis). This is suspected in offspring 4, who appears to have inherited HLA-A, and HLA-B27 from the father.

CLINICAL IMPORTANCE OF HLA TYPING

Transplantation

The most important application of HLA typing is to aid in organ matching for transplantation. When the donor graft and the recipient are more closely

TABLE 5-2
HLA Typing of a Family

	HLA PRODUCT DETECTED							PHENOTYPE		GENOTYPE	HAPLOTYPE
	A1	A2	A24	B7	B27	B44	B51	A	B		
Father	+	+	−	+	+	−	−	1, 2	7, 27	A1, B7/A2, B27	a/b
Mother	−	+	+	−	−	+	+	2, 24	44, 51	A2, B51/A24, B44	c/d
Offspring 1	+	+	−	+	−	−	+	1, 2	7, 51	A1, B7/A2, B51	a/c
Offspring 2	−	+	−	−	+	−	+	2	27, 51	A2, B27/A2, B51	b/c
Offspring 3	+	−	+	+	−	+	−	1, 24	7, 44	A1, B7/A24, B44	a/d
Offspring 4	+	−	+	−	+	+	−	1, 24	27, 44	A1, B27/A24, B44	b*/d

matched according to their HLA antigens, graft survival is better. Identical HLA matching, as seen in identical twins, is best. When donor cells and recipient cells are incubated together in a crossmatch, additional information about minor histocompatibility antigens is gathered. Transplantation is more fully discussed in Chapter 34.

HLA Paternity Testing

HLA typing is used as part of the genetic profile in paternity testing. By evaluating multiple markers, the cumulative effect is to exclude falsely accused men. It can never be said with absolute certainty that an alleged father is the biologic father. Because the HLA loci are highly polymorphic and recombination is rare, HLA has a high probability of excluding a falsely accused man; when combined with other markers, HLA is even more powerful.[12] When selected markers, including HLA, are measured using traditional techniques, a falsely accused father can be excluded with 99% confidence in whites and 98% confidence in blacks.

In paternity testing, the alleged father, mother, and offspring are typed. Consider the following HLA phenotypes:

Alleged father	A19, 28;	B8, 40
Mother	A10, 11;	B16, 35
Offspring	A10, 19;	B27, 35

Compare the phenotype of the offspring with that of the mother. In this example, the offspring must have inherited HLA-A10 and HLA-B35 from the mother. Therefore, HLA-A19 and HLA-B27 must have been inherited from the biologic father. Because the alleged father does not express HLA-B27, this supports the direct or first-order exclusion of this man as the biologic father.[13] It is important to remember that in this example the mother was assumed to be the true biologic mother.

HLA and Disease

Linkage disequilibria have been observed in HLA loci. This phenomenon is the difference between the observed frequency of two alleles occuring at two linked loci and the frequency of the two alleles occuring together because of random segregation. Certain pairs of alleles appear together more frequently than can be calculated based on the frequency of each allele in a population. For example, the frequency of the A1, B8 haplotype in the Caucasian population is observed to be 7% to 8%, whereas the expected haplotype frequency was 1.5%. The expected haplotype frequency is based on the observed frequency of individual specificities in a population. The frequency of A1 is 0.15 and the frequency of B8 is 0.10, yielding an expected haplotype frequency of 1.5%. The discrepancy between the expected and observed frequencies documents the linkage disequilibrium. Could there be a selective advantage when two alleles are in linkage disequilibrium?

The idea of selective advantage, coupled with finding immune response genes at the MHC in other species, encouraged the hunt for the association of some HLA antigens with specific diseases. In general, these diseases have an unknown cause, have a heritable pattern of distribution, and are associated with immunologic abnormalities. Not all individuals with a particular HLA antigen have the disease, but individuals with the disease have a higher frequency of expressing that particular antigen than that found in the control population. This is known as the relative risk. When the relative risk is greater than 1, it means that there is a positive association between the HLA antigen and the disease. The greater the relative risk value, the greater the association. It must be remembered that as the frequency of HLA antigens varies between races, the relative risk will also vary. The relative risk associated with selected diseases is listed in Table 5-3 (on p. 62); note that the greatest relative risk is associated with HLA-B27 and ankylosing spondylitis. The frequency of HLA-B27 in the Caucasian population without the disease is approximately 8%, while in those with clinical symptoms the frequency of HLA-B27 is approximately 87%. The relative risk is 87%. HLA-B27 is now used as a marker for ankylosing spondylitis.

SUMMARY

The major histocompatibility complex is a genetic region that is important in immune regulation, immune responsiveness, and transplant rejection. Class I antigens restrict the activity of cytotoxic T cells, and Class II antigens restrict the activity of helper T cells. Class III molecules are soluble complement components. The high degree of polymorphism and low incidence of recombination make MHC typing useful. MHC typing is performed to find the best match between a donor and recipient for tissue transplantation, to exclude alleged fathers in paternity testing, and to support a suspected diagnosis of a disease with a high relative risk.

TABLE 5-3
HLA Antigens Associated with Disease

DISEASE	HLA ANTIGEN	RELATIVE RISK
Ankylosing spondylitis	B27	87
Reiter's syndrome	B27	37
Goodpasture's syndrome	DR2	16
Insulin-dependent diabetes	DR3, DR4	8
Addison's disease	DR3	6

Review Questions

1. Which MHC Class is found on all nucleated cells and is necessary for cytotoxic T cell function?

   a. I
   b. II
   c. III
   d. I and II

2. On an activated T cell, what is the maximum number of HLA-DR specificities that can be expressed?

   a. one
   b. two
   c. four
   d. six

3. Which method detects HLA-DR?

   a. complement-mediated cytotoxicity using mononuclear cells
   b. complement-mediated cytotoxicity using enriched B cells
   c. one-way mixed-lymphocyte culture using mononuclear cells
   d. one-way mixed-lymphocyte culture using enriched B cells

4. Which pair demonstrates polymorphism?

   a. HLA-A2 and HLA-A28
   b. HLA-A2 and HLA-B27
   c. HLA-A2 and HLA-DR1
   d. HLA-DR1 and HLA-DQ1

5. Given the following HLA phenotypes, what are the haplotypes of the mother?

Father	A1,	A10;	B8,	B12
Mother	A2,	A10;	B27,	B38
Child 1	A1,	A10;	B8,	B27
Child 2	A10;	B12,	B27	

6. If an HLA designation is B5103, which statement most fully and correctly describes it?

   a. Its specificity is B51.
   b. Its specificity is B51 and there is more than one amino acid sequence that has been described.
   c. Its specificity is B51 and there is more than one gene sequence that has been described.
   d. Its specificity is B51 and there are more than two amino acid sequences and more than two gene sequences that have been described.

7. Which HLA specificity is helpful to diagnose ankylosing spondylitis?

   a. DR2
   b. DR3/4
   c. B8
   d. B27

References

1. Dausset H: Leukoagglutinins. IV. Leukoagglutinins and blood transfusion. Vox Sang 4:190, 1954
2. Dausset H: Iso-leuco-anticorps. Acta Haematol 20:156–166, 1959
3. Payne R, Rolfs MR: Fetomaternal leukocyte incompatibility. J Clin Invest 37:1756–1763, 1958
4. van Rood JJ, Eernisse JG, vanLeeuwen A: Leukocyte antibodies in the sera of pregnant women. Nature 181:1735, 1958
5. World Health Organization: Nomenclature for factors of the HL-A system. Bull WHO 39:483, 1968
6. Trowsdale J, Ragoussis J, Campbell RD: Map of the human MHC. Immunol Today 12:445, 1991
7. Bodmer JG, Marsh SGE, Albert ED, et al. WHO-HLA Nomenclature Committee. Nomenclature for factors of the HLA system, 1991. Vox Sang 63:142–157, 1992
8. Lotteau V, Teyton L, Peleraux A: Intracellular transport of class II MHC molecules directed by invariant chain. Nature 348:600, 1990

9. Germain RN: Antigen Processing and Presentation. In Paul WE (ed): Fundamental Immunology, 3rd ed, p 629. New York, Raven Press, 1993

10. National Institutes of Health. NIH Lymphocyte microcytotoxicity techniques. In NIAID Manual of Tissue Typing Techniques. Publication no. NIH 80-543. Atlanta, GA, Department of Health, Education and Welfare, 1979

11. Hansen JA, Mickelson EM, Choo SY, et al: Clinical bone marrow transplantation: Donor selection and recipient monitoring. In Rose NR, DeMacario EC, Fahey J (eds): Manual of Clinical Laboratory Immunology, 4th ed, p 850.

Washington, DC, American Society for Microbiology, 1992

12. Bauer MP, Danilovs JA: Population analysis of HLA-A, B, C, DR and other genetic markers. In Terasaki PI (ed): Histocompatibility Testing, pp 955–983. University of California Tissue Typing Laboratory, Los Angeles, 1980

13. Bias WB, Zachary AA, Rosner GL: Genetic and statistical principles of paternity determination. In Rose NR, DeMacario EC, Fahey J (eds): Manual of Clinical Laboratory Immunology, 4th ed, p 901. Washington DC, American Society for Microbiology, 1992

CHAPTER 6

Hypersensitivity

Anne E. Huot
Catherine Sheehan

Objectives

Upon completion of the chapter, the reader will be able to:

1. Describe the pathogenesis of the four types of hypersensitivity
2. List examples of each type of hypersensitivity
3. Distinguish between the preformed and newly formed mediators of type I hypersensitivity
4. Describe the process of immune complex deposition in tissues

Traditionally, immune responses were thought to develop only for the benefit of the host. It is now clear that the protective immune response can also have deleterious effects. Thus, immune responses may eradicate the infecting microorganism; at the same time, they can cause significant tissue damage. To distinguish between the beneficial and deleterious effects of the immune responses, the term *hypersensitivity* is used to describe an exaggerated response that causes tissue damage in a host. Such a response usually occurs in a sensitized host when it encounters the same antigen for the second time. Gell and Coombs classified the mechanisms of tissue injury resulting from hypersensitivity into four categories:[1]

1. Type I: anaphylactic
2. Type II: cytotoxic
3. Type III: immune complex disorders
4. Type IV: delayed hypersensitivity

The first three are antibody mediated, whereas type IV hypersensitivity involves T cells and macrophages. The major characteristics of four mechanisms of tissue injury are listed in Table 6-1 (on p. 66). This classification, however, is not absolute; frequently there is an overlap in the type of hypersensitivity response. Some substances can cause more than one type of reaction in a sensitive individual. For example, penicillin can cause a fatal type I anaphylactic reaction, type II hemolytic anemia, type III immune complex disorder, and a type IV delayed hypersensitivity reaction. These reactions may occur simultaneously or at different stages during a response.

TYPE I HYPERSENSITIVITY

Type I hypersensitivity is also known as immediate hypersensitivity because the reaction occurs within minutes of contact with the antigen or allergen. An allergic individual has circulating basophils or tissue mast cells

TABLE 6-1
Characteristics of Hypersensitivities

HYPERSENSITIVITY	EFFECTOR CELLS	IMMUNOGLOBULIN	COMPLEMENT ACTIVATION	EXAMPLE
Type I, anaphylactic hypersensitivity	Basophils Mast cells	IgE	No	Ragweed hay fever Insect allergy
Type II, cytotoxic antibody	—	IgG or IgM	Yes	Goodpasture's syndrome Graves' disease Myasthenia gravis
Type III, immune complex disorders	—	IgG or IgM	Yes	SLE, rheumatoid arthritis
Type IV, delayed-type hypersensitivity	T cells Macrophages	—	No	Contact sensitivity to poison ivy, PPD skin test

SLE, systemic lupus erythematosus; PPD 5, purified protein derivative from Mycobacterium tuberculosis.

that are sensitized by the cytotropic antibody, IgE (Fig. 6-1). Upon subsequent exposure to the allergen, these sensitized cells are triggered to release vasoactive amines that produce allergic symptoms (Fig. 6-2).

Allergy

The extent of an allergic response is partly influenced by the port of entry of the allergen. For example, a bee sting will introduce the allergen into the circulation, causing a systemic anaphylaxis, and an inhaled allergen can cause respiratory symptoms, such as rhinitis and asthma. Various clinical conditions, including asthma, eczema, and hay fever, are clinical symptoms associated with atopy. Atopy is a genetic predisposition to type I hypersensitivity and is associated with increased production of IgE antibody. If both parents are atopic for hay fever or asthma, there is a 75% chance that the child will be atopic. If one parent is affected, there is a 50% chance that the child will develop symptoms.[2] Approximately 5% to 10% of the population exposed to airborne allergens becomes sensitized.[3]

ALLERGENS AND TYPES OF DISEASE

Allergens are the antigens that are able to elicit IgE antibody responses in certain individuals. Most naturally occurring allergens have a molecular weight of 10,000 to 70,000 Da. Small antigens may not have sufficient numbers of epitopes to facilitate the Fc receptor crosslinking to trigger a basophil or mast cell, while a larger molecule may not be able to diffuse across the mucosal surface to reach the sensitized effector cells. The following modes of exposure to allergens have been identified:

1. The respiratory airway is constantly exposed to airborne particles that may cause allergic responses. The most common inhalant allergens are plant pollens, fungal spores, and animal danders.
2. Absorption of allergen from the digestive tract can also cause allergic responses.
3. Direct skin contact with pollen or another allergen can cause localized urticaria (hives) or even systemic symptoms in a highly sensitive individual.

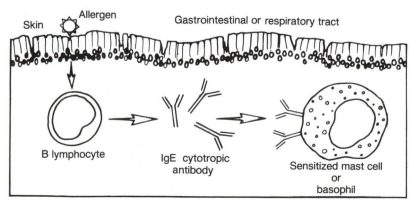

FIGURE 6-1
Mast cell or basophil sensitization.

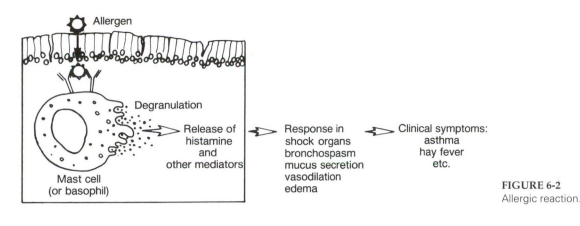

FIGURE 6-2
Allergic reaction.

Immediate hypersensitivity reactions occur most commonly in tissues rich in mast cells—the skin, nasal membranes, tongue, lungs, and gastrointestinal tract.[4] Inhaled allergens, such as animal danders, dust, pollen, and molds, are responsible for allergic rhinitis. Attacks occur only when the allergen is present. For some this is seasonal (when certain pollens are available), and for others it is perennial (when an offending allergen, such as house dust, is always available). If the immediate hypersensitivity reaction is localized in the nasal mucosa and conjunctiva, symptoms include rhinorrhea (runny nose), itching eyes and nose, sneezing, and nasal congestion. Elevated levels of eosinophils are present in the nasal secretions and blood. Serum IgE may or may not be elevated.

If the immediate hypersensitivity reaction is localized in the bronchus, allergic (intrinsic) asthma results. Symptoms of bronchial involvement are tightness of the chest, shortness of breath, and wheezing. Inhaled allergens may directly combine with IgE on bronchial mast cells, whereas ingested or injected allergens circulate to the lung and then combine with the mast cells. In either case, stimulation of the mast cells releases histamine and leukotrienes to contract bronchial smooth muscle. Frequently serum IgE is elevated.

Atopic dermatitis is commonly associated with allergic rhinitis, intrinsic asthma, eosinophilia, and very high levels of serum IgE. Skin testing does not generate useful information about the allergen. Patients with atopic dermatitis often have dry skin and pruritus (itching). Allergens such as pollen, house dust, animal dander, milk, and grains may be responsible for atopic dermatitis.

Food allergies or allergic gastroenteropathy is the least common form of atopy. Ingested food allergens can stimulate the local production of IgE, which can bind to mast cells in the gut. Local degranulation of mast cells and release of stored mediators promotes the food allergy. Signs and symptoms include nausea, vomiting, cramps, abdominal pain, and diarrhea, usually within 2 hours of allergen ingestion. Gastrointestinal loss of protein and blood may lead to anemia and hypoproteinemia. In infants the disease is transient; in adults it is uncommon.

Anaphylaxis is the systemic form of immediate hypersensitivity. It can affect more than one organ and is potentially life threatening when the allergic reaction causes shock or edema of the upper respiratory tract. Most often the precipitating allergen is food (peanuts, seafood, or egg albumin), insect venom (honeybee, wasp, or hornet stings), or drugs (vaccines, penicillin, or sulfonamides). Increased vascular permeability can result in leakage of plasma from the blood into the extravascular tissue, resulting in decreased blood volume; the resultant decreased cardiac output may contribute to hypoxemia and acidemia, leading to respiratory failure.[5]

CLINICAL AND LABORATORY EVALUATION OF ALLERGY

Skin Testing

If atopic allergy is suspected, skin testing with different allergens may identify the allergen responsible for the symptoms. Three skin testing techniques can demonstrate increased numbers of IgE-coated mast cells: scratch testing, prick testing (epicutaneous scratch), and intradermal testing. In each method, when the allergen is recognized by the IgE on the surface of mast cells in the skin, histamine is released within minutes, causing the characteristic wheal (localized edema) and flare (redness from vasodilation) with pruritus. The scratch test is performed by scratching the volar surface of the forearms or the back and then applying an allergen to the scratch. The prick test is accomplished by applying a drop of allergen to the skin surface and then pricking the skin directly beneath the drop. After 15 to 30 minutes, the areas are observed for the presence of wheal and erythema. If the results of the scratch or prick tests are equivocal, the intradermal test is performed. In the intradermal test a small volume of allergen is injected into the epidermis of the upper arm or forearm. After 20 minutes the area is observed for the wheal and erythema.

Total Serum IgE Levels

Another approach to assess atopic allergic individuals is to measure serum IgE in vitro. Methods to detect total IgE include competitive radioimmunosorbent test (RIST), noncompetitive RIST, double-antibody radioimmunoassay (RIA), and sandwich enzyme-linked immunosorbent assay (ELISA) and are shown in Figure 6-3. Competitive or indirect RIST is a competitive RIA based on the simultaneous incubation of radiolabeled IgE and reference or unknown IgE with an anti-IgE bound to a solid phase. The greater the concentration of the reference or unknown IgE, the fewer radiolabeled IgE that bind to the solid phase. There is a corresponding decrease in measured counts per minute (CPM).

Direct or noncompetitive RIST is a sandwich-type RIA in which solid-phase anti-IgE is incubated with reference or unknown IgE; the bound IgE then reacts with the radiolabeled anti–human IgE. The greater the concentration of the reference or unknown IgE, the greater the concentration of radiolabeled anti–human IgE that binds, which is indicated by a higher CPM.

The double-antibody RIA or radioimmunoprecipitation test involves the liquid-phase incubation of reference or unknown IgE and radiolabeled IgE with anti–human IgE. Resulting complexes are precipitated by adding a second, precipitating antibody. The greater the concentration of reference or unknown IgE, the fewer radiolabeled IgE present in the precipitate. This assay is sensitive and reproducible; however, ease of performance and commercial availability favors the use of direct RIST.[6] Modifications in testing procedures have included the development of enzyme-labeled assays in which enzyme activity is monitored by measuring the change in absorbance resulting from a change in the concentration of the substrate or product.[7,8] Rapid labeled immunoassays are now available in a dipstick or blot format.

Quantitation of Allergen-Specific IgE

The radioallergosorbent test (RAST) is the serologic quantitation of IgE antibodies directed against specific allergens.[9] This in vitro test yields information similar to skin testing. RAST testing may be preferred when skin testing is difficult to perform or interpret, when skin testing is negative, or when medication interference is suspected.[6] This test is a sandwich-type immunoassay in which the solid phase is coated with allergen. After incubation with reference or unknown sera, the specific allergen will capture IgE. Radiolabeled anti–human IgE is added to detect the bound IgE. The greater the amount of allergen-specific IgE bound, the greater the CPM of bound labeled IgE. When enzyme-labeled anti–human IgE replaces the radiolabeled antibody, the change in absorbance is measured.

There are a number of modifications of the RAST assay. The FAST (fluoroallergosorbent test) is a fluorescent enzyme immunoassay test in which total or specific IgE can be quantitated. FAST is a sandwich immunoassay in which the allergen is bound to the solid-phase membrane in the bottom of microtitration wells; following incubation with patient or reference serum, an enzyme-labeled anti–human IgE is added and the fluorescence is measured.[10] The MAST® (MAST® Immunosystems, Mountain View, CA) chemiluminescent assay (CLA) is a sandwich CLA in which a solid-phase cellulose thread is impregnated with a battery of allergens; after incubation with patient or reference serum, enzyme-labeled anti–human IgE is added.[11,12] The enzyme label reacts with photoreagents to produce light. When the light is exposed to photographic film, a permanent record is produced.

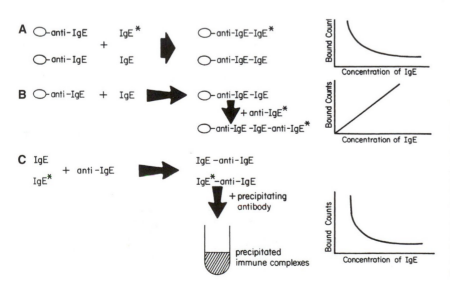

FIGURE 6-3
Methods to detect total serum IgE. (**A**) Competitive radioimmunosorbent test. Labeled IgE* and unlabeled IgE compete for the solid-phase anti-IgE. (**B**) Noncompetitive or radioimmunosorbent test. Immobilized anti-IgE captures IgE; radiolabeled anti-IgE is added and detects the bound IgE. (**C**) Double antibody RIA. Labeled IgE* and unlabeled IgE compete for soluble anti-IgE antibody; subsequently, precipitating antibody is added to precipitate bound IgE*.

TREATMENT

Treatment includes allergen avoidance, drug therapy, and immunotherapy. Ideally, once an allergen is defined, it should be avoided. Food and drug allergies can be best managed this way. Controlling household dust, avoiding pets, and preventing mold growth are other ways of controlling allergens.

Drug therapy is directed at controlling allergic symptoms. Antihistamines antagonize the effect of histamine by competing for the histamine H_1 receptors on target cells. Increased vascular permeability, vasodilation, itching, bronchial smooth muscle contraction, and gastrointestinal mucosal smooth muscle contraction can be blocked by antihistamine therapy. Antihistamine therapy is useful in allergic rhinitis. Cromolyn (disodium cromoglycate) protects asthmatic patients by preventing the release of mediators from mast cells. When it is administered prior to exposure to the allergen, bronchial spasm can be prevented. Asthma is often treated with theophylline, a methylxanthine that relaxes bronchial smooth muscle.

Immunotherapy or hyposensitization is the planned introduction of the allergen into a patient to reduce the IgE allergic response (Fig. 6-4). Allergic rhinitis, extrinsic asthma, and insect venom anaphylaxis may respond to this therapy. The allergen is injected weekly in gradually increasing doses. After an initial increase in circulating IgE, there is a decline. Allergen-specific IgG blocking antibody appears in the serum. This IgG binds to the allergen and prevents the allergen from stimulating mast cells, thus preventing the allergic reaction. The maximum tolerated dose or the maintenance dose is then administered less frequently to maintain sufficient IgG blocking antibody to prevent symptoms.

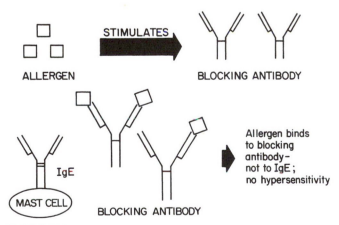

STIMULATES

ALLERGEN

BLOCKING ANTIBODY

IgE

Allergen binds to blocking antibody— not to IgE; no hypersensitivity

MAST CELL

BLOCKING ANTIBODY

FIGURE 6-4
Principles of immunotherapy. Injections of the offending allergen stimulate the production of blocking antibodies. When the allergen is encountered later, it will be neutralized by the blocking antibody and will not bind the IgE-sensitized mast cells.

Mechanism of Vasoactive Amine Release

The effector cells involved in an allergic response are basophils and mast cells. In general, basophils are found in the circulation, whereas mast cells are distributed in the tissue of shock organs. The two cell types are indistinguishable in many of their biologic characteristics: They express cell surface Fc receptors for IgE; they have cytoplasmic granules containing vasoactive amines; and they are triggered to release vasoactive amines by similar mechanisms.

IgE antibodies produced by the plasma cells are bound to the cell surface of a basophil or mast cell by way of Fcε receptors. Subsequent exposure to the same allergen will cause immune complex formation on the cell surface, leading to the release of vasoactive amines.[13,14] The crucial event appears to be crosslinking of the effector cell surface Fcε receptors.[15,16] It is possible to trigger the vasoactive amine release experimentally. For example, effector cells are triggered by crosslinking the Fcε receptors using an antibody to the Fcε receptor, or an antibody to the IgE heavy chain (Fig. 6-5 on p. 70). Thus, the physiologic conditions required for effector cell triggering are as follows: At least two IgE molecules are occupying the adjacent Fcε receptors on a effector cell and the allergen is multivalent, such that it is able to crosslink the two IgE molecules on the effector cell (see Fig. 6-5). Whereas the released vasoactive amines cause general symptoms of an allergic response, the IgE molecules convey the specificity of an allergic response. This is caused by the idiotype of the IgE antibody that binds to the allergen. One of the biologic events resulting from receptor crosslinking is the fusion of granular membranes and cell membranes, which leads to the release of stored, preformed granular contents. Therefore, the effector cells become degranulated. Receptor crosslinking also results in the synthesis of mediators from arachidonic acid.

Immunoglobulin E

Immunoglobulin E (IgE) is also known as reaginic antibody. The control mechanism for IgE synthesis by plasma cells is currently being investigated. IgE antibody differs from other immunoglobulin classes in that it has five heavy chain domains and is cytotropic for basophils and mast cells. The binding of IgE molecules to the Fc receptors is mediated by heavy-chain constant domains 3 and 4. The equilibrium of free (circulating) and bound IgE obeys the law of mass action; thus, the proportion is always the same. This cytotropic activity is heat sensitive; heating at 56°C for 30 minutes will abolish this activity. The serum half-life of IgE is approximately 2.5 days. However, once

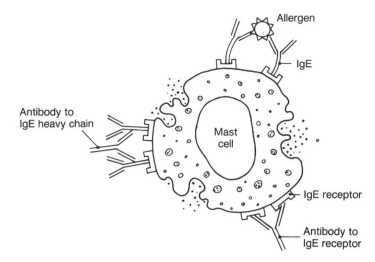

FIGURE 6-5
Granule release triggered by crosslinking of the cell surface Fc receptors.

bound to the effector cell surface by the Fc receptor, the half-life increases to 6 to 12 weeks.[17]

Pharmacologic Roles of the Mediators[16,18]

The primary role of the mediators appears to be defense against injury. For example, during nematode infection in rats, the sensitized tissue mast cells are triggered by the parasite antigen to release vasoactive amines. The increased vascular permeability causes the leakage of plasma proteins. Among these proteins are antibodies against the parasite. The antibodies neutralize the parasites, which are cleared from the host as a form of immune complex. Thus, in this case vasodilation is beneficial to the host. However, in an allergic response the similar normal defense mechanism is exaggerated, causing extensive tissue damages.

The mediators of allergic response may be divided into two categories: performed and newly synthesized mediators. Preformed mediators are stored in the granules, and the newly formed mediators are synthesized after the effector cells are triggered.

Preformed Mediators

HISTAMINE

Histamine (molecular weight 111 Da) causes contraction of the bronchioles and smooth muscle of blood vessels, increases capillary permeability, and increases mucus gland secretion in the airway. This preformed mediator is stored in the granules and can be released 1 to 2 minutes after allergen-antibody reaction. The duration of histamine activity is approximately 10 minutes.

EOSINOPHIL CHEMOTACTIC FACTOR OF ANAPHYLAXIS

Eosinophil chemotactic factor of anaphylaxis (ECF-A) has a molecular weight of 500 Da. This is a preformed mediator released during degranulation. It stimulates eosinophils to migrate to the site of an antigen-antibody reaction. Eosinophils are known to have several functions, including (1) phagocytosis and disposal of antigen-antibody complexes and (2) release of the enzymes histaminase and arylsulfatase. These enzymes dampen the allergic reaction caused by allergic mediators.

Newly Synthesized Mediators

Following activation, the newly synthesized mediators are derived from membrane lipids of basophils and mast cells. Arachidonic acid is liberated from the membrane lipid by the action of the enzymes phospholipase A or phospholipase C and diacylglycerol lipase. The freed arachidonic acid is then processed by one of two metabolic pathways, the cyclooxygenase (prostaglandin synthetase) pathway or the 5-lipoxygenase pathway. Whereas the former pathway leads to prostaglandin production, the latter leads to leukotriene production (Fig. 6-6).

PROSTAGLANDIN D_2

Prostaglandin D_2 causes vasodilation and increases vascular permeability. The clinical symptoms caused by this compound are similar to those seen with histamine—erythematous wheal and flare reaction. However, the prostaglandin D_2 effect can persist for as long as 2 hours; the histamine effect lasts approximately 10 minutes.

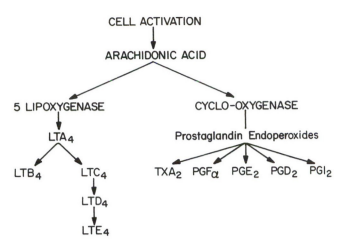

FIGURE 6-6
Pathway of oxidative metabolism of arachidonic acid.

LEUKOTRIENES

Leukotrienes C_4, D_4, or E_4 cause erythema and wheal formation. When inhaled, they cause bronchospasm. Furthermore, their bronchoconstrictive potency is 30 to 1000 times that of histamine. Leukotrienes C_4 and D_4 have also been shown to stimulate mucus secretion by human airway tissue.

TYPE II HYPERSENSITIVITY

Type II hypersensitivity involves IgG or IgM antibody against cell surface molecules or tissue components. The tissue damage may be mediated by one of the following mechanisms: (1) accelerated clearance of the antibody-sensitized target cells by the mononuclear phagocytic system (reticuloendothelial system), (2) blockade of normal cellular function because of antibody binding to the target cells, (3) complement-mediated lysis of the target cells, or (4) damage of innocent bystander cells or tissue by the lysosomal enzymes released by the neutrophils present at the site of antigen-antibody reactions.

Antibody-Mediated Tissue Damage

Hemolytic anemia from a warm antibody is frequently associated with antibody production against red cell antigen of the Rh system, such as C, D, and E antigen. The sensitized red blood cells are cleared by the macrophages at an accelerated rate, causing anemia in the afflicted individual. The etiology of this disease is unknown, but it is frequently associated with other autoimmune disorders.[19]

Patients with Graves' disease have circulating antibodies specific for thyroid stimulating hormone (TSH) receptor. When bound to the TSH receptors, these antibodies will stimulate the thyroid epithelial cells to produce thyroglobulin, independent of the normal feedback control mechanism. Persistent stimulation of the thyroid gland causes hyperthyroidism. These antibodies are known as long-acting thyroid stimulator (LATS).[20]

Antibodies against cell surface structure can also block the normal cellular activities. For example, the antibody against acetylcholine receptors prevents the neurotransmitter, acetylcholine, from binding to the receptor at the neuromuscular junction. This type of antibody is associated with myasthenia gravis, a disease with muscular paralysis as the clinical manifestation.[21]

Complement-Mediated Cell Lysis

When the antibody-antigen complex is able to activate the complement cascade, direct cell lysis occurs. Transfusion reactions are the most important clinical manifestation of this type of hypersensitivity. Transfusion of ABO-incompatible blood will result in lysis of the donor's red blood cells because the recipient has antibodies to non-self ABO antigens. For example, a recipient with type A blood will have antibody to the B antigen, a type B recipient will have antibody to A antigen, and a type O individual will have antibodies to both A and B antigens. These pre-existing antibodies against non-self ABO red cell antigens are also known as naturally occurring red cell antibodies. The production of such antibodies is thought to occur during bacterial infections because the infecting microorganisms coincidentally express antigens that are similar to the ABO blood group antigens.

Hemolytic disease of the newborn (HDNB) is due to maternal-fetal red cell incompatibility. The Rhesus D (RhD) antigen is the most frequently involved red cell antigen. An RhD-negative mother becomes immunized to the D antigen on fetal red blood cells because of maternal-fetal blood mixing during pregnancy or delivery. The mother synthesizes IgG antibodies against the D antigen. In a subsequent pregnancy with an RhD-positive fetus, the IgG antibodies cross the placenta and circulate in fetal circulation, causing complement-mediated lysis of the fetal red blood cells. Prophylactic RhD immune globulin treatment given to the mother immediately after delivery can prevent the HDNB in the subsequent pregnancy. The RhD antibodies in the Rh immune globulin will prevent maternal RhD antibody production by neutralizing the fetal RhD-positive red blood cells that leak into maternal circulation during delivery.[22]

Formed blood elements other than red blood cells can also be the target of cytotoxic antibody lysis. For example, antibody against platelets causes idiopathic thrombocytopenic purpura, antibody to neutrophils causes granulocytopenia, and antibody to T cells is associated with systemic lupus erythematosus.

Cytotoxic Antibodies to Tissue Components

Cytotoxic antibodies to tissue components frequently cause inflammatory responses. The sequence of events includes the antibody-antigen reaction, complement activation, generation of such chemotactic factors as C3a and C5a, infiltration of the tissue by neutrophils, and release of lysosomal enzymes by the neutrophils, which eventually leads to tissue damage. The classic example is Goodpasture's syndrome. The patient develops antibodies against glomerular and pulmonary basement membranes. Binding of these antibodies to the basement membrane initiates the sequence of events described earlier. Direct immunofluorescent study of a kidney biopsy shows linear deposition of antibodies and complement along the glomerular basement membrane. The inflammatory reactions produced by anti–basement membrane antibody deposition account for the clinical symptoms observed in these patients. The symptoms include hematuria, renal failure, and hemoptysis.[23]

TYPE III HYPERSENSITIVITY

Type III reactions are triggered by the deposition of circulating immune complexes in tissues, causing inflammation. The antibody involved is predominantly IgG or IgM, and the antigens can be infecting microorganisms, drugs, or self-antigens. Complement is usually activated, which greatly amplifies the inflammatory response.

Fate of Circulating Immune Complexes

Under normal conditions circulating immune complexes are rapidly cleared by the mononuclear phagocytic system, preventing tissue deposition and associated damage. The physicochemical property, especially the molecular size of immune complexes, appears to affect their clearance directly. Large immune complexes are cleared rapidly by the host, whereas small soluble complexes tend to have a prolonged plasma half-life and are associated with tissue deposition, which causes inflammatory responses. Various factors that affect the size of immune complexes are identified here; the principles of antibody-antigen binding are discussed in Chapter 10.

RATIO OF ANTIGEN TO ANTIBODY

The ratio of antigen (Ag) to antibody (Ab) has a direct effect on the size of immune complexes. Small immune complexes are usually formed in antigen excess (an excess of 5 to 60 times). These small complexes usually have an Ag/Ab ratio in the range of 1.2 to 1.25, and molecular formulas of Ag_1Ab_1, Ag_2Ab_2, or possibly Ag_2Ab_1. Studies of the rate of immune complex clearance in animals indicate that immune complexes with a density of less than 19S and an Ag/Ab ratio greater than 2:5 tend to have a prolonged plasma half-life. Conversely, immune complexes with a density greater than 19S and an Ag/Ab ratio of 2:5 or less are cleared rapidly by the animal (Fig. 6-7).[24–26]

ANTIGEN VALENCY

The number of antigenic determinants of an antigen may have an effect on the size of immune complexes. This is demonstrated experimentally using constructed hapten-protein conjugates. Conjugates with less than four hapten molecules form small soluble immune complexes with a density of less than 19S, an Ag/Ab ratio greater than 2:5, and a tendency to prolonged plasma half-life.[25]

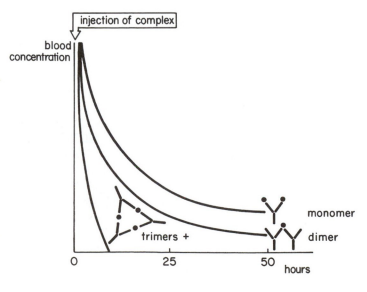

FIGURE 6-7
Immune complex clearance by the reticuloendothelial system. (From Roitt IM, Brostoff J, Male DK. Immunology. London, Gower Medical, 1985.)

ANTIBODY AFFINITY

Antibody with low affinity tends to form immune complexes that are easily dissociated and become small soluble immune complexes. The Fc receptors of phagocytic cells also play an important role in immune complex clearance because the receptors enable the phagocytic cells to attach to the immune complexes (opsonization), enhancing phagocytosis. Normally, the immune complex needs to have at least two IgG molecules to be cleared efficiently by the reticuloendothelial system. When the host is overloaded with a high concentration of immune complexes, the Fc receptors of the mononuclear phagocytic system can become saturated, which results in persistent circulating immune complexes.[24,25]

Complement activation by immune complexes also has an impact on their clearance. Complement receptors (C3b) on the mononuclear phagocytic cells appear to mediate immune adherence, promoting phagocytosis of the immune complexes that fix complement.[25]

Site of Immune Complex Deposition

The site of immune complex deposition is mainly determined by the hemodynamics and the concentration of the circulating immune complexes. The area of great blood flow and turbulence appears to have marked predilection for complex deposition; the arterial bifurcation of the heart valve and the renal glomeruli are frequently involved. The renal glomeruli seem to be the prime targets, and several factors may contribute to this predilection: (1) Filtration occurs in this site, (2) they are subjected to unusual hydrodynamic stress, and (3) glomerular endothelial cells have a high affinity for certain antigens, such as DNA.[24,26] Localized immune complex formation can also result in type III hypersensitivity. Inflammation of the joint seen in rheumatoid arthritis exemplifies the condition in which tissue damage occurs at the site of immune complex formation.

Pathogenesis

In experimental animals, systemically injected immune complexes do not always lead to tissue deposition. However, if histamine is injected with immune complexes, tissue deposition occurs. Furthermore, administration of antihistamine can abrogate the histamine effect, suggesting that increased vascular permeability plays an important role in immune complex deposition. There are several sources of vasoactive amines. These include basophils, mast cells, platelets, and complement fragments.

Inflammatory responses are triggered as a result of complement activation by immune complexes. Complement activation products, such as C3a and C5a, have anaphylatoxic activities (anaphylatoxins). These ana-

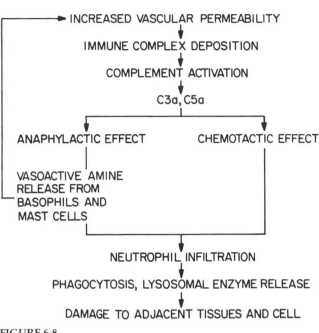

FIGURE 6-8
Pathogenesis of immune complex disorders.

phylatoxins will trigger vasoactive amine release from basophils and mast cells, leading to increased vascular permeability, which will enhance the immune complex deposition and neutrophil infiltration. Furthermore, neutrophils are attracted to the site of inflammation by C5a. Lysosomal enzymes are released by the neutrophils as they attempt to phagocytoze the immune complexes, leading to the damage to adjacent cells and tissues. The immune complexes can also interact with Fc receptors on platelets and trigger vasoactive amine release by the platelets, thus perpetuating the cycle described earlier (Fig. 6-8).

Examples of Type III Hypersensitivity

ARTHUS REACTION

The Arthus reaction is induced experimentally by intradermal injection of the antigen into a sensitized animal. The local antigen-antibody interaction (immune complex formation) results in destructive inflammation of small blood vessels, called vasculitis. Local swelling and erythema appear within 1 to 2 hours and subside within 10 to 12 hours. Microscopic examination of the tissue reveals neutrophil infiltration initially, followed by mononuclear cells and eosinophil infiltration. The mononuclear cells and eosinophils degrade the immune complexes.

Hypersensitive pneumonitis or extrinsic allergic alveolitis is probably the clinical counterpart of the Arthus reaction. The inhaled antigens may be fungal spores, avian proteins (the cause of bird handler's pneumonitis), or insect antigens. The clinical symptoms include chills, cough, dyspnea, and fever. Usually resolution of symptoms occurs in 12 to 18 hours once the source of antigen is eliminated.

IMMUNE COMPLEX DISORDERS

The term *immune complex disorder* is used to describe the diseases associated with clinical features secondary to immune complex deposition. The classic example is serum sickness, which frequently develops in patients who receive heterologous serum as a form of passive immunotherapy or immunosuppressive therapy. For example, horse antisera to diphtheria, tetanus, or other microorganisms were used in the past as a form of prophylactic immunotherapy, and heterologous antilymphocyte antibodies were given to renal transplant recipients to suppress tissue rejection. The patients make antibodies against the heterologous serum proteins and develop immune complex disorders.

GLOMERULONEPHRITIS

Deposition of immune complexes in the renal glomeruli causes inflammatory responses that present with clinical symptoms of glomerulonephritis. For example, systemic lupus erythematosus (SLE) is an autoimmune disorder in which autoantibody to double-stranded DNA plays an important role in pathogenesis. The pathogenic role of antibody-DNA immune complexes is indicated by experimental observations: Antibody-DNA immune complexes have been eluted from the diseased kidney, and immunofluorescent study of kidney biopsy demonstrates immunoglobulin and C3 deposition in the glomeruli. The immunofluorescent staining pattern of SLE kidney biopsy differs from that of glomerulonephritis associated with Goodpasture's syndrome. Whereas the latter demonstrates smooth, linear staining of the glomerular basement membrane, the SLE lesion shows granular or "lumpy" staining, which may be confined to the mesangium, extended to the subendothelium or the basement membrane.[24,27,28] Glomerulonephritis caused by immune complex deposition is also associated with such infections as streptococcal infection and hepatitis B viral infection.[29,30] Malignancies also appear to cause nephritis occasionally.

VASCULITIS

Vasculitis is a group of syndromes that have common clinicopathologic features associated with the inflammatory reaction in vessel walls. The classification of vasculitis is based on the type and size of affected vessels, the organs involved (lung, kidney, skin, etc.), the characteristic inflammatory reaction, and the clinical features. Polyarteritis nodosa is characterized by the inflammation of small and medium-sized arteries. Approximately 50% of the patients with polyarteritis nodosa are found to have hepatitis B infections. Hepatitis B surface antigens (HBsAg), either alone or with immunoglobulin and complement, have been demonstrated in the vessel walls in the patient with polyarteritis nodosa. Vasculitis is also seen in patients with rheumatoid arthritis. Immunofluorescent study of the lesion shows the deposition of immunoglobulin and C3 in the arterial walls in a granular pattern.[27,28]

Destruction of Innocent Bystanders

Circulating immune complexes can nonspecifically adhere to the elements of blood, initiating their destruction and that of innocent bystanders. Drug administration often elicits an antibody response that results in circulating antibody-drug immune complexes. These antibody-drug immune complexes become adsorbed onto the surface of red blood cells, causing intravascular hemolysis. The adsorption of immune complexes is thought to be mediated by the red blood cell surface C3b receptors. Quinidine, quinine, and phenacetin are known to cause red blood cell lysis by this mechanism.[24]

TYPE IV HYPERSENSITIVITY

Type IV hypersensitivity, the cell-mediated immune reaction or delayed hypersensitivity, is mediated by soluble factors or lymphokines released by the sensitized T lymphocytes. The characteristic histology of the lesion is a mononuclear cell infiltration. Such lesions appear 24 to 48 hours following antigen challenge and peak within 72 hours. Antibody and complement are usually not directly involved in type IV hypersensitivity.

Mechanisms of Pathogenesis

The response is initiated by interactions between the antigen and a small number of sensitized T lymphocytes. Lymphokines are produced by these T lymphocytes following activation. The lymphokines have biologic activities affecting various cell types, such as macrophages, neutrophils, and other lymphocytes. These secondary cells are recruited to the site of reaction. For example, macrophages that respond to the lymphokine, migration inhibition factor (MIF), are prevented from leaving the lesion and become activated.[31] The overall function of lymphokines is to amplify the response that is initiated by a small number of T lymphocytes. This is achieved by recruiting and directing the secondary cells, macrophages, neutrophils, and other lymphocytes, both T and B cells. Normal control mechanisms lead to resolution of the reaction; however, multiple antigenic challenges in a hypersensitive individual may lead to the ulceration and necrosis of the lesion. Usually the symptoms develop over a period of 24 to 48 hours after antigen exposure, and the histologic examination shows characteristic mononuclear infiltration.

Examples of Type IV Hypersensitivity

TUBERCULIN-TYPE HYPERSENSITIVITY

Tuberculin-type hypersensitivity is induced by subcutaneous injection of the antigen in a sensitized individual. The area of induration and swelling at the site of injection appears within 24 to 72 hours. Microscopic examination reveals intense mononuclear cell infiltration around the blood vessels and disruption of the organization of the collagen bundles in the dermis. The classic example is the tuberculin skin test, in which purified protein derivative (PPD) prepared from the culture filtrate of *Mycobacterium tuberculosis* is administered intradermally. A positive response consists of 10 mm or greater erythema and induration between 48 and 72 hours. A positive test indicates that the individual has been exposed to *M. tuberculosis* or related organisms. A negative test signifies either no infection or a false negative, caused by immunosuppression associated with severe infection. A false negative test result may also be caused by immune suppressive conditions, including corticosteroid therapy, lymphoid malignancies, viral infections, and sarcoidosis.[32]

CONTACT SENSITIVITY

Certain compounds can cause systemic sensitization through direct skin contact. A second encounter with the same antigen by skin contact results in edema of the epidermis with formation of microvesicles. The microscopic observation of the lesion indicates a mononuclear cell infiltrate that first appears at 6 to 8 hours and peaks at 12 to 15 hours after exposure to the antigen. The most common antigens that induce contact sensitivity are poison ivy and poison oak.[33] This sensitivity is caused by a hypersensitivity reaction to the hapten urushiol.

GRANULOMATOUS HYPERSENSITIVITY

Granulomatous hypersensitivity results from the persistent presence of microorganisms within the macrophages that the cell is unable to destroy. Inert substances, such as talc, may also cause granulomatous hypersensitivity. In both cases the macrophages are unable to digest the phagocytozed substance. The characteristic cells found in a granulomatous lesion are lymphocytes, macrophages, epithelioid cells, and multinucleated giant cells. Epithelioid cells are poorly understood. The giant cells are multinucleated with little endoplasmic reticulum, degenerated mitochondria, and lysosomes. Thus, it is likely a terminally differentiated macrophage. Granulomatous hypersensitivity is seen in tuberculosis, leprosy, and sarcoidosis.[34]

Review Questions

1. The portion of the IgE antibody that attaches to Fcε receptors is found on

   a. the idiotype of the antibody
   b. the variable regions of the epsilon heavy chain
   c. the Fab portion of the antibody
   d. the third and fourth domains of the constant region of the epsilon heavy chain

2. Anaphylactic reactions are mediated by

   a. mast cells
   b. lymphocytes
   c. macrophages
   d. natural killer cells

3. Type I hypersensitivity is characterized by

   a. cytotoxic reactions
   b. cell-mediated reactions
   c. immune-complex deposition
   d. immediate release of preformed mediators by mast cells

4. Type II hypersensitivity is characterized by

   a. cytotoxic reactions
   b. cell-mediated reactions
   c. immune-complex deposition
   d. immediate release of preformed mediators by mast cells

5. Type III hypersensitivity is characterized by

   a. cytotoxic reactions
   b. cell-mediated reactions
   c. immune-complex deposition
   d. immediate release of preformed mediators by mast cells

6. Type IV hypersensitivity is characterized by

   a. cytotoxic reactions
   b. cell-mediated reactions
   c. immune-complex deposition
   d. immediate release of preformed mediators by mast cells

References

1. Terr AI: Mechanisms of hypersensitivity. In Stite DP, Stobo JD, Terr AI, Parslow TG (eds): Basic and Clinical Immunology, 8th ed, p 315. Norwalk, CT, Appleton & Lange, 1994

2. Terr AI: The atopic diseases. In Stite DP, Stobo JD, Terr AI, Parslow TG (eds): Basic and Clinical Immunology, 8th ed, p 329. Norwalk, CT, Appleton & Lange, 1994

3. Marsh DG, Meyers DA, Bias WB: The epidemiology and genetics of atopic allergy. N Engl J Med 305:1551, 1981

4. Serafin WE, Austin KF: Mediators of immediate hypersensitivity reactions. N Engl J Med 317:30, 1987

5. Shatz GS: Anaphylaxis. In Korenblat PE, Wedner HJ (eds): Allergy: Theory and Practice. Orlando, Grune and Stratton, 1984

6. Hamilton RG, Adkinson NF Jr: Measurement of total serum immunoglobulin E and allergin-specific immunoglobulin E antibody. In Rose NR, Friedman H, Fahey JL, Macario EC, Penn GM (eds): Manual of Clinical Laboratory Immunology, 4th ed, p 703. Washington, DC, American Society for Microbiology, 1992

7. Hamilton RG, Adkinson NF Jr: Clinical laboratory methods for the assessment and management of human allergic diseases. Clin Lab Med 6:117, 1986

8. Hamilton RG, Adkinson NF Jr: Serological methods in the diagnosis and management of human allergic disease. CRC Crit Rev Clin Lab Sci 21:1, 1984

9. Wide C, Bennich H, Johansson SGO: Diagnosis of allergy by an in-vitro test for allergen antibodies. Lancet 2:1105, 1967

10. Rodriquez GE: A new IgE fluorescent allergosorbent test (FAST). Clin Immunol Newslett 9:81, 1988

11. Miller SP, Marinkovich VA, Riege DH, et al: Application of the MAST™ immunodiagnostic system to the determination of allergen-specific IgE. Clin Chem 30:1467, 1984

12. Brown CR, Higgins KW, Fazer K, et al: Simultaneous determination of total IgE and allergen-specific IgE in serum by MAST chemiluminescent assay system. Clin Chem 31:1500, 1985

13. Ishizaka T, Soto CS, Ishizaka K: Mechanisms of passive sensitization. III. Number of IgE molecules and their receptor sites on human basophil granulocytes. J Immunol 111:500, 1973

14. Schleimer RP, MacGlashan DW Jr, Shuiman FS, et al: Human mast cell and basophil—structure, function, pharmacology, and biochemistry. Clin Rev Allergy 1:327, 1983

15. Ishizaka T: Biochemical analysis of triggering signals induced by bridging of IgE receptors. Fed Proc 41:17, 1982

16. Schleimer RP, MacGlashan DW Jr, Peter SP, et al: Inflammatory mediators and mechanisms of release from purified human basophils and mast cells. J Clin Immunol 74:473, 1984

17. Bennich H: Structure of IgE. Prog Immunol 2:49, 1974

18. Serafin WE, Austin KF: Mediators of immediate hypersensitivity reactions. N Engl J Med 317:30, 1987

19. Petz LD, Garratty G: Specificity of autoantibodies: Specificity of autoantibodies associated with warm-antibody type autoimmune hemolytic anemia. In Acquired Immune Hemolytic Anemia, p 232. New York, Churchill Livingstone, 1980

20. Volpe R: Autoimmunity in the endocrine system, Vol 20, Monographs in Endocrinology. New York, Springer-Verlag, 1981

21. Lindstrom J: Autoimmune response to acetylcholine receptors in myasthenia gravis and its animal model. Adv Immunol 27:1, 1979

22. Donegan E, Bossom EL: Blood banking and immunohematology. In Stite DP, Stobo JD, Terr AI, Parslow TG (eds): Basic and Clinical Immunology, 8th ed, p 233. Norwalk, CT, Appleton & Lange, 1994

23. Briggs WA, Johnson JP, Teichnab S, et al: Antiglomerular basement membrane antibody-mediated glomerulonephritis and Goodpasture's syndrome. Medicine 58:348, 1975

24. Thaler MS, Klausner RD, Cohen HJ: Immune complex disease. In Medical Immunology, p 139. Philadelphia, JB Lippincott, 1977

25. Wells JV: Immune mechanisms in tissue damage. In Fudenberg HH, Stite DP, Caldwell JL, et al (eds): Basic and Clinical Immunology, 2nd ed, p 274. Los Altos, CA, Lange Medical, 1978

26. Roitt I: Hypersensitivity. In Essential Immunology, p 268. London, Gower Medical, 1991

27. Inman RD, Day NK: Immunologic and clinical aspects of immune complex diseases. Am J Med 70:1097, 1981

28. Inman RD: Immune complexes in SLE. Clin Rheum Dis 8:49, 1982

29. Gutman RA, Striker GE, Gillard BC, et al: The immune complex glomerulonephritis of bacterial endocarditis. Medicine 51:1, 1972

30. Shusterman N, London WT: Hepatitis B and immune-complex disease. N Engl J Med 310:43, 1984

31. Sergent JS: Vasculitis with hepatitis B antigenemia: Long-term observation in nine patients. Medicine 55:1, 1976

32. Snider DE: The tuberculin skin test. Annu Rev Respir Dis 125 (Suppl):102, 1982

33. Terr AI: Cell mediated hypersensitivity. In Stite DP, Stobo JD, Terr AI, Parslow TG (eds): Basic and Clinical Immunology, 8th ed, p 364. Norwalk, CT, Appleton & Lange, 1994

34. Roitt I: Hypersensitivity. In Essential Immunology, p 271. London, Gower Medical, 1991

CHAPTER 7

Tumor Immunology

Karen James

Objectives

Upon completion of the chapter, the reader will be able to:

1. Define the antigens associated with tumor immunity
2. Describe natural immunity to tumors, including the functions of macrophages, natural killer cells, and nonimmunologic changes to the environment associated with tumor invasiveness
3. Describe T-cell–mediated immunity to tumors, including cytokines and cytotoxic T-cell immune mechanisms
4. Recall the tumor markers that are useful in the diagnosis, prognosis, and monitoring of the effects of therapy for various forms of cancer
5. Describe the therapeutic approaches to eliminating tumor burden

Neoplasia means new growth. A neoplasm is "an abnormal mass of tissue, the growth of which exceeds and is uncoordinated with that of normal tissues, and persists in the same excessive manner after cessation of the stimuli that evoked the change."[1] The terms *tumor* and *cancer* are used by the general public when referring to neoplastic diseases. The word *tumor* actually refers to swelling or to a defined mass of tissue distinct from normal physiologic growth; thus, a scar would by definition be a tumor.[2] The Latin word for *tumor* is *oncos*, thus, the origin of the word *oncology*, the study and treatment of tumors or neoplasms. The commonly used term for all malignant tumors or neoplasms is *cancer*.

A neoplasm is essentially a parasite that establishes a relationship with the host, referred to as tumor-host interactions.[2] Benign tumors may cause clinical disease by interfering with the functions of normal tissues or by producing hormones with functional activity. Malignant tumors cause similar symptoms of disease; however, they also invade normal tissue, grow rapidly, and use nutrients that normal tissues need to survive. In contrast, the host also develops a response to the tumor, referred to as tumor immunity. Scientists have long hypothesized that the immune system has a role in tumor immunity. Key evidence is that solid tumors removed from humans during surgery invariably have a mononuclear cell infiltrate, implying an immune response to the cancer.

IMMUNE RESPONSIVENESS TO TUMORS

The study of the immunology of tumors originated in the 1950s when tumors induced by carcinogens (methylcholanthrene) were used to immunize inbred mice. These immunized mice could reject a graft of the same tumor, providing them protection from the same tumors, but no protection against other tumors.[3] Antigens on these chemically induced tumors were unique for the individual tumor and could be transferred in vivo or in vitro without loss of the antigens. Immunity to carcinogen-induced tumors could also be transferred to other mice with lymphocytes, suggesting that T cells were involved in the immune responsiveness to tumors. In the field of tumor immunology, any antigen may be used as an immunogen in efforts to control tumor growth; i.e., as potential therapeutic mechanisms.[4]

Tumor-Associated Antigens

Antigens on the surface of tumor cells were originally thought to be unique immunogens, recognized by the immune system as being different from molecules on the surfaces of normal cells. Chemically induced tumors were extensively studied to determine the nature of these antigens. Unfortunately, nearly every tumor had unique antigens, even when induced by the same carcinogen using the same strain of animals. After many frustrating years of investigations, four classes of tumor-associated antigens have been characterized to date:[4] (1) tumor-specific peptides that require major histocompatibility complex (MHC) interaction to stimulate an immune response; (2) virus-induced tumor antigens that must also be associated with MHC antigens on the surface of tumor cells to generate an immune response; (3) genome-encoded tumor antigens, in which point mutations of oncogenes induce uncontrolled cellular proliferation; and (4) expression of normally silent differentiation antigens.

TUMOR-SPECIFIC PEPTIDES

In the mid–1980s, the concept of immune surveillance broadened to include tumor-specific peptides derived from fragmented proteins presented by MHC products on the cell surface during antigen processing.[5] Antigen processing and presentation for T-cell recognition has been shown to follow two primary pathways: the exogenous protein presentation pathway and the endogenous protein pathway.[4] Exogenous protein presentation involves endocytosis of the foreign protein by professional antigen-presenting cells (APCs—macrophages and B cells), degradation of the protein into short peptides (eight to nine amino acids) within the APCs, and binding of these peptides to MHC Class II molecules within the APCs. When the MHC-peptide complexes reach the cell surface, they are recognized by T cells expressing the CD4 molecule.

Endogenous protein presentation involves loading the peptides into MHC Class I molecules within the endoplasmic reticulum of the cell. When these MHC-peptide complexes reach the cell surface, they are recognized by T cells expressing the CD8 molecule. Recognizing that there are two mechanisms of MHC-peptide interaction, it became clearer that intracellular proteins (not just surface antigens) could be displayed on the surfaces of tumor cells. This provides the mechanism for dysregulation in tumor cells to become visible to the immune system.[6]

VIRUS-INDUCED TUMOR ANTIGENS

The first antigenic structures detectable on tumor cells as targets for T-cell immunity were viral antigens on virus-induced murine neoplasms.[7] Virus-related-specific antigens have identical or crossreactive specificities, even if induced in different species of animals. Viruses known to be oncogenic in animals include the polyoma virus, Moloney virus, Gross virus, and simian virus (SV40). Human oncogenic viruses identified to date include Epstein-Barr virus (EBV) associated with Burkitt's lymphoma; papillomaviruses, which cause epithelial proliferative diseases (cervical cancer); human T-cell leukemia virus (HTLV-1), the causative agent of adult T-cell leukemia; and hepatitis B virus (HBV), associated with primary hepatoma. Peptides derived from EBV nuclear antigens (EBNA-3, EBNA-4, EBNA-6), when associated with specific HLA antigens, have been shown to elicit specific cytotoxic T-cell (CTL) responses.[8]

GENOME-ENCODED TUMOR ANTIGENS

Cancer-causing genes (oncogenes) result from single point mutations of protooncogenes (cellular genes that promote normal growth and differentiation) and/or tumor suppressor genes (TSG). These mutations result in single amino acid substitutions in the protein products of those genes, which transform them into genome-encoded tumor antigens that may induce specific immunity against cancer cells.[4] By definition, malignant cells have altered genes. It has been determined that multiple oncogenes and/or TSGs must be affected in order to transform normal tissue to a malignant tumor.[9] More than 10 TSGs and nearly 100 oncogenes have been defined. One TSG and three of the more common oncogenes are briefly reviewed.

Mutated p53 Proteins

The p53 protooncogene is a nuclear cellular gene that collaborates with the cytoplasmic ras gene in a complementary fashion to facilitate cell division, thus p53 is a nuclear regulatory protein. The most common genetic alteration seen in human cancers involves spontaneous mutations in the *p53* TSG cell cycle inhibitor.[4] Approximately 70% of colon cancers, 30% to 50% of breast cancers, 50% of lung cancers, and nearly 100% of small cell carcinomas of the lung have been shown to include *p53* mutations.[10] Mutations of the *p53* gene have been shown in a number of "hereditary cancers." Sixty-three peptides derived from observed point mutations on *p53* have been shown to induce CD8+ cytotoxic T lymphocyte (CTL) clones.

Ras Oncogenes

Mutations in *ras* oncogenes (Ki-*ras*, N-*ras*, or Ha-*ras*) are frequently found in human malignancies. Approximately 90% of pancreatic carcinomas, 50% of colorectal carcinomas, 25% of acute myelogenous leukemias (AML), but <5% of breast carcinomas show *ras* mutations.[4] *Ras* oncogenes are activated by single amino-acid substitutions in three specific codons; thus, these genetic alterations are well defined. Murine CD8+ CTL clones have been established using *ras* oncogenes. Human CTL clones, responsive to several *ras* oncogenes, have been detected by reacting lymphocytes from healthy donors with mutated peptides derived from *ras* oncogenes.[12]

Bcr/abl Oncogenes

The translocation of the *c-abl* oncogene on chromosome 9 to the *bcr* (breakpoint cluster region) on chromosome 22 produces the Philadelphia chromosome and leads to the production of the fusion gene termed *bcr/abl*. The *bcr/abl* gene is found in >95% of patients with chronic myelogenous leukemia (CML). A smaller proportion of acute lymphoblastic leukemia patients (10% of children and 25% of adults with a poorer prognosis) have a similar, but different, oncogene abnormality in which the *abl* gene is translocated to a different region of the *bcr* gene on the 22nd chromosome.[11] Synthetic peptides corresponding to the *bcr/abl* joining region, when used to immunize mice, have elicited peptide-specific CD8+ CTL clones.

c-Myc Oncogenes

c-*Myc* is strongly associated with lymphocyte activation and the proliferative capacity of cell populations. Deregulation of c-*myc* expression prevents cells from leaving the activation cycle, resulting in a state of continuous replication. c-*Myc* is one of several oncogenes translocated in lymphomas and lymphocytic leukemias.

ONCOFETAL ANTIGENS

Normally silent differentiation antigens that are expressed during malignant transformation are the oncofetal antigens. Examples of oncofetal antigens include α-fetoprotein (AFP), produced by human hepatomas, and carcinoembryonic antigen (CEA), expressed by col-orectal carcinomas. These oncofetal antigens were the first described human tumor-associated antigens, originally thought to be tumor specific. Laboratory quantitation of AFP and CEA is very useful in monitoring cancer patients for the effects of treatment. These antigens are described more fully in the tumor marker section of this chapter.

Natural Immunity to Tumors

Natural immunity is present spontaneously in normal individuals, analogous to the innate immunity of the acute phase response to inflammation. Natural immunity does not depend on previous exposure to tumor cells; its activity can be augmented very rapidly (within hours or a few days) and may be the first line of defense against tumors. Cells that are involved in natural immunity include macrophages, natural killer (NK) cells, killer (K) cells, lymphokine-activated killer (LAK) cells, and tumor-infiltrating lymphocytes (TIL).

MACROPHAGE-MEDIATED CYTOTOXICITY

The tumoricidal function of activated macrophages is macrophage-mediated cytotoxicity.[13] Resting macrophages (not activated) from normal individuals display only minimal levels of tumor cytotoxicity and have characteristic surface markers. Activated macrophages, however, can distinguish between tumor cells and normal cells and can selectively kill tumor cells, leaving normal cells unscathed. Macrophage tumoricidal activity is not dependent on recognition of MHC molecules or other self constituents and occurs independently of genetic factors, including species barriers.

A variety of factors or events activates macrophages, including infections with intracellular organisms, such as *Mycobacteria, Listeria,* and *Toxoplasma.*[14] Endotoxins (lipopolysaccharides), soluble products of bacteria, and the cytokine interferon (IFNγ) also can activate macrophages.[15] Immune complexes and complexes containing C-reactive protein have also been shown to stimulate macrophage-mediated cytotoxicity in vitro.[13]

Destruction of tumor cells by macrophages requires close physical contact between the macrophage and the tumor cell (Fig. 7-1). In vitro studies using labeled lysosomes indicate that the cytotoxic macrophage directly transfers its lysosomal contents to the tumor cell while the membranes of the two cells are fused.[14] Activated macrophages contain increased numbers of lysosomes and secrete copious amounts of the cytokine tumor necrosis factor (TNFα), further described in the cytokine section of this chapter.

One of the primary causes of death from malignancies is metastases (i.e., release of cells from the primary tumor site to initiate growth of a tumor). The metastasized cells have the same surface antigens and other

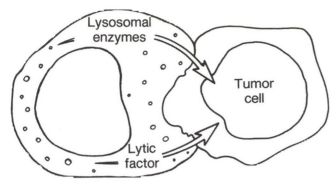

FIGURE 7-1
Macrophage-mediated tumor cytotoxicity.

characteristics that the primary tumor had when they relocate to a previously normal area of the body. The principal sites of metastases are the lymph nodes, lung, and liver. Activated macrophages have been shown in animal studies to be very effective at decreasing the incidence of metastases in several tumor models.[13]

NATURAL KILLER CELLS

Natural killer (NK) cells can recognize and lyse a number of tumor cells and other cell lines in vitro. There is a broad specificity for the NK effector function that may include target cells from the following sources:[16] syngeneic (e.g., identical twins), allogeneic (same animal species, different genetic background), and xenogeneic (different species with different genetic background). NK cells are also called large granular lymphocytes (LGL) because of the azurophilic granules in the cytoplasm and the high cytoplasm/nucleus ratio. NK cells have low-affinity FcγIII receptors, CD16, and NKH-1/Leu19 surface markers. Mice that are congenitally athymic or have been thymectomized as neonates and have no detectable T cells do have functional NK cells.

Similar to activation of macrophages, NK cells can also be activated by the cytokines IFNγ and interleukin-2 (IL-2), which are further described later in this chapter. In contrast to T cells and B cells, activation of NK cells does not induce immunologic memory. There is no primary or secondary response detectable for NK cells. Instead, activation and proliferation appear to be triggered by IL-1 during the acute inflammatory process. NK cells are also subject to suppression by certain factors known to be produced by tumor cells as well as by macrophages (e.g., prostaglandin E_2). NK activity changes with age, from low levels in the neonates, peaking at puberty, and steadily declining with advancing age. NK effector function appears to play no role in immunity to established solid tumors. The antitumor effects of NK cells are likely to be the first line of defense against developing tumors and metastases.

The sensitivity of tumor cells to NK cells in vitro is inversely proportional to the level of MHC Class I antigens expressed on the surface of the tumor cells. Thus it is postulated that MHC Class I expression can lead to escape from NK recognition in vivo.[4] The "missing self" hypothesis[18] states that NK cells constantly survey their environment for MHC Class I expression. Cells that have lost MHC will be recognized as targets and killed. One possible mechanism is that MHC molecules inhibit the lytic action of NK cells that have bound to target cells.

The lytic action of NK cells involves a complex sequence of events leading to the destruction of target cells and can be divided into at least four distinct stages,[17] as illustrated in Figure 7-2. The stages of NK effector function include: (1) target cell binding when physical contact is made between effector cells and target cells; (2) programming for lysis, during which the effector cell cytoskeletal components and Golgi apparatus move within the cytoplasm to the area of the ef-

Steps in NK cytotoxicity

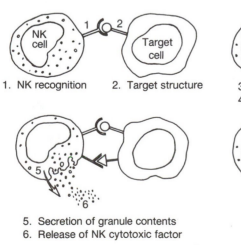

1. NK recognition
2. Target structure

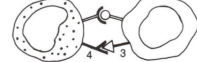

3. Stimulating target cell structure
4. Receptor for activation of NK effector

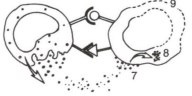

5. Secretion of granule contents
6. Release of NK cytotoxic factor

7. NKCF binding site
8. NKCF induced polymerization of PFP
9. Pore formation → lysis → killing

FIGURE 7-2
Stages of natural killer effector functions.

fector cell that has physical contact with the target cell; (3) secretion of factors such as NK cell cytotoxic factor (NKCF), granule cytolysin, and IL-1 by the NK cell; and (4) the cell-independent phase of the lytic event, where the NK cells are no longer needed because soluble factors complete the killing process.

Lymphokine-activated killer (LAK) cells, which specifically respond to IL-2, appear to have many of the same cell surface antigens as NK cells and may be unstimulated NK cells.[19] Like NK cells, LAK cells are LGLs that do not express the T-cell CD3 receptor. The LAK activity reflects the potent ability of IL-2 both to stimulate cytotoxic activity and to expand the population(s) of natural effector cells.

NONIMMUNOLOGIC CHANGES TO THE ENVIRONMENT

The process of tumor development and spread takes place in several steps: (1) transformation from normal/benign to malignant cells; (2) exponential, unrestricted growth of the malignant cells; (3) angiogenesis (development of blood vessels and blood supply to the tumor); (4) invasion by the tumor cells into the surrounding tissues; (5) intravasation/release of individual tumor cells into the blood and lymphatic system; (6) survival of individual tumor cells in the peripheral circulation; (7) arrest of the individual tumor cells in extraenvironmental locations (sites of metastasis such as the lung or the liver); (8) extravasation/invasion of these other environments by tumor cells (metastasis); and (9) growth/angiogenesis of the tumor at the sites of metastasis.[20] During each phase, non-immunologic mechanisms as well as immunologic mechanisms can influence the progression of the malignancy. Many of the interactions between cells are dependent upon integrins, a class of molecules that enables cells to adhere to other cells.[21] Proteolysis of tissue barriers is an essential mechanism of tumor cell invasion and metastasis. Enzymes such as metalloproteinases,[22] produced by tumor cells, degrade collagens and proteoglycans, thereby permitting tumor invasion.

T-Cell–Mediated Immunity to Tumors

T-cell-mediated immunity to tumor antigens is analogous to the body's response to other T-dependent antigens, such as transplantation antigens. In in-vitro experiments, tumor antigens provoke the proliferation of T cells of all subpopulations (helper, suppressor, and cytotoxic). The amplification of effector functions (Fig. 7-3) of these T lymphocytes requires the production and release of antigen-nonspecific, low-molecular weight, mediator molecules called cytokines. Cytokines are secreted by activated T cells (lymphokines) and macrophages (monokines).

CYTOKINES INVOLVED IN TUMOR IMMUNITY

Interleukin-1 (IL-1) and tumor necrosis factor (TNFα) are distinct cytokines that are secreted by APCs. IL-1 promotes the proliferation and activation of T cells, B cells, and NK cells. IL-1 is the endogenous pyrogen that elicits the fever response to inflammation.[23] TNFα has similar effects as IL-1, but also functions as a cytotoxin to cause necrosis of the tumor cells.[24] IL-2 is secreted by activated CD4+ T cells and NK cells, and stimulates the proliferation and further activation of T cells and NK cells, enhancing the cytotoxic activity of both cell types.

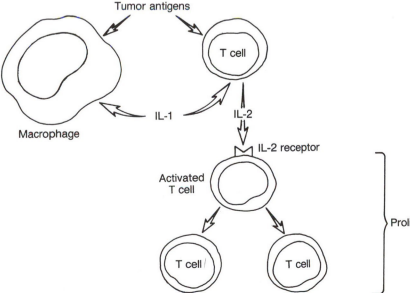

FIGURE 7-3
Amplification of effector functions of T cells.

Interferon (IFN-γ) is produced by activated CD4+ T cells and NK cells, and serves to activate macrophages and augment the cytocidal activities of NK cells. IL-6 is secreted by activated CD4+ T cells and APCs, and acts in synergy with IL-1 and TNF to stimulate T cells. IL-6, the production of which is stimulated by IL-1, is the primary cytokine that stimulates the acute phase response of the liver.[24]

Cytokines secreted by tumor cells that have immunosuppressive activity include transforming growth factor (TGFβ) and IL-10. TGFβ inhibits the activity of other cytokines, including IL-2, IL-4, IFNγ, and TNFα. TGFβ also blocks NK cytolytic activity, downregulates IL-2 receptor and MHC expression, and inhibits the proliferation of T cells, B cells, LAK, and CTL.[25] IL-10 blocks the proliferation of NK cells and inhibits the synthesis of cytokines by macrophages. IL-10 has been found in the supernatant of several human cancer cell lines,[26] as well as in the peritoneal fluid and serum of patients with ovarian cancer and other intraperitoneal cancers.[27]

CYTOTOXIC T-LYMPHOCYTE INVOLVEMENT IN TUMOR IMMUNITY

Cytotoxic T lymphocytes (CTL) have the capacity to directly lyse tumor cells that bear antigens to which these immune T cells have been previously exposed (also referred to as "primed"). The first step in the CTL response is recognition of the tumor antigens by cell surface interactions. The primary pathway of interactions between CTL and tumor cells involves the recognition of MHC Class II antigens, thereby identifying those tumor antigens or peptides as self through an interaction with the CD3 T-cell receptor (Fig. 7-4).

The second step in the T-cell–mediated response to tumors is specific proliferation of the previously activated (primed) CTL. Concomitant with this clonal proliferation is the production of cytokines. Simultaneously, the CTL seek out the tumor cells expressing the tumor-specific antigen/peptide and MHC, effecting lysis of the tumor cells.

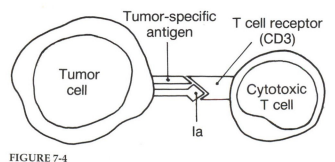

FIGURE 7-4
MHC involvement in recognition of tumor antigens as self.

Summary

The immune reaction against tumor cells is a two-step reaction: First, nonspecific effector cells, such as macrophages, eosinophils, neutrophils, and NK cells, are recruited into the environment and a local inflammatory reaction occurs. This nonspecific reaction facilitates the secondary, specific immune reaction by slowing the growth of the tumor and enhancing the level of tumor antigen presentation by the tumor through modulation of MHC molecule expression. In the secondary phase, CD8+ tumor-specific T cells arise, providing immune protection against the tumor growth.[4]

TUMOR MARKERS

α-Fetoprotein (AFP) and carcinoembryonic antigen (CEA) were the first tumor-associated antigens that, when quantitated in human serum, were useful to detect cancer and monitor therapy. Monoclonal antibodies specific for tumor markers have allowed additional tumor markers to be characterized. Tumor markers are rarely useful in detecting or diagnosing cancer because most tumor markers have also been found in benign conditions, but many tumor markers have a definite role in confirming diagnoses, detecting the recurrence of the cancer, monitoring responses to therapy, and estimating prognosis.[28] Useful tumor markers fall into four broad categories: glycoproteins, mucinous glycoproteins, hormones, and molecules of the immune system.

Glycoproteins

Glycoprotein tumor markers are derived from fetal or placental tissue and are found in small amounts in normal adult tissue; thus, they are not tumor specific. Although originally thought to be organ specific, most glycoprotein tumor markers have subsequently been found in more than one organ. Most glycoprotein tumor markers contain <20% carbohydrate (CEA is the exception, with 60%), contain N-linked glycosyl residues without repeating units, and express their antigenic determinants on polypeptide chains. Glycoprotein tumor markers include CEA, AFP, human chorionic gonadotropin (βHCG), and prostate-specific antigen (PSA).

CARCINOEMBRYONIC ANTIGEN

CEA was first identified in 1965 in extracts from human colon carcinoma and fetal colon cells. CEA is present in low levels on normal colon mucosa, lung, and breast tissue, and is found in serum in association with several malignancies. There is considerable heterogeneity of purified CEA attributed to varying amounts of sialic acid (n-acetyl neuraminic acid). CEA molecules are involved in cell recognition and intercellular adhesion, and may have a role in tumor metastasis.[28]

CEA is widely used in the management of gastrointestinal tumors, particularly colon cancer. CEA is normally synthesized and secreted by cells lining the gastrointestinal (GI) tract. In normal situations CEA is eliminated through the bowel. CEA can be found in the circulation in disorders of the GI tract where there has been damage to the mucosal surface that allows CEA into the blood stream. Such GI disturbances include inflammatory bowel disease, ulcerative colitis, Crohn's disease, multiple polyps, and tumors of the GI tract. Certain types of tumors have been shown to secrete CEA, including adenocarcinoma of the colon, pancreas, liver, and lung, especially when there is metastasis to the liver. In fact, the highest CEA levels are found in metastatic disease. CEA is elevated in 40% to 70% of patients with colon cancer. When present, CEA correlates with tumor histology and pathologic stage. Very high preoperative levels are prognostic for high recurrence rates and decreased survival. If the tumor is a CEA-secreting tumor, CEA can be used to monitor the effectiveness of surgical removal of the tumor as well as to monitor for recurrence of disease.[29]

Preoperative CEA levels are not useful in other cancers where CEA can be found, that is, breast, lung, and gastric cancers. Elevated postoperative CEA levels in other cancers, however, indicate recurrent or metastatic disease. CEA can be used to monitor for bone metastasis in breast cancer patients. CEA is not recommended for use as a screening test for cancer because of the incidence of CEA elevations in other inflammatory diseases.

α-FETOPROTEIN

AFP is a major plasma glycoprotein of the early human fetus, synthesized by the fetal liver, with levels peaking at 14 weeks gestation and falling to adult normal levels by 6 to 10 months of age. AFP is found in high concentrations in fetal serum, maternal serum, and serum of adults with hepatomas (liver cancer) and testicular teratoblastomas.[5] Not all hepatomas or teratoblastomas produce AFP, but those that do synthesize this glycoprotein do so in very large amounts. Elevated levels of AFP are not always associated with malignancy. AFP can be elevated in inflammatory diseases of the liver, such as viral hepatitis, chronic hepatitis, and cirrhosis. High levels of AFP can also occur in inflammatory diseases of the bowel, such as Crohn's disease and ulcerative colitis, that produce elevated levels of CEA as well. AFP is useful as a screening test for liver cancer only in patient groups at risk for developing hepatoma (Chinese, Japanese, and Alaskan Eskimos) but is not useful in most patient populations because of the significant elevations in benign conditions.

Measuring AFP levels is useful in obstetrics, where high levels are found in amniotic fluid associated with neural tube defects. Maternal serum can be screened for elevated levels of AFP in patients who are at higher risk for having a baby with certain forms of nephrosis or with neural tube defects, such as spina bifida.

β-HUMAN CHORIONIC GONADOTROPIN

βHCG is secreted by syncytiotrophoblasts of the placenta. The α-chain of HCG shares sequence homology with luteinizing hormone (LH), follicle-stimulating hormone (FSH), and thyroid-stimulating hormone (TSH). The non-covalently associated β-chain is unique for each molecule, confers the biological specificity, and contains the immunologically defined specificity. βHCG is normally found in serum and urine only during pregnancy but is found in 10% of patients with benign inflammatory bowel disease, duodenal ulcers, and cirrhosis. βHCG is also found in nearly 100% of trophoblastic tumors and in 10% to 40% of non–germ cell tumors, such as carcinoma of the lung, breast, gastrointestinal tract, and ovary. In patients with trophoblastic (germ cell) tumors (seminoma, teratoma, choriocarcinoma), βHCG is clinically very useful in diagnosis, correlating with the response to therapy, monitoring for metastasis, and predicting treatment failure or relapse.

βHCG, when used in combination with AFP, is particularly useful in seminomatous tumors. Increased βHCG indicates probable nonseminomatous elements and/or metastatic disease, while increased AFP signals the presence of yolk sac elements. The detection of AFP and/or βHCG correlates with the stage of nonseminomatous tumors.

SQUAMOUS CELL CARCINOMA ANTIGEN

Squamous cell carcinoma antigen (SCC-A) is a subfraction of tumor antigen 4 (TA-4), elevated in squamous cell carcinoma of the uterus, endometrium, and other genital tract carcinomas. TA-4 and SCC-A are also elevated in squamous cell tumors of the head/neck, lung, and cervix. SCC-A is useful for monitoring the effects of therapy in those squamous cell tumors but is not useful for diagnosis.[30]

PROSTATE-SPECIFIC ANTIGEN

Prostate-specific antigen (PSA) is a glycoprotein with proteolytic enzyme activity that dissolves seminal gel formed after ejaculation. PSA is found in normal, benign, and malignant prostatic tissue and seminal fluid. It is produced in the cytoplasm of prostatic acinar cells and ductal epithelium.[31] Other tissues of urogenital origin contain immunochemically detectable PSA.[32] In serum, PSA is bound to α-1 antichymotrypsin (ACT), which may influence the measurement of PSA in serum. Different vendors' PSA assays contain different molar proportions of PSA-ACT,[33] and antibody can detect PSA-ACT differently than free PSA. PSA is elevated in prostate cancer, the most common cancer in men over the age of 75. Elevated PSA levels are also found in benign prostatic hypertrophy and acute or chronic prostatitis. PSA levels correlate directly with prostate volume, with the stage of prostate cancer, and with the response to therapy.[30] PSA is not present in healthy men or women, and is not found in association with any form of cancer in women or in men other than prostate carcinoma. PSA assay is recommended to diagnose prostate cancer in conjunction with the digital rectal exam (DRE).[34]

Mucinous Glycoproteins

Mucinous glycoproteins are high molecular weight cell surface antigens with a polypeptide backbone attached to oligosaccharides by O-glycosidic linkages. They are 60% to 80% carbohydrate and are structurally similar to the Lewis blood group antigens A and B (Fig. 7-5).[35] Mucinous glycoprotein epitopes are expressed on epithelial surfaces and may be detected in serum, saliva, and other fluids, or adsorbed onto erythrocytes. CA 15-3, CA 19-9, and CA 125 epitopes are detected by bimonoclonal immunoassays in which one monoclonal antibody (MAb) captures the antigen and a second MAb detects the bound antigen by binding to the molecule at a different site from the capturing MAb. These cancer-associated antigens (CA) were defined by MAb from a particular vendor.

CA 15-3

CA 15-3 is expressed during mammary differentiation and detected on lactating mammary cells, lung epithelium, and carcinoma of the breast, ovary, pancreas, stomach, and liver. Low levels can be detected in nonmalignant conditions, such as chronic hepatitis, cirrhosis, sarcoidosis, tuberculosis, and systemic lupus erythematosus. High levels of CA 15-3 are found in epithelial malignancies, such as ovarian, lung, and liver carcinoma.[30] CA 15-3 levels provide no diagnostic discrimination and questionable prognostic ability. Levels of CA 15-3 are highest if bone or liver metastasis are present and decrease in response to chemotherapy. Serial measurements of CA 15-3 predicted relapses of breast cancer before clinical evidence of recurrence.[36] Recently another MAb (B27.29) from another vendor has been shown to be equivalent to CA 15-3. This B27.29 reagent has been more widely available to instrument manufacturers for assay development, thereby making the assay more accessible to the clinical laboratory.

CA 19-9

CA 19-9 is a very large mucinous glycoprotein, identical to sialated Lewis A antigen. The expression of CA 19-9 depends on Lewis antigen expression, except in pancreatic cancer.[37] CA 19-9 is found in acute and chronic pancreatitis, benign liver disease, and pancreatic cancer. CA 19-9 levels > 70 U/mL are the best serologic test for detecting pancreatic carcinoma. CA 19-9 decreases after curative resection and predicts recurrence 3 to 9 months before clinical symptoms.

CA-125

CA 125, a large mucinous glycoprotein with a low carbohydrate content, is expressed on embryonal urogen-

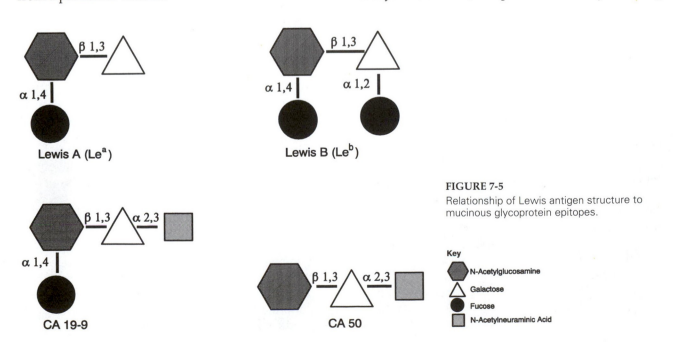

FIGURE 7-5
Relationship of Lewis antigen structure to mucinous glycoprotein epitopes.

ital epithelium, and is found in several nonmalignant diseases. CA 125 is most useful in detecting ovarian carcinoma in postmenopausal women, but has no diagnostic discrimination in premenopausal women.[38] CA 125 is, however, very useful in monitoring women of all ages during treatment for ovarian cancer.

Hormones Useful as Tumor Markers

CALCITONIN

Calcitonin, a peptide hormone produced by C cells of the thyroid, has a role in calcium regulation. Calcitonin is elevated in several nonmalignant diseases (hyperparathyroidism, Paget's disease, pernicious anemia) and pregnancy. Calcitonin is also elevated in certain malignancies (breast cancer, hepatoma, hypernephroma, and lung cancer) but is markedly elevated in medullary carcinoma of the thyroid (MCT).[30] As a tumor marker for MCT, calcitonin correlates with the extent of the disease, is useful for monitoring therapy, and is recommended as a screening assay for families with autosomal dominant transmission of MCT.

THYROGLOBULIN

Thyroglobulin is a glycoprotein produced by thyroid follicular cells, and is required for proteolysis and release of T3 and T4 into circulation. Thyroglobulin is elevated in nearly all thyroid disorders and is thus useless for discriminating benign from malignant diseases. It is useful as a tumor marker, however, after total thyroidectomy or radioiodine ablative therapy, when thyroglobulin levels can predict metastasis of thyroid cancer.[30]

CATECHOLAMINE

The catecholamine metabolites, vanillylmandelic acid (VMA) and homovanillic acid (HVA), are excreted into urine in pheochromocytoma and neuroblastoma. Pretreatment levels correlate with disease and serial determinations are useful in monitoring therapy.

Molecules of the Immune System as Tumor Markers

MONOCLONAL IMMUNOGLOBULINS (M PROTEINS)

Monoclonal immunoglobulins (M proteins) were the first known tumor markers. They are identified by serum or urine protein electrophoresis and are characterized by serum or urine immunofixation as IgG, IgA, IgM, IgD, IgE, or kappa or lambda free light chains. Ap-

proximately 1% of adults have M proteins, 25% of which are of undetermined significance.[39] Half of the M proteins identified will be diagnostic of multiple myeloma, a plasma cell malignancy of the bone marrow. Approximately 4% of patients with monoclonal immunoglobulins will be diagnosed with Waldenstrom's macroglobulinemia, a malignancy of activated B lymphocytes that secrete massive quantities of IgM. About 15% of patients with M proteins will have associated B-cell lymphoproliferative malignancies (chronic lymphocytic leukemia or lymphoma).

The detection of M proteins by serum protein electrophoresis (SPE) is not useful for screening for myeloma but is very useful for monitoring response to therapy in myeloma and macroglobulinemia. Detection and characterization of the Ig type by immunofixation is essential for diagnosis and prognosis. Patients with IgA myeloma have significantly shorter survival times, shorter durations, and more significant complications of their diseases than do patients with IgG myeloma or light chain disease. Monitoring response to therapy is best done using the SPE, integrating, serially following, and reporting the M-protein concentration. Monitoring M-protein levels by SPE is better than monitoring by nephelometry because M proteins frequently have altered antigenic components and do not react equally with antisera produced for quantitating polyclonal Igs.

β-2 MICROGLOBULIN

β-2 Microglobulin (β-2M) is found on the membrane surface of nearly all nucleated cells and is released into circulation during membrane turnover. β-2M is useful in predicting treatment failures and poor survival in patients with lymphoma.

THERAPEUTIC APPROACHES TO CANCER

There are basically four general approaches to cancer therapy: surgery, radiotherapy, chemotherapy, and immunotherapy. In many situations a combination of therapeutic approaches is necessary to eliminate or limit the tumor burden.

Surgery

Surgery is the first therapeutic modality to decrease the solid tumor burden in early stages of breast cancer, colon cancer, lung cancer, and prostate cancer—the four major cancers in humans, representing more than 50% of solid tumors.[40] In these and other types of cancers, the tumor may grow in an unnoticed "parasitic-type" of relationship with the host until it restricts a necessary function of the body and signals its presence. By then it may be necessary to remove the tumor surgically to prevent loss of function of a body part.

Radiotherapy

Radiotherapy can either be a primary therapy or an adjuvant (supplementary) therapy. Primary radiotherapy is most useful in cancers of the head and neck, and in Hodgkin's disease (HD). In HD the radiotherapy is targeted to affected lymph nodes in various portions of the body. Radiotherapy is less disfiguring and more efficacious for soft tissue tumors in areas adjacent to the jaw and nasal passages. In many other solid tumors, radiotherapy to draining lymph nodes after surgical excision of the primary tumor has been found to increase the 5-year survival rate.[41] The ultimate in radiotherapy, however, is whole body radiation, which is used prior to bone marrow transplantation as an effective treatment for certain types of acute leukemias that are refractory to chemotherapy and other solid tumors (e.g., breast cancer) that have recurred after several years of remission.

Chemotherapy

Chemotherapy generally consists of treatment with drugs that are antimetabolites (i.e., interfere with nucleic acid or protein synthesis). The approach to chemotherapy is to treat with as much of a single drug or combination of drugs as a person can tolerate. The rationale of chemotherapy is to kill the tumor cells, which are growing faster than normal cells.[42] The general approach is to give chemotherapy in "courses," allowing time for the normal body cells to recover before subsequent courses are administered. Leukemias are most effectively treated with chemotherapy. Acute leukemias of childhood are quite responsive to appropriate regimens of chemotherapy that are administered according to the cellular classification of the leukemia. Chemotherapy is also administered as adjuvant therapy to either surgery or radiotherapy in the treatment of solid tumors.

Most therapeutic regimens have been arrived at by trial and error of various combinations of drugs or therapies. Large study groups (oncology groups) have been formed, with regional institutions cooperating by submitting data.[43] The study groups can then generate a statistical approach to each combination. The cancer is "staged" prior to any therapy; that is, the extent of disease is ascertained by extensive evaluations that are consistently applied between institutions. Clinical trials are performed, randomly giving patients treatment A or treatment B. Within 2 years it is usually possible to determine which treatment is better. The statistically significantly "better" treatment is then later compared with treatment C and the process is repeated.

Immunoprophylaxis

Immunoprophylaxis with vaccines to certain viruses has been a successful therapeutic approach in animals.[44] Marek's disease, caused by a herpes virus, is a lymphoproliferative disease in chickens for which a vaccine has been highly successful. The incidence of feline leukemia has also been significantly decreased as a result of a vaccination program for cats. To date no vaccine is available to protect against any human tumors.

Immunotherapy

Immunotherapy of cancer attempts to destroy tumor cells using manipulations of the immune system to overcome the poor immune responses elicited by tumors. Several methods have been used to increase MHC expression on tumor cells, including chemical coupling, enzyme treatment, infection of tumor cell lines with vaccinia virus, and introduction of IFN-γ and other cytokine genes into tumor cells to upregulate the expression of self MHC molecules.[4] In murine tumor models, it is now generally accepted that defects in immune regulation, not the absence of tumor antigens, result in failure to mount an antitumor immune response. Investigators are now striving to modify the local tumor cell immunological environment to either enhance the presentation of tumor-specific antigens or to activate tumor-specific lymphocytes.[4]

Monoclonal antibodies (MAbs) to certain tumor antigens have been used to enhance the detection of metastatic lesions, facilitating their destruction by directed chemotherapy or radiotherapy. Radioimmunoguided surgery (RIGS) uses a gamma-detecting probe during second-look laparotomy to detect radiolabeled MAbs that bind to recurrent tumors.[45] Another method targets radiolabeled MAb to micrometastases of cancer patients.[46]

In Vitro Stimulation

In vitro stimulation of the patient's lymphocytes, NK cells, or macrophages has been developed as an alternative approach to chemotherapy. Rosenberg et al.[47] have shown limited success with systemic administration of autologous LAK cells plus recombinant IL-2 in achieving tumor regression in certain cancer patients. The toxic effects of this type of immunotherapy, however, may preclude its use in all but the most resistant forms of cancer that do not respond to conventional therapies.

Molecular Biology

Molecular biologic approaches to cancer will supplant tumor immunology in the future. The approach to cancer therapy is changing, largely as a result of the discovery of oncogenes. Several oncogenes found in various tumors were described previously. The oncogenic proteins appear to act on normal cells at different stages of differentiation, "freezing" their development to one specific stage. The protein products of oncogenes are helpful in identifying the stage at which differentiation of the abnormal cells was arrested. The therapy can then be specifically directed toward known susceptibilities of cells at that single stage of differentiation. As other protein products of oncogenes are identified and characterized, more rational approaches to cancer therapy can be developed.

Review Questions

1. Tumor-specific peptides are

    a. products of viral-induced tumors
    b. a degradation product of antigen processing by macrophages
    c. genome-encoded tumor antigens found in association with leukemias
    d. not associated with MHC products

2. Which of the following is an example of a tumor suppressor gene product?

    a. *p53* cell cycle inhibitor
    b. *bcr/abl* chromosomal translocation
    c. *ras* oncogenes
    d. c-*myc* deregulation

3. Natural killer (NK) cells have which of the following surface markers?

    a. FcγIII receptors
    b. CD3
    c. CD4
    d. C3b receptors

4. Which of the following cytokines are secreted by tumor cells?

    a. IFNγ
    b. TNFα
    c. IL-2
    d. IL-10

5. Which of the following tumor markers can be used to diagnose cancer?

    a. CEA
    b. PSA
    c. CA 19-9
    d. CA 125

6. Approximately half of adults with monoclonal immunoglobulin have which disease?

    a. myeloma
    b. macroglobulinemia
    c. lymphoma
    d. chronic lymphocytic leukemia

References

1. Willis RA: The Spread of Tumors in the Human Body. London, Butterworth, 1952
2. Robbins SL: Pathologic Basis of Disease, p 106. Philadelphia, WB Saunders, 1974
3. Prehn RT, Main JM: Immunity of methylcholanthrene induced sarcomas. J Natl Cancer Inst 18:69, 1957
4. Roth C, Rochlitz C, Kourilsky P: Immune response against tumors. Adv Immun 57:281, 1994
5. Babbit BP, Allen PM, Matsueda G, et al: Binding of immunogenic peptides to Ia histocompatibility molecules. Nature (London) 317:359, 1985
6. Kourilsky P, Jaulin C, Ley V: The structure and function of MHC molecules: Possible implication for the control of tumor growth by MHC-restricted T cells. Cancer Biol 2:275, 1991
7. Klein G: Immunovirology of transforming viruses. Curr Opinion Immunol 3:665, 1991
8. Gavioli R, Kurilla MG, DeCampos-Lima PO, et al: Multiple HLA-A11 restricted CTL epitopes of different immunogenicity in the Epstein-Barr virus (EBV) encoded nuclear antigen-4 (EBNA4). J Virol 67:1572, 1993
9. Fearon ER, Vogelstein B: A genetic model for colorectal tumorigenesis. Cell 61:767, 1990
10. Hollstein M, Sidransky D, Vogelstein B, Harris C: p53 mutations in human cancer. Science 253:49, 1991
11. Maurer J, Jannsen JW, Thiel E, et al: Detection of chimeric bcr-abl genes in acute lymphoblastic leukemia by the polymerase chain reaction. Lancet 337:1055, 1991
12. Jung S, Schluesener HJ: Human T lymphocytes recognize a peptide of single point-mutated oncogenic ras proteins. J Exp Med 173:273, 1991
13. Deodhar SD, Barna BP: Macrophage activation: Potential for cancer therapy. Clev Clin J Med 53:223, 1986
14. Adams DO, Nathan CF: Molecular mechanisms in tumor cell killing by activated macrophages. Immunol Today 4:166, 1983
15. Taramelli D, Holden HT, Varesio L: Endotoxin requirement for macrophage activation by lymphokines in a rapid microcytotoxicity assay. J Immunol Methods 37:225, 1980
16. Hersey P, Bolhius R: "Nonspecific" MHC-unrestricted killer cells and their receptors. Immunol Today 8:233, 1987
17. Wright S, Bonavida B: Studies on the mechanisms of natural killer cell cytotoxicity. III. Activation of NK cells by interferon augments the lytic activity of released natural killer cytotoxic factors (NKCF). J Immunol 130:2960, 1984
18. Ljunggren N, Karre K: In search of the "missing self": MHC molecules and NK recognition. Immunol Today 11:237, 1990

19. Herberman RB, Balch C, Golub S, et al: Lymphokine-activated killer cell activity: Characteristics of effector cells and their progenitors in blood and spleen. Immunol Today 8:178, 1987

20. Hart IR, Saini A: Biology of tumor metastasis. Lancet 339:1453, 1992

21. Hynes RO: Integrins: Versatility, modulation, and signaling in cell adhesion. Cell 69:11, 1992

22. Liotta LA, Steeg PS, Stetler-Stevenson WG: Cancer metastasis and angiogenesis: An imbalance of positive and negative regulation. Cell 64:327, 1991

23. Oppenheim JJ, Kovacs EJ, Matsushima K, et al: There is more than one interleukin 1. Immunol Today 7:45, 1986

24. Oppenheim JJ, Ruscetti FW, Faltynek CV: Cytokines. In Stites DP, Terr AI, Parslow TG (eds): Basic and Clinical Immunology, pp. 107–110. Los Altos, CA, Lange Medical, 1994

25. Sulitzeanu D: Immunosuppressive factors in human cancer. Adv Cancer Res 60:247, 1993

26. Gastl GA, Abrams JS, Nanus DM, et al: Interleukin-10 production by human carcinoma cell lines and its relationship to interleukin-6 expression. Int J Cancer 55:96, 1993

27. Gotlieb WH, Abrams JS, Watson JM, et al: Presence of interleukin 10 (IL-10) in the ascites of patients with ovarian and other intra-abdominal cancers. Cytokine 4:385, 1992

28. Seleznick MJ: Tumor markers. Primary Care 19:715, 1992

29. Martin EW, James KK, Minton JP: The use of CEA as an early indicator for gastrointestinal tumor recurrence and second-look procedures. Cancer 29:440, 1977

30. Jacobs EL, Haskell CM: Clinical use of tumor markers in oncology. Curr Probl Cancer Nov/Dec:301, 1991

31. Wang MC, Papsidero LD, Kuriyama M, et al: Prostatic antigen: A new potential marker for prostatic cancer. Prostate 2:89, 1981

32. Frazier HA, Humphrey PA, Burchette JL, Paulson DF: Immunoreactive prostatic specific antigen in male periurethral glands. J Urol 147:246, 1992

33. Graves HCB: Standardization of immunoassays for prostate-specific antigen. Cancer 72:3141, 1993

34. Gerber GS, Goldberg R, Chodak GW: Local staging of prostate cancer by tumor volume, prostate-specific antigen, and transrectal ultrasound. Urology 40:311, 1992

35. Virji MA, Mercer DW, Herberman R: New immunologic markers for monitoring of cancer. Ann Chir Gynaecol 78:13, 1989

36. Colomer R, Ruibal A, Genolla J, et al: Circulating CA 15-3 levels in postsurgical follow-up of breast cancer patients and in non-malignant diseases. Br Cancer Res Treat 13:123, 1989

37. Masson P, Palsson B, Andre-Sandberg A: Cancer-associated tumor markers CA 19-9 and CA-50 in patients with pancreatic cancer with special reference to the Lewis blood cell status. Br J Cancer 62:118, 1990

38. Malkasian GD, Knapp RC, Lavin PT, et al: Preoperative evaluation of serum CA 125 levels in premenopausal and postmenopausal patients with pelvic masses: Discrimination of benign from malignant disease. Am J Obstet Gynecol 159:341, 1988

39. Ameis A, Ko HS, Pruzanski W: M components: A review of 1242 cases. Can Med Assoc J 114:889, 1976

40. Silverberg E, Lubera J: Cancer statistics, 1987. CA Cancer J Clin 37:2, 1987

41. Harris JR, Hellman S, Kinne DW: Limited surgery and radiotherapy for breast cancer. CA Cancer J Clin 36:120, 1986

42. Krakoff IH: Cancer chemotherapeutic agents. CA Cancer J Clin 37:92, 1987

43. Bennett JM: Basic concepts in investigational therapeutics. In Rubin P (ed): Clinical Oncology, p 96. Rochester, NY, American Cancer Society, 1978

44. Jarrett W, Mackey L, Jarrett O, et al: Antibody response and virus survival in cats vaccinated against malignant lymphoma. Nature 253:71, 1975

45. LaValle GJ, Chevinsky A, Martin EW: Impact of radioimmunoguided surgery. Semin Surg Oncol 7:167, 1991

46. Goldenberg DM, Deland F, Kim E, et al: Use of radiolabeled antibodies to carcinoembryonic antigen for the detection and localization of diverse cancers by external photoscanning. N Engl J Med 198:1384, 1978

47. Rosenberg SA, Lotze MT, Muul LM, et al: Special report: Observations on the systemic administration of autologous lymphokine-activated killer cells and recombinant interleukin-2 to patients with metastatic cancer. N Engl J Med 313:1485, 1985

PART II

Immunologic Techniques

CHAPTER 8

Immunoglobulin Structure and Function

Dorothy J. Fike

Objectives

Upon completion of the chapter, the reader will be able to:

1. Diagram and label the basic unit of an immunoglobulin
2. Define the following terms: Fc component, Fab component, J chain, secretory component, heavy chain, light chain, constant region, variable region, isotype, allotype, and idiotype
3. Discuss the functional and structural differences between immunoglobulin classes
4. Discuss the differences between the subclasses of IgG
5. Describe the detection of the immunoglobulin classes
6. Define monoclonal antibody
7. Discuss the production of monoclonal antibodies
8. Describe the use of monoclonal antibodies in the laboratory
9. Explain the usefulness of quantitating immunoglobulins in body fluids other than serum

GENERAL STRUCTURE OF THE ANTIBODY MOLECULE

Overview

Antibody or immunoglobulin molecules are the major effector of the specific humoral response. All antibodies are proteins composed of amino acids and are divided into five different classes, designated IgG, IgA, IgM, IgD, and IgE. The classes are based on their molecular weight, amino acid sequence, and biological properties. The abbreviation Ig stands for *Immunoglobulin*.

Serum proteins are separated into five regions during electrophoresis; the order of migration from fastest to slowest fractions is albumin followed by the globulins: $\alpha1$, $\alpha2$, β, and γ. Immunoglobulins migrate to the $\alpha2$, β, or γ regions, as shown in Figure 8-1. IgG migrates to the γ region, IgA migrates to both the γ (predominant) and β globulin regions, and IgM migrates to the γ, β (predominant), and $\alpha2$ regions. IgD and IgE both migrate to the β globulin region.[1]

All immunoglobulins have the same basic structure, being composed of four polypeptide chains, two

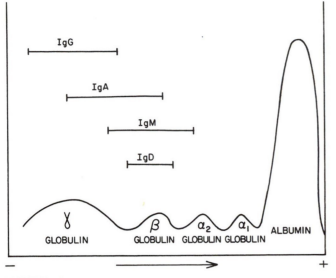

FIGURE 8-1
Serum proteins may be separated based on their electrical charge. Immunoglobulins may migrate to the α2, β, or γ regions.

region, some amino acid locations are more variable than others and are known as hypervariable regions.

Each light chain has one constant domain, and each heavy chain three or four domains. Each domain is coded for by a different exon of the immunoglobulin constant gene and is approximately 110 amino acids in length. The constant domains of the heavy chain are numbered beginning with the domain attached to the variable domain; these constant domains define the biologic function of immunoglobulin class.

The first and second constant domains of the heavy chain define the hinge region. This region allows an immunoglobulin molecule to change its configuration from a free immunoglobulin molecule with a T configuration to a Y configuration when the immunoglobulin binds to the antigen (Fig. 8-4). The Y configuration exposes the complement recognition site on the heavy chain of IgM and IgG; C1q attaches to the recognition site and initiates the classical pathway of complement.

Researchers used enzymes to degrade the immunoglobulin molecule to study the structure and function of specific areas of the immunoglobulin molecule. One enzyme, papain, splits the immunoglobulin molecule in the hinge region adjacent to the disulfide bonds that hold the two heavy chains together (Fig. 8-5 on p. 94).[2] This degradation yields three fragments: two Fab and one Fc. Two identical fragments bind to an epitope and are called Fab, Fragment *antigen binding,* to reflect their biologic function. They consist of an entire light chain attached to the variable domain and part of the constant domains of the heavy chain. The third fragment crystallizes and is called Fc for *Fragment crystallizable.* The Fc fragment is produced by papain cleavage and consists of the remainder of the constant domains of the two heavy chains linked by disulfide bonds. Fc receptors found on cells such as macrophages, B lymphocytes, and T lymphocytes will bind to this region of the immunoglobulin molecule.

heavy and two light, with attached carbohydrate. The amount of carbohydrate varies from 4% to 18% of the total composition of the immunoglobulin molecule (Fig. 8-2). The four chains are usually joined together by disulfide bonds; the number of disulfide bonds between heavy chains varies from 1 to 15. Only one disulfide bond joins a heavy chain to a light chain in most classes and subclasses of immumoglobulins.

Each heavy and light chain is composed of a variable domain and one or more constant domains. The amino acid sequences in the variable domains is diverse compared with the amino acid sequences in the constant domains. The variable domains of an antibody molecule define its unique specificity and dictate the epitope or antigenic determinant to which it can bind (Fig. 8-3). The variable region of the immunoglobulin molecule is encoded by a combination of genes. Within the variable

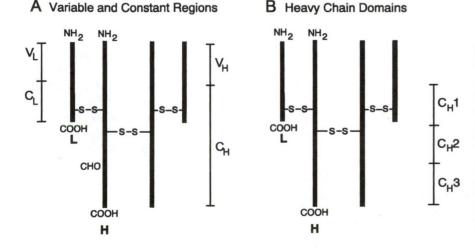

A Variable and Constant Regions

B Heavy Chain Domains

FIGURE 8-2
(**A**) The basic immunoglobulin structure is composed of two heavy and two light protein chains. Each chain has a variable and constant region. There are both intrachain and interchain disulfide bonds. (**B**) The heavy chain is composed of at least three constant domains. The specific number is cited in the text.
Key:
L, Light Chain; H, Heavy Chain; C_H, Constant Region of Heavy Chain; C_L, Constant Region of Light Chain; V_H, Variable Region of Heavy Chain; V_L, Variable Region of Light Chain; -s-s-, Disulfide Bond; CHO, Carbohydrate

Antibody Diversity

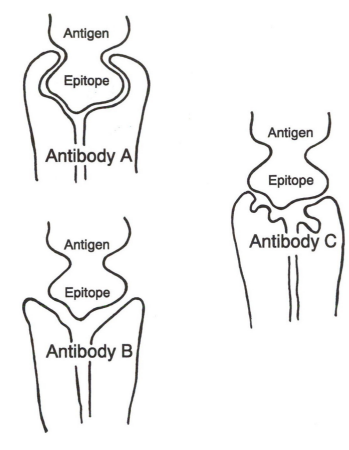

FIGURE 8-3

The variable domain of a heavy chain and of a light chain form the pocket in which the epitope can bind. Antibody A (**A**) is highly complementary for the epitope and binds tightly, as expected. Antibody B (**B**) is less complementary and binds weakly; this could be a cross-reacting antibody. Antibody C (**C**) is physically unable to bind to the epitope.

A second enzyme, pepsin, cleaves the molecule at a different location and yields different fragments. The two Fab fragments generated by papain cleavage are held together by a disulfide bond and are called F(ab')$_2$. The remaining pieces are two heavy-chain fragments, consisting of constant domains that are not joined together.[1,3]

Light Chains

There are two types of light chains, kappa (κ) and lambda (λ). For any immunoglobulin molecule, only one type, κ or λ chain, is present. For example, IgG may be either IgG κ or IgG λ, but it will never be IgG $\kappa\lambda$. Both types of light chains have a molecular weight of approximately 23 kilodaltons (kDa), although each is structurally different. It is interesting to note that both

chains have the amino acid threonine at position 5, glutamine at position 6, and glycine at position 16.[4] Approximately twice as many κ chains as λ chains are produced by most individuals in routine response to natural antigens.[3]

Of the 214 amino acids in the κ chain, the variable domain consists of the first 107 amino acids. There are three hypervariable (HV) regions in the κ chain, amino acid residues from 30 to 35, 50 to 55, and 95 to 100. Three allotypic variants, Km, are found in κ chains of humans; an individual can only have one or two of the Km allotypes. The other 107 amino acids constitute the constant domain.[3]

A Free Immunoglobulin

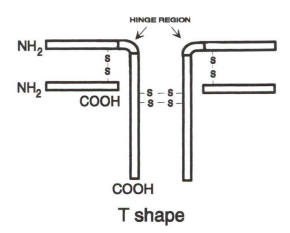

T shape

B Immunoglobulin with Attached Antigen

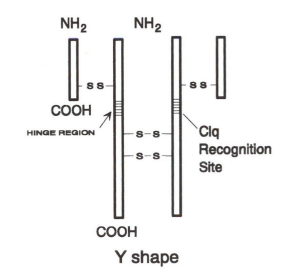

Y shape

FIGURE 8-4

(**A**) When the immunoglobulin is floating unattached to antigen in the plasma, it has a T shape. (**B**) When attached to an antigen, the immunoglobulin changes from the T shape to the Y shape.

A   Papain Cleavage

B   Pepsin Cleavage

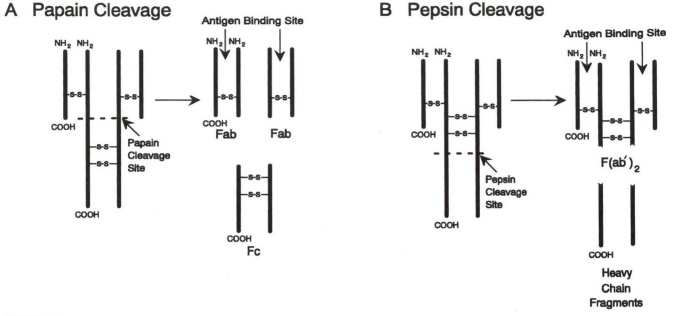

FIGURE 8-5
(**A**) Papain cleaves the immunoglobulin molecule above the interchain disulfide bonds. Two different cleavage products are obtained: Fab, which has the ability to combine with the antigen, and Fc, which is crystallizable. Compared with the Fc, twice as many Fab fragments are formed. (**B**) Pepsin cleaves the immunoglobulin below the interchain disulfide bond. Cleavage products are one F(ab')₂ and two heavy-chain fragments.

The number of amino acids in the λ light chain varies from 213 to 216 amino acids, although these differences are insufficient to be considered allotypic variants. The variable and hypervariable regions of the λ chain occur at approximately the same amino acid positions as the κ chain, depending on the exact number of amino acids in the λ chain.[3] The function of both types and allotypes is the same.[5]

Both the κ and λ chains have the amino acid cysteine in the constant domain that binds to a cysteine molecule on the heavy chain, forming the covalent disulfide bond. The cysteine molecule is the last amino acid of the κ chain and the penultimate (next to the last) amino acid of the λ chain. This disulfide bond creates the union of the heavy and light chains that creates the three-dimensional configuration essential for antibody-antigen interaction.

In some lymphoproliferative diseases, such as multiple myeloma, excess light chains are produced by B cells. These light chains do not polymerize with a heavy chain to form an immunoglobulin molecule; they may be free single light chain or may form light-chain polymers (dimers and trimers) using the cysteine molecule that would normally bind to the heavy chain. A κ chain will associate with a second κ chain, and a λ chain will associate with another λ chain only. Free light chains are secreted into the circulatory system and ultimately are eliminated by the kidney. Free light chains or Bence Jones protein have unique solubility properties because they precipitate at temperatures between 40°C and 60°C, and redissolve at 100°C. This unusual property is the basis of the Bence Jones test.[6]

Heavy Chains

Each class of immunoglobulins has a unique heavy chain that defines it: Gamma (γ) heavy chain is unique to IgG, mu (μ) to IgM, alpha (α) to IgA, delta (δ) to IgD, and epsilon (ε) to IgE. All heavy chains consist of three or four constant domains and one variable domain. Specific characteristics of each heavy chain are discussed later in this chapter.[1]

Antibody Heterogeneity

Immunoglobulin variability may be divided into three different types: isotypes, allotypes, and idiotypes (Table 8-1). Isotypes are the variations between heavy and light chains. These isotypes are the heavy chain classes and subclasses and light chain types. The constant domains of IgM, IgG (all subclasses), IgA, IgD, IgE, κ, and λ define the isotypes. All heavy and light chains are produced by healthy members of a species. Isotypes are species specific. For example, the constant domains of IgM produced by rabbits are different than those of human IgM.[1]

Allotypes are genetic variations in the constant domains of heavy or light chains within a species. The alleles are inherited in a simple Mendelian pattern and are codominant. There are three allotypic markers for the κ

TABLE 8-1
Antibody Heterogeneity

TYPE	DEFINES
Isotype	Heavy chain classes and subclasses (μ; γ_1, γ_2, γ_3, γ_4; α_1, α_2; δ; ε)
	Light chain types (κ and λ)
	Healthy individuals have all isotypes
Allotype	Allelic variation of a class or light chain type (Gm, Am, and Km variants)
	Healthy individuals may express one or more of these
Idiotype	Variation in the variable region that is unique for each specificity of immunoglobulin

chain (Km allotypes), two for the $\alpha 2$ heavy chain (A2m), and up to 25 for the γ heavy chain (Gm) class or subclass. Healthy individuals may express some allotypes.[1]

Idiotypes are the variation in the variable region of an immunoglobulin molecule. Each immunoglobulin molecule derived from a single clone is thought to express a unique idiotype.[1] A portion of the idiotype may be an antigenic determinant, an idiotope, against which anti-idiotype antibodies are produced. Anti-idiotype antibodies appear to have a role in the regulation of the immune response.[7,8] This response can be amplified or suppressed depending on the conditions. Anti-idiotype antibodies also have a role in some autoimmune diseases, such as myasthenia gravis, Graves' disease, and insulin-resistant diabetes mellitus.

Additional Components of Immunoglobulins

J CHAIN

IgM and IgA may be composed of more than one basic immunoglobulin unit. When multiple units are present, the polymers are held together by the J chain. The J chain is a small glycoprotein with a molecular weight of approximately 15 kDa that migrates electrophoretically to the pre-albumin region. The J chain attaches via a disulfide bond to the carboxyl end of the heavy chains. Only one J chain is required for each IgM or IgA polymer, and is believed to initiate polymerization.[3]

SECRETORY COMPONENT

The secretory component (SC) is a 70 kDa protein found on IgA and some IgM molecules present in external secretions. Secretory IgA or IgM is released from the plasma cells located in mucosal tissue of the respiratory, gastrointestinal, and genitourinary tracts. The immunoglobulin diffuses toward the epithelial surface, where SC on the epithelial surface acts as a receptor for IgA or IgM. The IgA or IgM is pinocytosed by the ep-

ithelial cell and transported across the cytoplasm in endocytic vesicles. The majority of secretory IgA or IgM is released from the epithelial cells into the lumen, where most secretory IgA or IgM is attached to the SC via disulfide bonds. The SC attachment is in the hinge region and other locations in the Fc region.[3] Secretory component facilitates IgA and IgM secretion, and makes the complex resistant to degradation by proteolytic enzymes present in secretions.[9]

IMMUNOGLOBULIN CLASSES

IgG

GENERAL CONSIDERATIONS

The basic four-chain unit of immunoglobulins is the basic structure of IgG. Two γ chains are present in all IgG molecules. Minor variation in the γ chain establishes the four IgG subclasses. Subclasses of immunoglobulins have structural and functional differences. The four subclasses of IgG vary slightly in the amino acid sequence (allotype) and the number of disulfide bonds between heavy chains. Gm allotypes define the variation in the chains in members of the same species. Carbohydrate content of IgG is 2.5% of its total molecular weight (Table 8-2). The IgG molecule has a sedimentation coefficient of 7S and a molecular weight of approximately 150 kDa. When serum is electrophoresed, most of the IgG migrates to the γ globulin region, which appears as a broad band because of the heterogeneity of IgG classes, subclasses, and variable regions. These differences in IgG molecule result in slight differences in charge and, therefore, in electrophoretic mobility. IgG, approximately 75% to 80% of all serum immunoglobulin, has a serum concentration range of 1000 to 1500 mg/dL (10 to 15 g/L) depending on age, sex, and race. This concentration reflects the high rate of synthesis and the long half-life (low catabolic rate) of IgG molecules.

The variable domain of the γ chain is the first 107 amino acids. Three hypervariable regions are located at nearly the same amino acid positions as the hypervariable regions of light chains: 30 to 35, 50 to 55, and 95 to 100. The constant region of the γ chain has three domains, designated CH1, CH2, and CH3, with CH1 adjacent to the variable domain. Each heavy chain domain contains an intrachain disulfide bond, and each constant domain has approximately 40% homology (same amino acid sequence) with the constant domain of the light chains. The hinge region of the chain is generally characterized by two interchain disulfide bonds, linking one heavy and one light chain.[3] The number of interchain disulfide bonds linking the two heavy chains depends on the subclass of IgG. This may vary from 2 to 15.[1]

TABLE 8-2
Properties of Immunoglobulins

PROPERTY	IMMUNOGLOBULIN CLASS				
	IgG	*IgM*	*IgA*	*IgD*	*IgE*
Serum concentration (approximate in mg/dL)	1000–1500	100–125	200–250	3	0.01–0.05
Half-life (days)	21–23	5–6	5–6.5	2–8	1–5
Molecular weight (approximate in kDa)	150	900–1000	150–350	150	150
Molecular formula	$\gamma_2\kappa_2$ or $\gamma_2\lambda_2$	Serum $(\mu_2\kappa_2)_5 \cdot J$ or $(\mu_2\lambda_2)_5 \cdot J$	Serum $\alpha_2\kappa_2$ or $\alpha_2\lambda_2$ Secretory $(\alpha_2\kappa_2)_2 \cdot J \cdot SC$ or $(\alpha_2\lambda_2)_2 \cdot J \cdot SC$	$\delta_2\kappa_2$ or $\delta_2\lambda_2$	$\varepsilon_2\kappa_2$ or $\varepsilon_2\lambda_2$
Valence	2	5	2, 4	2	2
Activation of the classical complement pathway	+	+++	–	–	–
Ability to cross the placenta	+	–	–	–	–
Subclasses	4	–	2	–	–
Alternative complement pathway	+ (IgG4)	–	+	+	–

IgG is the predominant antibody synthesized in the secondary antibody response. IgG is the exclusive antitoxin antibody. Both the intravascular and extravascular pools contain equal amounts of IgG. IgG is the only immunoglobulin class that crosses the placenta in humans. This allows maternal IgG to protect the fetus and newborn. If the mother is re-exposed to a microorganism, pre-existing specific IgG and newly synthesized specific IgG will protect the mother and fetus from infection by the microorganism. Because IgG has a relatively long half-life of 23 days, maternal antibodies present in the newborn at birth will continue to provide protection until the antibody is completely catabolized. Thus, maternal antibody provides the newborn with some protection for the first few months of life. Most IgG activates the classical pathway of complement. The C1q recognition unit attaches to the receptor in the hinge region, and when attached to two or more IgG molecules, the pathway is activated.

IgG SUBCLASSES

Slight variations in the amino acid sequence, the number of interchain disulfide bonds, and some biologic function were observed in IgG. These variations were insufficient to justify new immunoglobulin classes, so subclasses were defined. Properties of IgG subclasses are listed in Table 8-3.[10] IgG1 is found in the greatest serum concentration, approximately 900 mg/dL (9 g/L) of the total IgG. IgG2 has the next highest serum concentration of 300 mg/dL (3 g/L). IgG3 has a concentration of 100 mg/dL (1 g/L), and IgG4 has the least serum concentration with approximately 50 mg/dL (0.5 g/L). The molecular weight, number of interchain disulfide bonds, and electrophoretic mobility also show variability. IgG1, IgG2, and IgG4 have a molecular weight of approximately 146 kDa, but IgG3 has a molecular weight of 170 kDa because of the IgG3 heavy chain molecular weight of 60 kDa as compared with 52 kDa for the other subclass heavy chains.

IgG1 and IgG4 have two disulfide bonds between the heavy chains, but IgG2 has four and IgG3 has 11 interchain disulfide bonds. In addition to the greatest number of interchain disulfide bonds, IgG3 has the greatest number of Gm allotypes, 12 compared with IgG1 (4 Gm allotypes), IgG2 (1 Gm allotype), and IgG4 (2 Gm allotypes).[1] Under standard electrophoresis conditions, IgG2 and IgG4 migrate toward the anode, whereas IgG1 and IgG3 migrate toward the cathode. IgG3 has the shortest half-life, the lowest synthesis rate, and the highest catabolic rate of all the IgG subclasses.[1,3,4]

Macrophages have Fc surface receptors for IgG1 and IgG3 that can bind to the CH3 domain. This binding may lead to specific "arming" of the macrophage: First specific antibody binds to the macrophage Fc receptor, next antigen combines with the antibody, and finally antigen is phagocytozed by the macrophage.[11] Additional "arming" receptors on macrophages are the complement receptors.[1]

Functional variation between subclasses is also observed. All IgG subclasses are transported across the placenta, although IgG2 crosses the placenta poorly.

TABLE 8-3
Properties of IgG Subclasses

PROPERTY	SUBCLASS OF IgG			
	IgG1	*IgG2*	*IgG3*	*IgG4*
Serum concentration (approx., mg/dL)	900	300	100	50
Percentage of total IgG	65–70	25	4–7	3–4
Activation of the classical pathway of complement	++	+	+++	–
Placental transfer	+++	+	+++	++
Reactivity with staphylococcal protein A (binds with Fc portion of molecule)	+	+	–	+
Gm allotypes	4	1	13	2
Molecular weight (approx., kDa)	146	146	170	146
No. disulfide bonds linking heavy chains	2	4	11	2
Blocking activity in allergy	–	–	–	+

IgG3 activates the classical pathway of complement very well, whereas IgG4 fails to activate this pathway. The ranked order of IgG subclasses based on their ability to activate complement is IgG3 > IgG1 > IgG2 (Table 8-3).[1]

When exposed to a complex antigen, the antibody subclass response reflects the same proportion as the serum concentration. However, sometimes chemical classes of antigens preferentially stimulate the production of a selected IgG subclass. For example, spontaneously occurring antibodies to coagulation factors are only IgG4, certain polysaccharides stimulate IgG2 production, and DNA antibodies are primarily IgG2 and IgG3.[4]

In some disorders the ability to synthesize IgG subclasses is altered. Currently under investigation are recurrent sinopulmonary infections, in which some children are deficient in IgG2, some are deficient in IgG3, and a small percentage are deficient in both subclasses. The lack of IgG2 and/or IgG3 is an immune deficiency that allows repeated infections by *Streptococcus pneumoniae* and *Haemophilus influenzae*.[12-14] Increased IgG4 has been found in atopic individuals undergoing immunotherapy. It is postulated that IgG4 is a blocking antibody produced in response to the allergen. IgG4 binds to the allergen and prevents the allergen from binding to IgE on the surface of mast cells. Thus, mast cells do not release histamine and other mediators of the allergic response.[15] Measurement of IgG subclasses had been important for allergists to diagnose children, but the American Academy of Allergy and Immunology no longer recommends this.[16]

IgM

Immunoglobulin M (IgM) is a pentamer with a total molecular weight of 900 kDa and a molecular weight of 180 kDa for each basic unit. The J chain and the inter-chain disulfide bonds hold the basic units together (Fig. 8-6). Because IgM is so large, it has a sedimentation of 19S. Although it would appear that IgM has a valence of 10, experimentally IgM was able to bind only five epitopes because of steric hindrance.

IgM is 10% of the total serum immunoglobulin concentration or approximately 125 mg/dL (1.25 g/L). IgM migrates between the γ, β, and α2 regions. The mu (μ) heavy chain is composed of 576 amino acids arranged in four constant domains and one variable domain.[3] A secretory form of IgM has been found in body

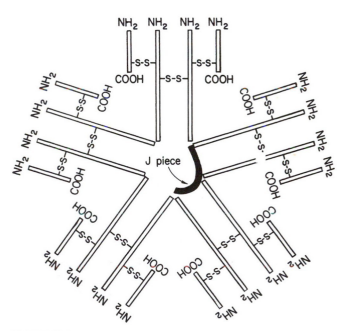

FIGURE 8-6
The IgM molecule is composed of five basic immunoglobulin units held together by the J piece at the carboxy terminus of the heavy chain.

fluids, and its transport through the epithelial lining is the same as that for secretory IgA.

In an immune response, IgM is the first antibody produced in response to an antigen and is produced in both the primary and secondary responses. During fetal development, IgM is the first antibody class to be produced. IgM is the most commonly found immunoglobulin on the surface of B cells; surface IgM is a monomer. IgM is the most efficient immunoglobulin class to activate the classical pathway of complement, requiring only one IgM molecule.

IgA

There are two forms of IgA, serum and secretory. Serum IgA is a single basic structure, with α heavy chains and a molecular weight of 160 kDa, that migrates to the slow β or fast γ globulin regions. The α chain consists of 472 amino acids organized into three constant domains and one variable domain. IgA has two subclasses. In IgA1, the disulfide bonds link the heavy and light chains, similar to those in other classes. No allotypes have been found in IgA1. IgA2, the second subclass of IgA, has no disulfide or other covalent bond between the heavy and light chains. Two allotypes (IgA2m1 and IgA2m2) have been described in IgA2.

The serum concentration of IgA is 15% to 20% of the total serum immunoglobulin concentration, with an approximate concentration of 250 mg/dL (2.5 g/L). Generally, the epitopes that stimulate the production of IgG and IgM will also lead to the production of IgA. Sometimes only IgA is produced.

The second form of IgA, secretory IgA (sIgA), is found in the external body secretions. External body secretions include the colostrum and early milk, mucus (nasal, respiratory, bronchial, and intestinal), saliva, tears, prostatic fluid, and vaginal secretions.[9,11] sIgA has a molecular weight of 400 kDa, which reflects its composition: two basic immunoglobulin units with a J chain and the secretory component attached (Fig. 8-7). Secretory IgA and serum IgA are under separate control mechanisms, as indicated by two supporting studies. First, when radiolabeled serum IgA is administered, it does not appear as secretory IgA. Second, when IgA is administered to an IgA-deficient patient, the serum IgA level increases but the secretory IgA level does not.

The synthesis of secretory IgA molecules begins with the production of IgA monomers by plasma cells present in the mucosa. After the J chain is attached, the dimers are released from the plasma cells. The dimer is selectively transported across the mucosal epithelium by binding to the secretory component (SC). The SC-IgA complex is endocytosed by the epithelial cell, moves through the cells, and is released into the secre-

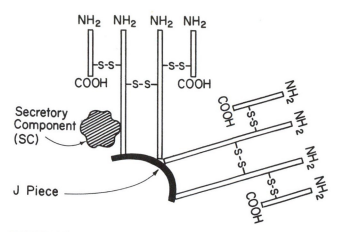

FIGURE 8-7
Secretory IgA is composed of two basic units held together by the J piece at the carboxy terminus of the heavy chain. In addition, there is a secretory component (SC) attached to the constant region of one heavy chain.

tion. SC may be cleaved from the dimer before its release into the secretions. Both sIgA and free SC are found in mucosal secretions (Fig. 8-8).[9]

The function of serum IgA is in antigen clearance and immune regulation. About 10% of the serum IgA is in the dimeric form.[9] The functions of secretory IgA are numerous compared with serum IgA. Because of its unique association with the SC, the IgA dimer is resistant to proteolysis. sIgA does not activate the classical pathway of complement, inhibits the complement-activating activity of IgG, and activates the alternative pathway of complement. Both the inhibitory effect on IgG complement activation and the IgA activation of the alternative pathway may provide protection and promote inflammation. Receptors for IgA have been found on inflammatory cells. IgA may help in the destruction of bacteria and other cellular pathogens by antibody-dependent cell-mediated cytotoxicity. sIgA can bind to some microorganisms and may inhibit their ability to move or to bind to the mucosal wall, preventing colonization. IgA-deficient individuals have increased mucosal infections, atopy, and autoimmune diseases.[9]

IgD

IgD molecules have the same basic unit as other immunoglobulin molecules. The δ heavy chains are joined by a single disulfide bond and are composed of four constant domains. Intact IgD has a molecular weight of 180 kDa. IgD migrates in the fast β region in serum protein electrophoresis. The immunoglobulin is degraded easily using proteolytic enzymes and heat. No subclasses or allotypes have been found.

The serum concentration of IgD is less than 1% of the total immunoglobulin or approximately 3 mg/dL

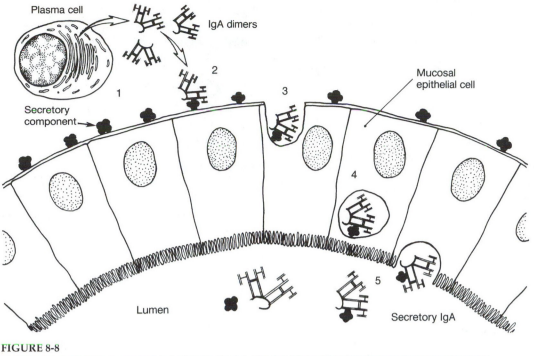

FIGURE 8-8

Step 1: The plasma cells secrete IgA dimers. Step 2: The IgA dimers bind to the secretory components (SC) located on the epithelial cell membrane. Step 3: The IgA-SC complex is endocytosed by the epithelial cell. Step 4: The endocytic vesicle moves through the epithelial cell to the cell membrane located on the lumen side. Step 5: The complexes are released into the lumen. The SC may be cleaved from the IgA dimer.

(0.03 g/L). The relatively short half-life (2 to 3 days) and low synthesis rate (0.4 mg/kg/day) contribute to the low serum concentration. The exact function of IgD has not been determined. IgD has been reported to have antibody activity to insulin, penicillin, nuclear antigens, and thyroid antigen. IgD in association with IgM is found on the surface of B lymphocytes. One theory suggests that IgD is important in B-lymphocyte differentiation.[3,9]

IgE

IgE, first called reagin, is responsible for allergy or Type I hypersensitivity. IgE has a molecular weight of approximately 190 kDa, and the ε heavy chain has four constant domains. The serum concentration of IgE is very low, about 0.004% of the total immunoglobulin concentration. The effects of IgE are considerable and are discussed in Chapter 6. The Fc portion of IgE binds to FcRε receptors on mast cells. When an allergen subsequently binds to the hypervariable region of the IgE molecule, the mast cell releases mediators (i.e., histamine and leukotrienes), which are responsible for the symptoms observed in allergic individuals. IgE receptors are also found on eosinophils, which may contribute to the regulation of allergies and helminth parasitic infections.

MONOCLONAL ANTIBODIES

When a complex antibody is encountered, the body responds by producing a diverse group of antibodies that may vary in class, subclass, idiotype, specificity, affinity, and avidity. This results from multiple clones of B lymphocytes expanding and producing different antibodies. An accident in nature has resulted in diseases (such as multiple myeloma) in which a single aberrant B-cell clone produces a monoclonal antibody. All antibody molecules are identical, with the same class, subclass, and specificity, although the stimulating antigen is unknown.

Technological developments and scientific knowledge have advanced so far that in the mid-1970s hybridomas were engineered that produced monoclonal antibodies of a desired specificity. This process requires the fusion of antigen-sensitized, splenic B lymphocytes and nonsecreting myeloma cells, creating an immortal cell line that secretes specific antibody. This was a significant advancement because it enabled the commercial development of large quantities of reproducible, consistent antibody.

The process begins with the immunization of a host (most often a mouse) with an antigen (Fig. 8-9). This step promotes the expansion of B-cell clones that respond to the antigen. The splenic B cells are harvested

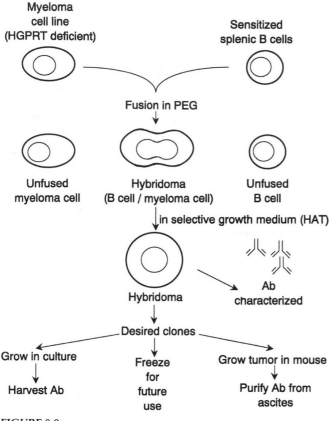

FIGURE 8-9
Myeloma cells are fused with sensitized B cells harvested from the spleen of an immunized mouse. Hybrid cells are grown in selective culture medium. Monoclonal antibody is characterized, and desired clones are grown in culture or as tumors in mice. The cell line can be frozen for use at a later time.

and provide an antigen-specific B-cell–enriched pool of cells. The second cell population is commonly derived from a nonsecreting mouse myeloma cell line. This myeloma cell line is also hypoxanthine guanine phosphoribosyl transferase (HGPRT) deficient.[17]

The splenic B cells and myeloma cells are incubated together in the presence of a fusion agent, such as polyethylene glycol. This agent increases the likelihood of forming hybrid cells. The hybrid cells are grown in a selective culture medium containing hypoxanthine aminopterin and thymidine. Only hybrid cells that contain genetic information from both splenic B cells and myeloma cells will survive and replicate. Splenic B cells do not survive because they have a limited ability to replicate in tissue culture. Myeloma cells would reproduce uncontrollably and would survive in tissue culture except for the fact that the enzyme deficiency and the selective culture medium do not provide the metabolic pathway to synthesize purines. Thus DNA replication is halted. The supernatant of the surviving hybrid cells is screened for antibody production; if antibody is present, the specificity and isotype are evaluated. Desired hybridoma cell lines can be propagated

in tissue culture (antibody in supernatant is harvested), grown in the peritoneum of a mouse (antibody in ascites is purified), or frozen for future use.

QUANTITATION OF IMMUNOGLOBULINS

Serum Quantitation

Quantitation of serum immunoglobulin provides important information about the functional status of humoral immunity. In deficiencies, individuals may lack a single class or subclass or multiple classes of immunoglobulin. For example, IgA deficiency is common and occurs with a frequency of 1 in 500 individuals. In some rare disorders, such as Bruton's agammaglobulinemia and severe combined immunodeficiency, little or no immunoglobulin is produced. At the other end of the spectrum, increased immunoglobulin production may be from a single clone of antibody-producing cells or may result from more general stimulation of many clones. Which class or classes are produced in excess determines the pattern seen in serum protein electrophoresis. A monoclonal increase, as seen in multiple myeloma, shows a single band with restricted mobility, whereas a polyclonal increase, as seen in virus infection, shows a broad band with diffuse mobility.

In the clinical laboratory IgG, IgM, and IgA may be quantitated using radial immunodiffusion (RID), nephelometry, or turbidimetry. IgD may be quantitated only by using RID techniques. IgE quantitation requires more sensitive labeled immunoassays, such as radioimmunoassay and enzyme immunoassay, because the serum levels are very low. Nonisotopic labeled immunoassays are gaining in popularity. Simultaneous measurement of total IgE and allergen-specific IgE by isotopic and nonisotopic methods is also available.

Quantitation of the IgG subclasses in the routine clinical laboratory may be carried out only using commercially available RID kits. There are no commercially available nephelometric assays. This presents a problem when total IgG is quantitated using nephelometry and the IgG subclasses are quantitated by RID. The sensitivity of nephelometry may allow the cumulative concentration of IgG subclasses measured by cumulative total RID to be less than the total IgG measured by nephelometry. Large centers have developed their own nephelometric methods to avoid this problem.[18,19]

Other Body Fluid Quantitation

In addition to serum, immunoglobulin quantitation may be performed on cerebrospinal fluid (CSF), saliva, urine, and synovial fluid by nephelometry as long as the fluid is clear. Quantitation of immunoglobulins in fluids other than serum may be indicated in diseases such as multiple sclerosis and B-cell dyscrasias. The concentrations of immunoglobulins in these fluids are generally much less than that found in serum. If CSF IgG quantitation is requested, the CSF is diluted less than the serum sample would normally be diluted. In nephelometry, the dilution needed depends on the instrument, and the instrument must be adjusted according to the manufacturers' directions. It is sometimes justified to do a CSF quantitation in patients with neurological disorders. Characterization of urine and CSF immunoglobulin may also be performed by high-resolution protein electrophoresis, immunoelectrophoresis, and immunofixation electrophoresis.[18,19]

Review Questions

1. The Fab is composed of
   a. the constant regions of both the heavy and light chains joined together by a disulfide bond
   b. the constant region of the heavy chain and the variable region of the light chain joined together by a disulfide bond
   c. the entire light chain and the variable region plus a portion of the constant region of the heavy chain joined together by a disulfide bond
   d. one entire light chain and one entire heavy chain joined together by a disulfide bond
   e. the variable regions of both the heavy and light chains joined together by a disulfide bond

2. The function of IgE is
   a. in the primary antibody response
   b. in the secondary antibody response
   c. unknown
   d. in the removal of immune complexes
   e. allergic reactions

3. What is the difference between IgG1 and IgG3?
   a. IgG3 has a higher serum concentration than IgG1.
   b. IgG3 crosses the placenta and IgG1 does not.
   c. IgG3 has more disulfide bonds than IgG1.
   d. IgG1 activates complement and IgG3 does not.
   e. IgG3 reacts with staphylococcal Protein A and IgG1 does not react.

4. Which of the following methods may not be used to quantitate immunoglobulins?
   a. enzyme immunoassay
   b. radial immunodiffusion
   c. nephelometry
   d. radioimmunoassay
   e. agglutination

5. Match the term with its definition:

Term	Definition
_____ a. Isotype	1. Component found on IgA
_____ b. Allotype	2. Found in papain cleavage
_____ c. Secretory component	3. All heavy chain classes
_____ d. Fc component	4. Variations in the variable region of immunoglobulins
	5. Allelic variation of a class

6. Monoclonal antibodies are less specific than polyclonal antibodies. (True or False)

References

1. Roitt IM, Brostoff J, Male DK: Immunology, 4th ed, p 4.1. St. Louis, CV Mosby, 1996
2. Roitt I: Essential Immunology, 6th ed, p 31. Oxford, Blackwell Scientific Publications, 1988
3. Barrett JT: Textbook of Immunology, 5th ed, p 103. St. Louis, CV Mosby, 1988
4. Bloch KJ: Antibodies and their functions. In Benacerraf B, Unanue ER (eds): Textbook of Immunology, 2nd ed, p 31. Baltimore, Williams and Wilkins, 1984
5. Abbas AK, Lichtman AH, Pober JS: Cellular and Molecular Immunology, 2nd ed, p 34. Philadelphia, WB Saunders, 1994
6. Ricardo MJ, Tomar RH: Immunoglobulins and paraproteins. In Henry JB (ed): Clinical Diagnosis and Management by Laboratory Methods, 17th ed, p 860. Philadelphia, WB Saunders, 1984
7. Kennedy RC: Anti-idiotype antibodies: Prospects in clinical and laboratory medicine. Lab Manag 23:19, 1985
8. Cerny J, Hiernaux J: Concepts of idiotypic network: Description and functions. In Cerny J, Hiernaux J (eds): Idiotypic Network and Diseases, p 13, Washington, DC, American Society for Microbiology, 1990
9. Ernst PB, Underdown BJ, Bienenstock J: Immunity in mucosal tissue. In Stites DP, Stobo JD, Wells JV (eds): Basic and Clinical Immunology, 6th ed, p 159. Norwalk, CT, Appleton & Lange, 1987
10. Hamilton RG: The human IgG subclasses. Calbiochem-Novabiochem International, San Diego, CA, 1994
11. Goodman JW: Immunoglobulins I: Structure and function. In Stites DP, Stobo JD, Wells JV (eds): Basic and Clinical Immunology, 6th ed, p 27. Norwalk, CT, Appleton & Lange, 1987
12. Umetsu DT, Ambrosino DM, Quinti I, et al: Recurrent sinopulmonary infection and impaired antibody response to bacterial capsule polysaccharide antigen in children

with selective IgG-subclass deficiency. N Engl J Med 313:1247, 1985

13. Lane P, Maclennan I: Impaired lung function in patients with IgA deficiency and low levels of IgG2 or IgG3. N Engl J Med 314:924, 1986

14. Matter L, Wilhelm JA, Anghern W, et al: Selective antibody deficiency and recurrent pneumococcal bacteremia in a patient with Sjögren's syndrome, hyperimmunoglobulinemia G and deficiencies of IgG2 and IgG4. N Engl J Med 312:1039, 1985

15. Aalberse RC, van der Zee J, Vlug A: IgG4 antibodies in atopic allergy. Lab Manag 23:19, 1985

16. AAAI Board of Directors: Position Statement: Measurement of specific and nonspecific IgG4 levels as diagnostic and prognostic tests for clinical allergy. J Allergy Clin Immunol 95:652, 1995

17. Fike DJ: Hybridomas: Their role in the clinical and research laboratories. Am J Med Tech 47:891, 1981

18. Check IJ, Piper M, Papadea C: Immunoglobulin quantitation. In Rose NR, DeMacario EC, Fahey JL, Friedman H, Penn GM (eds): Manual of Clinical Laboratory Immunology, 4th ed, p 71. Washington, DC, American Society for Microbiology, 1992

19. Caron J, Penn GM: Electrophoretic and immunochemical characterization of immunoglobulins. In Rose NR, DeMacario EC, Fahey JL, Friedman H, Penn GM (eds): Manual of Clinical Laboratory Immunology, 4th ed, p 84. Washington, DC, American Society for Microbiology, 1992

CHAPTER 9

Nature of Antigens

Dorothy J. Fike

Objectives

Upon completion of the chapter, the reader will be able to:

1. Describe the difference between antigens and immunogens
2. List five factors that contribute to immunogenicity
3. Discuss how each of the factors contributes to immunogenicity
4. Define the following terms: hapten, adjuvant, antigenic determinant, and epitope
5. List three different mechanisms for adjuvant action

IMMUNOGENS AND ANTIGENS

An immunogen is a substance that initiates a detectable immune response, whether humoral (antibody), cellular, or both. Immunogenicity is the ability of a substance to induce the immune response. Some immunogens elicit an allergic response and are known as allergens. An antigen is a substance that interacts with cells or molecules of the immune system. When an immunogen combines with an antibody molecule, it is an antigen-antibody reaction rather than an immunogen-antibody reaction.[1,2]

Generally, an immunogen is a substance of high molecular weight, greater than 10 kDa, a small portion of which can combine with antibody. This portion of the immunogen molecule is the antigenic determinant, or epitope. It is thought that an immunogen must have at least two epitopes per molecule to stimulate an antibody response. An epitope is approximately four to six amino acids or five to seven monosaccharides in length.[2]

For example, myoglobin, a muscle protein, has five different epitopes on the protein. Each epitope has a different amino acid sequence and location. Every immunogen will have unique epitopes; the number, chemical composition, and location are specific for each molecule. Generally the epitopes are located on the exposed portions of the molecules (Fig. 9-1). All epitopes of myoglobin are adjacent amino acids, as shown in Figure 9-2A. For other immunogens, the epitopes may consist of amino acids or monosaccharides that are not in sequence but are in close proximity to each other because of the folding of the molecule (Fig. 9-2B).[3]

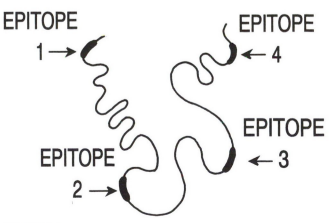

FIGURE 9-1
Antigenic determinants (or epitopes) are most likely to be located at either the amino or carboxyl terminals of the molecule (epitopes 1 and 4). Other epitopes are located on exterior portions of the molecule (epitopes 2 and 3).

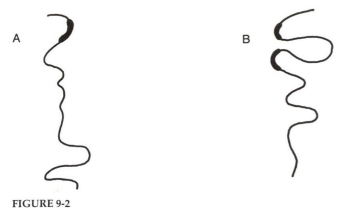

FIGURE 9-2
The epitope may have the amino acids or sugars located next to each other in a linear sequence (**A**) or located next to each other after folding of the molecule (**B**).

There are two major classes of immunogens: thymic-dependent immunogens and thymic-independent immunogens. The thymic-dependent antigens require antigens to be processed by antigen-presenting cells and presented to helper T cells, which then direct cellular and humor-specific immune responses. Most immunogens are thymic dependent.

Thymic-independent antigens stimulate antibody production without interacting with T cells. Structurally, thymic-independent antigens are composed of repetitive units. Some bacterial polysaccharides are thymic-independent antigens. In response to thymic-independent antigens, B cells synthesize IgM class antibodies, while generating little or no immunologic memory. This means that the same antibody response (class, lag phase, and plateau) occurs every time the immunogen is encountered. Some investigators found that limited T-cell interaction was required for the production antibody to T-cell–independent antigens, suggesting that thymus efficient, rather than thymus independent, is a more appropriate description.[2]

FACTORS AFFECTING IMMUNOGENICITY

What makes a substance immunogenic is unknown, but several characteristics of a molecule contribute to its immunogenicity. These characteristics are foreignness, size, and chemical composition and complexity. The genetic composition of the host, route and timing of exposure to the immunogen, and ability to degrade an immunogen also contribute to the level of immune response (Table 9-1). Both categories must be considered together when determining if there will be a response. One factor alone is not responsible for a response.[2]

An immunogen must somehow be recognized as "foreign" or "non-self" by the host. This important requirement encourages an immune response to potentially harmful substances rather than to substances normally found in that individual. If, for example, C3 is removed from an individual and then injected back into the same individual, there will be no response because the protein is recognized as "self." If that same human C3 is injected into a rabbit, the rabbit responds to the human C3 because rabbit C3 is antigenically different from human C3; the human C3 is recognized as "foreign." The extent of the response depends on the degree of "foreignness" of the substance. Generally, the greater the phylogenetic difference, the greater the immune response. The exact mechanisms by which a host recognizes self versus non-self immunogens are not completely understood, but major histocompatibility complex (MHC) antigens and clonal deletion or anergy play a role in this recognition.[2]

The size of an immunogen necessary to provoke a response is unknown. Generally, molecules with a molecular weight less than 10 kDa are poor immunogens, whereas complex substances with a molecular weight greater than 100 kDa are strongly immunogenic. Some small molecules (<10 kDa) may initiate an immune response, whereas other low-molecular-weight substances require a carrier protein be attached to induce a response. These low-molecular-weight substances are haptens; the mechanism of hapten-induced immune response will be discussed later in this chapter.[1–3]

Chemical composition and complexity contribute to immunogenicity. Under proper circumstances all classes of biochemical molecules can be immunogenic. Proteins and carbohydrates elicit the best response, while lipids and nucleic acids are weak immunogens.[1–3] For example, in systemic lupus erythematosus, antibodies may be found against histones (nuclear proteins), surface red blood cell antigens (protein and carbohydrate composition), cardiolipin (a phospholipid), and DNA (nucleic acid).

An immunogen must be diverse, composed of many different amino acids or monosaccharides. In fact, the more complex the molecule is, the better the immunogen. Aromatic amino acids, such as tyrosine, contribute more to the immunogenicity than nonaromatic amino acids.[2] The internal complexity also contributes to immunogenicity (Table 9-2). The primary, secondary, and tertiary structures of proteins define the internal complexity. Oligosaccharides, although sufficiently large, do not have internal complexity and are poor immunogens. Polysaccharides with extensive branching show more internal complexity and are good immunogens. Hydrophilicity, another factor in chemical composition and complexity, influences immunogenicity. Hydrophilic molecules are more immunogenic, and hydrophilic portions of immunogens are the epitopes.[1]

The genetic composition of the individual is critical to the ability to respond to an immunogen. For example,

TABLE 9-1
Factors Involved in Immunogenicity

FACTOR	DESCRIPTION
Foreignness	"Self" versus "non-self"; more unlike "self," more likely to have a response
Size	>10 kDa, best >100 kDa
Chemical composition and complexity	Proteins are best, complex carbohydrates are next, lipids and nucleic acids have a weak response
Genetic composition	HLA antigens are important to provide a "receptor" for the response to occur
Route, dose, and timing of administration	Variable; depends on the specific immunogen as to what the best response would be
Ability to be degraded	Some foreign particles, such as steel pins and plastics, cannot be degraded; the response is poor or absent

the mumps virus will be immunogenic when injected into humans but will not cause an immune response when injected into a guinea pig. To understand the genetic influence on responsiveness, intense research efforts to study MHC antigens and disease associations are ongoing. In humans, if a specific MHC antigen is absent, the host will not respond. In 85% of individuals expressing the HLA-A9 antigen, a high concentration of antibody was produced in response to tetanus toxoid, but in individuals with HLA-B5, 71% had a low response to the same tetanus toxoid.[4] HLA-Dw2 and HLA-Dw3 antigens are generally associated with the atopic response. Individuals allergic to cat dander frequently express HLA-B7 or HLA-B8. Individuals with ragweed allergy have a higher frequency of HLA-A2 or HLA-A28.[5]

Another factor of immune responsiveness is the route, dosage, and timing of immunogen exposure. As with other factors, the exact mechanisms by which immunogen exposure contributes to immune responsiveness are unclear. Immunogens may be encountered naturally or artificially. Research on immunogen exposure relies on artificial (or planned) exposure to evaluate differences in antigen exposure. Generally, soluble immunogens injected intramuscularly or intravenously elicit a better response than those same immunogens administered orally.[2] A notable exception is the polio vaccine; a better response is found when the vaccine is

administered orally than when the same dose is administered intramuscularly.[6] In the pathogenesis of poliovirus infection, resistance requires both mucosal and humoral immunity. Mucosal immunity prevents the virus from entering the body and eliminates the reservoir of virus, thus preventing carriers.

The dose response may partially depend on immunogen processing: T-cell dependent or T-cell independent. Generally, a small dose of immunogen will produce little or no response. (Consult Chapter 28 on immune tolerance for a discussion of dose response.)

The last factor in immunogenicity is the ability to degrade the immunogen because most immunogens must be presented to T and/or B cells. Some large, complex molecules, such as steel joint replacements or plastics, generally do not result in an immune response. These foreign bodies are too large to be ingested by the monocyte/macrophage and so cannot be "presented" to other cells of the immune system.[7]

HAPTENS

Haptens are low-molecular-weight substances (less than 10 kDa) that are not immunogenic but have the ability to combine with an antibody. When a hapten combines with a carrier molecule, the complex is immunogenic. In the early 1900s Karl Landsteiner used haptens to study the specificity and cross-reactivity of antibodies and epitopes. The haptens (substituted benzene) studied by Landsteiner were so small that essentially the variations he studied were epitopes. The carrier molecule, a protein, was immunogenic when injected alone into a mouse, whereas the hapten was not immunogenic when injected alone into the mouse. The hapten was covalently linked to the carrier molecule and the carrier-hapten complex was injected into a mouse. Three antibodies were produced: one that combined only with the hapten, one that combined only with the carrier, and a third that combined with the hapten-carrier junction (Table 9-3). Each antibody

TABLE 9-2
Factors Involved in Internal Complexity

FACTOR	COMMENT
Primary structure Secondary structure Tertiary structure	Oligosaccharides are poor immunogens, whereas polysaccharides, with their extensive branching, are good immunogens
Hydrophilicity	Those portions of the antigens that contain hydrophilic portions are the antigenic determinants

TABLE 9-3
Humoral Response with Hapten Injection

INJECTION	HUMORAL RESPONSE
Hapten alone	No antibodies produced
Carrier alone	Antibody to carrier produced
Hapten-carrier complex	Antibody to hapten produced
	Antibody to carrier produced
	Antibody to hapten-carrier junction produced
Free hapten and free carrier	Antibody to carrier produced

was specific for the hapten, the carrier protein, or the hapten-carrier junction. There was no crossreactivity between anti-carrier antibody and the hapten, nor between anti-hapten antibody and the carrier.[2]

In another set of experiments by Landsteiner, haptens with structures similar to the original hapten were reacted with the original hapten antibody (Fig. 9-3). In this set of experiments, aniline was monosubstituted in the ortho position with a carboxylic or sulfonic group. When specific antibody was produced against each hapten, only the homologous antibody reacted. That is, aniline*COOH reacted with anti-aniline*COOH and not with anti-aniline*HSO$_3$, whereas aniline*HSO$_3$ reacted only with anti-aniline*HSO$_3$ and not with anti-aniline*COOH. In a third set of experiments, the aniline molecule was conjugated with a carboxylic group in the ortho, meta, and para positions. As in the previous set of experiments, the specific homologous antibody reacted with its specific hapten. From these experiments,

it was concluded that antibody reactivity is very specific and recognizes the three-dimensional structure of the epitope or hapten.[2]

ADJUVANTS

Adjuvants are agents that potentiate an immune response; they are not immunogens and cannot evoke a response alone. The most frequently observed response is an increase in the amount of specific antibody produced, although activation of macrophages and cell-mediated immunity has also been observed.

There are several types of adjuvants that act by slowing the release of immunogen at the site of the immunogen injection (Table 9-4). The repository adjuvant enriches the antigen with aluminum and calcium salts. These salts combine with the immunogen to form an insoluble complex that slowly releases the immunogen from the subcutaneous or intramuscular site of injection and increases the time to which immune cells can react with the immunogen. Because the repository adjuvant also increases the size of the immunogen, phagocytosis is enhanced. Another type of adjuvant is the water-in-oil emulsifying agent. This type has had restricted use in humans. The emulsified adjuvants allow a slow release of immunogen from the oil droplets. The variation in droplet size allows the droplets to be degraded at different rates, resulting in the prolonged presence of immunogens. The oil droplets also aid in phagocytosis because immunogens in oil droplets are more easily phagocytosed than soluble immunogens.

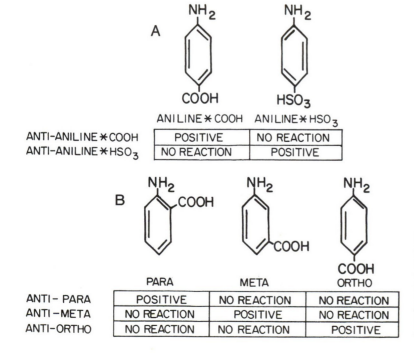

FIGURE 9-3
Hapten antibody reactions are very specific. (**A**) Anti-aniline*COOH reacts only with aniline*COOH and not with aniline*HSO$_3$, whereas anti-aniline*HSO$_3$ reacts only with aniline*HSO$_3$. (**B**) Aniline is substituted with –COOH in various positions; the antibody reacts only with the molecule that has the –COOH in the appropriate position (i.e., anti-para-amino-benzene carboxylate reacts only when the –COOH is in the para position).

TABLE 9-4
Adjuvants

I. Insoluble complex, salts (aluminum and calcium)
   Aluminum hydroxide
   Aluminum potassium tartrate (alum)
   Calcium phosphate
II. Slow release of antigen, oil in water
   Freund's incomplete, mineral oil
   Freund's complete, mineral oil with mycobacteria
III. Increase in IgM production
   Lipopolysaccharide (LPS)
   Endotoxins
   Bordetella pertussis
IV. Mobilizing T and B cells
   Bordetella pertussis
V. Lysosomal release
   Vitamin A
   Beryllium salts
   Toxic forms of silica
   Quaternary forms of ammonium salts

Freund's adjuvant is the classic example of a water-in-oil adjuvant. Freund's incomplete adjuvant is light mineral oil and an emulsifying agent. Freund's complete adjuvant contains light mineral oil, an emulsifying agent, and 0.5 mg/mL of killed mycobacteria. The mycobacteria induce granuloma formation at the site of injection. The granuloma further slows the release of the immunogen because it acts as a physical barrier.[8] Because Freund's complete adjuvant contains bacteria, macrophages and other antigen-presenting cells are stimulated.[9] Freund's complete adjuvant is not recommended for human use because the granuloma may be disfiguring.[8]

Lipopolysaccharides or endotoxins from gram-negative bacteria may also be used as adjuvants. These agents enhance the IgM response, although the exact mechanism for this increase of IgM is unknown. This adjuvant is not recommended for human use because it induces a high fever.[8]

Bordetella pertussis is another adjuvant that increases the amount of IgM produced. In addition, *Bordetella* has a lymphocytosis-promoting factor that mobilizes T and B cells to the site of injection, thereby enhancing the immune reaction.

Lysosomal enzyme release is another mechanism by which adjuvants may act. Vitamin A, beryllium salts, toxic forms of silica, and quaternary ammonium salts activate macrophages. These stimulated macrophages release lysosomal enzymes, which enhance the immune response.[8]

The previous discussion applies to experimental situations during immunization. The natural physio-logic adjuvant response may be affected by cytokines[10] and the C3d.[11]

The ultimate effect of an adjuvant is to blend the primary and secondary (booster) responses together. Theoretically, this activity may be accomplished by (1) increasing the number of cells involved in the immune response, (2) providing more efficient processing of the immunogen, (3) prolonging the presence of immunogen, or (4) increasing the rate of synthesis and release of antibody.[8]

Review Questions ✳

1. Which of the following is *not* a factor in immunogenicity?

   a. size greater than 5000 Da
   b. foreignness of the immunogen
   c. proteins being better than lipids
   d. HLA antigen being present as a receptor
   e. route of administration

2. An adjuvant

   a. is an immunogen
   b. does not activate macrophages
   c. may be a soluble complex with aluminum and calcium salts
   d. may slow the release of immunogen from a region

3. A substance that can combine with products of the immune response but cannot induce an immune response is a(n)

   a. adjuvant
   b. homologous antigen
   c. hapten
   d. thymic dependent antigen

4. A genetic association for immune responsiveness in atopy has been found in the expression of

   a. HLA-Dw2
   b. allotypic markers on immunoglobulin chains
   c. homozygous C3 deficiency
   d. HLA-B27

5. Which adjuvant is a water-in-oil adjuvant?

   a. Freund's
   b. alum
   c. *Bordetella pertussis*
   d. Vitamin A

6. Mucosal immunity is preferentially stimulated if the immunogen is administered

   a. intravenously
   b. intramuscularly
   c. intradermally
   d. orally

7. Which term may be used interchangeably with *epitope*?

   a. hapten
   b. thymic-dependent antigen
   c. homologous antigen
   d. antigenic determinant

References

1. Barrett JT: Textbook of Immunology, 5th ed, p. 29. St. Louis, CV Mosby, 1988
2. Goodman JW: Immunogenicity and antigenic specificity. In Stites DP, Stobo JD, Wells JV (eds): Basic and Clinical Immunology, 6th ed, p 20. Norwalk, CT, Appleton & Lange, 1987
3. Hammarstrom S, Perlman P: Antigens. In Hanson LA, Widgzell H (eds): Immunology. Boston, Butterworth, 1985
4. Sasazuki T, Kohno Y, Iwamoto I, et al: Association between an HLA haplotype and locus responsive to tetanus toxoid in man. Nature 272:359, 1978
5. Marsh DG, Meyers DA, Bias WB: Epidemiology and genetics of atopic allergy. N Engl J Med 305:1551, 1981
6. Benacerraf B, Unanue E: Textbook of Immunology, 2nd ed, p 12. Baltimore, Williams and Wilkins, 1984
7. Tizard IR: Immunology, An Introduction, 3rd ed, p 13. Philadelphia, WB Saunders, 1992
8. Barrett JT: Textbook of Immunology, 5th ed, p 146. St. Louis, CV Mosby, 1988
9. Abbas AK, Lichtman AH, Pober JS: Cellular and Molecular Immunology, 2nd ed, p 206. Philadelphia, WB Saunders, 1994
10. Roitt I, Brostoff J, Male D: Immunology, 4th ed, p 19.8. London, Mosby, 1996
11. Dempsey PW, Allison MED, Akkaraju S, Goodnow CC, Fearon DT: C3d of complement as a molecular adjuvant: Bridging innate and acquired immunity. Science 271:348, 1996

CHAPTER 10

An Overview of Antigen-Antibody Interaction and Its Detection

Catherine Sheehan

THE BASIS OF ANTIBODY STRUCTURE
FORCES BINDING ANTIGEN TO ANTIBODY
ELUTION
ANTIBODY AFFINITY
AVIDITY
SPECIFICITY AND CROSSREACTIVITY
HETEROPHILE ANTIBODIES
ASSAYS INVOLVING ANTIGEN-ANTIBODY INTERACTIONS
CONCLUSION

Objectives

Upon completion of the chapter, the reader will be able to:

1. Describe the four levels of protein structure applied to antibody molecules
2. Explain why antigen-antibody interactions are reversible
3. Describe the forces that work to keep antigen bound to antibody
4. Define elution, specificity, affinity, avidity, and heterophile antibody
5. Discuss four methods of antibody elution
6. Given the antibody-hapten affinity, select the pair with the greatest affinity
7. Explain why detecting heterophile antibody is important in clinical serology
8. Explain why assays involving unlabeled, soluble antigen and antibody are less sensitive analytically

When an antibody combines with an antigen, an antigen-antibody or immune complex is formed. The interaction is reversible and relies on non-covalent bonding to maintain the complex. When the three-dimensional structure and charge of the antibody are highly complementary for the antigen, the affinity of the antibody for the antigen is greatest and the complex will most likely be maintained. The specificity of the reaction is defined by the antibody and is related to the antigen that stimulated its production, the homologous antigen. This chapter discusses the protein structure related to antibody, the forces that contribute to antibody-antigen formation, elution, and general features of antigen-antibody assays.

THE BASIS OF ANTIBODY STRUCTURE

Antibody molecules are glycosylated proteins. The protein structure determines the isotypic, allotypic, and idiotypic variation of antibody molecules. The four levels of protein structure are as follows.

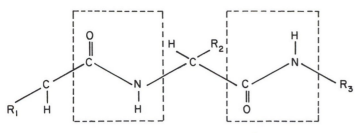

FIGURE 10-1
Primary structure of protein. The carboxyl group of one amino acid joins the amino group of a second amino acid to create a peptide bond (indicated by - - -). R = side chains of the amino acids.

1. *Primary:* The sequence of amino acids joined together by peptide bonds (Fig. 10-1).
2. *Secondary:* The shape of the amino acid chain resulting from interaction of amino acids in close proximity (Fig. 10-2).
3. *Tertiary:* The interaction of distant amino acids in the amino acid chain that are brought closer together by folding of polypeptide chains.
4. *Quaternary:* The association of polypeptide subunits to form a biologically active protein (Fig. 10-3).[1]

The primary structure of antibody as defined by the genetic code specifies the sequence of amino acids in a peptide chain. When amino acid sequences of monoclonal antibodies were studied, variation in the degree of substitution was observed. The similarity of amino acid sequences from one antibody molecule to another is the degree of homology. The constant domains within a single heavy-chain class or single light-chain type show greater similarity, thus more homology. Conversely, the variable domains of heavy and light chains show less similarity and less homology. Even within variable domains, some amino acid positions are more frequently substituted than other amino acid positions; these are the hypervariable regions. When the hypervariable regions are folded into their secondary, tertiary, and quaternary protein structures, they form a pocket or cleft in which the antigen can bind.

The secondary protein structure is the spatial arrangement of amino acids that results from the carbon-to-nitrogen linkage of the peptide bonds and amino acid interactions in close proximity. The result can be an α-helix, β-pleated sheet, or random structure. The β-pleated sheet structure is almost exclusively present in immunoglobulins.[2] The polypeptide chain folds back on itself, creating parallel linear areas; the close proximity of amino acids allows hydrogen bonding to stabilize the β-pleated structure.[3] The hinge region, a sequence rich in the amino acids proline and cysteine, does not display the same structure. The hinge region is thought to define the antibody subclass, to affect the flexibility of the molecule, to allow complement to be fixed, and to determine its susceptibility to proteolytic enzymes.

The tertiary structure of immunoglobulins allows the side chains of distant amino acids to interact. Hydrophilic side chains of amino acids are attracted to each other; likewise, hydrophobic side chains are attracted to each other. To promote solubility in aqueous environments (such as blood), most hydrophilic areas are located on the outside surface of the immunoglobulin molecule to be able to interact with water. Most hydrophobic areas are internal. An exception to this internal-external arrangement is in variable domains, where the hydrophilic pocket forms the antigen-combining site. An intradomain disulfide bond in the middle of the domain stabilizes the peptide chain. The tertiary structure of the constant domains is responsible for the biologic functions specific for each immunoglobulin class.

The quaternary structure is the association of polypeptides, two heavy chains and two light chains in

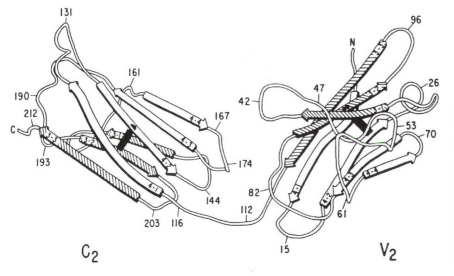

FIGURE 10-2
This schematic drawing of the constant (**C**) and variable (**V**) domains of a light chain illustrates the β-pleated structure. The striated arrows show a three-chain layer of β-pleated sheets; the white arrows show a four-chain layer. The intradomain disulfide bonds are shown with a black bar. (From Edmunson AB, Ely KR, Abola EE, Schiffer M, Panagiotopoulos N. Rotational allomerism and divergent evolution of domains in immunoglobulin light chains. Biochemistry 14:3954, 1975. Copyright 1975 American Chemical Society.)

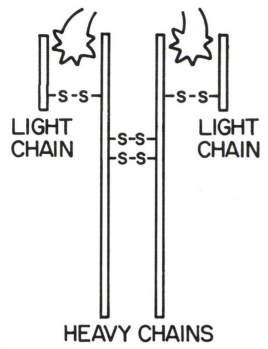

FIGURE 10-3

Quaternary structure of an immunoglobulin. The association of two heavy chains and two light chains forms a complete, biologically active molecule. Interchain disulfide bonds are shown by s-s.

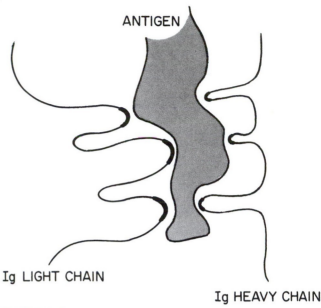

FIGURE 10-4

The hypervariable regions within the variable domains of the immunoglobulin (Ig) heavy chain and light chain form the antigen combining site. The darkened sections of the chains represent the hypervariable regions that interact with the antigen, which is the shaded area.

each basic immunoglobulin unit. For each chain, the tertiary folding of heavy and light chains positions the hypervariable regions within a chain to be close together. As seen in Figure 10-4, the quaternary structure finally brings the hypervariable region of one heavy chain in close proximity to the hypervariable region of one light chain.[4] The pocket that is created is the antigen-combining site in which an epitope can bind. Although each peptide chain contributes to primary, secondary, and tertiary structure, it is the quaternary structure that is required for antigen binding.

Each immunoglobulin basic unit or monomer has two antigen-combining sites, a valence of 2. IgG, IgD, and IgE exist exclusively as monomers. Circulating IgM is a pentamer (valence of 10), surface IgM is a monomer (valence of 2), serum IgA is a monomer (valence of 2), and secretory IgA is a dimer (valence of 4).

FORCES BINDING ANTIGEN TO ANTIBODY

The union of an antibody with an epitope is a reversible, biologic chemical reaction that obeys the physical principles of chemical bonding and equilibrium. An antigen-antibody complex will form only if sufficient free energy is released and the complex is stabilized. The goodness of fit and the complementary nature of the antibody for the epitope affect the speed and strength of this union. The forces that contribute to the stability of the complex are electrostatic force, hydrogen bonding, hydrophobic force, and Van der Waals force, as summarized in Table 10-1 and as shown in Figure 10-5.[5,6]

Electrostatic force or ionic bonding is the attraction of a positively charged portion of one molecule (e.g., the antibody) to a negatively charged portion of another molecule (e.g., the antigen). The ionization state of each reactant determines the charge of each and the strength of the electrostatic force. The pH and ionic strength of the environment (blood, tissue, or test tube) greatly affect the ionic state of each molecule, thus determining the complementary nature of the molecules

TABLE 10-1
Attractive Forces Between an Epitope and Antibody

ELECTROSTATIC FORCE OR IONIC BONDING

The attraction of one charge to the opposite charge

HYDROGEN BONDING

The mutual attraction of two electronegative atoms to an electropositive hydrogen atom

HYDROPHOBIC BONDING

The attraction between two nonpolar molecules

VAN DER WAALS FORCE

The weak attraction of the electron cloud of one atom to protons in the nucleus of another atom

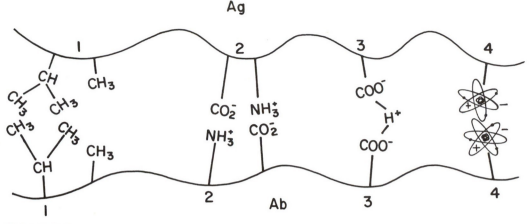

FIGURE 10-5

Forces of antigen-antibody binding. Site 1 shows the hydrophobic force, the complementary binding of a hydrophobic area of the antigen (Ag) with a hydrophobic area of the antibody (Ab). Site 2 shows the electrostatic force, the attraction of two charged areas. Site 3 shows hydrogen bonding in which two negatively charged groups attract hydrogen. Site 4 represents Van der Waals force, the weak attractive force between the electron cloud (–) of one atom and the nucleus (+) of another atom.

and the strength of the electrostatic force. As two complementary charged areas approach each other, the electrostatic force increases. The electrostatic force is inversely proportional to the square of the distance between the charges.

Hydrogen bonding is the attraction of two electronegative atoms for hydrogen. Though a weak bond, it is common in secondary and tertiary protein structures and contributes significantly to antigen-antibody reactions. Hydrogen bonding is an exothermic reaction, with maximum binding strength at lower temperatures, usually less than 37°C.[6] In laboratory procedures, hydrogen bonds can be dissociated in 8 M urea or 6 M guanine, unfolding the polypeptide chain.

The strength of hydrophobic forces is related to the attraction between nonpolar groups. In an aqueous environment, hydrophobic groups tend to associate together and to reduce the total surface area exposed to water. The resulting lowered energy state provides the force of attraction. When multiple antibody and antigen molecules bind together forming a large immune complex, the complex excludes water, becomes insoluble, and precipitates.

Van der Waals force is a weak, attractive force between the electron cloud of one atom and the nucleus of another atom. The force of attraction is inversely proportional to the seventh power of this distance. A slight decrease in the distance between an antigen and the antigen binding site greatly increases the strength of binding.

ELUTION

Given an immune complex, the process of separating antigen from antibody is known as elution and can be considered the opposite of antigen-antibody complex

formation. Elution is accomplished by creating an environment that discourages the union of antigen and antibody by altering the environmental factors, such as temperature, pH, polarity, ionic strength, and composition. Elution may be used to separate a complex to study the specificity of the antigen and the class of the antibody. The complex may be trapped in tissue, present in fluid, or present on the surface of red blood cells.

Several strategies can be used to elute antibody. The method chosen will depend on the methods sensitivity, the performance simplicity, the hazardous nature of reagents, and the degree of irreversible antibody denaturation. Acid or alkaline elution requires decreasing or increasing the pH, respectively, and affects the ionization of the antigen and antibody causing separation. High ionic strength buffers increase the ionic cloud surrounding the antibody and antigen, and prevent union of the antigen and antibody. Use of organic solvents, such as ether or chloroform, will alter the hydrophobic interaction, thus causing separation. Heat elution may dissociate the antibody by interfering with hydrogen bonding.

ANTIBODY AFFINITY

Consistent with other chemical reactions, the law of mass action describes the chemical equilibrium between an antibody molecule and a single binding site (hapten or ligand).[7,8] This reaction is reversible. In an aqueous solution, association of the hapten and antibody is related to the rate of diffusion of the two reactants and to the probability that a collision will result in binding. For binding to occur during a collision, each reactant must have sufficient energy and a favorable spatial orientation. Dissociation is related to the strength of the hapten-antibody bond; when this bond is strong, dissociation is low.

When the forward reaction rate (association) is faster than the reverse rate (dissociation), complex formation is favored and the likelihood of remaining together is high. At equilibrium, the rates of association and dissociation are constant, so that the amount of complex formed equals the amount of complex dissociated. The ratio of these two rate constants is the equilibrium constant or affinity constant, K_A, and is specific for each antibody-hapten pair. When the antibody is highly complementary for the hapten and tightly binds, the forward reaction is favored and the concentration of the antibody-hapten complex is high (Fig. 10-6).

If the concentration of the reactants and the environmental factors (pH, temperature, and ionic strength) are constant, then the ratio of the concentration of complex to the product of the concentration of reactants remains the same. In terms of concentration, the ratio of the concentration of the complex to the product of the concentrations of free antibody and free hapten is called the affinity constant. At equilibrium the ratio remains the same.

Another way to describe the affinity constant is as follows: When the concentration of free antibody equals the concentration of antibody complexed to the hapten, then 50% of the antibody is bound to the hapten. In the preceding equation, an equal concentration of free and complexed antibody allows these two terms to cancel each other. Thus, the affinity constant is the reciprocal of the concentration of free hapten when half of the total antibody is free. The affinity constant is expressed as liters per mole or molarity^{-1}. The smaller the hapten concentration needed to bind half of the total antibody, the greater the affinity of the antibody for the hapten. The antibody is highly complementary for the hapten, there is a good fit, and the antibody does not easily release the hapten. Complex formation is fa-

vored. For example, if the affinity constant for an antibody and hapten pair is 1×10^{10} L/mole, then the concentration of hapten needed to bind 50% of the antibody is 1×10^{-10} moles/L. This is an example of an antibody with high affinity for the hapten.

AVIDITY

The preceding discussion of antibody affinity is based on the interaction of a single epitope or a monovalent hapten with the combining site of an antibody. However, most naturally occurring antigens and all antibodies are polyvalent, and in a naturally occurring immune response antibodies with different specificities, affinities, and valences are synthesized. Avidity describes the tendency for multiple antibodies and multivalent antigens to combine and is the cumulative binding strength of all antibody-epitope pairs. Thus, avidity is related to the specific affinity constant of each antibody-epitope pair. The observed avidity is greater than the sum of individual affinity constants. Avidity is the bonus effect that promotes the stability of an antigen-antibody complex. For dissociation to occur, multiple bonds must be broken simultaneously (Fig. 10-7 on p. 114).[5,9]

SPECIFICITY AND CROSSREACTIVITY

The specificity of an antibody is most often described by the antigen that induced antibody production. In other words, during an immune response the homologous antigen promotes the production of antibody with the greatest affinity. Ideally, the antibody would react only with the homologous antigen, but this is not always the case. The interaction of an antibody with an antigen that is structurally similar to the homologous antigen is referred to as crossreactivity. Considering that an antigenic determinant can be five or six amino acids or one dominant sugar, it is not surprising that some antigen similarity and overlap exist in nature. The greater the similarity between the crossreacting antigen and the homologous antigen, the stronger the bond between the antibody and the crossreacting antigen. So there is a continuum of potential reactions of an antibody with similar antigens: There is the strongest binding with the homologous antigen, weaker binding with a similar antigen, and no binding with a dissimilar antigen (Fig. 10-8 on p. 114).

HETEROPHILE ANTIBODIES

A special group of crossreacting antibodies are heterophile antibodies. These antibodies are produced in response to one antigen and also react with a genetically

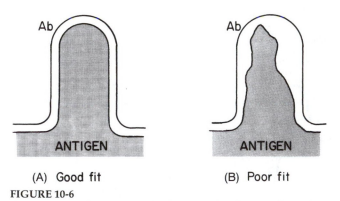

(A) Good fit   (B) Poor fit

FIGURE 10-6

The goodness of fit between the immunoglobulin molecule and an antigenic determinant determines the affinity. The shaded area in (**A**) represents an epitope that is highly complementary for the antibody; hence, there is a good fit or high affinity. (**B**) The poor fit between the antibody and the epitope results in lower affinity.

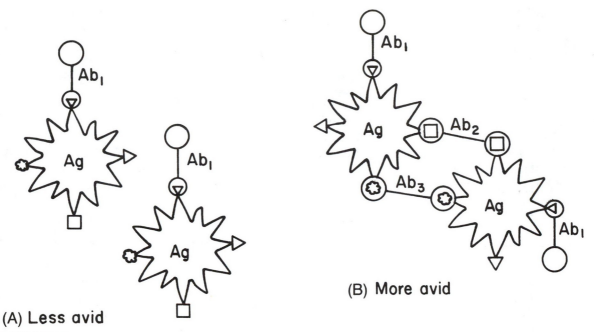

(A) **Less avid**

(B) **More avid**

FIGURE 10-7

The combined forces of multiple-antigen combining sites and multiple-antibody combining sites result in avidity. A multivalent antigen ( ) combines with a divalent antibody (O—O). In (**A**) there is only one antibody present and low avidity. In (**B**) the same multivalent antigen combines with several different antibodies, increasing avidity.

unrelated, yet structurally similar, antigen. For example, a group A streptococcal infection stimulates an antibody response to epitopes of the organism, one of which also reacts with a structurally similar antigen, human myocardium, and may result in rheumatic fever.

The prototypic heterophile antibody is associated with infectious mononucleosis. In this disease the Epstein-Barr virus is a polyclonal B-cell activator that stimulates the immune system to produce many antibodies. One of these antibodies is presumed to react with a viral epitope and is able to react with an epitope on the surface of sheep red blood cells. This is

useful clinically; by measuring the heterophile antibody reaction with sheep red blood cells, indirect evidence of a recent Epstein-Barr virus infection is easily demonstrated.

Other heterophile antibodies are also used to provide serologic evidence of recent infections. For example, antibodies produced in response to several rickettsial organisms react with *Proteus vulgaris* antigens. Therefore, one laboratory test strategy is to measure the antibodies that react with *Proteus* antigens and to interpret the titers in light of clinical findings of rickettsial infection. A second example of crossreactivity is the

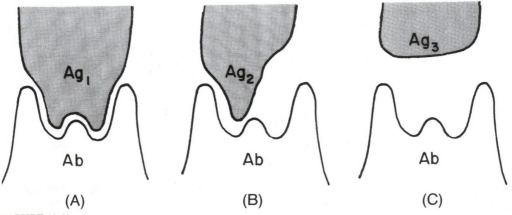

(A)   (B)   (C)

FIGURE 10-8

(**A**) The homologous antigen (Ag_1) stimulates the production of the antibody (Ab) and reacts with the antibody. (**B**) The same antibody reacts with another structurally similar antigen (Ag_2), showing crossreactivity. (**C**) The same antibody cannot react with the dissimilar antigen (Ag_3).

TABLE 10-2
Examples of Heterophile Antibodies

ANTIBODY TO	CROSSREACTS WITH
Group A streptococci	Human myosin
Epstein-Barr virus	Surface antigen on SRBC, HRBC
Selected rickettsia	Selected *Proteus vulgaris* antigen
Mycoplasma pneumoniae	I antigen on adult human RBC
Treponema pallidum	Cardiolipin-lecithin-cholesterol
Enterobacteriaceae	A and B antigens on human RBC
Forsmann	Guinea pig antigen

SRBC, Sheep red blood cells; HRBC, horse red blood cell; RBC, red blood cell.

TABLE 10-3
Assays Using Antigen-Antibody Interactions

PRECIPITATION—SOLUBLE ANTIGEN AND SOLUBLE ANTIBODY REACT

Agarose Gel

Double diffusion

Radial immunodiffusion

Immunoelectrophoresis

Immunofixation

Fluid Phase

Nephelometry

Turbidimetry

AGGLUTINATION—SOLUBLE ANTIBODY THAT CAN REACT WITH ANTIGEN ATTACHED TO A PARTICLE (OR VICE VERSA)

Latex particles

Red blood cells

Dye

Liposomes

LABELED IMMUNOASSAYS—A LABEL THAT CAN EMIT A MEASURABLE SIGNAL AND IS ATTACHED TO AN ANTIBODY OR ANTIGEN

Fluorochromes

Enzymes

Radionuclides

Chemiluminescent molecules

cold agglutinin produced in response to *Mycoplasma pneumoniae* infection. This antibody presumably reacts with the organism and also reacts with the I antigen on adult human red blood cells. When the titer of cold agglutinin is sufficient or increasing, it suggests a recent *Mycoplasma* infection.

Given the wide variety and complexity of antigens in nature, it is not surprising that crossreactivity between similar antigens and an antibody is seen. In clinical immunology, well characterized crossreactions are used to identify antibodies associated with a recent infection or with damage to the host. Table 10-2 summarizes common examples of heterophile antibodies.

ASSAYS INVOLVING ANTIGEN-ANTIBODY INTERACTIONS

The specificity of antibody makes it an attractive tool to use in in-vitro immunoassays to measure the concentration of antigen or antibody (Table 10-3). The affinity and avidity of the antibody influence the rate and quantity of antigen-antibody complex formation. In the simplest immunoassay, soluble antibody and soluble antigen are allowed to react; small complexes grow into larger complexes until precipitation can be visualized. This qualitative unlabeled immunoassay lacks analytic sensitivity. If soluble immune complexes were detected using the photodetector in an instrument (such as an endpoint nephelometer), the sensitivity improves. If the rate of complex formation is monitored using a rate nephelometer, the sensitivity continues to improve. Performing precipitation in agarose gel also improves the analytic sensitivity. All of these assays detect the secondary manifestation of antigen and antibody interaction.

A very popular format for immunoassays involves using a labeled reactant that enables the primary antigen-antibody interaction to be detected. The antibody determines the specificity, and the label (or the activity of the label) is what is measured. In agglutination, the labels are dyes, colored or white latex particles, liposomes, or red blood cells. When labels are brought into close proximity, which occurs when an antigen reacts with an antibody, the reaction is seen as a color or clumps. In labeled immunoassays, the label provides a signal that can be measured; the amount of signal generated is related to the concentration of the unknown. Examples of labels in immunoassays are fluorochromes, enzymes, radionuclides, and chemiluminescent molecules. The label and format of the assay determines the extent of improved analytic sensitivity. In general, precipitation assays have less analytic sensitivity than agglutination assays, which have less analytic sensitivity than labeled immunoassays.

CONCLUSION

The sequence of amino acids, defined by the genetic code, determines the structure and functions of all proteins, including antibody molecules. For full biologic activity of an antibody, all four levels of protein structure must be intact and unmodified. When the hypervariable regions of the variable domains of heavy and light chains are in close proximity, the antigen-combining site is created. The reversible association of antigen and antibody occurs through hydrogen bonding and electrostatic, Van der Waals, and hydrophobic forces. Affinity is the strength of an antibody-hapten or antibody-epitope bond, whereas avidity reflects the overall binding between multivalent antibodies and antigens. Antibody specificity is defined by the antigen that induced the production of that antibody; the opposite of specificity is crossreactivity, in which a second, structurally similar antigen can bind to the antibody. Heterophile antibodies are crossreacting antibodies that react with antigens from different species. The interaction of antigen and antibody in immunoassays provides a powerful, flexible, and sensitive strategy to measure analytes. Methods range from unlabeled to labeled and from visual inspection to automated detection.

Review Questions

1. What is the highest level of protein structure needed to have a functional antibody molecule?

    a. primary
    b. secondary
    c. tertiary
    d. quaternary

2. Heat elution disrupts

    a. ionic bonding
    b. hydrophobic bonding
    c. Van der Waals forces
    d. hydrogen bonding

3. The antigen combining site is created by the interaction of the

    a. variable domains of two heavy chains
    b. constant domains of two heavy chains
    c. variable domains of one heavy chain and one light chain
    d. variable domain of one heavy chain and the constant domain of one light chain

4. Which affinity constant indicates the greatest affinity between the antibody and the hapten?

    a. 1×10^8 moles/L
    b. 1×10^3 moles/L
    c. 1×10^{-3} moles/L
    d. 1×10^{-8} moles/L

5. The ability of an antibody to discriminate between the homologous antigen and any other antigen is the definition of

    a. sensitivity
    b. affinity
    c. specificity
    d. avidity

References

1. Danishefsky I: Biochemistry for Medical Sciences, p 24. Boston, Little, Brown, 1980
2. Carayannopoulos L, Capra JD: Immunoglobulins: Structure and function. In Paul WE (ed): Fundamental Immunology, p 283. New York, Raven Press, 1993
3. Edmunson AB, Ely KR, Abola EE, et al: Rotational allomerism and divergent evolution of domains in immunoglobulin light chains. Biochemistry 14:3953, 1975
4. Goodman JW: Immunoglobulins structure and function. In Stites DP, Terr AI (eds): Basic and Clinical Immunology, 7th ed, p 109. Norwalk, CT, Appleton & Lange, 1991
5. Roitt IM: Essential Immunology, 8th ed. Oxford, Blackwell Scientific, 1994
6. Howard PL: Principles of antibody elution. Transfusion 21:477, 1981
7. Berzofsky JA, Berkower IJ, Epstein Sl: Antigen-antibody interactions and monoclonal antibodies. In Paul WE (ed): Fundamental Immunology, p 421. New York, Raven Press, 1993
8. Steward MW, Steensgaard J: Antibody Affinity: Thermodynamic Aspects and Biological Significance, p 1. Boca Raton, FL, CRC Press, 1983
9. Eisen HN: Immunology, 2nd ed, p 298. New York, Harper & Row, 1980

CHAPTER 11

Precipitation

Dorothy J. Fike

Objectives

Upon completion of the chapter, the reader will be able to:

1. Define a precipitation reaction
2. Diagram and explain the precipitation curve
3. Compare and contrast the various types of precipitation reactions
4. Explain the advantages and disadvantages of each type of precipitation reaction

INTRODUCTION

The reaction between soluble antigen and soluble antibody may result in precipitation. Maximal precipitation occurs when the concentrations of antigen and antibody are in the zone of equivalence (Fig. 11-1). When the concentration of antigen is greater than that of the antibody, the amount of precipitate observed may be diminished or absent; this is the postzone. Likewise, when the antibody concentration is greater than that of the antigen, the precipitate may be diminished or absent; this is the prozone.

To develop a precipitate, the antigen must have at least two epitopes per molecule. Then bivalent antibody will combine with the multivalent antigen; the antigen becomes crosslinked and forms a lattice (Fig. 11-2). Lattice formation requires the antibody to combine with epitopes on two different antigens. A second antibody molecule combines with the second epitope on one of the antigen molecules and a third epitope on another antigen molecule so that a complex is formed. When repeated so many times, the complex continues to grow until it is sufficiently large to become insoluble and precipitate. Precipitation reactions can occur using polyclonal antibody or a mixture of monoclonal

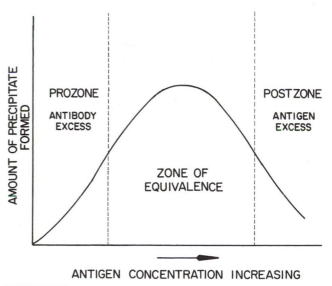

FIGURE 11-1
The precipitation curve shows the maximal amount of precipitation in the zone of equivalence. This reaction is obtained using several tubes, each with the same concentration of antibody. The tubes have an increasing amount of antigen added.

antibodies. If the antigen is monovalent or a single monoclonal antibody is used, no lattice will form; this requires a different methodology to detect the antigen or antibody. Precipitation reactions may require hours or days to become visible, depending on the type of precipitation reaction.

TYPES OF PRECIPITATION REACTIONS

Many different precipitation test systems (Table 11-1) are used in the clinical laboratory. Each system can detect antigens or antibodies, depending on the configuration of the assay. Moreover, each system has different sources of error that must be taken into account when performing a particular laboratory procedure. In all systems, optimal lattice forms in the zone of equivalence. In general, precipitation techniques are not as sensitive as other techniques because a sufficient number of antigen and antibody molecules must be crosslinked in order to see the precipitate.

Fluid-Phase Precipitation

One of the first precipitation reactions was the passive diffusion of fluid-phase antigen and antibody. This double diffusion method in a capillary tube layers an antigen solution over an antibody solution. Both the antigen and antibody will diffuse toward each other; at the interface, when antibody recognizes antigen, precipitate forms. The amount of precipitate is proportional to the concentration of both the antigen and antibody. In Figure 11-3, A and B show precipitation of antigen-antibody complexes. B shows more precipitate than A. In C no precipitate is formed. This procedure may be used to qualitatively detect either unknown antigen or unknown antibody. If an antigen is to be detected, a fixed amount of known reagent antibody is placed in the capillary

TABLE 11-1
Types of Precipitation Reactions

PASSIVE

Fluid

Double diffusion

Capillary tube precipitation

Gel

Double diffusion (Ouchterlony)

Single-diffusion radial immunodiffusion (RID)

ELECTROPHORESIS

Countercurrent immunoelectrophoresis (CIEP)

Immunoelectrophoresis (IEP)

Immunofixation electrophoresis (IFE)

Rocket technique (Laurell)

tube; the greater the amount of precipitate formed, the greater the concentration of antigen. If a double diffusion method is used to detect antibody, a fixed amount of known reagent antigen is used.

Precipitation Reactions in Gel

In other passive diffusion methods, gel is used as a semisolid medium. Gel is a gelatinous colloid in which a solid is dispersed in a liquid. Typically less than 1% of the total is the solid, and heat is required to dissolve the solid and to trap the liquid, creating the semisolid. The gel contains pores that allow the movement of molecules. In immunoprecipitation reactions, the gel is a derivative of agar and is called agarose. Agar is a complex sulfated polysaccharide derived from algae. Agar can be purified into agaropectin, containing carboxylic acid and acid sulfate side chains, and agarose, containing few ionizable groups. Agarose is preferred in immunologic reactions because its neutral nature does not interface with the antigen or antibody reactants, and it has low endos-

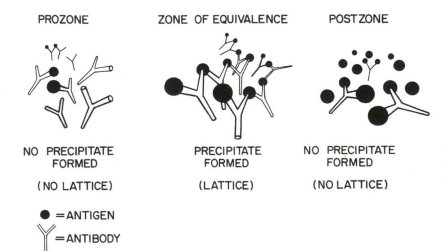

PROZONE   ZONE OF EQUIVALENCE   POSTZONE

NO PRECIPITATE FORMED   PRECIPITATE FORMED   NO PRECIPITATE FORMED

(NO LATTICE)   (LATTICE)   (NO LATTICE)

● =ANTIGEN

Y =ANTIBODY

FIGURE 11-2

The amount of precipitation in each of the zones of the precipitation curve is determined by the amount of lattice formed. In the prozone, little or no precipitate is formed; antibody excess prevents crosslinking of antigen molecules. In the zone of equivalence, precipitate is formed because the lattice is large and insoluble. In the postzone, little or no precipitate is formed because lattice formation does not occur in antigen excess.

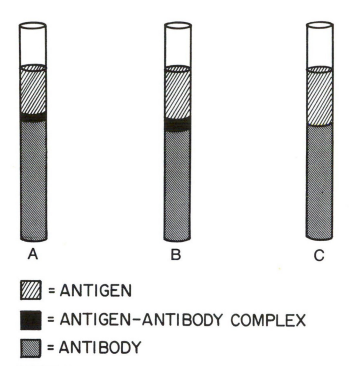

= ANTIGEN

= ANTIGEN–ANTIBODY COMPLEX

= ANTIBODY

FIGURE 11-3

The antigen and antibody solutions are placed on top of each other in a capillary tube. After diffusion the antigen and antibody precipitate in the zone of equivalence. In samples **A** and **B**, some precipitate is formed at the interface, with **B** having more than **A**. In sample **C** there is no precipitate.

mosis.[3] Agarose gel allows soluble antigen and/or antibody to diffuse through the pores until the antigen and antibody reach the optimal concentration for lattice formation. The molecular size determines the rate of diffusion through the gel. In general, smaller molecules move through the gel faster than larger molecules. A mixture of antigens and/or antibodies may result in several precipitin lines; each antigen and the corresponding antibody will form a lattice in its zone of equivalence. The diffusion rate also depends on temperature, gel viscosity and hydration, electroendosmotic effect, and the interactions between the gel matrix and reactants.

DOUBLE DIFFUSION

The Ouchterlony technique is a double diffusion method in which both the antigen and antibody diffuse in a gel. Agarose gel is placed on a solid surface

(such as a petri dish, glass slide, or plastic plate) and allowed to solidify. Wells are cut into the gel and the agarose plug is removed. Typically a central well is surrounded by multiple wells. If antigen is to be detected, a known reagent antibody is placed in the center well and the unknown samples are placed in the surrounding wells. If antibody is to be detected, unknown antigen is placed in the center. After each of *wrong.* the samples and reagent have added to the appropriate wells diffusion occurs, and a line of precipitation forms at the zone of equivalence. If multiple wells of antigen are positioned around an antibody well on the same plate, several patterns of reactivity may be observed (Fig. 11-4). In Figure 11-4A, if antigen a is the same as antigen b, the reaction of each with the antibody will be the same. The result is a solid, continuous, smooth line of identity between the antigen wells and the antibody well. If antigen a is different from antigen b and both react with the antibody, as shown is Figure 11-4B, the precipitin lines cross and a double spur is formed; this is a line of nonidentity. Each antigen-antibody lattice forms its own distinct precipitin line. Because both antigens and antibodies are diffusing in all directions, the two lines cross where each antigen-antibody complex is in its own zone of equivalence. If antigen a and antigen b share a common element but are not exactly the same, a single spur is formed. This is the line of partial identity, as seen in Figure 11-4C. If antigen a and antigen b share amino acids or sugars in a particular sequence, the antibody can react with both antigens. The spur is formed when the antibody reacts with the more simple antigen to form a precipitin line; additional antibodies react with the more complex (or "true") antigen as it migrates through this line. In Figure 4C the "spur" points to the well containing antigen a, which is the simple antigen.[1]

This technique has been used in the clinical laboratory to detect antibodies to specific nuclear components in autoimmune diseases such as systemic lupus erythematosus. This can be used to qualitatively detect the presence of the antibody, and serial dilutions can react to establish a titer.

Sources of error in the double diffusion technique include irregular patterns caused by the overfilling of wells, irregular well punching, and nonlevel incuba-

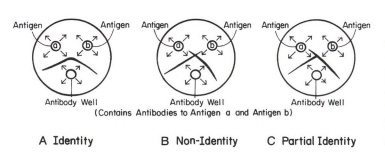

A Identity   B Non-Identity   C Partial Identity

FIGURE 11-4

(**A**) Antigens a and b are identical. Where the lines of precipitate come together on the plate, a smooth curve is formed. (**B**) Antigens a and b are not the same. In the area on the plate where the two antigens may react with antibody, the lines of precipitate will cross through each other. (**C**) Antigens a and b are similar but not completely identical. Where the lines of precipitate join, the line is not completely smooth. The spur points to the simpler antigen.

tion. Other problems may include gel drying, so that the gel is not as porous, and increased room temperature, which causes greater diffusion. Antigen or antibody degradation caused by bacterial or fungal contamination will result in diminished precipitation. Considering the lattice theory, antigen or antibody excess may yield false negative results. This may be partially overcome by using several concentrations of both antigens and antibodies, so that the combination will be in the zone of equivalence.

RADIAL IMMUNODIFFUSION

A commonly used gel precipitation technique is that of radial immunodiffusion (RID) (Fig. 11-5). In this technique antiserum is added to the liquified gel, which is poured into a plate and allowed to solidify by cooling to room temperature. The antiserum should be monospecific, have high affinity and avidity, and excellent precipitating ability; generally, IgG antibodies are best. The antigen is added to wells cut into the agar. The antigen diffuses in all directions from the well, and the precipitate is a concentric ring. The incubation time for the diffusion depends on the molecular weight of the antigen; larger molecules diffuse more slowly, requiring more time for full diffusion and maximum precipitin ring formation.

Radial immunodiffusion can be constructed with one of two incubation times—the kinetic diffusion, or Fahey,[4] method and the endpoint diffusion, or Mancini,[5] method. Regardless of which method is performed, three standards are used—generally a high concentra-

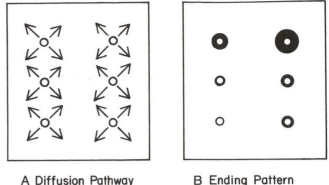

A Diffusion Pathway   **B Ending Pattern**

FIGURE 11-5
(**A**) The antigen is placed in the well; it diffuses into the agarose in all directions. (**B**) The area around the well where precipitation occurs is the area of the zone of equivalence between the antigen and antibody. The diameter of the area of precipitation (including the well diameter) is measured to determine the concentration of antigen.

tion, a normal concentration, and a low concentration. In the kinetic diffusion method, the diameter of the precipitin rings is measured at 18 hours. The logarithm of the concentration of the standards is proportional to the diameter of the precipitin ring. Using semilogarithmic paper, the y axis is the analyte concentration and the x axis is the diameter of the ring (including the well diameter). The standard values are plotted and a line is drawn point to point. The analyte concentration of the patient and the control sera may be read from the graph. Figure 11-6 is an example of a kinetic diffusion graph.

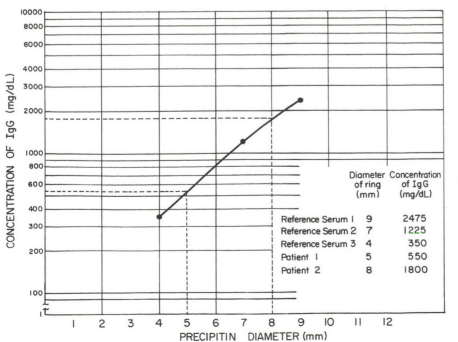

	Diameter of ring (mm)	Concentration of IgG (mg/dL)
Reference Serum 1	9	2475
Reference Serum 2	7	1225
Reference Serum 3	4	350
Patient 1	5	550
Patient 2	8	1800

FIGURE 11-6
In the kinetic radial immunodiffusion method, the diameter of the ring is plotted versus the concentration on semilogarithmic graph paper. Values of high, normal, and low reference samples are plotted, and the points are connected. Concentrations of unknown samples may be determined using this graph. For example, if the patient sample has a diameter of 5 mm, the sample contains 550 mg/dL of IgG. If the patient sample has a diameter of 8 mm, the sample contains 1800 mg/dL.

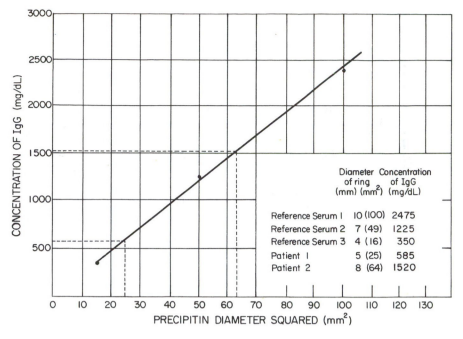

	Diameter of ring (mm) (mm²)	Concentration of IgG (mg/dL)
Reference Serum 1	10 (100)	2475
Reference Serum 2	7 (49)	1225
Reference Serum 3	4 (16)	350
Patient 1	5 (25)	585
Patient 2	8 (64)	1520

FIGURE 11-7

In the endpoint method, the square of the diameter of the ring is plotted against the concentration of antigen on linear graph paper. Values of high, normal, and low reference samples are plotted and the line of best fit is drawn. Concentrations of unknown samples may be determined using this graph. For example, if the patient sample has a diameter of 5 mm, the sample contains 585 mg/dL of IgG. If the patient sample has a diameter of 8 mm, the sample contains 1520 mg/dL of IgG.

In the endpoint method the antigen is allowed to diffuse fully to achieve maximal precipitation. The time needed varies, depending on the molecular weight of the protein being measured. For example, IgG quantitation requires a 48-hour incubation, whereas IgM requires a 72-hour incubation. Using linear graph paper, the concentration of antigen is plotted on the y axis and the diameter squared of the precipitin ring is plotted on the x axis. The points are connected by the line of best fit (Fig. 11-7). The concentration of the unknown sera is read from this graph.

Patient values can be obtained only if the precipitin ring of the patient sample is within the range of measured rings for the standard sera. Only valid readings are obtained between the highest and lowest standards. If the patient results are outside of these limits, the assay must be repeated. If the diameter of the precipitin ring of the patient sample is greater than that of the highest reference serum, the line should not be extended to obtain the patient concentration, since linearity above the reference line cannot be guaranteed. It is recommended that the serum be diluted with normal saline and the assay repeated. The result obtained should be multiplied by the dilution factor. If the diameter of the precipitin ring of the patient sample is below the lowest reference standard, the results should be reported as less than the standard value or the sample should be assayed on a low-level plate. A low-level plate contains less antibody in the gel so that lower concentrations of antigen are detected.[7]

Sources of error include overfilling or underfilling the wells, spilling the serum on the gel, nicking the side of the well when filling, and improper incubation time and temperature. These will all lead to inaccurate quantitation, requiring the sample to be reassayed (Fig. 11-8).

COUNTERCURRENT IMMUNOELECTROPHORESIS

A third precipitin reaction in gel is countercurrent immunoelectrophoresis (CIEP). Gel is poured onto a plate and cooled. Two columns of wells are cut and evacuated; antigen is place in one well and the antibody is placed in the other well. The plate is placed in an electric field, causing migration of the antigen and antibody based on charge. At pH 8.6 the antigen will migrate toward the anode and the antibody toward the cathode.

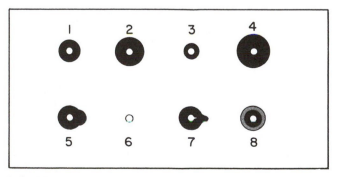

FIGURE 11-8

Ring patterns on a RID plate should be equal around the well. In this figure, wells 1 through 4 are normal. Well 5 has more precipitate on one side, which indicates that some of the sample spilled on the gel. There is no precipitate around well 6, which indicates that the well was not filled, was underfilled, or that the sample contained little or no analyte. Well 7 has an irregular shape on one side, which indicates that the well was nicked during filling. Well 8 is an example of double precipitin rings.

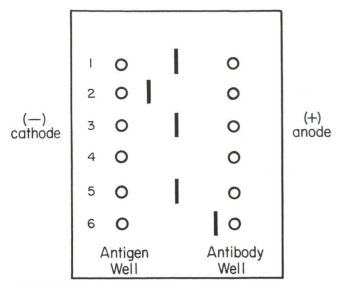

FIGURE 11-9

In countercurrent electrophoresis, antigen and antibody wells are placed opposite each other. In this figure, unknown antigen is detected using known reagent antibody. The plate is electrophoresed and a precipitin line is formed at the zone of equivalence, which may not always be midway between the two wells. Samples 1, 3, and 5 have antigen present and in equal concentration to the known antibody. Sample 2 has antigen present, but at a lower concentration than the antibody. Sample 4 has no antigen present. Sample 6 has antigen present at higher concentration than the antibody.

At equivalence, precipitation occurs (Fig. 11-9). The electric field increases the rate of migration of the antigen and antibody, thereby accelerating the visibility of the precipitate. This qualitative procedure is used to detect autoantibodies, antibodies to infectious agents, and certain microbial antigens.[3,8]

This method can be semiquantitative by using serial dilutions. If the antigen is diluted and the concentration of antibody is constant, the precipitin line moves closer to the antibody well as the concentration of antigen increases. The antibody may be diluted instead of the antigen, with the line of precipitation moving toward the antigen well.

Sources of error are related either to electrophoresis or precipitation. One electrophoresis error is the reversal of the wells so that the current is applied in the wrong direction. The antigen and antibody migrate to the edge of the plate rather than the center. Other problems associated with the electrophoresis technique are improper pH of the buffer, which may alter the net charge of the antigens and antibodies, thus affecting migration, and insufficient electrophoresis time, which will not allow complete migration to occur. As with other precipitation methods, there will be no or reduced precipitate in the prozone or postzone. When the plate is prepared, it is important that the two lines of wells are parallel so that the antigen and antibody migration paths meet.

IMMUNOELECTROPHORESIS

Immunoelectrophoresis (IEP) is another gel electrophoretic technique commonly performed in the clinical immunology laboratory. This procedure uses both electrophoresis and double diffusion (Fig. 11-10). Patient serum is placed in a well and electrophoresed. The parameters of IEP are the same as serum protein electrophoresis so that the separation is the same. Albumin migrates toward the anode and the immunoglobulins migrate to the α_2, β, and γ globulin regions.[2,9] Anti-human serum is place in the trough, and the antiserum and the separated patient proteins diffuse toward each other.

Precipitin arcs form at the zone of equivalence between the antigen and specific antisera. Anti–total human serum is a mixture of antibodies against all serum proteins and produces many precipitin arcs. If a nonspecific antiserum is place in the trough, then only one arc will be formed if the particular serum component is present. The plate may be stained and photographed. The precipitation patterns of identity, nonidentity, and partial identity are observed. A normal control serum is performed simultaneously, so that the two may be compared.

This procedure is relatively insensitive to the antigen/antibody ratio, so it has been used to detect free light chains in antigen excess. It can also be used to

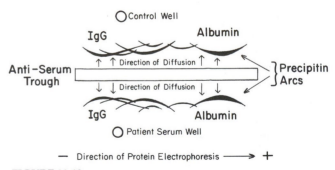

FIGURE 11-10

The first step required to form a precipitin arc in immunoelectrophoresis is to separate proteins in patient and control sera. The proteins migrate to the same area as in routine protein electrophoresis (Fig. 8-1). The second step requires total anti-human serum, which contains specific antibodies to different serum proteins to be added to the trough and allowed to diffuse through the gel. Wherever the patient or control sera and each specific antibody in the total anti–human serum are in the zone of equivalence, a precipitin arc is formed. The relative serum protein concentration determines the size of the arc. For example, the anti-albumin in the trough diffuses toward the albumin of the patient control serum. Where the two meet, the precipitin arc forms. Because more albumin is present than IgG in normal serum, the size of the arc for albumin is larger than that for IgG.

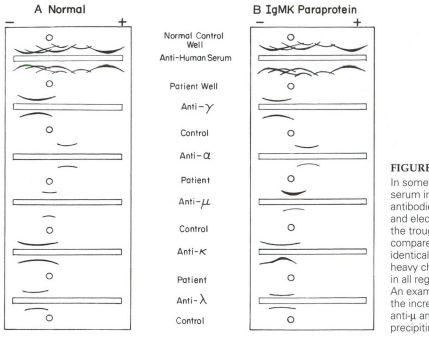

A Normal   B IgMK Paraprotein

Normal Control
Well
Anti-Human Serum

Patient Well

Anti-γ

Control

Anti-α

Patient

Anti-μ

Control

Anti-κ

Patient

Anti-λ

Control

FIGURE 11-11

In some cases more information may be obtained from serum immunoelectrophoresis by using monospecific antibodies. In each case, the sample is placed in the well and electrophoresed; monospecific antiserum is placed in the trough. (**A**) An example of normal patient serum compared with the control serum. The two patterns are identical. Because the κ and λ chains are found on all heavy chains, the arc formed with κ and λ antisera will be in all regions where IgG, IgM, IgA, and IgD are found. (**B**) An example of a patient with the IgM κ paraprotein. Note the increase in the precipitin arc of the patient serum with anti-μ and anti-κ antiserum when compared with the precipitin arcs of the control.

screen for abnormalities in immunoglobulin classes (Fig. 11-11). Because the size of the arc indicates the amount of immunoglobulin present, the procedure is semiquantitative.[3,9] The shape and position of precipitin arcs provide clues as to the monoclonality of a protein. Sources of error associated with this procedure include prolonged diffusion, which results in artifacts, especially at the anode and cathode. Excess antibody may result in multiple concentric arcs that could be mistaken for multiple antigen reactions.

IEP may also be used to identify urine proteins. Urine is placed in the well and electrophoresed, troughs are filled with antisera, and diffusion occurs. Free light chains and intact immunoglobulin molecules can be characterized (Fig. 11-12).

IMMUNOFIXATION ELECTROPHORESIS

Immunofixation electrophoresis (IFE) is another gel electrophoretic technique useful in the clinical laboratory.

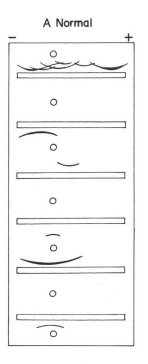
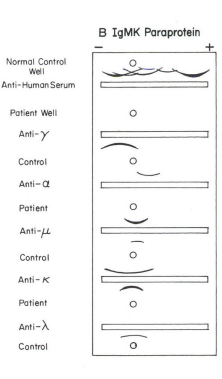

A Normal   B IgMK Paraprotein

Normal Control
Well
Anti-Human Serum

Patient Well

Anti-γ

Control

Anti-α

Patient

Anti-μ

Control

Anti-κ

Patient

Anti-λ

Control

FIGURE 11-12

Urine immunoelectrophoresis from the same two patients whose sera were evaluated in Figure 11-11 are shown here. (**A**) Normally urine contains little protein; therefore, no precipitin arcs are formed. The control used in this procedure is normal human serum. (**B**) The patient urine has increased μ and κ precipitin arcs compared with the control. This is consistent with the serum findings in Figure 11-11. No other arcs are formed because no other urine proteins are present in detectable quantities.

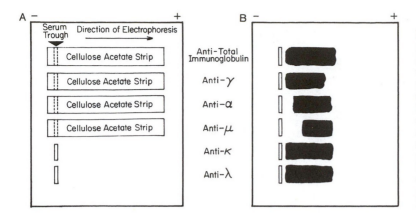

FIGURE 11-13

(**A**) After gel electrophoresis on the serum, urine, or cerebrospinal fluid, cellulose acetate strips impregnated with antiserum are placed on the gel. There should be no bubbles between the strip and the gel so that the antiserum can completely diffuse into the gel. (**B**) After incubation to allow for diffusion, the cellulose acetate strips are removed and the precipitin bands are stained. As with other electrophoresis procedures, the stained area identifies the location of the specific protein as it would be found on routine protein electrophoresis. Because the κ and λ light chains are usually associated with all heavy-chain classes, the anti-κ and anti-λ reactions will occur in all regions where immunoglobulin has been electrophoresed.

Serum, urine, or cerebrospinal fluid (CSF) are electrophoresed, followed by the application of antisera. A cellulose acetate strip impregnated with the antiserum is placed on the separated proteins (Fig. 11-13). The antiserum diffuses into the gel rapidly, resulting in the precipitation of antigen-antibody complexes.[10] The resolution of IFE is greater than that of IEP. Compared with IEP, the IFE technique is more sensitive to the antigen/antibody ratio. In IFE serum dilution or antiserum dilution is necessary to produce the precipitin reaction. The dilution depends on the size of the monoclonal band in high-resolution protein electrophoresis. Urine and CSF must be concentrated to be in the zone of equivalence; typically urine is concentrated 25 times and CSF is concentrated 50 to 100 times. If there are air bubbles when the cellulose acetate is applied to the gel, diffusion cannot occur at these points and a precipitation reaction may be missed.

ROCKET TECHNIQUE

Another electrophoretic precipitation technique, used primarily in research and coagulation laboratories, is the rocket, or Laurell, technique. This technique is used to quantitate antigens other than immunoglobulins. Antiserum is incorporated into the gel. The unknown antigen is placed in the well and electrophoresed. As the antigen migrates through the gel, it combines with antibody. Precipitation occurs along the lateral boundaries and resembles a rocket (Fig. 11-14). The total distance of antigen migration and precipitation is directly proportional to the antigen concentration.[9]

As previously discussed, a variety of procedures may be used in the clinical and research laboratories using precipitation techniques. The specific methodology used depends on the concentration of the antigen and whether quantitation is necessary. Table 11-2 summarizes some of these tests and which procedure may be used for each. Table 11-3 summarizes the advantages and disadvantages of each procedure.

APPLICATIONS

Radial Immunodiffusion

RID procedures may be used for the quantitation of immunoglobulins, including subclasses of IgG, complement components, and other serum proteins. Many

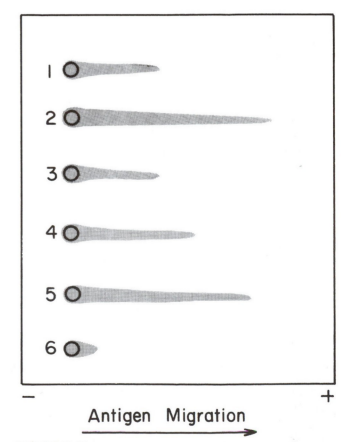

Antigen Migration

FIGURE 11-14

In the Laurell rocket technique, the gel contains a specific antiserum. The samples are electrophoresed. The area where the antigen and antibody are in the zone of equivalence will show precipitation. The rocket area may be quantitated. Sample 2 has the highest concentration of antigen; sample 6 has the least amount.

TABLE 11-2
Test Procedures Using Precipitation Techniques

TEST	METHOD
Antibodies to nuclear antigens	Double diffusion
Immunoglobulin quantitation	RID
IgG, total and subclasses	
IgA	
IgM	
IgD	
Complement proteins	RID
C3	
C4	
Microbial antigens	CIEP
Monoclonal proteins	IEP and IFE
(serum, urine, and cerebrospinal fluid)	
Coagulation factors	Rocket technique

RID, radial immunodiffusion; CIEP, countercurrent immunoelectrophoresis; IEP, immunoelectrophoresis; IFE, immunofixation electrophoresis.

small laboratories use this quantitative method because no capital equipment is needed. The only problem is the time required for the assay and the additional time needed if the results are outside of the standard limits.[7] Currently, the majority of IgG subclasses are performed using RID. In larger institutions, RID has been replaced by nephelometry. Immunoglobulin classes and complement component concentrations may be obtained in minutes rather than the hours or days required for RID. Both methods are accurate and reproducible.

Immunoelectrophoresis

The IEP procedures may be used to qualitatively identify monoclonal proteins, including free κ and λ chains. In this procedure, the antigen and antibody ratios are not critical. In addition to free κ and λ chains, all immunoglobulin classes may be detected in both serum and urine. This test is especially useful to evaluate hypergammaglobulinemia, such as in multiple myeloma. Some indications of an immunoglobulin disorder are increased sedimentation rate, the presence of rouleaux or immature plasma cells on the peripheral smear, proteinuria, and increased CSF protein without evidence of inflammation.[10] This test is semiquantitative because the concentration of the protein is proportional to the amount of precipitate formed in the arc. The patient serum or urine results are compared with the normal control results.

Immunofixation Electrophoresis

Like IEP, IFE may be used to detect the presence of immunoglobulins in serum and urine. This procedure is also used to determine if an immunoglobulin disorder exists. In many laboratories, IEP or IFE is performed, although some laboratories perform both procedures.[10]

TABLE 11-3
Advantages and Disadvantages of Precipitation Techniques

TECHNIQUE	ADVANTAGES	DISADVANTAGES
Capillary tube precipitation	Easy to set up	Insensitive
		Reaction time long
		Semiquantitative
Radial immunodiffusion (RID)	Sensitive	Reaction time long (kinetic: 18 hr; endpoint: 48 hr)
	Quantitative	Can detect only one antigen/plate
Double diffusion (Ouchterlony)	Can detect similarities among antigens	Semiquantitative
		Reaction time long
Countercurrent immunoelectrophoresis (CIEP)	More rapid reaction than other tests	Semiquantitative
Immunoelectrophoresis (IEP)	Sensitive	Semiquantitative
	Less problem with antigen/antibody ratio	
Immunofixation electrophoresis (IFE)	Sensitive	Semiquantitative
	Can detect genetic variations among antigens	Antigen/antibody ratio important
Rocket technique (Laurell)	Rapid reaction time	Can detect only one antigen/plate
	Quantitative	

Review Questions

1. The precipitation reaction is a serologic method in which

   a. soluble antigen reacts with solid-phase antibody
   b. soluble antibody reacts with solid-phase antigen
   c. lattice formations result from soluble antigen and soluble antibody
   d. electrophoresis is required

2. Which procedure is quantitative?

   a. CIEP
   b. IEP
   c. IFE
   d. RID

3. Why must urine be concentrated 25-fold in order for the IFE technique to be accurate?

   a. to prevent prozone
   b. to provide the appropriate salt concentration
   c. to allow better electrophoretic separation
   d. to minimize the volume of antiserum needed

4. In a double diffusion reaction in gel, structurally similar antigens react with monospecific antibody. The expected pattern is

   a. identity
   b. partial identity
   c. nonidentity
   d. double identity

5. Which statement describes the endpoint RID assay?

   1. The antigen fully diffuses.
   2. Timing is critical: 18 hours.
   3. d² versus concentration on linear graph paper.
   4. Establish the line by connecting the points plotted from the standards.
      a. 1 and 3 are correct.
      b. 2 and 4 are correct.
      c. 1, 2, and 3 are correct.
      d. All are correct.

References

1. Barrett JT: Textbook of Immunology, 5th ed, p 292. St Louis, CV Mosby, 1988
2. Stansfield WD: Serology and immunology: A clinical approach, p 1335. New York, Macmillan, 1981
3. Karcher RE, Epstein E: Electrophoresis. In Burtis CA, Ashwood ER (eds): Tietz Fundamentals of Clinical Chemistry, 4th ed, p 98. Philadelphia, WB Saunders, 1996
4. Johnson AM: Immunoprecipitation gels. In Rose NR, Friedman H, Fahey JL (eds): Manual of Clinical Laboratory Immunology, 3rd ed, p 14. Washington, DC, American Society for Microbiology, 1986
5. Fahey JL, McKelvey EM: Quantitative determination of serum immunoglobulins in antibody-agar plates. J Immunol 94:84, 1986
6. Mancini G, Carbonara AO, Heremans JF: Immunochemical quantitation of antigens by single radial diffusion. Immunochemistry 2:2335, 1965
7. Check IJ, Piper M, Papadea C: Immunoglobulin quantitation. In Rose NR, DeMacario EC, Fahey JL, Friedman H, Penn GM (eds): Manual of Clinical Laboratory Immunology, 4th ed, p 71. Washington, DC, American Society for Microbiology, 1992
8. Roitt I: Essential Immunology, 6th ed, p 69. Oxford, Blackwell Scientific Publications, 1992
9. Stites DP, Rodgers RPC: Clinical laboratory methods for detections of antigens and antibodies. In Stites DP, Stobo JD, Wells JV (eds): Basic and Clinical Immunology, 6th ed, p 241. Norwalk, CT: Appleton & Lange, 1987
10. Caron J, Penn GM: Electrophoretic and immunochemical characterization of immunoglobulins. In Rose NR, DeMacario EC, Fahey JL, Friedman H, Penn GM (eds): Manual of Clinical Laboratory Immunology, 4th ed, p 84. Washington, DC, American Society for Microbiology, 1992

CHAPTER 12

Agglutination

Dorothy J. Fike

Objectives

Upon completion of the chapter, the reader will be able to:

1. Compare and contrast agglutination and precipitation reactions
2. Describe the phases of the agglutination
3. Discuss the types of agglutination reactions
4. Discuss why enhancement media may be needed in agglutination reactions
5. List five enhancement media
6. Explain how each type of enhancement media enhances the agglutination reaction
7. Explain how anti–human serum is prepared
8. Discuss the use of anti–human serum
9. Compare and contrast direct and indirect antiglobulin techniques

GENERAL CONSIDERATIONS

Agglutination is the crosslinking of a particulate or insoluble antigen with the corresponding antibody and is observed as clumping. If the particles are red blood cells, the reaction is hemagglutination. If latex particles are the insoluble particle, the reaction is latex agglutination. As in precipitation, this serologic reaction results when antigen and antibody molecules complex and form a lattice (Fig. 12-1).

Excess antibody or antigen in agglutination reactions results in the prozone and postzone, as observed in precipitation. For lattice formation to occur, the antigen must have at least two antigenic determinants.[1] Lattice formation is more rapid in agglutination than in precipitation, requiring minutes or hours compared with hours or days. Because there is an insoluble particle in the agglutination reaction, fewer antigen-antibody complexes are required to detect the reaction. Agglutination and precipitation are compared in Table 12-1.

The antibody class is also important in agglutination reactions. IgM class antibody is most effective because its large size allows the attachment of up to five antigens.[2] IgG can also agglutinate.[2] In some cases, IgG fails to agglutinate under the same conditions as IgM reactions. Altering incubation conditions allows IgG class molecules to produce an agglutination reaction.

PHASES OF AGGLUTINATION

Agglutination requires two phases: (1) specific binding of antibody to antigen and (2) lattice formation (see Fig. 12-1). Although agglutination reactions are faster

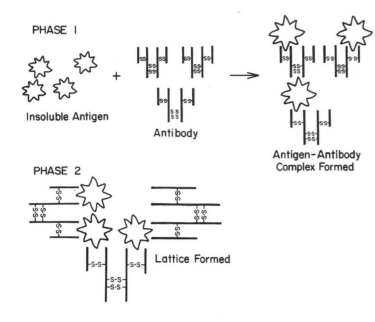

FIGURE 12-1

Agglutination reactions result in lattice formation. The lattice formation occurs in two phases. Phase 1 is the attachment of the antibody molecule to the insoluble antigen and the formation of individual antigen-antibody complexes. Phase 2 is the formation of the lattice.

than precipitation reactions, they are still qualitative tests. In qualitative test procedures, the presence of an antigen or antibody is detected, but the concentration of the analyte is not determined. Semiquantitative results are obtained from a titration. The results give the relative concentration of antigen or antibody present in the sample. Detection of a fourfold increase in antibody titer between two patient samples suggests recent antigenic stimulation. If it is necessary to know the exact concentration of antigen or antibody, other methodologies must be used. In many instances, detection of the presence of antigen or antibody and/or a rough estimate of the concentration is sufficient for diagnosis; the agglutination procedure is adequate.

Agglutination procedures may be performed in slide, tube, or microtiter formats. Figure 12-2 demonstrates the appearance of agglutination in each format.[1] In slide test procedures, the antigen-antibody reaction occurs on a glass or paper slide. Reaction time for the slide procedures is short, with most procedures requiring slide rotation for 2 to 3 minutes at room tempera-

ture. The maximum time required for a slide test procedure is the rapid plasma reagin (RPR) test for syphilis, which requires slide rotation for 8 minutes. Because the volume of antigen and antibody are small, the relatively long mixing time may lead to drying of the reactants. This drying may look like weak agglutination. In the RPR test, the card is rotated with a moist lid to prevent drying of the reactants. Although the results in the RPR test appear as clumping, this is a flocculation procedure. In flocculation antigen-antibody complexes are in suspension due to the lipid nature of the antigen. In the RPR procedure, charcoal is used to aid in the detection of the flocculent, as the antigen-antibody lattice traps the charcoal particles.

Tube test reactions generally require a longer incubation period and may be incubated at 4°C, room temperature, or 37°C. The incubation time ranges from 15 minutes to overnight. Microtiter techniques are generally adaptations of tube test procedures. The major advantage of microtiter techniques is that small volumes of sample and reagents are required.

TABLE 12-1
Comparison of Agglutination and Precipitation Reactions

AGGLUTINATION	PRECIPITATION
Insoluble or particulate antigen or antibody	Soluble antigen and antibody
Antigen must have at least two antigenic determinants	Antigen must have at least two antigenic determinants
Antigen excess results in a postzone reaction	Antigen excess results in a postzone reaction
Antibody excess results in a prozone reaction	Antibody excess results in a prozone reaction
Reaction time: minutes to hours	Reaction time: hours to days
Test results: qualitative or semiquantitative	Test results: qualitative, semiquantitative, or quantitative

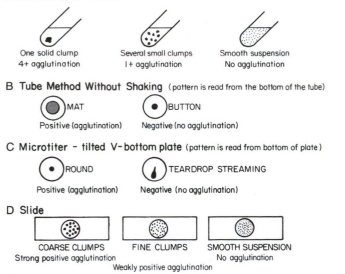

A Shaken Tube Method

One solid clump
4+ agglutination

Several small clumps
1+ agglutination

Smooth suspension
No agglutination

B Tube Method Without Shaking (pattern is read from the bottom of the tube)

MAT
Positive (agglutination)

BUTTON
Negative (no agglutination)

C Microtiter - tilted V-bottom plate (pattern is read from bottom of plate)

ROUND
Positive (agglutination)

TEARDROP STREAMING
Negative (no agglutination)

D Slide

COARSE CLUMPS
Strong positive agglutination

FINE CLUMPS
Weakly positive agglutination

SMOOTH SUSPENSION
No agglutination

FIGURE 12-2

Agglutination reaction procedures may be performed using test tubes, microtiter plates, or slides; reaction patterns for each are shown. **(A)** Test tubes may be shaken and the amount of agglutination observed. In some reactions the antigen-antibody lattice formation results in one solid clump, a 4+ reaction. In other reactions, more than one clump results when the tube is shaken. If there are many small clumps, this is a 1+ reaction. A negative reaction is a completely smooth suspension of the particles or cells. **(B)** In some procedures, the tube is not shaken and the pattern of reactivity is read from the bottom of the tube. If a mat is formed, agglutination has occurred. If there is a button, no agglutination has occurred. **(C)** When a V-bottom microtiter plate is tilted, a round pattern indicates the presence of agglutination; a teardrop shape indicates that no agglutination has occurred. **(D)** Coarse clumps in a slide procedure indicate strong positive agglutination. Fine clumps occur in a weak agglutination, and a smooth suspension of particles indicates that no agglutination has occurred.

CLASSIFICATION OF AGGLUTINATION REACTIONS

Direct Agglutination

There are three major types of agglutination reactions: direct, passive (indirect), and viral hemagglutination.[3] Direct agglutination uses naturally occurring antigens on the surface of cells, such as red blood cells or bacteria. Human red cell antigens (blood groups) are very diverse, with more than 600 antigens that have been identified. The ABO and Rh systems contain the most important red blood cell antigens. ABO antigens are found on all cells in the body. If the individual lacks a particular ABO antigen, antibodies against that antigen will develop in response to naturally encountered antigens that share a similar epitope as the human ABO antigen. The detection of antigens of the ABO system and the corresponding antibodies is important in blood and tissue transplantation (Table 12-2). The Rh antigen is important because it is highly antigenic and the antibody can be a major cause of hemolytic disease in the newborn.

Red blood cells may be used to detect antibodies to infectious agents. One serologic test, the cold agglutinin test, uses adult human group O red blood cells to detect antibodies produced in response to *Mycoplasma pneumoniae*. Following a recent infection, antibodies to *M. pneumoniae* will react with the I antigen found on human red cells with a titer >32. This is an example of a heterophile antibody. Heterophile antibodies are produced in response to one antigen yet can react with a second antigen from a phylogenetically different species.

Another direct hemagglutination test uses the antigens expressed on horse, sheep, or beef red blood cells to detect another type of heterophile antibody in human serum. In infectious mononucleosis and serum sickness, heterophile antibodies react with horse, sheep, or beef blood cells. If not specified differently, heterophile antibodies refer to those associated with infectious mononucleosis.

Bacterial natural antigens have been used to demonstrate a recent infection by measuring the titer of antibody against a specific species of microorganism.[3] Febrile agglutinins are antibodies produced in response to bacterial infections in which fever is a prominent feature. The Widal test uses *Salmonella* bacteria to detect antibodies in typhoid and paratyphoid fevers. In this

TABLE 12-2
ABO Antigens and Antibodies

GROUP	ANTIGEN PRESENT	ANTIBODIES PRESENT	ABLE TO RECEIVE TRANSPLANT FROM
O	None	Anti-A Anti-B	Group O
A	A	Anti-B	Group O Group A
B	B	Anti-A	Group O Group B
AB	A and B	None	All blood groups

test procedure, antibodies to both H antigens (flagellar antigens) and O antigens (somatic antigens found in the cell wall) are detected. Other febrile agglutinins are detected following infection with *Brucella*, *Francisella*, and *Bordetella*. The Weil-Felix reaction has been used to detect antibodies in rickettsial diseases, such as Rocky Mountain spotted fever. Rickettsial antibodies crossreact with and agglutinate subspecies of *Proteus vulgaris*. (This is another type of heterophile antibody.) Because these direct agglutination tests lack sensitivity and specificity, other procedures are recommended to provide serologic evidence of a recent infection.[1,4]

Antibodies to a specific bacterial antigen may be used to identify the bacteria. In this procedure, known specific bacteria antisera are used to detect the bacterial antigen in a patient specimen or culture.[1,4,5]

Viral Hemagglutination

Viral hemagglutination, a natural phenomenon, occurs when a virus, such as the rubella or influenza virus, agglutinates red blood cells by binding to receptors on the red blood cell surface. Most commonly, viral hemagglutination inhibition tests are used to detect the presence of patient antibody. In this reaction, antibody inhibits the virus from agglutinating the red blood cells.[5]

Passive and Reverse Passive Agglutination

The third type of agglutination reaction is passive agglutination (or indirect agglutination), in which the antigen is attached to a particle. When antibody is attached to a particle, the technique is reverse passive agglutination.

Particles used in clinical laboratory tests are charcoal, latex particles, gelatin particles, and red blood cells. Some antigens, such as lipopolysaccharide, endotoxin, DNA, and penicillin, attach to the red cell membrane spontaneously. Other antigens, especially proteins, adsorb onto red cells only after the cells have been treated to increase the cell membrane reactivity. Most often, red cells are treated with tannic acid or chromic chloride, so that additional protein will adhere to the cell. Antigens adsorbed onto the surface of the red cell membrane must not be released during the antigen-antibody reaction. Generally, this problem has been evaluated and is controlled by the manufacturer.[1]

Latex particles and charcoal are inert substances that must have a minimum size for agglutination reactions. This is controlled in the manufacturing process. For clinical testing latex is a 0.81-μm diameter polystyrene polymer sphere. Polystyrene is an inert colloid with a negative charge that adsorbs protein. Because different proteins adsorb onto latex particles in varying degrees, optimal coating of the particle is necessary to yield maximal agglutination. Charcoal consists of inert carbon molecules onto which protein may adsorb.[1]

Passive agglutination procedures can be used to detect rheumatoid factor, rubella antibody, and thyroglobulin antibody. In each specific test procedure, the particle with adsorbed antigen is used to detect antibody semiquantitatively or qualitatively. As in direct agglutination, the test format may be slide, tube, or microtiter techniques. These tests are summarized in Table 12-3.

Latex particles and red cells may also be used to detect antigen in the reverse passive agglutination procedure. Antibody is attached to the particle, and agglutination occurs when specific antigen is present.

TABLE 12-3
Tests Using Agglutination Techniques

TEST	DETECTING ANTIGEN OR ANTIBODY	INSOLUBLE PARTICLE	TYPE OF TECHNIQUE
Rapid plasma reagin (syphilis)	Antibody	Charcoal with lecithin—cardiolipin–cholesterol antigen	Flocculation (passive)
Cold agglutinin (primary atypical pneumonia)	Antibody	Human group O red cells (natural I antigen on red cells)	Agglutination (direct)
Febrile agglutinins Widal Weil-Felix (*Rickettsia*) *Francisella* *Brucella*	Antibody	Bacteria (natural antigens) *Salmonella typhi* and *S. paratyphi* *Proteus vulgaris* *Francisella tularensis* *Brucella abortus*	Agglutination (direct)
Infectious mononucleosis (heterophile)	Antibody	Sheep, horse, or beef red cells (natural heterophile antigens)	Agglutination (direct)
Rheumatoid factor	Antibody	Latex particle with human IgG attached	Agglutination (passive)
Rubella	Antibody	Tanned red cells with rubella antigen attached	Agglutination (passive)
Thyroglobulin	Antibody	Red cells with thyroglobulin attached	Agglutination (passive)
C-reactive protein	Antigen	Latex particle with anti-CRP attached	Reverse passive agglutination

C-reactive protein (CRP) may be detected by the reverse passive latex agglutination. Because high levels of CRP are produced during acute inflammation, the postzone is a serious source of error.

Sources of error in passive or reverse passive techniques include those stated for direct agglutination: prozone reactions, postzone reactions, and crossreactivity. In addition, false negative results are obtained if test reagents are not at the appropriate pH, the antigen or antibody is released from the particle, or the red cells are fragile. It is important for the particle to bind a high concentration of antigen or antibody so that maximal agglutination is observed.

Column Agglutination Technology

Column agglutination technology (CAT) is a new technology that enhances the reading of tube agglutination techniques. The reactants are placed in a special tube that contains glass bead microparticles, and the reactants are placed above the beads. After the reaction, the CAT tube is centrifuged. If no agglutination has occurred, the red cells are at the bottom of the CAT tube; if agglutination has occurred, the antigen-antibody complex is located between the reaction chamber and the bottom of the tube. The extent of agglutination can be semiquantitated (Fig. 12-3).[6]

Agglutination Inhibition ✳

Sometimes the direct or reverse passive agglutination procedure is inappropriate to detect the presence of an antigen. In these cases, a two-step agglutination inhibition procedure may be used. When red cells are used, the procedure is hemagglutination inhibition; if latex particles are used, it is latex agglutination inhibition. In the first step, soluble antigen in the patient sample is incubated with the antibody reagent. If the soluble antigen is present, it combines with the antibody. In the second step, a particulate antigen (a natural antigen, a red blood cell, or latex particle with an antigen attached) is added. If the antigen is present in the patient sample, it binds to the reagent antibody and prevents agglutination of the particulate antigen. This means that agglutination was inhibited and the test is positive. If no antigen is in the patient sample, reagent antibody is available to agglutinate the particulate antigen. This means that agglutination was not inhibited and the test is negative (Fig. 12-4 on p. 132).[1]

Agglutination inhibition has been used to detect soluble A, B, and H substances in body fluids for problem solving in blood banks, forensic studies involving crime scenes, and anthropologic studies of mummies. Eighty percent of the Caucasian population secretes soluble A, B, or H substances in body fluids, such as the urine, saliva, and semen. In step 1, the body fluid is incubated with known anti-A, anti-B, or anti-H antibodies. In step 2, red cells with the corresponding antigen

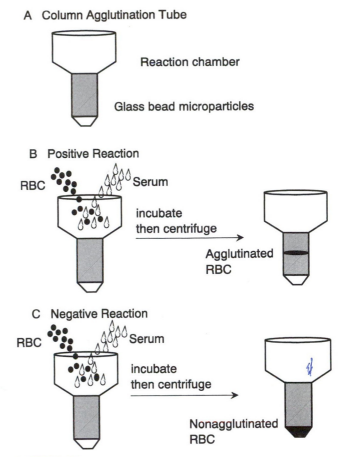

FIGURE 12-3
(A) The column agglutination technology (CAT) tube has a reaction chamber, a glass bead microparticle area, and a space for unreacted red blood cells. (B) A patient sample containing antibody, reagent red blood cells, and enhancement media is added to the reaction chamber, incubated, and centrifuged. When the lattice is too large to filter through the glass bead microparticles, a complex forms in the bead region. This is a positive reaction. (C) A patient sample without antibody, reagent red blood cells, and enhancement media is added to the reaction chamber, incubated, and centrifuged. The unagglutinated red blood cells are small enough to filter through the glass bead microparticles to the bottom of the tube. This is a negative reaction.

are added. If the soluble substance is present in the body fluid, agglutination is inhibited in step 2. If no soluble substance is present, agglutination is observed after the addition of the red cell antigens.[7] Sources of error in agglutination inhibition are the same as those found in other agglutination procedures. It is important that controls be used to identify sources of error, especially those related to reagent failure.

ADDITIONAL REAGENTS USED IN AGGLUTINATION PROCEDURES

Sometimes an agglutination reaction must be enhanced to visualize the reaction. Because red cells have a net negative charge, they repel each other (zeta potential)

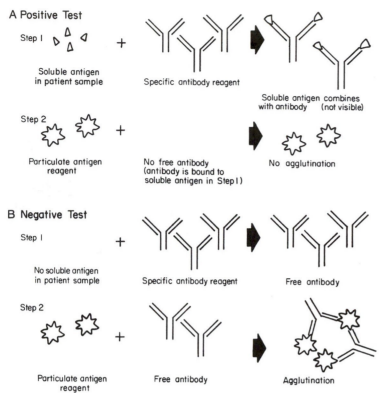

FIGURE 12-4

(A) In a positive test for agglutination inhibition, soluble antigen in the patient sample combines with the specific antibody reagent in step 1 to form soluble antigen–antibody complexes that are not visible. In step 2, when particulate antigen reagent is added there is no free antibody to react, so no agglutination occurs. (B) In a negative test, there is no antigen in the patient sample to react with the specific antibody reagent in step 1. In step 2, when particulate antigen reagent is added, the antibody from step 1 is free to react with the particulate antigen reagent to form a lattice. Agglutination will be observed.

(Fig. 12-5). IgG molecules are small and cannot link one epitope on one cell with an epitope on a second red cell. No lattice is formed, and the reaction is not visible. To overcome this spatial deficiency, enhancement media and anti–human IgG may be used to detect the presence of antibodies in the serum. Note that even with enhancement media and/or anti–human IgG reagent, an antibody-antigen reaction may still not be visible.

Enhancement Media

Enhancement media may be used to affect the first or second phase of the antigen-antibody reaction during an incubation.[8] Enhancement media include bovine albumin, low ionic strength solutions, proteolytic enzymes, polyethylene glycol, and polybrene.[9]

BOVINE ALBUMIN

Bovine albumin (22% or 30%) has been used to enhance antigen-antibody reactions since 1945. At first it was thought that albumin enhanced the uptake of antibody in phase 1 of the reaction, but it is now thought to affect the second phase of the reaction.[9]

LOW IONIC STRENGTH (SALT) SOLUTIONS

When red cells are suspended in normal saline, the sodium and chloride ions partially neutralize the charges on the antigen and antibody molecules. This shielding effect hinders the association of antibody with the antigen. When the ionic concentration is de-creased, the ability of an antibody to bind to the antigen is increased (phase 1 of the reaction).[8,9]

PROTEOLYTIC ENZYMES

Four major enzymes are used to enhance hemagglutination reactions: papain, trypsin, ficin, and bromelin. Proteolytic enzymes may be used in two different enhancement techniques. In the first technique, the enzyme is added to the patient sample and red cells, and everything is incubated together. In the second technique, the red cells are treated with the enzyme. After treatment with the enzyme, the red cells are washed to remove the enzyme. The patient sample is added to the treated red cells and incubated. The proteolytic enzymes act at phase 2 of the agglutination reaction. The enzyme removes some of the charge between the cells (reducing the zeta potential), and thus the cells are closer together and the second bond can form.[8,9]

POLYETHYLENE GLYCOL

Polyethylene glycol (PEG) is a neutral polymer that is water soluble. This potentiator appears to enhance the rate of antibody uptake.[8,9]

POLYBRENE

Polybrene is a cationic polymer that causes aggregation of red cells. This aggregation of red cells, after incubation with a low ionic solution, brings the red cells closer

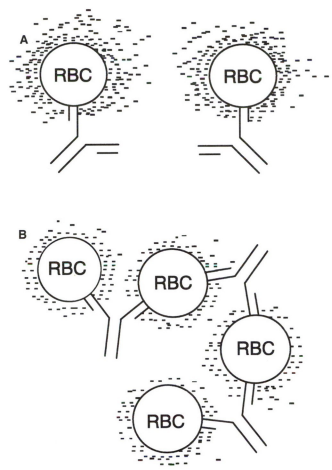

FIGURE 12-5

(A) Natural charges keeps the red blood cells apart. Some antibodies can form the first bond but cannot bridge the distance between the red blood cells for lattice formation. The charge on other antibodies prevents them from reacting in the first phase. (B) The distance between red blood cells is changed by enhancement media so lattice formation occurs.

together so that the second antigen-antibody bond can form in the second phase of the reaction. Table 12-4 provides a summary of the mode of action of enhancement media.[8,9]

TABLE 12-4
Enhancement Media

MEDIA	MODE OF ACTION
Albumin	Changes charge for phase 2 enhancement
Low ionic strength solution	Increases antibody uptake in phase 1
Polyethylene glycol	Increases antibody uptake in phase 1
Proteolytic enzyme	Decreases the distance between cells by decreasing the zeta potential; phase 2 is enhanced
Polybrene	Decreases the distance between cells by causing aggregation; phase 2 is enhanced

Anti–Human Globulin

Sometimes even the presence of enhancement media does not cause an agglutination reaction, even though both the antigen and antibody are present. Anti–human globulin can be used to detect sensitized red blood cells. Usually the antiglobulin reagent used in red cell agglutination reactions is prepared in rabbits, but anti–human globulin used in other tests may be prepared in goats, horses, or any other animal to produce a potent anti–human globulin. Rabbits (or other animals) are injected with purified human γ chains; following an immune response, rabbit anti–human IgG serum is harvested (Fig. 12-6).[10] If anti-IgM is desired, the μ chains are injected into the animal. If anti-IgA is desired, the α chains are injected into the animal and harvested. The anti–human Ig reagent may also be used in fluorescence immunoassays, radioimmunoassays, and enzyme immunoassays.

Anti–Globulin Procedures

Two specific agglutination procedures use anti–human globulin: direct and indirect. In the direct anti–human globulin test, the antigen-antibody reaction has occurred in vivo, whereas the indirect anti-globulin technique requires an in vitro incubation to sensitize the red blood cells. In both procedures the red cells are washed with isotonic saline to remove any unbound antibody. The anti–human immunoglobulin reagent is added and will bind to the human immunoglobulin on the surface of the red cell; a lattice forms and agglutination is observed (Fig. 12-7).[10]

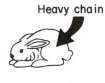

A Specific heavy chain injected into an animal

Heavy chain

B After an immune response, specific antibody is produced. The animal is bled to harvest the antibody.

Serum with antibody

RBC

C After purification, specific antiserum is available for diagnostic testing.

Anti- human heavy chain antiserum

FIGURE 12-6

(A) Anti–human globulin is prepared by injecting the IgG heavy chain (γ chain) into a rabbit or another animal. (B) After the immune response, a specific antibody is produced, and the animal is bled to obtain the antibody. (C) After purification, the specific antibody may be used for diagnostic procedures.

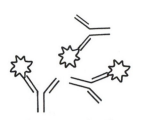

Antibody–coated antigen
without visible agglutination
(No lattice formation)

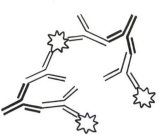

Anti–human globulin is added
which reacts with the antibody
on the antigen.

Visible agglutination occurs.
(Lattice formation)

FIGURE 12-7
(A) In some agglutination reactions, the antigen-antibody complex will not form a lattice. (B) When anti–human globulin (AHG) is added, the AHG will react with the antibody on the surface of the particle and form a lattice. Agglutination will be observed.

DIRECT ANTIGLOBULIN TECHNIQUE

The direct antiglobulin technique is performed to detect in vivo attachment of a red cell antibody to the individual's red cells. This occurs in four disease states or conditions: hemolytic disease of the newborn (HDN), autoimmune hemolytic anemia, hemolytic transfusion reactions, and drugs binding to the red cell membrane. Premature red cell destruction results in anemia. In hemolytic disease of the newborn, maternal IgG crosses the placenta; if the IgG binds to fetal red cell antigen, the cells will be destroyed. Several red cell antibodies, such as anti-D, anti-A, and anti-B, cause HDN. In autoimmune hemolytic anemia, the individual produces antibodies to autologous red cells. Generally, in hemolytic transfusion reactions, the patient has produced antibodies to previously transfused red cell antigens. When the antigen is encountered again, the antibody attaches to the cells. In drug reactions, the drug attaches to the red cell membrane; the individual now produces antibody to the drug-membrane complex. The cell will then be prematurely removed from the circulation and destroyed.[10]

INDIRECT ANTIGLOBULIN TECHNIQUE

The indirect antiglobulin procedure is performed to detect red cell antigens, to detect red cell antibodies, or to determine compatibility between the unit of blood and the patient. In these procedures, the red cells are incubated in vitro with patient serum or known antiserum to allow the antibody to bind to the antigen. After an incubation period of 10 to 60 minutes at 37°C, the red cells are washed with isotonic saline to remove any unbound antibody; anti–human Ig is added. If antigen-antibody binding has occurred during incubation, agglutination will be observed.[10]

Review Questions

1. What is the major difference between agglutination and precipitation?

   a. Agglutination detects only antigen.
   b. Precipitation is more sensitive.
   c. Agglutination requires a particle.
   d. Precipitation is quantitative.

2. Which enhancement medium acts to decrease the zeta potential by neutralizing surface charge?

   a. bovine albumin
   b. polyethylene glycol
   c. low ionic strength solution
   d. polybrene

3. In passive hemagglutination, the _____ is attached to _____.

   a. antigen; red blood cells
   b. antigen; latex particles
   c. antibody; red blood cells
   d. antibody; latex particles

4. The direct antiglobulin test detects

   a. circulating antibody
   b. antibody bound to red blood cells
   c. antiglobulin
   d. red blood cell antigens

5. Which agglutination method uses latex particles coated with anti–human CRP to detect patient CRP?

   a. passive
   b. reverse passive
   c. inhibition
   d. antiglobulin enhanced

References

1. Nicols WS, Nakamura RM: Agglutination and agglutination inhibition. In Rose NR, Friedman H, Fahey JL (eds): Manual of Clinical Laboratory Immunology, 3rd ed, p 49. Washington, DC, American Society for Microbiology, 1986

2. Barrett JT: Textbook of Immunology, 5th ed, p 313. St. Louis, CV Mosby, 1988

3. Stites DP, Rodgers MPC: Clinical laboratory methods for detection of antigens and antibodies. In Stites DP, Stobo JD, Wells JV (eds): Basic and Clinical Immunology, 6th ed, p 275. Norwalk, CT: Appleton & Lange, 1987

4. Bryant NJ: Laboratory Immunology and Serology, 3rd ed, p 171. Philadelphia, WB Saunders, 1992

5. Stansfield WD: Serology and Immunology: A Clinical Approach, p 168. New York, Macmillan, 1981

6. Reis KJ, Chachowski R, Cupido A, Davies D, Jakway J, Setcavage TM: Column agglutination technology: The antiglobulin test. Transfusion 33:639, 1993

7. Walker RH (ed): Technical Manual, 11th ed, p 625. Bethesda, MD American Association of Blood Banks, 1993

8. Walker RH (ed): Technical Manual, 11th ed, p 167. Bethesda, MD, American Association of Blood Banks, 1993

9. Walker RH (ed): Technical Manual, 11th ed, p 319. Bethesda, MD, American Association of Blood Banks, 1993

10. Walker RH (ed): Technical Manual, 11th ed, p. 175. Bethesda, MD, American Association of Blood Banks, 1993

CHAPTER 13

Assays Involving Complement

Dorothy J. Fike

Objectives

Upon completion of the chapter, the reader will be able to:

1. Discuss the tests that evaluate the function of the complement systems
2. Discuss the procedures for detecting complement component levels
3. List the approximate normal ranges for complement components
4. Discuss complement levels in disease states
5. Describe the complement fixation test

The complement system is a collection of proteins that work together to lyse cells, mediate inflammation, and aid in phagocytosis. Background information about the components, pathways, control mechanisms, and deficiencies is discussed in Chapter 4. In this chapter assays that quantitate complement components and indicate pathway activation and assays that use complement as a reagent will be presented.

EVALUATION OF COMPLEMENT

Complement components in patient serum or body fluid can be quantitated immunologically when the component reacts with monospecific antiserum. The functional activity of the complement cascade can be measured by lysing red blood cells. Some complement components—C1q, C3, C4, and C5—are heat labile, so that proper sample handling is critical. Prolonged exposure to heat will decrease complement activity and produce different complement fragments. To preserve complement activity, blood should clot for 1 hour at room temperature, and the serum should be removed and stored at $-70°C$ in small aliquots.[1,2]

Functional Assays

The CH_{50} assay (also known as the total hemolytic complement assay) measures the functional ability of serum complement components of the classical pathway to lyse sheep red blood cells (SRBCs) coated with rabbit anti-SRBC antibody. When the antibody-coated (sensitized) SRBCs are incubated with patient serum, the classical pathway of complement is activated and hemolysis results. If a complement component is absent, the CH_{50} level will be zero; if one of more components of the classical pathway are decreased, the CH_{50} will be decreased. An initial serum dilution of 1:50 or 1:60, depending on the specific method used, is serially diluted.[1,2] A fixed volume of optimally sensitized SRBCs is added to each serum dilution. After incubation, the mixture is centrifuged and the hemolysis is quantitated by measuring the absorbance of the supernatant at 540 nm.

A typical sigmoid curve obtained can be seen in Figure 13-1. Because these results do not yield a straight line, the CH_{50} titer may be obtained graphically by plotting the reciprocal of the serum dilution versus the percent lysis on semilog graph paper or by using the von Krogh transformation (Fig. 13-2). The von Krogh transformation is a graphic representation of the log of milliliters of serum versus the log of $Y/(1 - Y)$, where Y is the percent hemolysis. When $Y/(1 - Y) = 1$, 50% of the SRBCs are hemolyzed. The reciprocal of the corresponding volume of serum when $Y/(1 - Y)$ is the CH_{50} unit. The reference range of CH_{50} units varies with the analytical method used in the laboratory. If the method described by Mayer is used, the reference range is 25 to 50 U/mL; but if the method of Kent and Fife is used, the reference range is 125 to 300 U/mL. Variation in these methods and reference ranges is caused by the volume of SRBCs used, the concentration of SRBCs, and the total volume of the test solution. The method of Mayer uses 1.0 mL of 5% SRBCs in a total volume of 7.5 mL, whereas the method of Kent and Fife uses 0.6 mL of a 1% SRBCs suspension in a total volume of 1.5 mL. Regardless of the method used, each laboratory performing this test should establish its own reference range.[1]

The CH_{50} assay is a labor-intensive, demanding procedure subject to many interferences. Some SRBCs are more fragile than others, resulting in spontaneous hemolysis unrelated to the complement activity. It has been suggested that the SRBCs be from the same sheep every time the assay is performed in order to minimize this problem. The affinity of the rabbit antibody varies

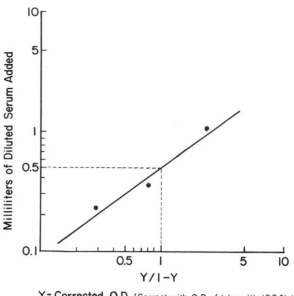

FIGURE 13-2

Because the CH_{50} cannot be calculated from the absorbance curve, a von Krogh transformation must be plotted. Y is the corrected optical density (O.D.), as corrected with the optical density of the tube with 100% lysis.

from lot to lot and from one manufacturer to another; this affects the amount of antibody that binds to the SRBCs. Also, the process of sensitizing SRBCs results in cells with differing amounts of antibody coating the SRBCs. Specimen collection and storage are important potential sources of error. To detect as many sources of error as possible, it is critical to test a control serum with a known CH_{50} value every time the assay is performed and to reproduce the accepted value of the known serum control. The total hemolytic complement assays are useful to detect inherited deficiencies or pathway activation.[1,2]

An innovative rapid method to measure CH_{50} uses liposomes that contain the enzyme glucose-6-phosphate dehydrogenase (G6PDH) and have antigen on the liposome surface (Autokit CH50, Wako Chemicals USA, Richmond, VA). The patient sample (which is the source of complement to be measured) is mixed with the reagent (which contains the liposomes nicotinamide adenine dinucleotide [NAD], and reagent antibody). The reagent antibody binds to the antigen on the liposome. Complement in the patient sample is activated by the antigen-antibody complexes and damages the liposome, releasing the enzyme. G6PDH reacts with NAD and glucose-6-phosphate in the reagent to produce NADH and β-gluconolactone-6-phosphate, respectively. The absorbance of NADH is measured at 340 nm using a spectrophotometer. The measured NADH is directly proportional to the total hemolytic complement in the sample. The results compare well with Mayer's method. This homogeneous liposome

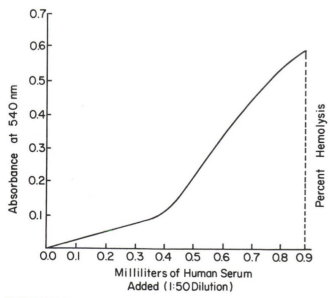

FIGURE 13-1

The CH_{50} absorbance curve. The absorbance of the hemolysis of various concentrations of a 1:50 serum dilution is read at 540 nm.

immunoassay is designed to be used on commercially available automated analyzers and, as such, is categorized as a moderately complex text.[3]

The activity of the alternative or properdin pathway of complement may be measured by modifying the CH_{50} procedure. Rabbit red blood cells are capable of initiating the alternative complement pathway. When they replace the sensitized SRBCs in the traditional CH_{50} assay, the hemolysis reflects the functional ability of the alternative pathway. Antibody and C1q are not required for activation of this pathway.[1]

Component Assays

All assays that measure individual complement components require specific antisera to react with the complement protein. Methodologies include radial immunodiffusion (RID), nephelometry, turbidimetry, radioimmunoassay, and latex agglutination photometric assay. Routinely RID or nephelometry is used to measure complement components.

Sample collection and handling are extremely important. Care must be taken to prevent activation of the complement cascade prior to the assay. In some cases, plasma is used instead of serum to ensure that the classical pathway of complement is not activated during blood coagulation. Heating and prolonged storage at 2 to 8°C will produce smaller fragments of some components.

All complement components (except Factor D) may be measured by RID. The quantity of Factor D present in the blood is too low to be measured by RID. In RID, agarose gel contains the specific antibody for the complement protein to be measured. Patient serum or plasma is placed in the well and diffuses in all directions, producing a concentric ring. The reference range of selected complement components is presented in Table 13-1.[4,5] All laboratories are advised to establish their own reference ranges because geographic and methodologic variations are known.[1] C3 and C4 levels are frequently measured using RID and may appear elevated when the component is split into smaller fragments that diffuse faster than intact molecules. The antibody in the agarose reacts with these fragments and produces a larger precipitin diameter, thus falsely elevating the results.

Nephelometry is another method commonly used to quantitate C3 and C4. The amount of C3 or C4 present is proportional to the amount of light scattered. All nephelometric systems have a high degree of automation, with sample handling and data analysis under instrument control. Nephelometric methods can detect all components of complement, including Factor D.[1]

Detection of complement activation or degradation products provides a more sensitive index of complement activation than a loss of concentration during a disease process. Radioimmunoassay is used to detect the anaphylatoxins, C3a, C4a, and C5a. Patients with rheumatoid arthritis and gout have increased levels of C3a in their synovial fluid.[1] Currently these assays are for research use only, and the measurement of the majority of complement components is limited in diagnostic value.

COMPLEMENT COMPONENTS IN DISEASE

Most frequently in disease, C3, C4, and CH_{50} are increased. C3 and C4 are acute phase reactants and are increased during acute inflammation. This increase is associated with the diseases listed in Table 13-2. In rheumatoid arthritis, systemic lupus erythematosus and other rheumatic diseases, complement is increased in the acute phase of the disease and may be decreased when complement is activated in vivo. Other conditions in which complement levels are increased during an acute phase response are myocardial infarction, viral hepatitis, cancer, and pregnancy. The increase is generally not more than twofold, which is less than the dramatic hundred-fold increase of C-reactive protein.[1,6]

TABLE 13-1
Reference Range of Some Complement Components

COMPONENT	REFERENCE RANGE
C1q	11–21 mg/dL
C3	80–180 mg/dL
C4	15–50 mg/dL
C5	7–17 mg/dL
Properdin	1.0–2.0 mg/dL
Factor B	17.5–27.5 mg/dL

TABLE 13-2
Some Disorders Associated with Increased Complement Levels

AUTOIMMUNE DISORDERS	OTHER
Rheumatoid arthritis	Gout
Ulcerative colitis	Obstructive jaundice
Diabetes mellitus	Thyroiditis
Systemic lupus erythematosus	Acute myocardial infarction
	Pregnancy
INFECTIOUS DISORDERS	Oral contraceptives
Acute rheumatic fever	
Typhoid fever	
Acute viral hepatitis	

Decreased CH_{50} levels can be related to a congenital component deficiency, in vivo consumption by antigen-antibody complexes, decreased synthesis of one or more components, increased catabolism of components, or the presence of an inhibitor (Table 13-3). Although the CH_{50} test assesses the overall function of the pathway, it is less sensitive than immunologically based component assays. The immunologic measurement of individual components better reflects changes in the serum concentration. Slight decreases in the CH_{50} value have been associated with a reduction of up to 50% in the C1, C2, or C3 levels.[6]

Complement deficiencies are rare; however, they are valuable for studying and understanding the function of the component. In general, deficiency of a specific component causes an autoimmune disease or increased infections. Most important is a deficiency of C1 inhibitor (C1INH), which causes hereditary angioedema. These individuals have repeated, potentially life-threatening episodes of edema, especially of the skin, upper respiratory tract, and gastrointestinal tract.[2,7]

Decreased serum concentrations of complement components, other than a deficiency, may be caused by hyposynthesis. Most complement components are synthesized in the liver, so that severe liver disease results in decreased complement production. Likewise, in protein calorie malnutrition, such as anorexia nervosa, complement production is decreased.

Hypercatabolism is associated with diseases that have circulating immune complexes, such as systemic lupus erythematosus, acute glomerulonephritis, malaria, rheumatoid arthritis, and pneumonococcal infections. C3 and C4 both are decreased because the classical pathway is activated by immune complexes. C4 levels are reduced first, followed by a decrease in C3 levels; this pattern occurs most frequently in systemic lupus erythematosus. The decreased complement levels reflect immune complex-mediated activation in renal disease; in rheumatoid arthritis, the component levels are decreased when immune complex-mediated vasculitis is present. The serum levels of C3 and C4 may also be normal or increased in rheumatoid arthritis when the acute phase synthesis exceeds the consumption; synovial fluid levels are usually decreased (Table 13-4).[1,2,4]

Decreased C3 levels are also found in diseases that activate the alternative pathway of complement, such as membranoproliferative glomerulonephritis, paroxysmal nocturnal hemoglobinuria, and circulating endotoxin. C4 levels are normal because this component is not activated in the alternative pathway. Some diseases can activate both pathways, thereby decreasing both C3 and C4. To distinguish activation of the classical and alternative pathways from activation of the classical pathway only, Factor B should be measured. Factor B is decreased only if the alternative pathway is activated.[1,2,4]

Two conditions deserve special consideration with respect to complement levels. In disseminated intravascular coagulation, a decreased C3 concentration is caused by the catabolism of C3 by enzymes involved in fibrinolysis, whereas C4 is unaffected. Sepsis, trauma, surgery, and neoplasm may cause disseminated intravascular coagulation. A deficiency of C1 inhibitor (C1INH), either inherited or acquired, may cause a decrease in the C4 concentration.[1,4] In normal individuals, once the classical cascade is activated, activated C1 cleaves C4 into C4a and C4b until activated C1 is inactivated by the regulatory protein, C1INH. A deficiency of C1INH prevents inactivation of C1. In the inherited form of C1INH deficiency, the C4 concentration is low, even when the patient is asymptomatic, and may become undetectable during an acute episode. The acquired form of C1INH deficiency may develop in lymphoproliferative diseases and autoimmune disease when the regulatory protein is consumed or destroyed. In either inherited or acquired C1INH, the C3 levels are normal.

TABLE 13-3
Some Disorders Associated with Decreased CH_{50} Levels

AUTOIMMUNE DISORDERS

Systemic lupus erythematosus with glomerulonephritis
Myasthenia gravis

IMMUNE DEFICIENCY DISORDERS

Severe combined immunodeficiency
Hereditary angioedema (C1INH deficiency)
Hereditary C2 deficiency

INFECTIOUS DISORDERS

Acute glomerulonephritis
Infected ventriculoarterial shunts
Infective hepatitis with arthritis

OTHER

Disseminated intravascular coagulation (DIC)
Paroxysmal cold hemoglobinuria
Allograft rejection

COMPLEMENT FIXATION

In the complement fixation technique, the test system and indicator system compete for complement binding. If complement is bound (fixed) by the antigen-antibody complex in the test system, then complement will not be available to react in the indicator system. If no antigen-antibody complex is formed in the test system, complement will be available to bind in the indicator system. The complement fixation technique can be useful in viral, rickettsial, and fungal serology. Some diseases that may be diagnosed by complement fixation are Rocky Mountain spotted fever, herpes simplex infection, and

TABLE 13-4
Diseases Associated with Decreased Levels of Complement Components

DISEASE	C3 LEVEL	C4 LEVEL
CLASSICAL PATHWAY ACTIVATION WITH CIRCULATING IMMUNE COMPLEXES	D	D
Systemic lupus erythematosus		
Glomerulonephritis		
Rheumatoid arthritis		
Pneumococcal infections		
Malaria		
ALTERNATIVE PATHWAY ACTIVATION OF C3	D	N
Membranoproliferative glomerulonephritis		
Paroxysmal nocturnal hemoglobinuria		
Circulating endotoxins		
OVERT IMMUNOLOGIC ACTIVATION: BOTH PATHWAYS ACTIVATED	D	D
TISSUE INJURY: C3 CLEAVAGE BY PROTEOLYTIC ENZYMES	D	N
Disseminated intravascular coagulation		
HEREDITARY ANGIOEDEMA (C1 INHIBITOR DEFICIENCY)	N	D

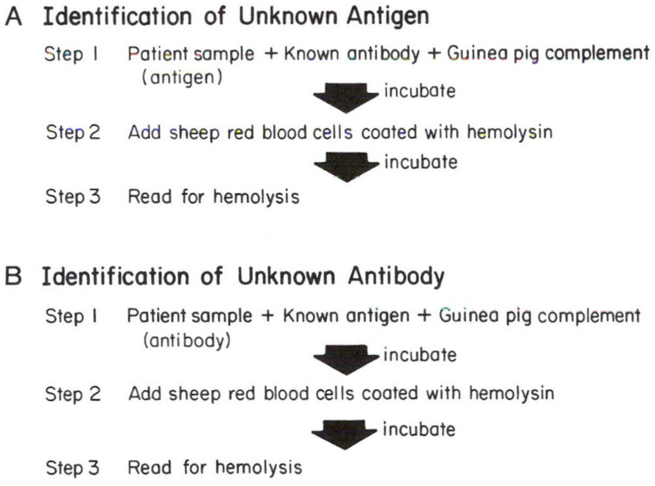

influenza. Prior to the development of radioimmunoassays and enzyme immunoassays, complement fixation procedures were the most sensitive available.

Before performing this technique, the complement present in the patient sample must be inactivated by heating at 56°C for 30 minutes. This critical step ensures that only the fresh guinea pig complement is available to react in the complement fixation test.

The complement fixation technique may be used to detect an unknown antigen or an unknown antibody in the patient sample. As seen in Figure 13-3, the procedure for antibody detection requires two steps. In the first step of the test system the test antigen is incubated with the patient serum or control serum, and fresh guinea pig complement. If the serum contains the homologous antibody, it will bind to the test antigen. Complement will then bind to the antigen-antibody complex. The second step is the incubation of the test mixture with the indicator system, sensitized SRBCs. In the presence of free complement, the indicator system results in hemolysis. The extent of hemolysis is proportional to the degree of inhibition by the specific complex formation. Sensitized SRBCs are prepared by incubating SRBCs with an amboceptor (anti–SRBC hemolytic antibody).

As shown in Figure 13-4A, guinea pig complement is activated because of antigen-antibody complex formation (step 1). Complex formation and complement activation are not visible. Because there is no unreacted complement, no hemolysis occurs in the indicator step (step 2). If hemolysis does not occur, the serum contains the antigen.

As shown in Figure 13-4B, no antigen-antibody complex is formed. When the sensitized SRBCs are added, complement is available to react with the sensitized SRBCs. The complement pathway is activated, resulting in detectable hemolysis. If hemolysis is observed, the serum does not contain the antigen.

The complement fixation test can be modified to detect antibody, as shown in Figure 13-4C. In this case a known antibody is used in the test system to complex with the antibody to be detected. The indicator system is the same as that described earlier. No hemolysis indicates the presence of the antibody, and hemolysis indicates the absence of the antibody.

Some reagents are tested prior to the complement fixation procedure and are additionally controlled during the complement fixation test. The SRBCs are washed prior to use, and the supernatant from the second wash is examined for visible hemolysis. If hemolysis is present, the cells are fragile and should be discarded; a new lot of cells should be washed and used. Prior to SRBC sensitization, the hemolysin is titered to determine the optimal concentration of antibody. Complement is also titered prior to use; generally, a 1:400 dilution is sufficient to produce adequate hemolysis. The antigen or antibody reagent is also titered to obtain its optimal concentration in the test system.

A Identification of Unknown Antigen

Step 1 Patient sample + Known antibody + Guinea pig complement (antigen) — incubate

Step 2 Add sheep red blood cells coated with hemolysin — incubate

Step 3 Read for hemolysis

B Identification of Unknown Antibody

Step 1 Patient sample + Known antigen + Guinea pig complement (antibody) — incubate

Step 2 Add sheep red blood cells coated with hemolysin — incubate

Step 3 Read for hemolysis

FIGURE 13-3
(**A**) Complement fixation procedures may be used to detect the presence of unknown antigen in patient serum. In step 1 a known antibody is incubated with the patient sample. (**B**) Unknown antibody may also be detected. In step 1 a known antigen is incubated with the patient sample. For both techniques, steps 2 and 3 are identical.

A Positive Reaction

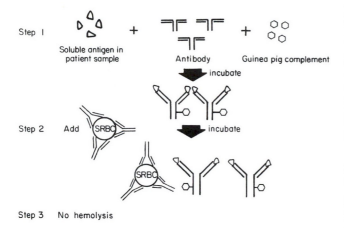

Step 1 — Soluble antigen in patient sample + Antibody + Guinea pig complement — incubate

Step 2 — Add SRBC — incubate

Step 3 — No hemolysis

B Negative Reaction for Unknown Antigen

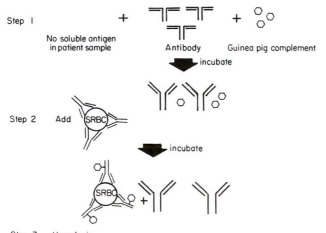

Step 1 — No soluble antigen in patient sample + Antibody + Guinea pig complement — incubate

Step 2 — Add SRBC — incubate

Step 3 — Hemolysis

C Negative Reaction for Unknown Antibody

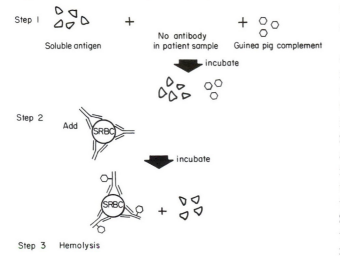

Step 1 — Soluble antigen + No antibody in patient sample + Guinea pig complement — incubate

Step 2 — Add SRBC — incubate

Step 3 — Hemolysis

FIGURE 13-4

(**A**) A positive result is shown. An antigen-antibody reaction has occurred in step 1, and guinea pig complement binds to this complex. There is no free complement to bind with the anti–sheep antibody in step 2. No hemolysis will be observed. (**B, C**) There is no antigen (**B**) nor antibody (**C**) present in the patient sample. There is no antigen-antibody complex formed in step 1, so complement is free to bind with the anti–sheep red blood cell antibody added in step 2. Hemolysis will occur.

The complement fixation technique is a titration procedure with many controls. In the clinical laboratory, the procedure is usually performed in a microtiter tray, as shown in Figure 13-5. Controls include a known positive serum, a known negative serum, an antigen control, a patient serum control, a cell control, and a complement control. These controls are used to detect the instability of complement, the variability of SRBCs, the immunochemical variation of hemolysin, and the narrow optimal range of diluted components.[7]

In the complement fixation assay, both positive and negative control sera are titered in parallel with the patient serum, and the titer produced must be within the acceptable limit. The cell control is a mixture of sensitized SRBCs and buffer incubated under test conditions. To be acceptable, no hemolysis should be seen. Hemolysis would most likely be caused by fragile cells. The complement (hemolytic) control contains all reagents except the patient serum. It is used to indicate the ability of the complement to function by lysing the sensitized SRBCs; total hemolysis is expected.[7]

The serum control is the test system (without the test antigen) and the indicator system. It is a check on the ability of the patient serum to bind complement nonspecifically or to inhibit complement activity in the absence of the test antigen and should show hemolysis. When it does not, it is anticomplementary; complement appears to be neutralized by the patient serum.

The antigen control is the test system (without the patient serum) and the indicator system. It is used to determine if the test antigen can nonspecifically bind complement or to inhibit the complement activity and should show hemolysis. If it shows no or little hemolysis, it is anticomplementary; the complement is neutralized by the test antigen. If any control is unacceptable, the assay results are invalid and must be repeated.

False positive reactions occur if the serum control or antigen control are anticomplementary, the complement is inactive, the antigen or antibody is not added to the test system, or the patient serum is too concentrated. A summary of the sources of error is presented in Table 13-5. False negative results may occur if the SRBCs are fragile, if the SRBCs are mechanically damaged, or if the patient serum is incompletely heated to inactivate endogenous complement prior to testing. In the latter situation, more complement will be present; the extra complement will react with the sensitized SRBCs, thus causing a falsely negative result. If the patient serum has too little analyte, only one antibody molecule will attach to the antigen and complement will not be activated in step 1, causing a false negative.

CONCLUSION

Complement components and functional activity can be measured in patient samples; decreased levels indicate in vivo activation, in vitro activation during coagulation, or

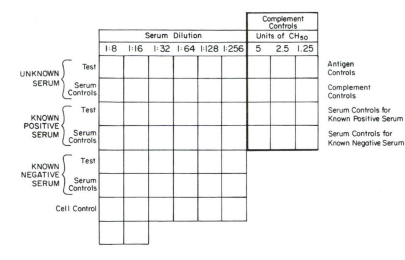

FIGURE 13-5

The complement fixation technique is performed using a microtiter plate. Serum dilutions are performed on the unknown sample, the known positive serum, and the known negative serum. Cell controls, complement controls, and antigen controls are also performed.

a component deficiency. Specific assays are used to pinpoint the pathway or component that is decreased in activity or concentration. The CH_{50} assay is the functional assay used to evaluate the ability of the classical pathway to lyse sensitized SRBCs. When rabbit red blood cells are used in the modified CH_{50} assay, it evaluates the ability of the alternative pathway to be activated. Individual components are quantitated by immunologic methods.

Complement can be used as a reagent in the complement fixation technique. Most often, patient serum antibody reacts with a known antigen, forming a complex that is capable of fixing guinea pig complement. When the indicator, sensitized SRBCs, is added, unreacted complement will lyse the sensitized SRBCs. This sensitive assay has largely been replaced by other assays that have comparable or better sensitivity and are easier to perform.

TABLE 13-5
Sources of Error in Complement Fixation Tests

FALSE POSITIVE (NO OR DECREASED LYSIS)

Inactive complement

Patient serum insufficiently diluted

Anti-complementary components in patient serum

Anti-complementary antigen

FALSE NEGATIVE

Fragile sheep red cells

Failure to heat-inactivate the serum

Failure to add antigen or antibody

Patient serum overdiluted

Review Questions

1. A decreased CH_{50} test result is associated with

   1. classical pathway activation
   2. alternate pathway activation
   3. hereditary angioedema
   4. acute phase of rheumatoid arthritis

      a. 1 and 3 are correct
      b. 2 and 4 are correct
      c. 1 only is correct
      d. 1, 3, and 4 are correct

2. In the complement fixation test, which control is unacceptable?

   a. The hemolytic control shows 50% hemolysis.
   b. The antigen control shows hemolysis.
   c. The cell control shows no hemolysis.
   d. The negative serum control shows hemolysis at all dilutions.

3. A decreased CH_{50} test result with normal serum C3 and C4 concentrations is most likely to be caused by

   a. alternative pathway activation
   b. C2 deficiency
   c. gout
   d. disseminated intravascular coagulopathy

4. The source of complement in the complement fixation test is

   a. pooled human serum
   b. endogenous patient complement
   c. guinea pig complement
   d. sheep complement

5. Which is the best indicator of acute phase reactions?

   a. C-reactive protein
   b. C3
   c. C4
   d. fibrinogen

References

1. Ruddy S: Complement. In Rose NR, DeMacario EC, Fahey JL, Friedman H, Penn GM (eds): Manual of Clinical Laboratory Immunology, 4th ed, p 114. Washington, DC, American Society for Microbiology, 1992

2. Gaither TA, Frank MM: Complement. In Henry JB (ed): Clinical Diagnosis and Management by Laboratory Methods, 18th ed, p 830. Philadelphia, WB Saunders, 1991

3. Yamamoto S, Kubotsu K, Kida M, et al: Automated homogeneous liposome-based assay system for total complement activity. Clin Chem 41:586, 1995

4. Luskin AT, Tobin MC: Alterations of complement components in disease. Am J Med Technol 48:749, 1982

5. Satoh P, Yonker TC, Kane DP, et al: Measurement of anaphylatoxins: An index for activation of complement cascade. BioTechniques 1:90, 1983

6. Frank MM: Complement in the pathophysiology of human disease. N Engl J Med 316:1525, 1987

7. Palmer DF, Whaley SD: Complement fixation test. In Rose NR, Friedman H, Fahey JL, (eds): Manual of Clinical Laboratory Immunology, 3rd ed, p 57. Washington, DC, American Society for Microbiology, 1986

CHAPTER 14

Labeled Immunoassays

Catherine Sheehan

Objectives

Upon completion of the chapter, the reader will be able to:

1. Compare and contrast binding reagents
2. In the context of immunoassays, define ligand, tracer, homogeneous, heterogeneous, competitive, noncompetitive, ELISA, RIST, and RAST
3. For each method of separation, explain its mechanism of separation and how it contributes to error in an assay
4. Given parameters of an assay, classify the assay as heterogeneous or homogeneous, and competitive or noncompetitive, and state the analyte, label, signal measured, and conjugate
5. State the principle of enzyme multiplied immunoassay, fluorescence polarization immunoassay, rapid flow-through immunoassay, and optical immunoassay
6. State the clinical use for measuring total IgE, allergen-specific IgE, and human chorionic gonadotropin
7. Explain why luteinizing hormone can be an interference when measuring human chorionic gonadotropin

In labeled immunoassays, a labeled reactant (either the antibody or antigen) will bind to the analyte and generate a simple antigen-antibody complex. The antibody contributes specificity to the assay, and the label generates the signal that indicates antigen-antibody complex formation.

In more general terms, a binding reagent combines with the ligand (derived from the Latin term *ligare*, meaning "to bind"). In practical terms, the binder can be a receptor, transport protein, or antibody, all of which demonstrate specificity in binding. Table 14-1 summarizes the different binding reagents. The ligand is the analyte (usually the antigen or hapten to be measured). Depending on the design of the assay, hormones, therapeutic drugs, antibodies, autoantigens, infectious disease antigens, tumor markers, or isoenzymes may be measured. In this chapter, *antibody* will refer to the binding reagent, and *antigen* or *hapten* will refer to the ligand. Several parameters contribute to the overall design of an assay: the label (particle, enzyme, fluorophore, radionuclide), signal measured, source of antibody, method of separation, competitive versus noncompetitive assays, antibody or antigen (hapten) measured, and data reduction. These variables in methodology contribute to the diversity of assays currently available for use in the clinical laboratory.

GENERAL CONSIDERATIONS

The modern era of immunoassays began in the 1960s following the work of Yalow and Berson, who developed a radioimmunoassay to measure insulin.[1] In this

TABLE 14-1		
Types of Binding Reagents		
BINDING REAGENT	**TYPICAL K_A (L/MOLE)**	**EXAMPLES**
Receptor	10^8–10^{11}	Human chorionic gonadotropin
Transport protein	10^7–10^8	Thyroid binding globulin
		Transcortin
Antibody	10^9–10^{11}	Monoclonal antibodies
		Polyclonal antibodies

competitive assay, radiolabeled insulin and unlabeled insulin in the patient sample competed for human insulin antibody binding sites, thus quantitating patient insulin. This research method sparked the innovation and development of the numerous commercial clinical immunoassays available today.

Under favorable conditions in a labeled immunoassay, the antigen and antibody bind together quickly and strongly, forming a complex. The reversible reaction can be summarized as

Antigen + antibody $\longleftrightarrow$ Antigen-antibody complex

The degree of complex formation is related to the attractive, stabilizing forces between the antigen and antibody. These forces include hydrogen binding, electrostatic forces, hydrophobic forces, and Van der Waal's forces. (For further discussion of these forces, consult Chapter 10.) At equilibrium, the rate of the forward reaction (k_1) equals the rate of the reverse reaction (k_{-1}), so that the ratio of free to bound antigen is constant.

Free Ag + free Ab $\longleftrightarrow$ Bound Ag-Ab

When a single binding site on a hapten (Hp) is considered, the binding obeys the law of mass action and can be expressed mathematically as

$$Ka = \frac{k_1}{k^{-1}} = \frac{[Hp \text{-} Ab]}{[Hp] [Ab]}$$

Ka is the affinity or equilibrium constant and represents the reciprocal of free hapten concentration when 50% of the binding sites are occupied. The affinity constant is expressed in L/mole or moles/L^{-1}. The greater the affinity of the Hp for the antibody, the smaller the concentration of hapten required for 50% saturation. For example, if the affinity constant of a monoclonal antibody reagent is 3×10^{11} L/mole, it means that a hapten concentration of 3×10^{-11} moles/L is needed to occupy half of the binding sites. Typically, the affinity constant for antibodies used in radioimmunoassay procedures

ranges from 10^9 to 10^{11} L/mole, whereas the affinity constant for transport proteins ranges from 10^7 to 10^8 L/mole and the affinity constant for receptors ranges from 10^8 to 10^{11} L/mole.[2]

CLASSIFICATION OF IMMUNOASSAYS

Each immunoassay can be described based on six considerations: (1) the label, (2) which reactant is labeled, (3) the relative concentration and source of the antibody, (4) the method to separate free from bound labeled reagent, (5) the signal measured, and (6) the method used to assign the analyte concentration in the unknown sample.

Labels

The simplest way to identify an assay is by the label used. Table 14-2 lists the labels commonly used and their detection method for assays performed in the routine clinical laboratory.

RADIOACTIVE LABELS

Radioactive labels are atoms with unstable nuclei that spontaneously emit radiation.[3] The emission is known as radioactive decay and is independent of chemical or physical parameters, such as temperature, pressure, or concentration. Three forms of radiation can be emitted: alpha, beta, and gamma. Alpha particles are the nuclei of helium atoms consisting of two protons and two neutrons. They are positively charged, large particles from heavy radioactive nuclides. These particles are of little significance in the clinical laboratory.

In beta decay, the nucleus can emit negatively charged electrons or positively charged particles called positrons. The emitted electrons are also known as beta particles. A specific spectrum of energy levels is associated with each beta-emitting radionuclide. Tritium (^{3}H)

TABLE 14-2
Labels and Detection Methods

IMMUNOASSAY	COMMON LABELS	DETECTION METHODS
RIA	^{3}H	Liquid scintillation counter
	^{125}I	Gamma counter
EIA	Horseradish peroxidase	Photometer, fluorometer, luminometer
	Alkaline phosphatase	Photometer, fluorometer, luminometer
	β-D galactosidase	Fluorometer, luminometer
	Glucose-6-phosphate dehydrogenase	Photometer, luminometer
CLA	Isoluminol derivative	Luminometer
	Acridinium esters	Luminometer
FIA	Fluorescein	Fluorometer
	Europium	Fluorometer
	Phycobiliproteins	Fluorometer
	Rhodamine B	Fluorometer
	Umbelliferone	Fluorometer

RIA, radioimmunoassay; EIA, enzyme immunoassay; CLA, chemiluminescent assay; FIA, fluorescent immunoassay

is the commonly used radionuclide in cellular immunology assays for diagnostic and research applications.

Gamma emission is a portion of the electromagnetic radiation spectrum. Gamma rays have very short wavelengths originating from unstable nuclei; the properties of gamma rays are similar to those of x-rays and light waves. Radionuclides emitting gamma rays are the most common radiolabel used in the clinical laboratory.

As a radionuclide releases its energy and becomes more stable, it disintegrates or decays, releasing energy. The standardized unit of radioactivity is the becquerel (Bq), which is equal to one disintegration per second. The traditional unit is the curie (Ci), which equals 3.7×10^{10} Bq; 1 μCi equals 37 kBq. The half-life of the radionuclide is the time needed for 50% of the radionuclide to decay and to become more stable. The longer the half-life, the more slowly it decays, thereby increasing the length of time it can be measured. For those radioactive substances used in diagnostic tests, it is preferable that the emission have an appropriate energy level and that the half-life be relatively long; ^{125}I satisfies these requirements and is the most commonly used gamma-emitting radionuclide in the clinical laboratory.

Gamma-emitting nuclides are detected using a crystal scintillation detector (also known as a gamma counter). The energy released during decay excites a fluor, such as thallium-activated sodium iodide. The excited fluor releases a photon of visible light, which is amplified and detected by a photomultiplier tube; the amplified light energy is then translated into electrical energy. Detectable decay of the radionuclide is expressed as counts per minute (CPM).

In immunoassays, one reactant is radiolabeled. In competitive assays the antigen is labeled and is called the tracer, and in noncompetitive assays the antibody is usually labeled. The radiolabel must allow the tracer to be fully functional and to compete equally with the unlabeled antigen for the binding sites. When the antibody is radiolabeled, the antigen-combining site must remain biologically active and unhindered.

ENZYME LABELS

Enzymes are commonly used to label the antigen/hapten or antibody.[4,5] Enzymes are biologic catalysts that increase the rate of conversion of substrate to product and are not consumed during the reaction. As such, an enzyme catalyzes many substrate molecules and thus amplifies the signal. Listed in order of frequency of use, horseradish peroxidase, alkaline phosphatase, and glucose-6-phosphate dehydrogenase are the enzymes used most often. The enzyme activity may be monitored directly by measuring the product formed or by measuring the effect of the product on a coupled reaction. Depending on the substrate used, the product can be photometric, fluorometric, or chemiluminescent. For example, a typical photometric reaction using horseradish peroxidase–labeled antibody (Ab-HRP) and the substrate, a peroxide, generates the product, oxygen; this reaction is then coupled to a second reaction, producing a colored product. The oxygen oxidizes a reduced chromogen (reduced orthophenylenediamine [OPD]), producing a colored compound (oxidized OPD), which is measured using a photometer.

$$Ab\text{-}HRP + peroxide \rightarrow Ab\text{-}HRP + O_2$$
$$O_2 + reduced\ OPD \rightarrow Oxidized\ OPD + H_2O$$

FLUORESCENT LABELS

Fluorescent labels or fluorophores are compounds that absorb radiant energy of one wavelength and emit radiant energy of a longer wavelength in less than 10^{-4} seconds. Generally, the emitted light is measured at a 90° angle from the path of excitation light using a fluorometer or a modified spectrophotometer. The difference between the excitation wavelength and emission wavelength is the Stokes shift and usually ranges between 20 and 80 nm for most fluorophores. Some fluorescence immunoassays simply substitute a fluorescent label (such as fluorescein) for an enzyme label and quantitate the fluorescence.[6] Another approach, time-resolved fluorescence immunoassay, uses a highly efficient fluorescent label, such as a europium chelate,[7,8] which fluoresces approximately 1000 times more slowly than the natural background fluorescence and has a wide Stokes shift. The delay allows for measurement of the fluorescent label without interference from background fluorescence. The long Stokes shift facilitates separating the emission wavelength (to be measured) from the excitation wavelength. The resulting assay is highly sensitive, is time resolved, and has little background fluorescence.

CHEMILUMINESCENT LABELS

Chemiluminescent labels emit a photon of light in response to a chemical reaction.[9] Some organic compounds become excited when oxidized and will emit light as they revert to their ground states. Oxidants include hydrogen peroxide, hypochlorite, and oxygen. Sometimes a catalyst, such as peroxidase, alkaline phosphatase, or metal ions, is needed. The two popular systems for luminescent immunoassays use luminol or luciferase.

Luminol is a cyclic diacylhydrazide that emits light energy under alkaline conditions in the presence of peroxide and peroxidase. Because peroxidase can serve as the catalyst, assays may use this enzyme as the label. The chemiluminogenic substrate, luminol, will produce light that is directly proportional to the amount of peroxidase present.

$$Luminol + 2H_2O_2 + OH^- \xrightarrow{\text{peroxidase}} 3\text{-Aminophthalate} + light$$

A second system of chemiluminescent labels is acridinium esters. Acridinium is a triple-ringed organic molecule linking an ester bond to an organic chain. In the presence of hydrogen peroxide and under alkaline conditions, the ester bond is broken and an unstable molecule (N-methylacridon) remains. Light is emitted as the unstable molecule reverts to its more stable ground state.

$$Acridinium\ ester + 2H_2O_2 + OH^-$$
$$\rightarrow N\text{-}Methylacridon + CO_2 + H_2O + light$$

Assay Design

COMPETITIVE IMMUNOASSAYS

In the earliest immunoassays, the antigen was labeled and the assay was based on competition between the labeled antigen (Ag*) and unlabeled antigen (Ag) for a limited number of binding sites (Ab). The concentration of unlabeled antigen is inversely related to the concentration of bound labeled antigen. These limited reagent assays were very sensitive because low concentrations of unlabeled antigen yielded a large measurable signal from the bound labeled antigen. If the competitive assay is designed to reach equilibrium, often the incubation times are long. The antigen-antibody reaction can be done in one step, in which labeled antigen, unlabeled antigen, and reagent antibody are simultaneously incubated together.

Simultaneous Competitive Assay

$$Ag^* + Ag + Ab\ \text{(limited reagent)}$$
$$\rightarrow Ag^*Ab + AgAb + Ag^*$$

Alternatively, there may be two sequential steps to accomplish the antigen-antibody reaction: (1) Unlabeled antigen is incubated with the reagent antibody and (2) labeled antigen is then added.

Sequential Competitive Assay

Step 1 $Ag + Ab \rightarrow AgAb + Ab$

Step 2 $AgAb + Ab + Ag^* \rightarrow AgAb + Ag^*Ab + Ag^*$

A relatively small, yet constant, number of Ab combining sites is available to combine with a relatively large, constant amount of Ag* (tracer). When Ag is added, it will displace or prevent the tracer from binding. The displacement of the tracer will be proportional to the amount of Ag present. Consider the example in Table 14-3. The amount of tracer and antibody are constant, and the amount of tracer exceeds the antibody binding sites. The only variable in the test system is the amount of unlabeled antigen. The greater the concentration of unlabeled antigen, the greater the concentration of free tracer or the greater the percentage of free tracer.

TABLE 14-3
Competitive Binding Assay Example:

Ag	+	Ag*	+	Ab	→	AgAb	+	Ag*Ab	+	Ag*

CONCENTRATION OF REACTANTS			CONCENTRATION OF PRODUCTS		
Ag	*Ag**	*Ab*	*AgAb*	*Ag*Ab*	*Ag**
0	200	100	0	100	100
50	200	100	20	80	120
100	200	100	34	66	134
200	200	100	50	50	150
400	200	100	66	34	166

SAMPLE CALCULATIONS

Dose of [Ag]	%B	B/F
0	$\dfrac{100}{200} = 50$	$\dfrac{100}{100} = 1$
50	$\dfrac{80}{200} = 40$	$\dfrac{80}{120} = .67$
100	$\dfrac{66}{200} = 33$	$\dfrac{66}{134} = .49$
200	$\dfrac{50}{200} = 25$	$\dfrac{50}{150} = .33$
400	$\dfrac{34}{200} = 17$	$\dfrac{34}{166} = .20$

By using different concentrations of standards (known concentrations of unlabeled antigen) in an assay, a dose-response or standard curve is established. As the concentration of unlabeled Ag increases, the concentration of tracer that binds to the Ab decreases. The amount of either free tracer or bound tracer can be measured. In the example presented in Table 14-3, if the amount of unlabeled antigen is 0, maximum tracer will combine with the antibody. When the amount of unlabeled antigen is the same as the tracer, each will bind equally to the antibody. As the concentration or dose of unlabeled ligand increases in a competitive assay, the amount of labeled antigen (tracer) that complexes with the binding reagent decreases. Most separation techniques allow the bound tracer to be measured. When no unlabeled antigen is present, maximum binding by the tracer is possible; this is referred to as B_0, B_{max}, or maximum binding. The data are plotted in one of three ways: bound/free versus the arithmetic dose of unlabeled antigen, percent bound versus the log dose of unlabeled antigen, and logit bound/B_0 versus the log dose of the unlabeled antigen (Fig. 14-1 on p. 150).

The bound fraction can be expressed in several different formats. Bound/free (B/F) is the counts per minute (CPM) of the bound fraction compared with the CPM of the unbound fraction. Bound/total (B/T) is the CPM of the bound fraction compared with the CPM of maximum binding by the tracer (B_0) added to each tube.

Percent bound (%B) is B/T times 100. Logit B/B_0 transformation is the natural log of $(B/B_0)/(1 - B/B_0)$.

When using special logit graph paper on which B/B_0 is plotted on the ordinate and the log dose of the unlabeled antigen is plotted on the abscissa, a straight line with a negative slope is produced.[2]

Several graphic representations, shown in Figure 14-1, can be used to relate the dose of known unlabeled antigen (standard) to the measurable tracer. When a patient sample is assayed, the unlabeled antigen in the patient sample competes with the tracer and the amount of bound tracer is measured. When compared with the dose-response curve, the concentration of the unlabeled antigen is assigned.

To determine the amount of free or bound tracer, competitive assays require that free tracer be separated from bound tracer. Separation techniques are discussed later in this chapter.

A representative protocol for simultaneous incubation of tracer and unlabeled antigen is summarized here. A schematic is shown in Figure 14-2 (on p. 150).

1. Pipet serum (control, standard, or patient sample) into test tubes.
2. Pipet tracer into each tube.
3. Pipet antibody reagent into each tube.
4. Incubate to allow binding to occur.
5. If necessary, separate free tracer from bound tracer.
6. Measure the amount of bound tracer.

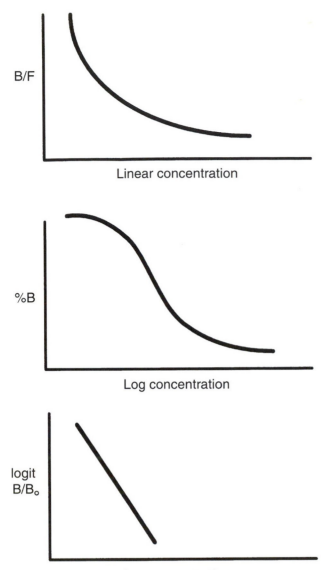

FIGURE 14-1
Dose-related curves in competitive immunoassay. B = bound counts per minute; F = free counts per minute; B_0 = maximum binding.

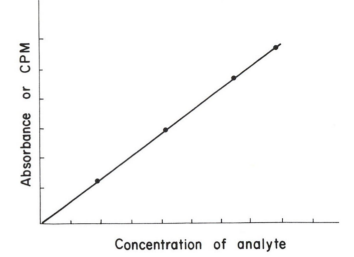

FIGURE 14-3
Noncompetitive dose response curve. As the concentration of the unlabeled antigen increases, the amount of label that is measured increases.

NONCOMPETITIVE IMMUNOASSAYS

This group of immunoassays, also known as immunometric immunoassays, uses a labeled reagent antibody to detect the antigen. Excess labeled antibody is required to ensure that it does not limit the reaction. The concentration of the antigen is directly proportional to the signal generated by the bound labeled antibody, as shown in Figure 14-3. The relationship is linear up to a limit and then is subject to the high-dose hook effect.

Commonly the format is the "sandwich" type. In the sandwich assay to detect antigen (also known as an antigen capture assay), immobilized unlabeled antibody captures the antigen. After washing to remove unreacted molecules, the labeled detector antibody is added. After washing to remove unreacted labeled antibody, the signal from the bound labeled antibody is proportional to the antigen captured. This format relies on the ability of each antibody reagent to react with different epitopes on the antigen. The

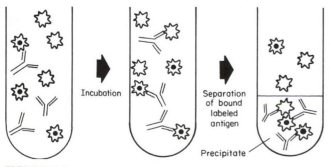

FIGURE 14-2
Competitive immunoassay. During simultaneous incubation, labeled antigen (✿) and unlabeled antigen (✿) compete for the antibody binding sites (✁). The bound label in the precipitate is measured.

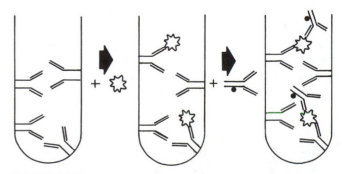

FIGURE 14-4
Noncompetitive assay to detect antigen. In sequential incubation, unlabeled antigen (✿) binds to immobilized antibody, followed by incubation with labeled antibody (✆). The bound label is measured.

specificity and quantity of monoclonal antibodies has allowed the rapid expansion of diverse assays. A representative protocol for a sandwich assay to detect antigen is summarized here. A schematic is shown in Figure 14-4.

1. Pipet serum (control, standard, or patient sample) into test tubes.
2. If the tube is not coated with the antibody, add the antibody-coated solid phase.
3. Incubate to allow the antigen to bind to the solid-phase antibody.
4. Wash to remove unbound serum components.
5. Add labeled antibody; incubate.
6. Wash to remove unbound labeled antibody.
7. Measure the bound antibody.

Especially important in the serology laboratory is the sandwich assay to detect antibody. Here the immobilized antigen reacts with serum containing an unknown amount of specific antibody. After washing, the labeled detector antibody is added and binds to the captured antibody. When all classes of bound antibody are to be measured, then the detector antibody is labeled anti–human globulin. The amount of bound labeled antibody is directly proportional to the amount of specific antibody present. This assay can be modified to determine the immunoglobulin class of the specific antibody present in serum. For example, if the detector antibody were labeled and monospecific (such as a rabbit anti–human IgM [μ-chain specific]), it would detect and quantitate only human IgM captured by the immobilized antigen.

A schematic is presented in Figure 14-5. A sample protocol to detect antibody is summarized following.

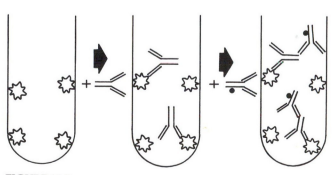

FIGURE 14-5
Noncompetitive assay to detect antibody. Unlabeled antibody () is incubated with immobilized antigen (✿). In a second step, labeled anti–human globulin (✁) is added. The bound label is measured.

1. Pipet serum (control, standard, or patient sample) into the test tubes.
2. If the antigen is not bound to the tube, add the antigen-coated solid phase.
3. Incubate to allow the specific antibody to bind to the solid-phase antigen.
4. Wash to remove unbound serum components.
5. Add the labeled anti–human globulin; incubate.
6. Wash to remove unbound labeled antibody.
7. Measure the bound labeled antibody.

Distinguishing Between Free and Bound Labeled Reactant

All immunoassays require that free labeled reactant be distinguished from bound labeled reactant. In heterogeneous assays, physical separation is necessary and is achieved by adsorption, precipitation, or interaction with a solid phase. This is in contrast to homogeneous assays, in which the activity or expression of the label depends on whether the labeled reactant is free or bound. In most homogeneous assays, when the labeled reagent is bound, the signal is absent. Thus no physical separation step is needed in homogeneous assays.

In heterogeneous ligand assays, the better the separation of bound from free reactant, the more reliable the assay will be. Separation techniques—adsorption, precipitation, and use of the solid phase—are summarized in Table 14-4 (on p. 152).[10]

ADSORPTION

Adsorption techniques use particles to trap the small antigens, labeled or unlabeled.[2] Most commonly, a mixture of charcoal and crosslinked dextran is used. Charcoal is porous and readily combines with small molecules to remove them from solution; dextran prevents nonspecific protein binding to the charcoal. The size of the dextran influences the size of the molecule that can be adsorbed; the lower the molecular weight of dextran used, the smaller the molecular weight of free ligand that can be adsorbed. Other adsorbents include silica, ion exchange resin, and sephadex. After adsorption and centrifugation, the free labeled antigen is found in the precipitate.

PRECIPITATION

Nonimmune precipitation occurs when the environment is modified to alter the solubility of protein. Compounds such as ammonium sulfate, sodium sulfate, polyethylene glycol, and ethanol precipitate protein

TABLE 14-4
Characteristics of Separation Techniques

SEPARATION TECHNIQUE	EXAMPLES	ACTION
Adsorption	Charcoal and dextran	Traps free labeled antigen
	Silica	Separation by centrifugation
	Ion exchange resin	
	Sephadex	
Precipitation		
Nonimmune	Ethanol	Denatures bound labeled antigen
	Ammonium sulfate	Separation by centrifugation
	Sodium sulfate	
	Polyethylene glycol	
Immune	Second antibody	Primary antibody is recognized
	Staph protein A	and forms an insoluble complex
Solid phase	Polystyrene	Separation by centrifugation
	Membranes	One reactant is adsorbed or
		covalently attached to the
		inert surface
	Magnetized particles	Separation by washing

nonspecifically; both free antibody and antibody-antigen complexes will precipitate. Ammonium sulfate and sodium sulfate "salt out" free globulins and antibody-antigen complexes. Ethanol denatures protein and antibody-antigen complexes, causing precipitation. Polyethylene glycol precipitates larger protein molecules with or without the antigen attached. To facilitate separation of the precipitate, centrifugation is used. Ideally, all antibody-bound labeled antigen will be in the precipitate, leaving free labeled antigen in the supernatant.

Soluble antigen-antibody complexes can be precipitated by a second antibody that recognizes the primary antibody in the soluble complex. The result is a larger complex that becomes insoluble and will precipitate. Centrifugation is again used to aid in the separation. This immune precipitation method is also known as the double-antibody or second-antibody method. For example, in a growth hormone assay, the primary or antigen-specific antibody is produced in a rabbit and recognizes growth hormone. The second antibody, produced in a sheep or goat, would recognize rabbit antibody. Labeled antigen-antibody complexes, unlabeled antigen-antibody complexes, and free primary antibodies are precipitated by the second antibody. This separation method is more specific than nonimmune precipitation because only the primary antibody is precipitated. A similar separation occurs when staphylococcal protein A (SpA) replaces the second antibody. SpA selectively binds to human IgG, causing precipitation.

SOLID PHASE

Solid-phase immobilization of reagent antibody or antigen provides a method to separate free from bound labeled reactant by washing. The solid-phase support may be, but is not limited to, polystyrene surfaces, membranes, and magnetic beads. The immobilized antigen or antibody may be adsorbed or covalently bound to the solid-phase support; covalent linkage prevents spontaneous release of the immobilized antigen or antibody. Immunoassays using solid-phase separation are easier to perform, require less manipulation, require less time to perform than other immunoassays, and are easily automated. However, relatively large amounts of antibody or antigen are required to coat the solid-phase surfaces, and consistent coverage of the solid phase is difficult to achieve. Solid-phase assays are more expensive to produce and require greater technical skill to perform to minimize intra-assay and interassay variability. Insufficient washing is a common source of error.

EXAMPLES OF IMMUNOASSAYS

Table 14-5 is a summary of some currently available immunoassays. Most of these assays are automated. A brief discussion of each is presented here.

The *particle enhanced turbidimetric inhibition immunoassay (PETINIA)* is a homogeneous competitive immunoassay in which low molecular weight haptens bound to particles compete with unlabeled analyte for the specific antibody. The extent of particle agglutination is inversely proportional to the concentration of unlabeled analyte and is assessed by measuring the change in transmitted light in a DuPont Automated Chemistry Analyzer.[11]

Enzyme linked immunosorbent assays (ELISAs) are very popular heterogeneous immunoassays that all have an enzyme label and use a solid phase as the separation

TABLE 14-5
Labeled Immunoassay Methods

ASSAY	LABEL	COMPONENT LABELED	SIGNAL MEASURED	COMPETITIVE	NONCOMPETITIVE	HOMOGENEOUS	HETEROGENEOUS	SEPARATION TECHNIQUE
PETINIA	Polystyrene particles	Antigen (hapten)	Agglutination	✓		✓		
ELISA 1	Enzyme	Antigen or antibody	Enzyme activity	✓			✓	Solid phase
ELISA 2	Enzyme	Antigen or antibody	Enzyme activity		✓		✓	Solid phase
EMIT	Enzyme	Hapten	Enzyme activity	✓		✓		
MEIA 1	Enzyme	Antigen	Fluorescence	✓			✓	Solid phase
MEIA 2	Enzyme	Antibody	Fluorescence		✓		✓	Solid phase
CEDIA	Enzyme donor	Hapten	Enzyme activity	✓		✓		
SPFIA 1	Fluor	Antigen or antibody	Fluorescence	✓			✓	Solid phase
SPFIA 2	Fluor	Antigen or antibody	Fluorescence		✓		✓	Solid phase
PCFIA	Fluor	Antigen or antibody	Fluorescence	✓			✓	Solid phase
FETI	Two fluors	Antigen or antibody	Fluorescence	✓		✓		
SLFIA	Enzyme	Antigen (hapten)	Fluorescence	✓		✓		
FPIA	Fluor	Antigen (hapten)	Polarized light	✓		✓		
DELFIA 1	Fluor	Antigen	Fluorescence	✓			✓	Solid phase
DELFIA 2	Fluor	Antibody	Fluorescence		✓		✓	Solid phase
RIA 1	Radionuclide	Antigen	Decay	✓			✓	Physical adsorption precipitation, solid phase
RIA 2	Radionuclide	Antibody	Decay		✓		✓	Precipitation, solid phase
CLA 1	Chemicals/enzyme	Antigen	Light emission	✓			✓	Solid phase
CLA 2	Chemicals/enzyme	Antibody	Light emission		✓		✓	Solid phase

153

technique. Four formats are available: a competitive assay using labeled antigen, a competitive assay using labeled antibody, a noncompetitive assay to detect antigen, and a noncompetitive assay to detect antibody. In the competitive ELISAs using labeled antibody, bound antigen and test antigen compete with labeled antibody; the bound labeled antibody is inversely proportional to the concentration of test antigen.

One of the earliest homogeneous assays was an enzyme immunoassay named the *enzyme multiplied immunoassay technique (EMIT™)*, which is currently produced by Syva Corporation.[12] As shown in Figure 14-6, the reactants in most test systems include an enzyme-labeled antigen (in this example, a drug), an antibody directed against the drug, the substrate, and test antigen. The enzyme is catalytically active when the labeled antigen is free (not bound to the antibody). It is thought that when the antibody combines with the labeled antigen, the antibody sterically inhibits the enzyme. The conformational changes that occur during antigen-antibody interaction inhibit the enzyme activity. The unlabeled antigen in the sample competes with the labeled antigen for the antibody binding sites; as the concentration of unlabeled antigen increases, less enzyme-labeled antigen can bind to the antibody. Therefore, more labeled antigen is free and the enzymatic activity is greater.

The *cloned enzyme donor immunoassay (CEDIA)* is a competitive, homogeneous assay in which the genetically engineered label is β-galactosidase.[13] The enzyme is in two inactive pieces: the enzyme acceptor and the enzyme donor. When these two pieces bind together, the enzyme activity is restored. In the assay, the antigen labeled with the enzyme donor and unlabeled antigen in the sample compete for specific antibody binding sites. When the antibody binds to the labeled antigen, it prevents the reconstitution of the enzyme. More unlabeled antigen in the sample results in more enzyme activity.

The *microparticle capture enzyme immunoassay (MEIA)* is an automated assay available on the Abbott IMx. The microparticles serve as the solid phase and a glass fiber matrix separates the bound labeled reagent. Both competitive and noncompetitive assays are available. Although the label is an enzyme (alkaline phosphatase), the substrate (4-methyllumbelliferyl phosphate) is fluorogenic; thus the product is measured with a fluorometer.

Solid phase fluorescence immunoassays (SPFIAs) are analogous to the ELISA methods except that the label fluoresces. Of particular note is FIAX® (Carter Wallace/Wampole Laboratories, Cranbury, NJ). In this assay fluid-phase unlabeled antigen binds to capture antibody on the solid phase; after washing, the detector antibody (with a fluorescent label attached) reacts with the solid-phase captured antigen.

The *particle concentration fluorescence immunoassay (PCFIA)* is a heterogeneous, competitive immunoassay in which particles are used to localize the reaction and to concentrate the fluorescence. Labeled antigen and unlabeled antigen in the sample compete for antibody bound to polystyrene particles. The particles are trapped and the fluorescence is measured. The assay can also be designed so that labeled antibody and unlabeled antibody compete for antigen fixed onto particles.

The *fluorescence excitation transfer immunoassay (FETI)* is a competitive, homogeneous immunoassay using two fluorophores (such as fluorescein and rhodamine).[14] When the two labels are in close proximity, the emitted light from fluorescein is absorbed by rhodamine. Thus the emission from fluorescein is quenched. Fluorescein-labeled antigen and unlabeled antigen compete for rhodamine-labeled antibody. More unlabeled antigen lessens the amount of fluorescein-labeled antigen that binds; thus, more fluorescence is present (less quenching).

The *substrate level fluorescence immunoassay (SLFIA)* is another competitive, homogeneous assay. This time the hapten is labeled with a substrate; when catalyzed by an appropriate enzyme, a fluorescent product is generated. The substrate-labeled hapten and unlabeled hapten in the sample compete with the antibody. The bound labeled hapten cannot be catalyzed by the enzyme.

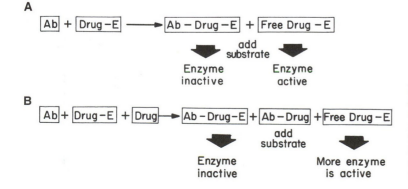

FIGURE 14-6
Enzyme-multiplied immunoassay technique. (**A**) Without unlabeled drug, the enzyme-labeled drug (Drug-E) binds maximally to the antibody (Ab). In the Ab-Drug-E complex, the enzyme is inactive. Only free enzyme-labeled drug is enzymatically active. (**B**) In the test system, the unlabeled drug in a patient sample competes with the labeled drug, thereby increasing the amount of free enzyme-labeled drug.

The *fluorescence polarization immunoassay (FPIA)* is another assay that uses a fluorescent label.[15,16] This homogeneous immunoassay uses polarized light to excite the fluorescent label. Polarized light consists of parallel light waves oriented in one plane and is created when light passes through special filters. When polarized light is used to excite a fluorescent label, the emitted light can be polarized or depolarized. As depicted in Figure 14-7, small molecules, such as free fluorescent-labeled hapten, randomly rotate rapidly and emit light in many directions, thus producing depolarized light. Large molecules, such as those created when the fluorescent-labeled hapten binds to an antibody, rotate more slowly and emit polarized light parallel to the excitation polarized light. The polarized light is measured at a 90° angle compared with the path of the excitation light. In a competitive FPIA, fluorescent-labeled hapten and unlabeled hapten in the sample compete for limited antibody sites. When no unlabeled hapten is present, the labeled hapten binds maximally to the antibody, creating large complexes that rotate slowly and emit a high level of polarized light. When hapten is present, it competes with the labeled hapten for the antibody sites; thus, as the hapten concentration increases, more labeled hapten is displaced and is free. The free labeled hapten rotates rapidly and emits depolarized light. The degree of labeled hapten displacement is inversely related to the amount of unlabeled hapten present.

The *dissociation-enhanced lanthanide fluorimmunoassay (DELFIA)* is an automated system (Pharmacia) that measures time-delayed fluorescence from the label europium. The assay can be designed as a competitive, heterogeneous assay or a noncompetitive (sandwich), heterogeneous assay.[17]

The classic *radioimmunoassay (RIA)* is a heterogeneous, competitive assay with labeled antigen (referred to as a tracer). When bound tracer is measured, the signal from the label (counts per minute) is inversely related to the concentration of the unlabeled antigen in the sample. Various separations may be used. Noncompetitive, heterogeneous assays are usually sandwich assays to detect antigen or antibody in which the bound labeled reagent is proportional to the concentration of the analyte.

Rapid Immunoassays

The sensitivity and specificity of automated labeled assays and the trend of decentralized laboratory testing have led to the development of assays that are easy to use, simple (many are classified as waived or moderately complex, according to the Clinical Laboratory Improvement Amendments of 1988), fast, site-neutral, and require no instrumentation. Those to be discussed here are representative of available commercial kits, but this is not intended to be an exhaustive discussion. Three categories emerge: (1) latex particles to visualize the reaction, (2) fluid flow and labeled reactant, and (3) changes in a physical or chemical property following antigen-antibody binding.

The earliest rapid tests were those in which a latex particle suspension was added to the sample; if the immunoreactive component attached to the particle recognized its counterpart in the sample, macroscopic agglutination occurred. Colored latex particles are now available to facilitate reading the reaction.

Self-contained devices that use the liquid nature of the specimen have evolved. In flow-through systems, a capture reagent is immobilized onto a membrane, the solid phase. The porous nature of membranes increases the surface area to which the capture reagent can bind. The more capture antibody or capture antigen that binds to the membrane, the greater the potential sensitivity of the assay. After the capture reagent binds to the membrane, other binding sites are saturated with a nonreactive blocking chemical to reduce nonspecific binding by substances in the patient sample. In the assay, the sample containing the analyte is allowed to pass through the membrane and the analyte is bound to the capture reagent. Commonly the liquid is attracted through the membrane by an absorbent material. The analyte is then detected by a labeled reactant, and the signal from the labeled reactant is detected.

The next step in the development of self-contained, single-use devices was to incorporate internal controls. One scheme, ICON© (Hybritech, Inc.),[19,20] to detect human chorionic gonadotropin, creates three zones in which specifically treated particles are deposited. In the assay zone, particles are coated with antiserum specific

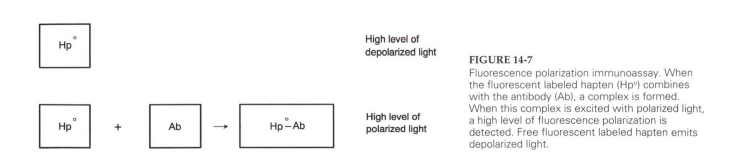

FIGURE 14-7
Fluorescence polarization immunoassay. When the fluorescent labeled hapten (Hp°) combines with the antibody (Ab), a complex is formed. When this complex is excited with polarized light, a high level of fluorescence polarization is detected. Free fluorescent labeled hapten emits depolarized light.

for the assay; in the negative control zone, particles are coated with nonimmune antibody; and in the positive control zone, particles are coated with an immune complex specific for the assay. The patient sample (serum or urine) passes through the membrane, and the analyte attaches to the specific antibody in the assay zone. Next, a conjugated antibody passes through the membrane, which fixes to the specific immune complex formed in the assay zone or in the positive control zone. Following color development, a positive reaction is noted when the assay and positive zones are colored.

A second homogeneous immunoassay involves the tangential flow of fluid across a membrane. The fluid dissolves and binds to the dried capture reagent; the complex flows to the detection area where it is concentrated and visualized.

A third homogeneous immunoassay, enzyme immunochromatography, involves vertical flow of fluid along a membrane.[21] This is quantitative and does not require instrumentation. A dry paper strip with immobilized antibody is immersed in a solution of unlabeled analyte and an enzyme-labeled analyte; the liquid migrates up the strip by capillary action. As the labeled and unlabeled analyte migrate, they compete and bind to the immobilized antibody. A finite amount of labeled and unlabeled analyte mixture is absorbed. The migration distance of the labeled analyte is visualized when the strip reacts with a substrate reagent and develops a colored reaction product. Comparing the migration distance of the sample with the calibrator allows the concentration of the unlabeled ligand to be assigned.

The next generation of rapid immunoassays involves change in physical or chemical properties after an antigen-antibody interaction occurs. One example is the optical immunoassay (OIA®).[22] A silicon wafer is used to support a thin film of optical coating; this is then topped with the capture antibody. Sample is applied directly to the device. If an antigen-antibody complex is formed, the thickness of the optical surface increases and this changes the optical path of light. The color changes from gold to purple. Some studies suggest that this method has better analytic sensitivity than immunoassays, which rely on fluid flow.

INTERFERENCES AND SOURCES OF ERROR

For quantitative immunoassays, the sensitivity suggests that minor variations in technique can be a significant source of error. Therefore, when quantitative immunoassays are performed manually, it is recommended that each patient sample, control, and standard be tested in duplicate to minimize technical variation, especially in pipetting.

In heterogeneous assays, the separation step is critical. In solid-phase assays, washing is the separation step; incomplete washing fails to completely remove free labeled reagent. The detected signal increases and results in a falsely elevated reaction in a noncompetitive assay or a falsely decreased reaction in a competitive assay. Likewise, when centrifugation is used, the speed and time of centrifugation and completeness of decanting contribute to the effectiveness of separation. The hook effect occurs in noncompetitive assays when the concentration of the analyte exceeds the linear range of the assay.

Each laboratory develops confidence in an immunoassay procedure by adequately evaluating each method to ensure its accuracy, analytic sensitivity, and precision prior to its adoption. The source, purity, affinity, avidity, and specificity of the antibody are important in an immunoassay. The design of the assay, including the requirement for separation, the ease of separation if needed, the number and length of incubations, and the number of pipetting steps influence the sensitivity and reproducibility of the assay.

APPLICATIONS

The list of analytes that are measured by immunoassay continues to grow. In this section, in vitro allergy testing and detection of human chorionic gonadotropin are discussed.

In Vitro Allergy Testing

QUANTITATION OF TOTAL SERUM IgE

Total serum IgE is measured to assess atopic allergic individuals. The concentration of total serum IgE in nonatopic individuals is low and varies with age. During the first year of life, total serum IgE concentration is less than 10 IU/mL. The level rises during childhood, peaks in adolescence, and declines after age 65.[23] In the majority of nonatopic North American adults, the serum IgE level ranges from 30 to 80 IU/mL; the mean adult level is 40 IU/mL.[23,24] Variation in the serum IgE concentration between individuals of the same age exists, including an overlap in serum IgE levels between atopic and nonatopic individuals. Generally, when the level of total IgE is greater than 100 IU/mL (95th percentile), IgE-mediated disease is present. Total serum IgE concentration may predict the risk of developing allergic disease in asymptomatic infants in whom there is a family history of allergy.[23,25]

Methods to detect total IgE include competitive radioimmunosorbent test (RIST), noncompetitive RIST, double-antibody radioimmunoassay (RIA), and sandwich enzyme-linked immunosorbent assay (ELISA), and are shown in Figure 6-3. Competitive or indirect RIST is a competitive RIA based on the simultaneous incubation of radiolabeled IgE and reference or unknown IgE with an anti-IgE bound to a solid phase. The greater the concentration of the reference or unknown IgE, the fewer the radiolabeled IgE that bind to the solid phase. There is a corresponding decrease in measured counts per minute (CPM).

Direct or noncompetitive RIST is a sandwich-type RIA in which solid-phase anti-IgE is incubated with reference or unknown IgE; the bound IgE then reacts with radiolabeled anti–human IgE. The greater the concentration of the reference or unknown IgE, the greater the concentration of radiolabeled anti–human IgE that binds, which is indicated by higher CPM.

The double antibody RIA or radioimmunoprecipitation test involves the liquid-phase incubation of reference or unknown IgE and radiolabeled IgE with anti–human IgE. Resulting complexes are precipitated by adding a second, precipitating antibody. The greater the concentration of reference or unknown IgE, the fewer radiolabeled IgE present in the precipitate. At one time the double-antibody method was preferred because of its sensitivity and reproducibility. Currently, ease of performance and commercial availability favors the use of noncompetitive RIST.[26] Modifications in testing procedures have included the development of enzyme-labeled assays in which enzyme activity is monitored by measuring the change in absorbance resulting from a change in concentration of the substrate or product.[27,28]

Total serum IgE is reported in international units (IU) per milliliter; 1 IU is equivalent to 2.4 ng of IgE protein.[26,29,30] Standardization of the total IgE immunoassay against a reference preparation is necessary to ensure the accuracy and comparability of interlaboratory assay results. In 1981 the second International Reference Preparation (75/502) of human serum IgE became available from the World Health Organization. A U.S. Reference Preparation is available from the National Institutes of Health and contains 900 IU/mL of IgE.[31] A trilevel Canadian IgE Reference Preparation is available through the Canadian Society for Allergy and Clinical Immunology.[30]

Total IgE is generally, although not always, elevated in atopic individuals. In children, an elevated serum IgE concentration suggests the likelihood of developing an allergic disease, especially if one or both parents have allergic disease. A normal IgE concentration, however, does not exclude the possibility of allergic disease in infancy or later in life. In older children or adults, some patients with atopic disease have elevated serum IgE levels; others do not. Again, low serum levels do not exclude the presence of IgE-mediated hyper-

sensitivity. IgE may also be elevated in diseases other than allergy, such as Wiskott-Aldrich syndrome, hyper-IgE syndrome, and parasitic infections.

QUANTITATION OF ALLERGEN-SPECIFIC IgE

The radioallergosorbent test (RAST) is the serologic quantitation of IgE antibodies directed against specific allergens.[32] This in vitro test yields information similar to skin testing. In fact, RAST testing may be preferred when skin testing is difficult to perform (in a young child) or interpret (when a second skin condition exists), when skin testing is negative, or when medication interference is suspected.[26] This test is a noncompetitive immunoassay in which the solid phase is coated with allergen. After incubation with reference or unknown sera, the specific allergen will capture IgE. Radiolabeled anti–human IgE is added to detect the bound IgE. The greater the amount of allergen-specific IgE bound, the greater the CPM of bound labeled IgE. When enzyme-labeled anti–human IgE replaces the radiolabeled antibody, the change in absorbance is measured.

There are two classifications to score and evaluate the results of the RAST method. In the first, the average patient counts per minute are compared with the average counts per minute of the reference sera. The reference serum is a standardized pool of human serum containing a high content of IgE directed against specific allergens. The greater the IgE content, the greater the CPM that are measured. A standard curve establishes the relationship between the concentration of several reference sera and the CPM or absorbance; from this the IgE concentration in patient or control sera is assigned. The patient results are graded from 0 to 4, indicating an increasing amount of specific IgE.

The second classification is a modification of the RAST scoring system. The patient counts are expressed as a percentage of the time control or positive control. The time control is the time required for the IgE standard (with a concentration of 25 IU/mL) to record 25,000 counts; all specimens are then counted for that period of time. The reading of the negative serum control is the second point to be plotted. A straight line is drawn between the readings of the negative control and the 25 IU/mL standard. The line is divided into five sections, defining classes 0 to 5; the higher the class, the greater the level of allergen-specific IgE that is present.[27,28] The time control minimizes variation in allergen, antibody affinity, and radioactive decay rates, so that more reliable results are generated.[33] Procedural modifications for better low-end sensitivity include a longer incubation time with the labeled anti–human IgE, and transferring the solid phase to a clean tube prior to quantitation.

New methodologies continue to emerge. The FAST (fluoroallergosorbent test) is a fluorescent enzyme immunoassay test in which total or specific IgE can be quantitated. FAST is a sandwich immunoassay in which the allergen is bound to the solid-phase membrane in the bottom of microtitration wells; following incubation with patient or reference serum, an enzyme-labeled anti–human IgE is added. The fluorescent substrate is added, and the intensity of fluorescence is measured.[34] The MAST® (MAST® Immunosystems, Mountain View, CA) chemiluminescent assay (CLA) is a noncompetitive CLA in which a solid-phase cellulose thread is impregnated with a battery of allergens; after incubation with patient or reference serum, enzyme-labeled anti–human IgE is added.[35,36] The enzyme label reacts with photoreagents to produce light. When the photographic film is exposed to light, a permanent record, an immunograph, is produced. Most recently, enzyme immunoassay dipstick methods have been introduced as screening tests for total IgE and for some common allergens. The short time required to perform the tests and the visual endpoint are advantages of these screening tests.

Detection of Human Chorionic Gonadotropin

The following discussion about human chorionic gonadotropin (hCG) highlights the development and progression of immunoassays.[37,38] The first molecular marker of pregnancy, hCG is produced by trophoblastic cells of the placenta. The first assay to detect hCG was a bioassay in which the biologic effect of hCG, its ability to induce the formation of corpus luteum in female mice, was observed. In the 1960s, agglutination immunoassays, which are faster and easier to perform, replaced the bioassays.[39] Examples of agglutination assays include hemagglutination inhibition, latex agglutination inhibition, hemagglutination, and latex agglutination. The agglutination inhibition methods require the premixing of patient urine with hCG antiserum; then particles (erythrocytes in the hemagglutination inhibition method or latex particles in the latex agglutination inhibition method) coated with hCG are added. Patient hCG, if present, will neutralize the antiserum, which prevents it from agglutinating hCG-coated particles; therefore, lack of agglutination with the hCG-coated particles indicates the presence of hCG in the patient sample (a positive test). In the latex agglutination or hemagglutination methods, the particle is coated with hCG antibody. When a patient sample containing hCG is added, it binds to the antibody and crosslinks the particles, resulting in macroscopic agglutination.

The specificity of all immunoassays is controlled by the specificity of the antibody used in the assay. It must be remembered that the four glycoprotein hormones (thyroid-stimulating hormone, luteinizing hormone, follicle-stimulating hormone, and hCG) have the same dimeric structure: All have identical α subunits and differ only in their β subunit. The β subunit of luteinizing hormone, structurally the most similar to hCG, shows 80% homology with the β subunit of hCG. The similarity of glycoprotein hormones, especially luteinizing hormone, may permit the glycoprotein hormones to crossreact in an assay designed to measure hCG, depending on the antiserum used. To develop an assay specific for hCG, the antibody must recognize the unique section of the β subunit or recognize an epitope present only on an intact hCG molecule.

Monoclonal antibody technology has allowed easier production of well-characterized antibodies; thus, specific assays with little or no crossreaction with the glycoprotein hormones have been developed. Improved specificity has made available assays with greater sensitivity, mostly RIA and EIA methods (Table 14-6). Some assays detect hCG by using two different antibodies, one recognizing an epitope on the α chain and the other on the β chain, whereas other assays are engineered to recognize an epitope present only on the intact molecule. Protein does not interfere in these RIA and EIA methods, so urine or serum may be used. Methods include double-antibody precipitation RIA and sandwich ELISA antigen assay.

Recently developed antigen capture assays using membranes are popular because they are easier to perform, have better sensitivity, and require less time to perform. Urine or serum containing hCG is passed through a filter membrane on which specific antibody is immobilized; hCG is captured. After applying the enzyme-labeled second antibody and the appropriate substrate, the color developed in the patient test is compared with the intensity of color generated by the standard. Some assays are read by viewing colored circles or a symbol such as a plus "+" (indicating the presence of hCG) or a minus "–" (indicating the asence of hCG).

TABLE 14-6
Analytic Sensitivity of Selected Methods to Measure hCG

ASSAY	ANALYTIC SENSITIVITY (mIU/mL)
Radioreceptor assay	20
Latex agglutination inhibition	500
Hemagglutination inhibition	150
Rapid immunoassays	25
Automated labeled assay	5

The hCG concentration is expressed in mIU/mL, IU/mL, or ng/mL, where 1 ng/mL = 9–11 mIU/mL.[38] The First International Reference Preparation of Human Chorionic Gonadotropin for Immunoassay made available in 1975 from the World Health Organization serves as the reference for all hCG immunoassays; the concentration of the reference preparation is 650 IU/ampoule. The sensitivity of several commercially available methods appears in Table 14-6.[38]

The level of hCG in normal pregnancy changes during gestation. The detectable level of hCG increases sharply during the first trimester, peaks at approximately 100,000 mIU/mL between 60 and 80 days after the last menstrual period, declines to a plateau of 10,000 to 20,000 mIU/mL at about 15 to 16 weeks gestation, and remains constant for the second and third trimesters. Generally, urine levels of hCG are sufficient to diagnose normal pregnancy; however, in the event that a urine hCG test is negative and pregnancy is still suspected, a second specimen should be collected and tested. In early pregnancy, up through 10 weeks gestation, hCG levels double every 2 days.

hCG is also measured to diagnose ectopic pregnancy and to evaluate a threatened spontaneous abortion. In ectopic pregnancy the hCG level is less than that in uterine pregnancy, in the range of 150 to 800 mIU/mL; those tests with lower sensitivity are particularly useful to diagnose this potentially life-threatening condition. The doubling time is longer than expected. Lower than expected levels or decreasing levels of hCG in the first trimester are also associated with spontaneous abortion.

hCG is measured to evaluate trophoblastic tumors, testicular tumors, and some nontrophoblastic tumors. Trophoblastic tumors, such as hydatidiform mole and choriocarcinoma, secrete high levels of hCG in the range of 5000 to 6,000,000 mIU/mL. To quantitate these levels, it may be necessary to dilute the specimen and perform a quantitative EIA or RIA method. High levels of hCG may also be associated with multiple pregnancies, eclampsia, polyhydramnios, and erythroblastosis fetalis. Testicular choriocarcinomas, seminomas, teratomas, and embryonal carcinomas are associated with elevated levels of hCG. When monitoring tumor activity, quantitating the β subunit is preferred because tumors may produce free β chains as well as intact hCG molecules.

Review Questions

An ELISA assay to detect rubella antibody requires that diluted patient sample react with rubella antigen coated onto a microtitration well. After washing the well, alkaline phosphatase–labeled rabbit anti–human IgM (μ chain specific) is added. After washing, paranitrophenol phosphate is added. The reaction is stopped and the absorbance of the product is read at 405 nm.

1. What does ELISA stand for?

2. What analyte is quantitated in this method?

3. Is this assay homogeneous or heterogeneous?

4. Is this assay competitive or noncompetitive?

5. What is the label?

6. What is the conjugate?

7. What is the purpose of para-nitrophenol phosphate?

8. When compared with the low positive control, will the high positive control have more or less absorbance?

9. How will incomplete washing affect the absorbance values?

References

1. Yalow RS, Berson SA: Assay of plasma insulin in human subjects by immunological methods. Nature 184: 1648–1669, 1959
2. Travis JC: Fundamental of RIA and Other Ligand Assays: A Programmed Text, p 48. Anaheim, CA, Radioassay Publishers, Division of Scientific Newsletters, 1979
3. Powsner ER: Basic principles of radioactivity and its measurement. In Burtis CA, Ashwood ER (eds): Tietz Fundamentals of Clinical Chemistry, 4th ed. Philadelphia, WB Saunders, 1996
4. Engvall E, Perlmann P: Immunochemistry 8:871, 1971
5. Van Weemen BK, Schuurs AHWM: Immunoassay using antigen-enzyme conjugates. FEBS Lett 15:232, 1971
6. Nakamura RM, Robbins BA: Fluorescence immunoassays. In Rose NR, DeMacario EC, Fahey JL, et al (eds):

Manual of Clinical Laboratory Immunology, 4th ed. Washington, DC, American Society for Microbiology, 1992

7. Alpert NL: Time-Resolved Fluorescence Immunoassay. Clinical Instrument Systems 9:1, 1988

8. Déchaud H, Bador R, Claustrat F, et al: New approach to competitive lanthanide immunoassay: Time-resolved fluoroimmunoassay of progesterone with labeled analyte. Clin Chem 34:501, 1988

9. Kricka LJ: Chemiluminescent and bioluminescent techniques. Clin Chem 37:1472–1481, 1991

10. Weiss AJ, Blankenstein LA: Membranes as a solid phase for clinical diagnostic assays. Am Clin Prod Rev June: 8, 1987

11. Litchfield WJ: Shell-core particles for the turbidimetric immunoassays. In Ngo TT (ed): Nonisotopic Immunoassay. New York, Plenum Press, 1988

12. Rubenstein KE, Schneider RB, Ullman EF: "Homogeneous" enzyme immunoassay, a new immunochemical technique. Biochem Biophys Res Commun 47:846, 1972

13. Henderson DR, Freidman SB, Harris JD et al: CEDIA, a new homogeneous immunoassay system. Clin Chem 32:1637, 1986

14. Ullman EF, Schwartzberg M, Rubinstein KD: Fluorescent excitation transfer assay: A general method for determination of antigen. J Biol Chem 251:4172, 1976

15. Tiffany TO: Fluorometry, nephelometry, and turbidimetry. In Burtis CA, Ashwood ER (eds): Tietz Fundamentals of Clinical Chemistry, 4th ed. Philadelphia, WB Saunders, 1996

16. Buhles WC: Fluorescence immunoassays. In Rippey JH, Nakamura RM (eds): Diagnostic Immunology: Technology Assessment and Quality Assurance, p 59. Skokie, IL, College of American Pathologists, 1983

17. Soini E, Kojola H: Time resolved fluormeter for lanthanide chelates: A new generation of nonisotopic immunoassays. Clin Chem 29:65–68, 1983

18. Hesterberg LK, Crosby MA: An overview of rapid immunoassay. Lab Med 27:41–46, 1996

19. Valkirs RF, Barton R: Immunoconcentration©: A new format for solid phase immunoassays. Clin Chem 31:1427, 1985

20. Rubenstein AS, Hostler RD, White CC, et al: Particle entrapment: Application to ICON© immunoassay. Clin Chem 32:1072, 1986

21. Zuk RF, Ginsberg VK, Houts T, et al: Enzyme immunochromatography: A quantitative immunoassay requiring no instrumentation. Clin Chem 31:1144, 1985

22. Harbeck RJ, Teague J, Crossen GR et al: Novel, rapid optical immunoassay technique for detection of group A streptococci from pharyngeal specimens: Comparison with standard culture methods. J Clin Microbiol 31: 839–844, 1993

23. Halpern GM: Markers in human allergic disease. J Clin Immunoassay 6:131, 1983

24. Barbee RA, Halonen M, Lebowitz M, et al: Distribution of IgE in a community population sample: Correlations with age, sex and allergen skin test reactivity. J Allergy Clin Immunol 68:106, 1981

25. Orgel HA: Genetic and development aspects of IgE. Pediatr Clin North Am 22:17, 1975

26. Hamilton RG, Adkinson NF Jr: Measurement of total serum immunoglobulin E and allergen-specific immunoglobulin E antibody. In Rose NR, DeMacario EC, Fahey JL, et al (eds): Manual of Clinical Laboratory Immunology, 4th ed. Washington, DC, American Society for Microbiology, 1992

27. Hamilton RG, Adkinson NF Jr: Clinical laboratory methods for the assessment and management of human allergic diseases. Clin Lab Med 6:117, 1986

28. Hamilton RG, Adkinson NF Jr: Serological methods in the diagnosis and management of human allergic disease. CRC Crit Rev Clin Lab Sci 21:1, 1984

29. Homburger HA: Current status of laboratory tests for allergic disease. In Rippey JH, Nakamura RM (eds): Diagnostic Immunology: Technology Assessment and Quality Assurance, p 195. Skokie, IL, College of American Pathologists, 1983

30. Mandy FF, Perelmutter L: Laboratory measurement of total human serum IgE. J Clin Immunoassay 6:140, 1983

31. Evans R: A U.S. reference for human immunoglobulin E. J Allerg Clin Immunol 68:79, 1981

32. Wide C, Bennich H, Johansson SGO: Diagnosis of allergy by an in-vitro test for allergen antibodies. Lancet 2:1105, 1967

33. Ali M, Nalebuff DJ, Fadal RG, et al: Allergy testing: From in vivo to in vitro. Diagn Med May/June, 5:3, 1982

34. Rodriquez GE: A new IgE fluorescent allergosorbent test (FAST). Clin Immunol Newslett 9:81, 1988

35. Miller SP, Marinkovich VA, Riege DH, et al: Application of the MAST© immunodiagnostic system to the determination of allergen-specific IgE. Clin Chem 30:1467, 1984

36. Brown CR, Higgins KW, Fazer K, et al: Simultaneous determination of total IgE and allergen-specific IgE in serum by the MAST chemiluminescent assay system. Clin Chem 31:1500, 1985

37. Sheehan C. Current status of pregnancy testing. Am J Med Technol 49:485, 1983

38. Flynn SD, Seifer DB: Clinical application of human chorionic gonadotropin. In Henry JB (ed): Clinical Diagnosis and Management by Laboratory Methods, 19th ed. Philadelphia, WB Saunders, 1996

39. Wide L, Genzell CA: An immunological pregnancy test. Acta Endocrinol 35:261, 1960

40. Speroff L, Glass RH, Kase NG: Clinical Gynecologic Endocrinology and Infertility, 5th ed. Baltimore, Williams and Wilkins, 1994

CHAPTER 15

Immunofluorescence

Catherine Sheehan

Objectives

Upon completion of the chapter, the reader will be able to:

1. Define fluorescence, direct immunofluorescence, indirect immunofluorescence, substrate, biotin, and avidin in the context of diagnostic immunology
2. Compare and contrast direct immunofluorescence and indirect immunofluorescence with respect to substrate, steps in the procedure, and conjugate
3. Compare and contrast transmitted light and epi-illumination fluorescence microscopes
4. State the absorption and emission maxima of fluorescein isothiocyanate
5. For the following sources of error associated with indirect immunofluorescence, discuss what each is and how to monitor it: increased nonspecific staining, increased background staining, decreased specific fluorescence, and increased autofluorescence
6. Describe two applications of indirect immunofluorescence to include the substrate used, analyte detected, and expected patterns

Immunofluorescence combines immunologic and histochemical or cytochemical methods to demonstrate the presence of antigen or antibody on the surface of cells or microorganisms, in tissues or cells, or circulating in serum. This technique uses a conjugate, reagent antibody labeled with a fluorescent dye (fluorochrome) to detect the antigen or antibody. The intensity and location of the fluorescence is then visualized using a specially adapted fluorescence microscope.

There are two commonly performed fluorescent antibody techniques: direct and indirect. In the direct method, conjugated reagent antibody reacts with the test antigen, forming an antigen-antibody complex. In the indirect method, the test antigen (the substrate) is allowed to react with unlabeled antibody (usually found in patient serum), and subsequently this antigen-antibody complex is layered with the conjugate, creating an antigen-antibody-antibody complex. Either complex (antigen-antibody or antigen-antibody-antibody) is rendered visible when excitation light strikes the fluorochrome and produces light emission of a longer wavelength in the visible spectrum. More recently, improved sensitivity and specificity have been achieved using biotin-avidin immunofluorescence, in which the biotin-labeled antibody is followed by avidin-labeled fluorochrome.

Immunofluorescence assays are both sensitive and reliable. The method sensitivity allows detection of soluble antibodies and protein antigens in concentrations as low as 10^{-4}/mL.[1] Moreover, insoluble antigens in

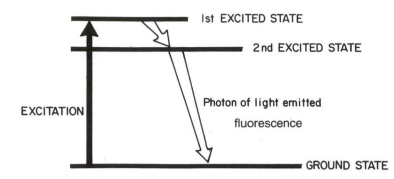

FIGURE 15-1
The movement of an electron that produces fluorescence.

tissues can be directly tested by using immunofluorescence. Confidence in the specificity of the assay is achieved by observing a predictable staining pattern in tissues and cells. In addition, flexibility in the method is possible when multiple antibodies or antigens are detected simultaneously and are distinguished by the location and staining pattern seen in tissue or cells, or by using reagent antibodies conjugated with fluorochromes that emit different colors.

FLUORESCENCE

Molecules capable of absorbing electromagnetic radiation or light energy become excited, altering the electron configuration of that molecule. The absorbed energy is dissipated, usually in the form of heat; however, some molecules emit a photon of light as the electron reverts to the stable ground state. This is luminescence.[2,3]

There are two types of luminescence: fluorescence and phosphorescence. In fluorescence the length of time between excitation and emission of light energy is short ($\leq 10^{-8}$ seconds). In phosphorescence the length of time is longer ($>10^{-4}$ seconds). The light energy is emitted in all directions, regardless of the direction of the excitation light.

Fluorescence occurs when a molecule absorbs light energy, causing an electron to move from the stable ground state to an excited state; thus, the electron moves from one orbital to another. Some energy will be lost as heat when the electron shifts to a second excited state, with lesser energy. Finally, as the electron returns to its original orbital, the ground state, a photon of light is emitted. This is fluorescence (Fig. 15-1). The amount of energy emitted is always less than the amount of excitation energy; hence, the wavelength of the emitted light is always longer than the wavelength of the excitation light (Fig. 15-2).

The intensity of fluorescence is influenced by some environmental factors. The pH may enhance fluorescence; use only fresh mounting media developed for the specific fluorochrome. Cooler temperatures, such as 4 to 8°C, will slow the spontaneous loss of fluorescence. Avoid exposure to electromagnetic radiation from artificial or natural light by storing slides in the dark, ideally in the refrigerator. This will help to maintain the intensity of the specific fluorescence. Some fluorochromes (such as fluorescein) are photosensitive and are subject to photobleaching when exposed to intense excitation light. Some fluorochrome molecules participate in chemical reactions; thus the fluorescence lessens.

A fluorescent label may be called a fluorochrome, fluorophore, or fluor; in immunofluorescence, the term *fluorochrome* is preferred. In general, the fluorochrome is attached to a specific antibody and its purpose is to visualize the location and pattern of specific antibody binding. The most commonly used fluorochrome is fluorescein isothiocyanate, a derivative of fluorescein that more readily covalently bonds to protein.

METHODS

Two major immunofluorescence methods are commonly performed in clinical immunology: direct immunofluorescence (DIF, also known as the direct fluorescence assay [DFA]) and indirect immunofluorescence (IIF, also known as the indirect fluorescence assay [IFA]).

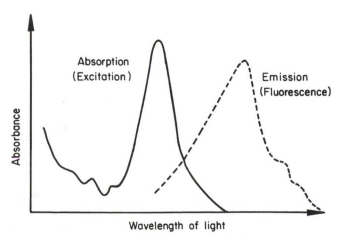

FIGURE 15-2
Absorption and emission spectra of a fluorescent compound.

DIF is used to detect an antigen that is part of the tissue, cell, or microorganism. IIF is used to detect circulating antibody in a patient sample. A modification, biotin-avidin immunofluorescence, improves analytic sensitivity and specificity.

Direct Immunofluorescence

The sample to be evaluated (thin frozen section of tissue biopsy, bacterial suspension, or cell suspension) is fixed onto a microscope slide. A conjugate specific for the antigen to be detected is overlaid onto the sample. The labeled antibody binds to the antigen. Excess conjugate is washed away. The slide is covered with a nonfluorescing mounting medium and coverslip, and is examined for specific staining using a fluorescence microscope. This method is used to detect organisms (viral, fungal, or parasitic) in host tissue, lymphocyte surface markers, and immune complexes in tissue biopsies (most commonly in skin and kidney biopsies) (Fig. 15-3).

Indirect Immunofluorescence

Indirect immunofluorescence is a two-step test. In the first step, patient sample containing unlabeled antibody is incubated with an antigen attached to a slide. This antigen, also known as the substrate, expresses known antigens to capture the patient antibody. Washing removes unreacted patient antibody. The remaining antigen-antibody complex (antigen in the substrate and antibody from the patient sample) is detected using a conjugate, a labeled anti–human globulin reagent. The slide is washed to remove excess conjugate, a coverslip is mounted with buffered glycerol, and the preparation is viewed for a specific pattern of fluorescence. Thus a specific, known antigen (or substrate) captures an antibody from a patient sample and that antibody is then visualized by a fluorochrome-labeled antibody. Most often this method is used to detect autoantibodies to nuclear antigens (Fig. 15-4).

Biotin-Avidin Immunofluorescence

Modification of the detection system in indirect immunofluorescence with biotin-avidin improves the specificity by reducing nonspecific, background fluo-

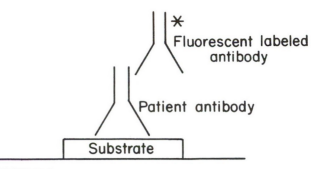

FIGURE 15-4
Schematic of indirect immunofluorescence.

rescence, and thus improves the lower detection limit of the assay. Immobilized substrate is incubated with patient antibody. After washing, reagent antiglobulin or monospecific antibody coupled with biotin is allowed to react. Excess antibody reagent is washed away. Avidin labeled with a fluorochrome is added. After washing, the complex is viewed microscopically. The avidin has a very strong affinity for biotin and a low affinity for the immobilized substrate; thus, background staining is minimized. Also, many biotin molecules attached to an antibody allow many avidin molecules to bind. More avidin binding results in more fluorochrome binding and increased fluorescence.

FLUOROCHROMES

Fluorochromes are organic dyes that fluoresce when exposed to short-wavelength light energy. Each has an excitation spectrum in which there is one wavelength that optimally excites the fluorochrome. The emission spectrum of each fluorochrome identifies the wavelength at which maximum fluorescence is emitted. To ensure that the optimal excitation wavelength interacts with the fluorochrome and that the optimal emission wavelength is viewed, filters are employed in the fluorescence microscope. The filters must be matched for the fluorochrome used. A summary of the absorption and emission wavelengths of commonly used fluorochromes is found in Table 15-1.[4]

Fluorescein is the most commonly used fluorochrome in clinical immunofluorescence (Fig. 15-5). To increase its efficiency for labeling antibody molecules, the more reactive fluorescein derivative, fluorescein isothiocyanate (FITC), is used. The molar fluorescein-to-protein ratio (F/P ratio) is an indication of the relative number of fluorescein molecules per antibody molecule. This molar ratio relates to a weight ratio by a factor of approximately 0.6 (i.e., a molar ratio of 5 will have substantially more activity than a weight ratio of 5). In IIF the molar ratio should be between 1 and 6, although the usual ratio is between 2 and 4.[1,5]

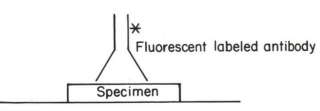

FIGURE 15-3
Schematic of direct immunofluorescence.

TABLE 15-1
Absorption and Emission Wavelengths of Commonly Used Fluorochromes

FLUOROCHROME	ABSORPTION (nM)	EMISSION (nM)
COVALENT LABELING OF PROTEIN		
Fluorescein isothiocyanate	490	514
R-phycoerythrin	480–565	578
Quantum Red™	488	670
Tetramethyl rhodamine isothiocyanate	540	578
Texas red	596	615
Phycocyanin	620	650
Allophycocyanin	650	660
NUCLEIC ACIDS		
Acridine orange		
+RNA	440–470	650
+DNA	480	510
Propidium iodide	493	630

Two factors influence the lower limit of detection and the specificity in immunofluorescence testing: the F/P and the titer of reagent antibody. Fluorescein is strongly electronegative and may bind nonspecifically to the substrate. If the F/P ratio is too high, the fluorescein, rather than the antibody, binds to the tissue or substrate, causing increased nonspecific fluorescence. This nonspecific fluorescence may be difficult or impossible to distinguish from the desired specific fluorescence. If the ratio is too low, specific staining will be diminished, causing the test results to be falsely decreased or negative. Secondly, the titer and affinity of

antibody in the conjugate must be sufficient to ensure acceptable sensitivity. In DIF the conjugate should contain approximately 100 to 200 µg antibody/mL. In IIF the concentration of conjugate should be 25 to 50 µg antibody/mL.[1]

FLUORESCENCE MICROSCOPY

A fluorescence microscope creates darkfield illumination and then, using special components, produces the conditions to separate excitation and emission wavelengths. The special components are the light source, the excitation filter, and the barrier filter.

Light sources for fluorescence microscopes must emit light rich in the wavelength necessary for excitation of the fluorochrome. The two common light sources are the tungsten halogen lamp and the mercury vapor arc lamp. The tungsten halogen lamp produces a continuous spectrum, has a short life span (about 30 hours), maintains its intensity until it burns out, and can be used in a standard lamp housing. The mercury vapor arc lamp produces a discrete spectrum, has a long life span (about 200 hours), loses intensity as the lamp ages, and requires a special protective lamp housing. When the fluorochrome is fluorescein, the mercury vapor arc lamp produces a more intense light emission at 577 nm than the tungsten halogen lamp, thereby producing stronger fluorescence.

The excitation or primary filter is placed between the light source and the specimen, and allows the wavelength of light that can be absorbed by the fluorochrome to reach the specimen and removes undesired wavelengths of light. The barrier or secondary

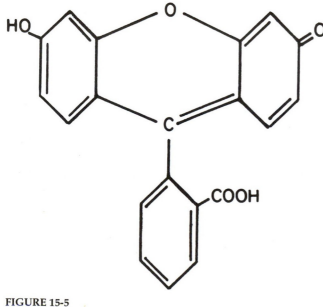

FIGURE 15-5
Structure of fluorescein.

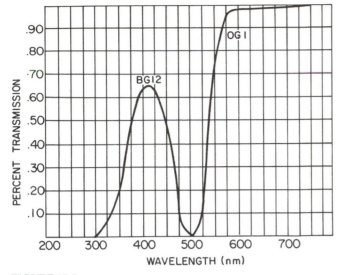

FIGURE 15-6
An example of a filter system that can be used with fluorescein. The BG 12 filter is the excitation filter and allows the optimal excitation wavelength (490–495 nm) to be transmitted to the specimen. The OG 1 filter is the barrier filter, can transmit the emission wavelength of fluorescein (520 nm), and does not transmit the excitation wavelength.

filter is placed between the specimen and the ocular lens. It allows the light emitted from the fluorochrome to pass through the filter while preventing undesired wavelengths from passing. Most commonly, these filters are glass (Fig. 15-6).

There are two configurations for fluorescence microscopes: the transmitted light microscope and the epifluorescence microscope. In the transmitted light fluorescence microscope, the light travels from the light source through the excitation filter, a darkfield condenser, and the specimen. The light emitted from the fluorochrome passes through the barrier filter to the ocular lens to be viewed by the observer. Because the light beam is transmitted from below and then passes through the specimen, some light is diffused, thereby decreasing the fluorescence (Fig. 15-7).

The epifluorescence microscope, described by Ploem in 1967, uses vertical illumination and a dichroic mirror. In this system, light travels from the light source through the excitation filter and is reflected by the dichroic mirror at a 45° angle to pass through the objective (which serves as the condenser) to the surface of the specimen. The fluorescence emitted from the fluo-

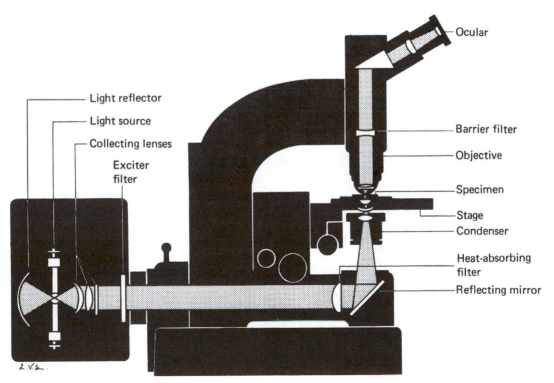

FIGURE 15-7
Fluorescence microscope with transmitted light. The light beam is generated by a mercury vapor lamp, reflected by a concave mirror, and projected through collecting lenses to the exciter filter, which emits a fluorescent light beam. A reflecting mirror directs the beam from underneath the stage, through the condenser, into the specimen. A barrier filter removes wavelengths other than those emitted from the fluorescent compound in the specimen, and the fluorescent pattern is viewed through magnification provided by the objective and ocular lenses. (Reproduced with permission from Stites DP, Stobo JD, Wells JV: Basic and Clinical Immunology, 6th ed. ©Appleton and Lange, 1987.)

rochrome enters the objective and passes through the dichroic mirror and the barrier filter to the ocular lens. The dichroic mirror is an interference filter that allows specific wavelengths of light to be reflected (the excitation light) and other wavelengths of light to be transmitted (the emitted light). Because the excitation light is passed down through the objective and stops on the specimen, a darkfield is created. Also, because the excitation light travels through optics to the surface of the specimen and does not pass through the specimen, the specimen does not interfere with the intensity or clarity of fluorescence. The filter systems are easily changed, so that viewing more than one fluorochrome is simple. Epi-illumination may be combined with transmitted light from brightfield or phase-contrast microscopes (Fig. 15-8).

The objectives in fluorescence microscopy must be nonfluorescent and should have the highest numerical aperture (N.A.) possible. The higher the N.A. of an objective lens, the greater the light-gathering capability of the objective; therefore, the fluorescence is brighter. The immersion oil must be nonfluorescing.

In immunofluorescence the mounting medium must be water soluble. When the fluorochrome is fluorescein, most often buffered glycerol is used (nine parts glycerol to one part of 0.2 M carbonate buffer, pH 9.0).[6] The pH should be greater than 8 to enhance fluorescence and retard fading on exposure to ultraviolet light. Stored buffered glycerol mounting medium may absorb CO_2, resulting in a decrease in pH.

STANDARDIZATION

Types of Fluorescence

Specific staining (both desired and undesired) is the result of an immunologic reaction between the conjugate and an antigen. Desired specific staining detects the analyte of the test. Undesired specific staining may be caused by a crossreaction with a heterologous antigen or an impure antibody preparation. Nonspecific staining is a nonimmunologic interaction of the conjugate with the sample or substrate. This may be caused by the presence of free (unconjugated) fluorochrome or of

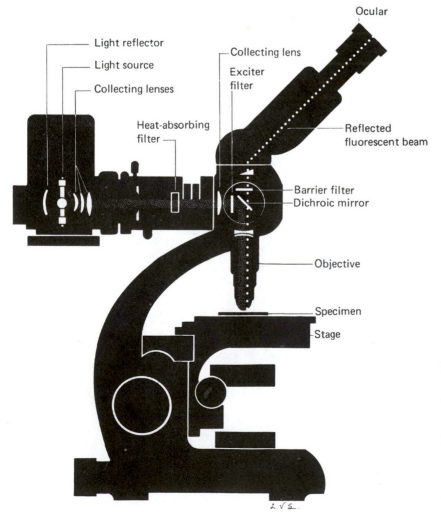

FIGURE 15-8
Fluorescence microscope with epi-illumination. The light beam is directed through the exciter filter and down onto the specimen. A dichroic mirror allows passage of selected wavelengths in one direction but not another. After reaching the specimen, the light is reflected through the dichroic mirror and emitted fluorescent light is visualized at the ocular. (Reproduced with permission from Stites DP, Stobo JD, Wells JV: Basic and Clinical Immunology, 6th ed. ©Appleton and Lange, 1987.)

labeled serum protein other than immunoglobulin (such as globulin), or it may result when the specimen dries out during the staining procedure. Nonspecific staining can be decreased or eliminated by appropriate dilution of the conjugate and by control of the reaction time and temperatures.

Autofluorescence is the natural fluorescence of tissue or substrate. The color of autofluorescence depends on the filter system used and may appear blue to blue-green, to yellow, to red. Proper filter selection allows sufficient contrast between autofluorescence and specific fluorescence. Autofluorescence is increased by formalin fixation, embedding in paraffin, and long storage time.

Optimal Conjugate Dilution

To determine the proper dilution of conjugated antiserum to be used in a particular IIF test, a chessboard titration must be performed.[5] For this titration, slides containing the appropriate substrate are incubated with serial dilutions of a known positive control serum and are then tested with a serial dilution of the conjugate. The performance of conjugate will be constant for several conjugate dilutions for a specific control serum dilution (the plateau titer) and is related to the F/P ratio. One twofold dilution less than the highest conjugate dilution (plateau endpoint) to generate this constant fluorescence is the optimal dilution of conjugate to be used in the assay.

If a commercial diagnostic kit is used, the manufacturer will supply the conjugate at its optimal dilution. For reproducible test results, it is imperative that the manufacturer's instructions be strictly followed and that components of one lot number not be used with components of other lot numbers.

Quality Control

Positive control serum and negative control serum must be run in every IIF assay and should produce the expected specific fluorescence pattern, intensity, and titer. These are used to evaluate sources of error in the assay run that may be related to the function of the microscope, the integrity of the reagents, the performance of the assay, and subjectivity when reading the slide. In antinuclear antibody testing, the World Health Organization 66/233 Reference Preparation provides a standard preparation to which a positive control serum can be referenced for the pattern and intensity. Defined sera are available through the Centers for Disease Control and Prevention by the Arthritis Foundation.[6] Manufacturers may state the expected pattern and intensity for the control sera supplied in their diagnostic kits as demonstrated using a specific microscope configuration. Some control sera also have a stated endpoint titer,

which can be useful when monitoring the assay sensitivity. By running serial dilutions of the control serum, the endpoint can be determined and then compared with the stated value. Deviation greater than one twofold dilution suggests a shift in the assay sensitivity and the need to evaluate the reason for this shift.

While the positive and negative serum controls are primarily intended to evaluate the fluorescent pattern, the FITC Quality Control Slideslide™ (Immuno Concepts, Sacramento, CA) and Optical Standard Slide (Behring Diagnostics, Westwood, MA) more specifically evaluate the fluorescent microscope. Five levels of fluorescent microbead standards are immoblilized onto a slide. For a given level, all beads demonstrate a uniform level of fluorescein fluorescence, and absorption and emission spectra are comparable with those expected with cellular fluorescence. The intensity of fluorescence is evaluated, and the endpoint is established. This reflects the type and condition of the light source, alignment of the light path, correctness of the filters, numerical aperture of the objective, and consistency in reading.

APPLICATIONS

Anti-Nuclear Antibodies

Antibodies to nuclear antigens (ANA) are antibodies directed against components of the cell nucleus, such as nucleoproteins and nucleic acids. ANA are associated with many systemic diseases, including systemic lupus erythematosus, mixed connective tissue disease, and rheumatoid arthritis. ANA can be used as a diagnostic indicator, a prognostic indicator, or a means of monitoring the effectiveness of therapy.

Indirect immunofluorescence is the method of choice to screen for ANA. A representative protocol follows: Fixed substrate containing nuclei (rodent liver or tissue culture cells) is incubated with patient or control serum. After washing, the tissue is incubated with anti–human immunoglobulin conjugated with fluorescein; following a second wash, the slide is viewed with a fluorescence microscope. The pattern and titer are recorded.

Several patterns of nuclear fluorescence can be described, depending on the substrate used. When rodent (mouse or rat) liver cells are used, the patterns are diffuse, peripheral, speckled, and nucleolar. The diffuse, or homogeneous, pattern evenly stains the nuclei and is associated with deoxyribonucleoprotein; the peripheral, or rim, pattern appears as bright fluorescence near the edge of the nuclei and is associated with native DNA; the speckled pattern appears as numerous evenly distributed speckles of fluorescence within the nuclei and is associated with many saline-extractable

PATTERN	NUCLEAR ANTIGEN
Homogeneous	ds-DNA, histone
Peripheral	ds-DNA
Speckled	Sm, Ul-RNP
	SS-A, SS-B
	Scl-70
Nucleolar	4-6S RNA
Centromere	Centromere

DIRECT IMMUNOFLUORESCENCE	
Skin biopsy	Bullous pemphigoid
	Pemphigus vulgaris
	Dermatitis herpetiformis

INDIRECT IMMUNOFLUORESCENCE	
Smooth muscle Ab	Autoimmune chronic active hepatitis
Mitochondrial Ab	Primary biliary cirrhosis
Thyroglobulin Ab	Hashimoto's thyroiditis Graves' disease
Thyroid peroxidase Ab	Hashimoto's thyroiditis Graves' disease
Parietal cell Ab	Chronic atrophic gastritis with pernicious anemia

Ab, antibody.

nuclear antigens; and the nucleolar pattern appears as two or three large, nearly round fluorescent areas within the nucleus and is associated with nucleolar RNA. If a human epithelial tissue culture cell line (HEp-2 or KB cells) is used as the substrate, the antigens present are those found in rodent liver cells plus the SSA/Ro antigen and the centromere antigen. The centromere antigen is present in actively replicating cells and produces a characteristic discrete speckled pattern when the centromere fluoresces. A summary of the immunofluorescence patterns and nuclear antigens is presented in Table 15-2.[7]

Thus, from the indirect immunofluorescence procedure, not only can the presence and titer of an ANA be demonstrated, but the pattern of fluorescence can also be described. Positive ANA are seen in a variety of diseases. The pattern, although not a diagnostic marker for any specific disease, may suggest the specificity of the antibody(ies) present. Multiple ANAs can be present in a patient specimen, and further testing can confirm the antibody specificity.

Double-Stranded DNA Antibodies

Antibodies to double-stranded DNA (ds-DNA) can be detected by indirect immunofluorescence (IIF).[7] Sometimes these antibodies are referred to as native DNA (nDNA). The IIF method uses *Crithidea luciliae* as the substrate, because the hemoflagellate possesses ds-DNA in its kinetoplast. After incubating the substrate with patient serum, washing, incubating with fluorescent-labeled anti–human globulin, and final washing, the slide is viewed with a fluorescence microscope. Specific fluorescence of the kinetoplast at the base of the flagellum indicates the presence of ds-DNA antibodies. Measuring the titer of ds-DNA antibodies is important in patients with systemic lupus erythematosus to assess the level of disease activity and as a prognostic indicator of renal disease.

Although the ANA and ds-DNA antibodies are the most common IIF assays, many other immunofluorescence applications are available in the clinical laboratory. Table 15-3 describes the clinical significance of some common procedures.

Review Questions

1. Which of the following CANNOT be detected by direct immunofluorescence?

   a. Circulating antibody
   b. DNA–anti-DNA complexes in the glomeruli
   c. Surface immunoglobulin on B lymphocytes
   d. *Treponema pallidum* in lesional exudate

2. Which statement best describes the conjugate in indirect immunofluorescence?

   a. It is the fluorescent dye.
   b. It is the antibody-fluorescent dye complex.
   c. It is the specific antibody.
   d. It is the antigen-antibody complex.

3. Which quality control measure will best identify a change in the quality of the microscope?

   a. Negative control serum
   b. Positive control serum
   c. Standardized particle slide
   d. Comparing results with another laboratory

4. Compared with the excitation light energy, the wavelength of light emitted is _____ and the energy level is _____ .

   a. shorter; lower
   b. shorter; higher
   c. longer; lower
   d. longer; higher

5. An increase in background, nonspecific staining in an indirect immunofluorescence assay to detect anti-nuclear antibodies could be caused by

   a. a prozone effect
   b. photobleaching
   c. an increased F/P
   d. autofluorescence

References

1. Kwapinski G: The Methodology of Investigative and Clinical Immunology, p 245. Malabar, Robert E. Krieger Publishing, 1982

2. Cleveland BJ: Emission and absorption spectroscopy. In Ward KM, Lehmann CA, Leiken AM (eds): Clinical Laboratory Instrumentation and Automation: Principles, Applications, and Selection. Philadelphia, WB Saunders, 1994

3. Skoog DA, West DM: Fundamentals of Analytical Chemistry, 2nd ed, p 638. New York, Holt, Rinehart and Winston, 1969

4. Givan AL: Flow Cytometry: First Principles, p 64. New York, Wiley-Liss, 1992

5. Cavallaro JJ, Palmer DF, Bigazzi PE: Immunofluorescence Detection of Autoimmune Diseases, p 128. Atlanta, GA, U.S. Department of Health Education and Welfare, 1976

6. Tan EM, Fritzler MJ, McDougal JS, et al: Reference sera for antinuclear antibodies. Arthritis Rheum 25:1003–1005, 1982

7. Nakamura RM, Peebles CL, Molden DP, et al: Autoantibodies to Nuclear Antigens, 2nd ed. Chicago, American Society of Clinical Pathologists Press, 1985

CHAPTER 16

Nephelometry

Alice K. Chen

Objectives

Upon completion of the chapter, the reader will be able to:

1. Describe the nature and type of light scattering due to immunoprecipitation
2. Describe the kinetics of immunoprecipitation formation
3. Describe the difference between endpoint and rate nephelometry
4. Describe nephelometric or turbidimetric inhibition immunoassay and particle-enhanced immunoassay
5. Identify the major components of instruments for nephelometry and turbidimetry
6. Describe the performance characteristics and limitations of nephelometry
7. Name the most commonly used analyzers for immunonephelometry and immunoturbidimetry
8. Give examples of common applications of nephelometry and turbidimetry

Nephelometry is a direct method of measuring light scattered by particles suspended in solution. Nephelometry, based on the classic antigen-antibody precipitation reaction first described by Heidelberger and Kendall,[1] is now routinely used to quantitate specific proteins. With automated commercial analyzers and reagents readily available, nephelometry provides great advantages over the standard techniques of radial immunodiffusion (RID) and immunoelectrophoresis (IEP). Quantitation of specific protein by nephelometry is now accurate, precise, fast, easy to perform, and fully automated. It is most commonly used to measure plasma proteins such as immunoglobulins, complement components, coagulation factors, acute-phase proteins, and drugs. This chapter discusses the basic principles of nephelometry and its application to immunology. For more detail, manuals and review articles are readily available in the literature.[2,3]

PRINCIPLES OF NEPHELOMETRY

Nature of Light Scattering

The interaction of light with particles in solution can be measured by nephelometry or turbidimetry. When light strikes a solution containing particles, the light is transmitted through the solution and absorbed, reflected, or scattered by the particles. Nephelometry is a direct measurement of light scattered by the particles; the instrument detects the scattered light at an angle different from the incoming light source (incident light). The low intensity of scattered light, sometimes not visible to the eye, is measured by a sensitive detector. Turbidimetry is the measurement of light transmitted through a suspension of particles and can be measured by a sensitive spectrophotometer or photometer. For nephelometry and turbidimetry to be useful methods to measure specific proteins, the solutions must negligibly absorb and reflect incident light.

In immunonephelometry, a soluble antigen and soluble antibody bind and form immune complexes, particles capable of scattering light. The nature of light scattering can be classified into two types, depending on the diameter (d) of the particles relative to the wavelength (λ) of incident light. As shown in Figure 16-1, small particles, such as albumin, IgG, and IgM ($d < .1\lambda$), produce Rayleigh light scattering that is symmetrical in the forward and backward directions. A minimum scatter is observed at 90° from the incident light. Larger molecules and antigen-antibody complexes, with diameters comparable with the wavelength, produce Rayleigh-Debye light scattering. In this case, the light scattered has greater intensity in the forward direction when the detection angle, θ, approaches zero.

For both types of light scattering, the intensity of scattered light is proportional to the intensity of incident light and concentration of the light scattering particles, and is inversely related to the fourth power of the wavelength of light. Using light in the blue-green region (λ = 400 to 500 nm), immune complexes and serum lipoprotein produce Rayleigh-Debye and Rayleigh scattering, depending on particle size. A laser light source and forward angle detection of scattered light produces greater signals and, hence, greater sensitivity in nephelometry. Immunoturbidimetry measures the reduction in light intensity after the incident light passes through the light-scattering suspensions of immunoprecipitation. If light absorbance is insignificant, turbidity is expressed as absorbance and is proportional to the concentration of suspended particles and to the path length of the reaction sample.

Kinetics of Fluid-Phase Precipitation

The interaction of antigen and antibody in solution depends on many factors, most important of which is their relative concentrations. The initial interaction is the primary binding of antigen to antibody molecules. This reaction is reversible. Polyvalent antigens and a polyclonal antibody mixture encourage the secondary rearrangement, and crosslinking of the antigen-antibody complexes slowly forms a lattice. At this stage, the complex is large enough to produce Rayleigh-Debye scattering of visible light. If the antibody concentration remains in excess and the secondary rearrangement continues, eventually aggregates form and appear as visible precipitation that settles out of the solution. As shown in Figure 16-2, maximal lattice is formed when the reaction is in the zone of equivalence. If more antigen or antibody is added to the lattice, the additional antigen or antibody will break up the lattice, producing a large amount of smaller antigen-antibody complexes. For a single antibody dilution, two different antigen concentrations, one in the antibody excess zone and one in the antigen excess zone, can produce the same amount of lattice and light-scattering signal. Nephelometry is often used to quantitate antigen concentrations in the presence of excess antibody so that the size of the lattice scatters light optimally for the wavelength of incident light and is directly proportional to the anti-

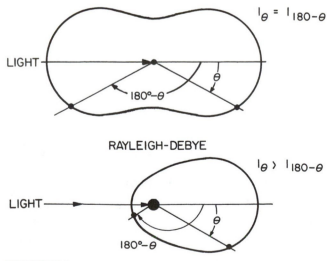

FIGURE 16-1
Angular distribution patterns for Rayleigh light scattered from small particles, and Rayleigh-Debye scattering from somewhat larger particles. (From Sternberg JC: Rate nephelometry. In Rose NR, Friedman H, Fahey JL (eds): Manual of Clinical Laboratory Immunology, 3rd ed, p 34. Washington, DC, American Society for Microbiology, 1986. Used by permission.)

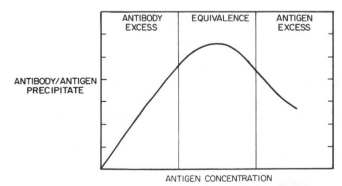

FIGURE 16-2
The quantitative precipitin curve generated by adding increasing amounts of antigen to a solution of antibody and measuring antibody-antigen complexes by nephelometry. (Reprinted from Whicher JT, Perry DE: Nephelometric methods. In Butt WR (ed): Practical Immunoassay: The State of the Art. Clin Biochem Anal 14:123, 1984, courtesy of Marcel Dekker, Inc.)

gen concentration in the test sample. To prevent a reaction in antigen excess, a check of free antibody is included in the assay.

Figure 16-3 shows a typical immunoprecipitation reaction monitored by nephelometry under the optimal antibody excess condition. When the specimen is diluted with buffer and added to the cuvette, a small background light scattering is detected. This serves as the sample blank. The sources of this background scattering are proteins and lipoproteins in the sample, particles or dust present in the reagents, or stray light. The small background signal is usually independent of the detection angle and can be minimized by using nephelometric grade antisera and a high dilution of the samples. The addition of antiserum into the cuvette initiates the antigen-antibody binding reaction. Over a short period of time, complexes form slowly, which is reflected in the slow increase of scatter intensity. This is followed by a rapid increase in scatter intensity when antigen-antibody complexes crosslink. The amount of scattered light reaches a plateau and then declines when the precipitate starts to aggregate and settle out of the solution. The rate of increase of scattered light and the height of the plateau are directly related to the antigen concentration and the dilution of the antiserum.

Similar to other chemical reactions, the antigen-antibody interaction is controlled by the antiserum affinity and avidity, the buffer, pH, ionic strength, and mixing of the assay solution. The reaction can be greatly enhanced by the presence of a nonionic, hydrophilic

polymer. Because the polymer is more hydrophilic than the antigen or antibody molecules, it attracts water molecules away from the antigen and antibody, and subsequently increases the rate and amount of antigen-antibody reaction. Polyethylene glycol (PEG) is now routinely used in nephelometry assays. It speeds up the reaction rate, increases the slope of the precipitation curve in the antibody excess zone, and shifts the equivalence zone to a higher antigen concentration. This results in nephelometry of considerably greater sensitivity, wider detection range, and faster assay. The PEG is especially effective with low-avidity antisera. Microparticles conjugated with immune complex components have been used successfully to enhance the antigen-antibody reactions in microparticle enhanced immunonephelometry or immunoturbidimetry.

METHODS

Endpoint Nephelometry

In the immunoprecipitation reaction, the time to reach the plateau of light scattering may vary from a few minutes to 1 hour, depending on reaction conditions. After correction for background light scattering, the plateau for each sample is often directly proportional to its antigen concentration. The steps in an assay include the following: (1) reagents, buffer, sample, and antisera are first mixed together; (2) the background signal is measured; (3) incubation of the mixture continues until the plateau is reached; (4) the plateau or endpoint signal is measured; (5) a final signal is generated after correcting for background signal; and finally, (6) the antigen concentration is determined using a calibration curve. Because samples vary considerably, the background light scatter must always be corrected in endpoint nephelometry. The background interference in the sample blank limits the sensitivity of endpoint nephelometry. The antisera avidity and affinity determine the incubation time and the height of the plateau reached for each assay. Instruments using endpoint analysis are more susceptible to specimen matrix interference and require a long incubation time (10 minutes to an hour) but can handle a greater number of samples per hour. The long incubation time necessitates a longer turnaround time, making endpoint nephelometry impractical for stat analysis.

Rate Nephelometry

For most nephelometric immunoassays, the maximum or peak rate of light scattering usually occurs in less than 1 or 2 minutes. The kinetics of the antigen-antibody complex formation are shown in Figure 16-3. The velocity of a reaction depends on the concentration of

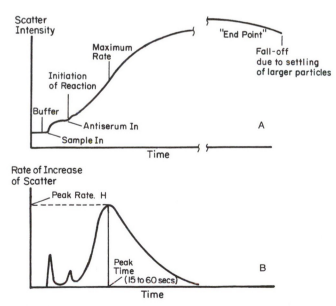

FIGURE 16-3
Time course of the immunoprecipitation reaction. (**A**) Variation of intensity of scattered light versus time. (**B**) Rate of increase of scatter versus time. (From Sternberg JC: Rate nephelometry. In Rose NR, Friedman H, Fahey JL (eds): Manual of Clinical Laboratory Immunology, 3rd ed, p 34. Washington, DC, American Society for Microbiology, 1986. Used by permission.)

antigen and the affinity and titer of the antiserum. In antibody excess, the peak rate increases as the antigen concentration increases, though not necessarily in a linear relationship. To establish the relationship between antigen concentration and peak rate, multiple standards, each with a known concentration, are assayed and the reference curve is prepared. This nonlinear relationship can be stored in the instrument and used to determine the concentration of antigen in a sample. The time required to reach the peak reaction rate is inversely proportional to the sample antigen concentration. Rate assays, also called kinetic, nephelometric, or turbidimetric assays, need continuous monitoring of the reaction, starting when antiserum is added and continuing through the antigen excess check. The rate assay bypasses the problem of background interference and requires a short incubation time to reach the peak rate of immune complex formation. It generally requires antiserum of higher affinity and avidity than that needed in the endpoint method. The rate method is more sensitive to adequate mixing and factors such as pH, buffer, and polymer enhancement. In the rate method, a light source with a wider bandwidth produces reaction rates that are more reproducible than rates measured with a laser. This is caused by the fact that scattering signals from a single-wavelength laser source is more susceptible to the changing size of the immune complex during its initial formation.

Nephelometric Inhibition Immunoassay

Although the basic principles of nephelometric inhibition immunoassay (NIIA) were first reported by Pauling in 1942,[6] application of this immunoassay for haptens and drugs was only developed when automated analyzers became available in the 1970s.[5] Haptens with a molecular weight less than 4000 Da cannot be measured directly by light scattering because haptens are monovalent. They form soluble complexes with the hapten antiserum but cannot form the lattice. When haptens are covalently conjugated to carrier proteins, they can react with hapten antiserum and will form a lattice of sufficient size to be easily detected. In NIIA, sample containing hapten is added to a mixture of a fixed amount of hapten conjugate and a limited amount of hapten antiserum; the sample hapten will bind to the antibody and inhibit the lattice formation between hapten conjugate and hapten antiserum. Under conditions near the zone of equivalence and with the addition of enhancers, NIIA has been used in endpoint and rate assays to measure therapeutic drugs. The competition of sample hapten and hapten conjugate for antibody binding in NIIA results in a homogeneous (no separation) immunoassay. As in all competitive binding assays, the amount of light scattered is inversely related to the concentration of hapten in the sample and produces a classic sigmoidal standard curve with a negative slope.

Microparticle-Enhanced Immunoassay

Latex particles were the first microparticles to be used in serologic testing. The latex agglutination method described by Singer and Plotz[6] in 1956 allowed visualization of an antigen-antibody reaction with greater sensitivity than could be achieved with precipitation methods. Similarly, using a microparticle in nephelometric and turbidimetric assays can increase method sensitivity. The sensitivity of these methods depends on the size of immune complexes that will scatter sufficient light to be measured. For some analytes the immune complexes are too small; microparticles are used to add "bulk" to the immune complex, creating more light scatter. As the sensitivity improves, the sample can be diluted further; thus, sample interference is reduced and sample blanks or pretreatment are eliminated.

In the simplest assays, polymers of latex ranging from 0.07 to 0.2 μm in diameter are covalently linked to a reagent antibody. The corresponding antigen in a sample binds to the antibody particle and forms a complex; the scattered light can then be measured with a nephelometer or turbidimeter. The sensitivity approaches enzyme immunoassay and other labeled methods, and for serum proteins is reported to be as low as 1 μg/L.[7] A second approach using microparticles is in a competitive inhibition assay. Similar to NIIA, the sample antigen competes with a microsphere coated with antigen to bind to an antibody reagent. A sigmoidal calibration curve with a negative slope is produced.[8] Test results are typically calculated by the analyzer using logit-log function and linear regression analysis. Compared with other immunoassays that require washing or separation, the particle-enhanced turbidimetric or nephelometric immunoassays are simpler, faster, and can be run on many automated analyzers readily available in the clinical laboratories.

INSTRUMENTATION

The basic components of a nephelometer are shown in Figure 16-4. Typically, the instrument includes a light source, a collimating system to focus the light, a monochromator, a cuvette, and a photomultiplier tube. The light source varies from simple, inexpensive tungsten lamps to mercury lamps, xenon arc lamps, and high-intensity lasers. The nephelometer requires the same components as a fluorometer, except in nephelometry the wavelength of the incident light does not need a very narrow bandwidth. In fact, a fluorometer can be used

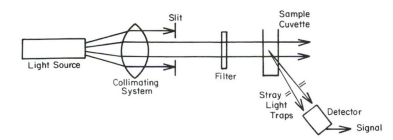

FIGURE 16-4
Schematic of basic components of a nephelometer. (Reproduced by permission from Pesce AJ, Frings CS, Gauldie J: Spectral techniques. In Kaplan LA, Pesce AJ (eds): Clinical Chemistry: Theory, Analysis and Correlation, 3rd ed, p 102. St. Louis, CV Mosby, 1995.)

for nephelometric measurement simply by using the same filter or wavelength for the incident light and the scattered light. A high-quality spectrophotometer can be used directly for turbidimetric assay or the detection angle can be modified for use in nephelometric assays.

Nephelometers with the highly intense, single-wavelength, narrowly focused laser light source allow a greater signal to be measured and do not require the collimating system, but the scattered light is more susceptible to fluctuations of particle size, because the antigen-antibody complex size changes with reaction time. An instrument with a conventional lamp, such as a tungsten light source, has light of a wider bandwidth, produces signals proportional to the average size of the complex, and is therefore less susceptible to particle size change and produces a more reproducible kinetic or rate measurement. As shown in Figure 16-1 for Rayleigh and Rayleigh-Debye scattering, front angle detection can more than double the amount of light scattering compared with an instrument with a 90° angle of detection.

Some clinical instruments dedicated to nephelometric assays and automated analyzers capable of nephelometric or turbidimetric analysis are listed in Table 16-1. All instruments are highly automated, integrated with a microcomputer for tasks such as calibration, calculation, check of antigen excess, and quality control. In the 1989 CAP proficiency survey, 75% of laboratories surveyed used nephelometry to quantitate immunoglobulins. Among these laboratories, over 70% of the nephelometers used for IgA determinations were Beckman Array 360 or Beckman ICS nephelometer, followed by the Behring and Sanofi (formerly Kallestad Diagnostics) nephelometers.[9] For laboratories where automated, random-access, spectrophotometric-based analyzers are available, nephelometric or turbidimetric immunoassay can be performed with little difficulty.

LIMITATIONS OF LIGHT-SCATTERING METHODS

As shown in Figure 16-2 for each antibody dilution, two different antigen concentrations, one in prozone and the other in postzone, will produce the same amount of antigen-antibody lattice and, thus, intensity of light scattered. Antigen excess is most frequently encountered in monoclonal immunoglobulins, C-reactive protein, and β_2 microglobulin. To validate assay results, antigen excess must be checked in all light-scattering immunoassays, typically programmed into a nephelometer. One way to check for antigen excess is to assay the sample at two different dilutions. Alternatively, assays can be checked for antigen excess by adding more antibody to the assay mixture and monitoring the reaction rate or plateau response. Samples with antigen excess are then reassayed at a greater dilution. It is possible to extend the range of an immunoturbidimetric assay to the antigen excess range. For example, using complex multiparameters and data manipulation, the working range of albumin assay was extended by three- to fourfold.[10] Nephelometry or turbidimetry based on sample analyte inhibition eliminates the risk of antigen excess.

Interferences in light scattering caused by endogenous particles, such as lipoproteins, proteins, or dust particles, may limit the assay sensitivity of the endpoint method but often are eliminated using clearing or supplementary precipitation reagents. Turbid specimens may need to be filtered or centrifuged before they can be assayed. PEG can nonspecifically precipitate macromolecules in samples. Freezing and thawing of samples

TABLE 16-1
Automated Clinical Instruments for Light-Scattering Immunoassay

NEPHELOMETERS	AUTOMATED ANALYZERS
Beckman Array 360, ICS II	Abbott TDx
Behring BNII, BNA, BN100	Beckman Synchron CX4,5,7
Sanofi Diagnostic Pasteur QM300, N600	Boehringer Mannheim Hitachi 704, 717, 911
Bayer Technicon DPA I	Ciba Corning 550 Express
	DuPont ACA
	IL Multistat
	Roche COBAS® Bio, Fara, Mira, Integra
	Bayer Technicon RA 1000

often causes protein denaturation or aggregation of immunoglobulins, and produces high sample blanks or background light scattering.

Nonspecific side reactions can be initiated by rheumatoid factor (RF) or C1q. Rheumatoid factor, an IgM antibody directed against the Fc portion of an IgG molecule, will react with any IgG and decrease the IgG concentration in the patient sample and antibody reagent. The nonspecific interference by RF can be minimized by using F(ab')$_2$ fragments instead of whole antibodies. C1q has six sites that recognize a binding site on IgG and IgM. When IgG or IgM is to be quantitated, C1q can bind to the analytes as well as the nephelometric antiserum reagent, hence decreasing the specific reaction measured.

The detection limit of nephelometric immunoassay is approximately 0.1 mg/L, comparable with the sensitivities of RID, IEP, enzyme immunoassay, and fluorescence immunoassay. A sensitivity of 1 μg/L was reported by the microparticle-enhanced nephelometric immunoassays based on competitive inhibition.[7] With automation, the precision or coefficient of variation of nephelometry has improved to 2% to 4%. Accuracy is more difficult to achieve. For each analyte to be measured, accuracy is determined by the availability of acceptable reference material or calibrator, the quality of antisera, and the quality of samples. There is an urgent need for improved standards for protein measurement. Although common to all immunoassays, calibrators or standards may be difficult to obtain, even if available. Whenever available, calibrators or standards certified by international or professional organizations, such as the World Health Organization (WHO) and the College of American Pathologists (CAP), are strongly recommended. A new international secondary reference preparation for proteins in human serum (RPPHS) has been released by the Community Bureau of Reference of the Commission of the European Communities. It has been approved by the U.S. Food and Drug Administration and is distributed by the CAP.[11]

A recent study of six antiserum reagents used in immunonephelometry of human IgG revealed significant differences in protein content, composition, and functional performance.[10] Therefore, fundamental and classical criteria for testing antisera remain valid; specificity and sensitivity studies and precipitation in the prozone and postzone should be performed. Antiserum reagent evaluation is valid only in the system in which it was performed.

APPLICATIONS

Measurement of immunoglobulins, complement components, C-reactive protein, and many other serum proteins is now routinely performed by automated nephelometry or turbidimetry in many clinical laboratories. Commercial kits are readily available for IgG, IgA, IgM,

C3, C4, and other specific proteins using polyclonal or mixtures of monoclonal antibodies. The antisera used should be nephelometric grade with affinity higher than that required for RID. The titer and avidity of the antisera determine the dilution of antisera for sensitive standard curves and the useful range of the assay. Monoclonal antibodies will not precipitate antigens because crosslinking of multivalent antigens does not occur. This can be overcome by using a mixture of monoclonal antibodies against different antigenic determinants.

Accuracy in immunoassays depends on the homogeneity of the calibrator and the antigen tested. Because immunoglobulin class can be extremely heterogeneous, with variations in size and subclass, accuracy is difficult to acheive. The WHO International Reference Preparation of human immunoglobulins IgG, IgA, and IgM, and the CAP Reference Preparation for Serum Proteins (RPSP), are accepted as standards against which many commercial calibrators are calibrated.[2]

Serum Immunoglobulin

Numerous commercial reagents are available for nephelometric or turbidimetric determination of serum IgA, IgG, and IgM. The serum concentration of IgD and IgE is often too low to be detected by nephelometry. Because nephelometry is precise, accurate, easy to perform, cost effective, has a short turnaround time, and can be automated, it has replaced RID and is more commonly used.[2] In addition, the data indicate a good correlation between nephelometry and RID because the correlation coefficient is greater than 0.9. Rate nephelometric determination of the κ/λ ratio can distinguish between monoclonal and polyclonal hypergammaglobulinemia; this distinction may be difficult using serum immunoelectrophoresis.[12]

Although nephelometry has been accepted as a standard laboratory procedure against which to compare new tests, problems may occur in nephelometric detection and characterization of immunoglobulin in immunoproliferative diseases. Abnormalities in light-chain disease; polymeric IgG, IgD, and IgE; and antigen excess lead to inaccurate measurement. Nephelometric quantitation is limited by the subclasses of immunoglobulins in the calibrator and the specificity of the antisera used. Myeloma proteins and polymeric IgA of high molecular weight can be underestimated by a factor of 10. Suspicious nephelometric results may be identified by comparing the immunoglobulin quantitation with the appearance of the serum protein electrophoresis. When an inaccurate result is suspected, confirmation by IEP or isoelectric focusing is recommended.

Cerebrospinal Fluid Immunoglobulin Synthesis

While quantitation of serum immunoglobulins is used to detect changes in primarily systemic B-cell function, evaluation of immunoglobulin concentration in cerebrospinal fluid (CSF) is used to detect localized immunoglobulin production. When immune activation occurs in the central nervous system, the immunoglobulin concentration increases and specific antibodies may become detectable. Immune activation may occur in infectious diseases (such as neurosyphilis and viral meningitis), in neoplastic diseases (such as metastatic lymphoma), or in autoimmune diseases (such as multiple sclerosis). It is important to distinguish immunoglobulin that leaked across the blood-brain barrier from local immunoglobulin synthesis. The CSF IgG index can be used to make this distinction. The CSF IgG index is defined as the ratio of CSF IgG/albumin to serum IgG/albumin. The normal range of this index is 0.26 to 0.58; an index greater than 0.70 is considered elevated and an indication of local IgG production. Measuring this index is very useful in the diagnosis of multiple sclerosis because this is one of the few diagnostic parameters in this disease. The index is elevated in approximately 90% of patients with multiple sclerosis.[13]

In addition to clinical applications, nephelometry has become an important research and manufacturing tool to monitor the quality of immunoreagents, to determine antisera titer and avidity, and to characterize modified antisera.

CONCLUSIONS

Nephelometry has replaced RID as the most common routine clinical laboratory method to quantitate immunoglobulins and complement components. Nephelometric and turbidimetric immunoassays are nonisotopic, fast, and easily automated. Nephelometry instruments are generally expensive, but many automated spectrophotometric analyzers are readily available for nephelometric and turbidimetric immunoassays. With a good quality control program and the use of high-quality calibrators and reagents, nephelometric and turbidimetric immunoassays produce reliable results.

Review Questions

1. Which of the following does not apply to intensity of light scattered by immunoprecipitation?

   a. It is proportional to the particle concentration.
   b. It is independent of angle of detection.
   c. It is wavelength dependent.
   d. Identical intensity can be produced by antigen at two different concentrations.

2. Light scattering caused by immunoprecipitation can be measured by which of the following instruments?

   a. nephelometer
   b. fluorometer
   c. turbidimeter
   d. high-quality spectrophotometer
   e. all of the above

3. In immunonephelometry, which of the following statements are true?

   a. Separation of bound and free antibodies is not required.
   b. The reaction rate is very sensitive to the conditions of the Ag-Ab reaction.
   c. A laser is the best light source for nephelometry.
   d. Calibrators and reagents from different vendors can be used for all analyzers.

4. Particle-enhanced immunoassay is typically used to quantitate

   a. haptens or drugs
   b. immunoglubulins
   c. hormone binding proteins
   d. RF

5. Nephelometry or turbidimetry based on analyte inhibition provides which of the following advantages?

   a. Light scattered is not angle dependent.
   b. A linear calibration between intensity of scattered light and Ag concentration occurs.
   c. Antigen excess does not occur.
   d. Less sample matrix interference because a higher sample dilution can be used.

6. The CSF IgG index is defined as

   a. the concentration of IgG in the CSF sample.
   b. the ratio of IgG/albumin in the CSF
   c. the ratio of IgG/albumin in serum
   d. the ratio of CSF IgG/albumin to serum IgG/albumin

References

1. Heidelberger M, Kendall FE: A quantitative study and a theory of the reaction mechanism. J Exp Med 61:563, 1935
2. Check IJ, Piper M, Papadea C: Immunoglobulin quantitation. In Rose NR, DeMacario E, Fahey JL, Friedman H, Penn G (eds): Manual of Clinical Laboratory Immunology, 4th ed, p 71. Washington, DC, American Society for Microbiology, 1992
3. Tiffany TO: Fluorometry, nephelometry, and turbidimetry. In Burtis CA, Ashwood ER (eds): Tietz Textbook of

Clinical Chemistry, 2nd ed, p 151. Philadelphia, WB Saunders, 1994

4. Pauling L, Pressman D, Campbell DH, et al: The serological properties of simple substances II: The effects of changed conditions and of added haptens on precipitation reactions of polyhaptenic simple substances. J Am Chem Soc 64:3003, 1942

5. Cambiaso CL, Riccomi H, Masson PL, et al: A new technique for the immunoassay of haptens: Nephelometric inhibition immunoassay (NINIA). Protides Biol Fluids Proc Colloq 21:585, 1973

6. Singer JM, Plotz RM: The latex fixation test—applications to rheumatoid arthritis. Am J Med 21:888, 1956

7. Montagne P, Laroche P, Bessou T, Cuilliere M, Varcin P, Duheille J: Measurement of eleven serum proteins by microparticle-enhanced nephelometric immunoassay. Eur J Clin Chem Clin Biochem 30:217, 1992

8. Cuilliere M, Montagne P, Bessou T, et al: Clin Chem 37:20, 1991

9. College of American Pathologists: Special Diagnostic Immunology Surveys. Skokie, IL., College of American Pathologists, 1978–1989.

10. Tillyer C: Calibration in three dimensions: Optimizing a two-parameter calibration technique to extend the range of an immunoturbidimetric urinary albumin assay into antigen excess. Clin Chem 36:307, 1990

11. Baudner S, Bienvenu J, Blirup-Jensen S, et al: The certification of a matrix reference material for immunochemical measurement of 14 human serum proteins. CRM 470, Brussels: Community Bureau of Reference, Commission of the European Communities, pp 1–172, 1993

12. Renckens AL, Jansen MJ, van Munster PJ, et al: Nephelometry of the kappa/lambda light-chain ratio in serum of normal and diseased children. Clin Chem 32:2147, 1986

13. Mehta P: Diagnostic usefulness of CSF in MS. CRC Crit Rev Clin Lab Sci 28:233, 1991

CHAPTER 17

Cellular Assays

Denise R. Zito

Objectives

Upon completion of the chapter, the reader will be able to:

1. Define the derivation of the terms *T cell* and *B cell*
2. Describe the use and basic operating principles of flow cytometry
3. List the most important leukocyte markers to enumerate in monitoring HIV-infected patients
4. Describe the classic method of separating mononuclear cells from whole blood
5. List the four most common mitogens used in the immunology laboratory
6. Define the term *stimulator cell* as used in the mixed-lymphocyte culture
7. Describe the method used for identifying MCH Class I antigens in histocompatibility testing
8. Define the term *cytokine*
9. Name the most common functional abnormality of neutrophils
10. Describe the principle of the nitroblue tetrazolium test

Immunological testing has developed as a tool for assessing the health and integrity of the immune system as well as a marker for specific disease processes. Knowledge of cellular immunity has increased tremendously over the last two decades since the development of monoclonal antibodies (MAb) for more definitive classification of the various lymphocytes and through the use of the flow cytometer, which allows both the enumeration and sorting of defined cells. These two scientific advancements have led to an enormous increase in clinical research and have aided in the development of new treatment modalities for many diseases of the cellular immune system.

Cellular assays are used to monitor both quantitative and qualitative aspects of the immune system. This chapter describes the most common method of enumerating the various white cell types and the assays available to help the clinician to determine if a patient's immune system is functioning normally. Cellular assays are essential in matching donors and recipients in transplantation. Although the histocompatibility system is not fully defined, improved matching techniques and the discovery of better drugs for immunosuppression have allowed a dramatic increase in the number and variety of organ and tissue transplants. While the majority of the tests described in this chapter are still performed mostly in large laboratories in research and teaching hospitals, many have been simplified and are now able to be performed in medium-sized hospital clinical laboratories.

LYMPHOCYTE SUBSET ENUMERATION

Lymphocyte analysis begins with the straightforward counting procedures performed in the hematology laboratory. White blood cell counts, performed by manual microscopy in a counting chamber or by automation using electrical impedance or light scatter techniques, plus differential analysis, either automated or using a 100-cell count of a Wright-stained blood smear, are the first steps in lymphocyte enumeration. Subset analysis developed later, with the discovery of the two major classes of lymphocytes: the T cell, named because it matured in the thymus,[1] and the B cell, for the bursal equivalent cell described in chickens.[2] Today, clinical laboratories use monoclonal antibodies to differentiate the various lymphocyte subsets. These subsets cannot be differentiated by visual microscopy, but only through identification of cell surface antigens.

Murine (mouse) monoclonal antibodies against human leukocyte antigens are the reagents used for cell staining and enumeration. Kohler and Milstein produced the first hybridoma by fusing a human myeloma cell with a mouse B cell.[3] A mouse is first immunized with a human lymphocyte (the source of antigens); weeks later the mouse is sacrificed and the spleen removed. The splenic B cells produce antibodies of many specificities, including those against which the mouse was immunized. These B cells can be kept in culture for a short time, long enough to test which B cell is producing the desired antigenic specificity. This B cell is then fused with the human myeloma cell. The resulting daughter cell (the hybridoma) has characteristics of both parent cells: the immortality of the tumor cell and the single specificity of the B cell. This technology has contributed to the vast knowledge of the cellular immune system developed over the past 20 years.

Commercial production of monoclonal antibodies increased rapidly in the 1980s. Several vendors produced various antibodies against T cells, B cells, and other lymphocytes and monocytes, with each vendor identifying the various antibodies with proprietary trade names. Publication in the scientific literature became cumbersome because researchers were using different vendors' antibodies, making comparison difficult. A consensus conference was held in 1982 to standardize the nomenclature of the monoclonal antibodies for white blood cell identification. The resulting standardization gave each antibody a cluster of differentiation (CD) designation, which referred to a specific antigenic epitope against which antibodies from different vendors would react.[4] Note that two manufacturers' CD antibodies may carry the same number but may not be absolutely identical. Leukocyte antigens, like all antigens, are composed of several epitopes, that is, antigen binding sites. The CD designation only specifies the epitope specificity. Thus two antibodies may have different specificities and CD designations, but may bind to the same antigen. Table 2-1 is a partial listing of CD designations for lymphocytes.

During the same time period as the commercial development of monoclonal antibodies, a second technological improvement was underway: Clinical flow cytometers first appeared in hospital laboratories. These instruments provided a means of counting the lymphocytes labeled with monoclonal antibodies, providing the first automated counting of human lymphocyte subsets. This was also the time period when the acquired immune deficiency syndrome (AIDS) emerged as a recognizable clinical entity.

Once a monoclonal antibody has been produced and characterized, it can be conjugated with a fluorescent compound, the same as those compounds used to label the secondary antibody reagents in indirect immunofluorescence (see Chapter 15). Fluorescein is the most common fluorescent dye used, followed by phycoerythrin. This dye combination is advantageous because both are excited by light with a wavelength of 488 nm but each emits at a different wavelength. By using a series of filters and reflectors that block one wavelength but allow another to pass through, one can establish a detection system for identifying different cells based on which dye is detected. These cells can be visualized using a fluorescence microscope or quantitated using a flow cytometer (Fig. 17-1).

FLOW CYTOMETRY

The flow cytometer measures the light scatter of cells as they pass one by one through a laser beam. Cells scatter the laser light in a small-angle, forward direction according to their size, that is, small cells scatter a small amount of light and larger cells scatter more light. Cellular granularity is directly proportional to the amount of laser light scattered at a 90° angle (also referred to as side scatter). Data are displayed graphically by plotting forward versus side scatter to produce a two-parameter histogram or scattergram (Fig. 17-2). The instrument operator electronically selects the desired cell population for analysis by drawing a gate or window around the population of interest, for example, lymphocytes.

Besides detectors for forward angle scatter and side scatter, there are detectors to measure the fluorescence emitted from labeled monoclonal antibodies that have previously been incubated with cells. These data are displayed as single-parameter histograms that plot number of cells versus fluorescence (Fig. 17-3 on p. 182). A tube containing cells stained with a mouse antibody, not specific for human cells but the same isotype as the MAb in use (isotype control), is analyzed first to establish

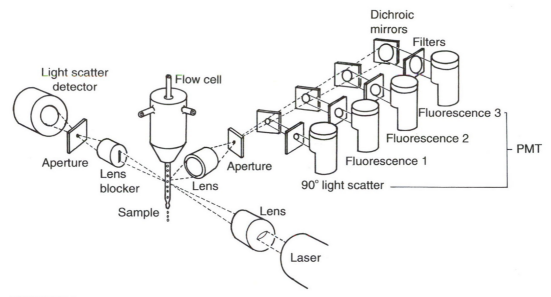

FIGURE 17-1

In the flow cytometer the cells flow through a laser light source one by one. The light is scattered by the presence of the cell. The amount of light scattered may be detected using a photomultiplier (PMT). Other photomultiplier tubes are used to detect the presence of fluorescence if a particular fluorescent-labeled antiserum is used to detect a specific cell marker.

the background fluorescence. An electronic cursor is positioned to distinguish negative from positive cells. Cells can be stained with two antibodies simultaneously, each of which is labeled with an MAb with different emission wavelength so that two membrane markers can be measured on a given cell population.

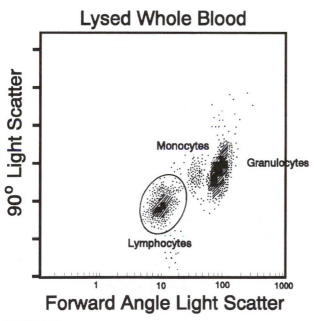

FIGURE 17-2

When the two parameters of 90° light scatter and forward light scatter are used together, a dot display is obtained. Lymphocytes, monocytes, and granulocytes are found in a particular area of the dot display based on their size and granularity. A gate is drawn around the lymphocytes.

Routine analysis involves receipt of the specimen with a brief patient clinical history that details the reasons for the analysis. Specimens may be peripheral blood or bone marrow preserved in EDTA or heparin. Solid tumors may also be analyzed by mechanically removing cells and suspending them in nutrient medium. Most clinical laboratories have defined antibody panels that are performed according to the patient's clinical history. For example, patients with suspected or confirmed human immunodeficiency virus (HIV) infection will be tested for total T cells, T-helper cells, and T-suppressor cells. Specimens from patients with suspected leukemia would be tested using several B-cell, T-cell, and myelomonocytic markers. It is important to have a complete patient history because it is not cost effective to use extensive antibody panels on every patient.

After the appropriate antibody panel is selected, a series of test tubes are labeled, one for the isotype control(s), one for the gating tube, and one for each of the other antibodies to be tested. The gating tube is prepared by staining an aliquot of cells with a two-color preparation of CD45, a pan-leukocyte marker, and with CD14, a monocyte marker. An aliquot of patient specimen and appropriate reagent MAb(s) is added to each tube. After 15 to 20 minutes of incubation at room temperature, the red cells are lysed and the specimens are ready for analysis. There are several commercial lysing kits available, and this process can also be automated.

After staining the cell aliquots are ready for analysis. The gating tube is analyzed first; a population of cells, usually lymphocytes, is selected based on light scatter properties (see Fig. 17-2). When the gate is se-

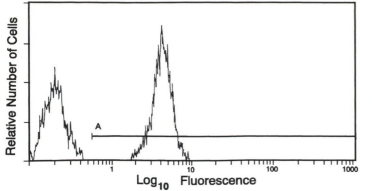

FIGURE 17-3
Whole blood stained with a monoclonal antibody conjugated with fluorescein, for example CD4, with data displayed as a single-parameter histogram. The first peak represents background staining. An electronic cursor is placed by the operator to distinguish positive events from negative events. The CD4-positive events are enumerated in the second peak observed in the histogram.

lected, all cells will stain with CD45 and only the contaminating monocytes will stain with CD14. There may be monocytes in the lymphocyte gate, and these must be distinguished because a significant numbers of monocytes could artificially lower the number of lymphocytes counted. If there is significant monocyte contamination, the gate can be redrawn until the monocytes are no longer included. When analyzing bone marrow specimens, it may be useful to stain an aliquot of specimen with an antibody against red cell antigens, such as anti-glycophorin. This antibody will detect any nucleated red cells that are not lysed in the lysing step. Red cells in the lymphocyte gate will artificially lower

the percentage of positive lymphocytes. If nucleated red cells are detected, the technologist can either redraw the gate to attempt to exclude the red cells or report the percent of red cells in the lymphocyte gate.

Today, most laboratories analyze cells using two antibodies labeled with fluorochromes that are excited by the same laser wavelength but emit light at different wavelengths (Fig. 17-4). Many laboratories use three-color and even four-color fluorescence so that a given cell can be analyzed for the presence of three or four different cell surface antigens. By permeabilizing the cell membrane, internal antigens can also be detected. This can be a very useful technique, enabling

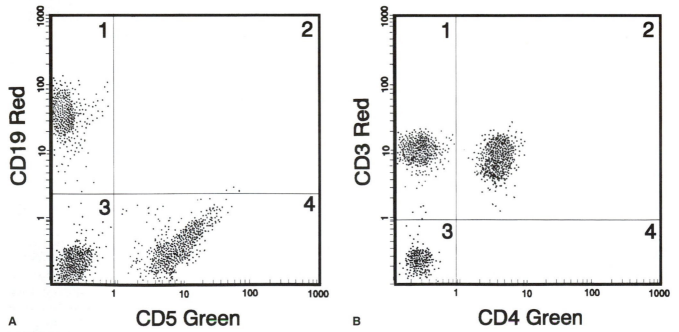

FIGURE 17-4
(**A**) A two-color histogram of whole blood staining for CD19 and CD5. Events in quadrant 3 represent background staining. Events above the horizontal cursor are CD19 positive. Events to the right of the vertical cursor are CD5 positive. (**B**) A two-color histogram of whole blood staining for CD3 and CD4. Quadrant 3 events are the unstained cells and background staining. Quadrant 1 are the CD3 + CD4-negative cells. Because some CD3 (T cells) also carry the CD4 antigen (T helper cells), cells will stain with both antibodies and will be shown in quadrant 2. Quadrant 4 are the CD4 + CD3-negative cells. This quadrant is empty because there are no cells in the electronic gate that are CD4 positive but CD3 negative.

the technologist to measure intracellular and one or two cell membrane antigens simultaneously.

A schematic diagram of the flow cytometer is shown in Figure 17-1. Cells enter the flow cell and pass by the laser beam one by one. This is accomplished through a process called laminar flow. Cells are forced through a donut-shaped fluid stream. The pressure of the cell stream and the pressure of the fluid stream are different, causing the cells to pass in single file. This is an important feature that allows each cell to pass in front of the laser so that the various detectors can collect data on each individual cell and send it to the instrument computer. As a cell passes through the laser beam, the two light scatter detectors measure laser light that is scattered based on cell size and granularity. If the cell is labeled with an MAb, the fluorescent dye on the MAb will be excited by the laser light and will emit light of a longer wavelength, which is then detected by the photomultiplier tubes. Data from each detector are sent to the instrument computer, where histograms are generated for examination by the instrument operator. Instrument calibration consists of analyzing uniform suspensions of fluorescent beads that allow the operator to align the laser beam and optimize the light scatter and fluorescence detectors.

T-CELL SUBSET ANALYSIS

The classical test for enumerating T lymphocytes is the E-rosette assay, in which isolated lymphocytes are incubated with sheep erythrocytes (SRBCs).[5] The SRBCs bind to the T cells, producing a "rosette" pattern of a T lymphocyte in the center surrounded by SRBCs. The assay is read using a brightfield microscope to count 200 lymphocytes and to calculate the percent of rosettes. It has been determined that the SRBCs bind to the receptor now identified as CD2 by the MAb. Using a variety of MAbs that recognize different CD, T cells can be identified in leukemias and lymphoma using bone marrow, bronchial lavage, cerebrospinal fluid, and solid organ specimens.

Monoclonal antibodies are commercially available to characterize T lymphocytes during maturation (Fig. 17-5).[6] From the stem cell, T cells express CD7 and CD2, then CD5, and later CD1, CD4, and CD8. Following thymic development the cells further differentiate and lose CD1. Those cells expressing CD3 plus CD4 are the helper/inducer phenotype, and those expressing CD3 plus CD8 are the suppressor/cytotoxic phenotype.

It is important to note that a given CD is not always found *exclusively* on the cell that the antibody identifies. For example, CD4 identifies the helper T cells subclass of T lymphocytes. However, CD4 is also found on monocytes. It is therefore important to exclude the monocytes from the lymphocyte gate during flow cytometric analysis. Otherwise, the CD4 count may be erro-

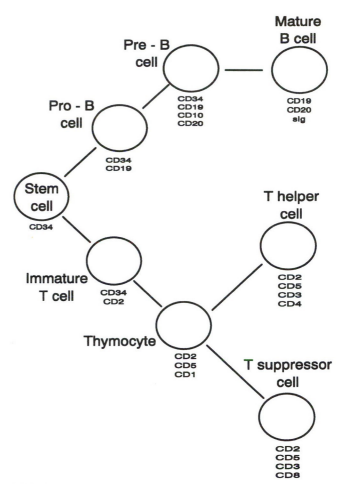

FIGURE 17-5
Simplified schematic of lymphoid development as identified by monoclonal antibodies. CD34 = bone marrow progenitor cells; CD19 = B cells; CD10 = common acute lymphoblastic leukemia antigen, immature B cells; CD20 = B cells; SIg = surface immunoglobulin; CD2 = E-rosette receptor; CD5 = T cells, B-cell subset of chronic lymphocytic leukemia; CD1 = thymocyte; CD3 = T cells; CD4 = T helper cells; CD8 = T cytotoxic/suppressor cells.

neously elevated if the gate also contains monocytes. Most laboratories avoid this problem by analyzing lymphocytes using two-color fluorescence with CD3 (pan T cell) and CD4 (helper T cell). The helper T cells are those defined by positivity with both markers, thus eliminating monocytes, which would be negative for CD3.

Similarly, CD5, a pan T-cell marker, is also found on a subset (2% to 3%) of normal B cells. However, in chronic lymphocytic leukemia (CLL), this B-cell subset expands as part of the malignant process, resulting in a population of cells (up to 80% to 90%) that express CD19 (a pan B-cell marker) and CD5.

B-CELL ANALYSIS

The classic method for identifying B lymphocytes used labeled antibody to detect integral surface membrane immunoglobulin.[7] The assay was performed by isolating lymphocytes, incubating them with fluorescein-labeled anti–human immunoglobulin, and counting the number of cells that stained using a fluorescence microscope. The test was tedious, subjective, and prone to monocyte interference. This problem has been resolved by using MAbs and flow cytometry. B lymphocytes are identified by incubating an aliquot of whole blood with an appropriate marker, usually CD19 or CD20. Following red cell lysis, the fluorescent cells are counted.

For many testing applications, if the percentage of B lymphocytes is increased, it is essential to know if the B-cell population is monoclonal, that is, if all cells carry the same light chain, or if the population is polyclonal, that is, if some have kappa and some have lambda light chains. A monoclonal population usually suggests malignancy, while a polyclonal expansion of B cells in peripheral blood may indicate an infection. Determining B-cell clonality is still a challenge. There are no B-cell subsets equivalent to the helper and suppressor T cells; clonality must be established by the presence of a single light chain type (kappa or lambda) on the surface immunoglobulin.

Attempts to make MAbs against light chains have been relatively unsuccessful. Light chains, especially lambda light chains, are not very immunogenic, and the allotypic variation in the human light chain makes the use of monoclonal reagents unreliable. Thus, polyclonal reagents continue to be used for detecting B-cell surface immunoglobulin light chains. Occasionally, a B-cell population weakly or negatively stains for kappa and lambda light chains. This is most often caused by the failure of the polyclonal reagent to recognize the light chain on the B-cell population. To resolve this finding, many laboratories maintain several kappa and lambda light chain antisera from various manufacturers and animal sources. It may take several attempts before the light chain and antibody specificities "match."

Another testing strategy to determine B-cell clonality uses two- or three-color staining. Cells can be stained simultaneously with fluorescein-labeled anti-kappa and phycoerythrin-labeled anti-lambda. Dual-color CD19/kappa and CD19/lambda can be used. A third color-staining technique involves CD19, kappa, and lambda staining, each with a different fluorochrome in the same tube.

LYMPHOCYTE PHENOTYPING IN HIV INFECTION

The discovery of the human immunodeficiency virus and its effect on the immune system have increased our understanding of cellular immunity. Although the mechanism is still unclear, it is generally accepted that HIV leads to the death of circulating T helper cells and that the viral receptor for cell infection is the CD4 anti-

gen. Thus, the focus of HIV monitoring is to enumerate the helper T cells in the peripheral circulation. There are national testing panels used for individuals participating in investigational drug-treatment protocols.[8] These testing panels are extensive and use defined procedures and two-color antibody preparations. Consistent methodology and reporting methods are essential in this setting so that interlaboratory comparisons can be easily made.

In the routine hospital laboratory setting, economics play an important role in deciding on the extent and frequency of testing. Physicians are most concerned with monitoring the absolute CD4 count because patients are most susceptible to opportunistic infections when the absolute CD4 count falls below 200/μL.[9] However, it is unadvisable to test and report simply the CD4 count because it is important to know both the total T-cell count and the T-helper count. Most laboratories report the CD3, CD4, and CD8 numbers; these three results can be obtained by testing only two aliquots of blood (CD3 plus CD4 and CD3 plus CD8), or by testing one aliquot if three-color analysis is available.

ENUMERATION OF OTHER CELLS

Table 17-1 lists the MAbs available for identifying other cells in peripheral blood. Enumeration of natural killer (NK) cells, monocytes, and granulocytes may be important in certain malignancies. There are also antibodies available for defining red cells and platelets, which are useful for characterizing erythroid and megakaryocytic leukemias, respectively. Antibodies directed against the HLA-DR antigen may be useful for determining the maturation of a cell or the activation state.

CELL SEPARATION AND VIABILITY VERIFICATION TECHNIQUES

The development of flow cytometric techniques has eliminated the need for physical separation of cells from whole blood for routine phenotyping. However, there are still tests that require purified preparations of mononuclear cells, that is, lymphocytes and monocytes. Density gradient separation is the method of choice. Diluted, anticoagulated whole blood is carefully layered onto the separation medium, Ficoll-Hypaque (specific gravity of 1.077).[10] The tube is centrifuged; gentle deceleration is essential to prevent disturbing the separated cell layers. This results in four layers, as illustrated in Figure 17-6. Red blood cells and granulo-

TABLE 17-1
Non–Lymphoid-Specific Markers

CD DESIGNATION	MOLECULAR WEIGHT (kDa)	CELLULAR DISTRIBUTION	ANTIBODY CLONE*
CD16	50–80	NK cells, macrophages, neutrophils	Leu-11a
CD34	105–120	Immature hematopoetic cells	HPCA-1
HLA-DR (no cluster designation)	33–35	B cells, monocytes, myeloid and erythroid precursors	HLA-DR
Glycophorin A (no cluster designation)		Erythroid cells	JC159
CD14	53–55	Myelomonocytic cells	Leu-M3 Mo2
CD45	180–240	All hematopoetic cells except erythrocytes	KC56
CD41	114	Platelets, megakaryocytes	Plt-1

*The antibody clones are representative of those that are commercially available and are not intended to be comprehensive.

cytes are on the bottom of the tube. The mononuclear cells (lymphocytes and monocytes) appear at the interface between the separation medium and the plasma, and the plasma and platelets are in the top layer.

Following separation, cells are washed and counted using standard hemocytometer technique or an automated cell counter. The wash solution is removed and enough buffer or nutrient medium is added to adjust the cell concentration. The cell viability should be verified before the cells are used in a clinical assay. This is done by adding trypan blue dye to an aliquot of cells. Viable cells will exclude the dye and appear clear under brightfield microscopy. Dead cells have damaged cell membranes that prevent dye exclusion and appear blue under brightfield microscopy. One hundred cells are counted and the percentage of viable cells is calculated. Cell viability should be greater than 90% for use in the cellular assays described following.

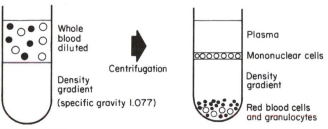

FIGURE 17-6
The separation of lymphocytes using a density gradient is performed by adding the diluted whole blood to a tube containing a density gradient with a specific gravity of 1.077. The tube is centrifuged and four layers are obtained. The lightest layer is plasma, which is on top. The mononuclear layer is located between the plasma layer and the density layer. Red cells and granulocytes are the most dense and are located on the bottom of the tube.

ASSAYS TO ASSESS CELL FUNCTION

A clinical evaluation of a patient's immune system usually begins with immunoglobulin quantitation followed by lymphocyte subset enumeration. If the number of cells and concentration of immunoglobulins are not depleted and an immune system defect is still suspected, the clinician may opt for further studies, including lymphocyte function testing. These tests are recommended when there is the suspicion of a disorder in cellular immunity, which manifests as unusual skin disorders, repeated viral illnesses, and fungal infections. Although there may be adequate numbers of lymphocytes, the cells may not be fully functional. These tests are performed in large clinical and academic laboratories and are not considered to be routine assays. Fortunately, the functional immune deficiencies are relatively rare.

Lymphocyte Transformation

The classic test for evaluating cell function is the lymphocyte transformation test. Cells are "challenged" with at least three separate mitogens (plant or bacterial derivatives that stimulate mitosis). Transformation refers to the appearance of the cells as they are stimulated to mitosis. The four most widely used mitogens are phytohemagglutinin (PHA), concanavalin A (Con A), pokeweed mitogen (PWM), and staphylococcal protein A (SpA). PHA and Con A stimulate T cells, while PWM stimulates both T and B lymphocytes.[11] SpA stimulates B cells by binding the Fc receptor (Table 17-2). When normal lymphocytes are exposed to any of these substances, the cells begin to divide.

TABLE 17-2
Mitogens for Lymphocyte Transformation

MITOGEN	RELATIVE SPECIFICITY
PHA	T cells
Con A	T cells (different subset from PHA)
PWM	B cells, T-cell dependent
SpA	B cells, T-cell independent

PhA, phytohemagglutinin; Con A, concanavalin A; PWM, pokeweed mitogen; SpA, staphylococcal protein A

The test is performed using separated mononuclear cells from the patient and normal control whole blood specimens. The cells are suspended in a nutrient medium and are placed in the wells of a 96-well culture plate, with 1×10^6 cells in each well. Three wells of patient cells and three wells of control cells are incubated with each mitogen. One set of three wells is left as an unstimulated control. The plate is then incubated for 4 days at 37°C. On day 5, the plate is removed from the incubator and a preparation of tritiated thymidine is added to each well. This reagent incorporates radioactive hydrogen (^{3}H) into the purine base, thymidine. When this radioactive DNA base is added to the cell preparation, dividing cells will incorporate the radiolabeled base into the DNA in the daughter cells. The plate is incubated for one more day and then the cells are harvested using an instrument that aspirates the liquid from the culture wells, trapping the cells onto filter paper. The paper can then be assayed using a beta scintillation counter (Fig. 17-7). The counts from the patient wells are compared with those from the normal control and the unstimulated cells. The normal cells are stimulated by all four mitogens; patient counts that are similarly elevated indicate normal lymphocyte reactivity, while lower counts indicate a decreased response to normal stimuli. Lymphocyte transformation assays can be modified and can employ specific antigens such as *Candida* to determine the patient's ability to respond to specific antigens.

The problems associated with employee risk and radioactive waste disposal have encouraged laboratory scientists to seek alternatives to radioisotopes for this test. One alternative has been the use of flow cytometry.[12] The cells are prepared and stimulated as usual. Instead of adding radiolabeled thymidine, the cells are incubated with a DNA stain such as propidium iodide. In transformed cells, the amount of DNA is increased, and, therefore, the amount of propidium iodide staining the DNA is increased. The histograms of the normal and control cells can be compared to determine whether the patient cells respond similarly to the control.

Mixed-Lymphocyte Culture

The mixed-lymphocyte culture is used to detect HLA-Dw on the surface of cells.[13] Most often it is used as an indication of the compatibility of donor cells with recipient cells. This is a critical parameter for compatibility for bone marrow transplantation. The goal is to determine if the recipient cells respond to the donor cells; if there is no response, this suggests that the recipient and donor cells share HLA-Dw antigens and that acceptance of the transplanted graft is favored. The test uses fresh, purified mononuclear cells from the donor and recipient. The donor cells are the stimulator cells because they are first irradiated to render them unresponsive to antigenic stimuli. The recipient cells are the responder cells. Stimulator and responder cells are suspended in nutrient medium and incubated for 4 days in a CO_2 environment. Tritiated thymidine is then added to each well and the plates are incubated for 6 more hours. If the responder cells share the HLA-Dw antigens on the stimulator cell, they will *not* be induced to respond or transform. However, if the stimulator cells have different HLA-Dw antigens than the responder cells, the latter will transform and react to the stimulator cells. After the cells have incubated with the tritiated thymidine, the cells are harvested as described in the lymphocyte transformation assay described earlier. Counts of responder cells are compared with unstimulated cells and control cells (Fig. 17-8); the radioactive count is proportional to the response. Each laboratory must establish its own criteria for making the decision to transplant or not based on HLA-Dw compatibility. It is important to note that because of the length of time needed to perform this assay, it can be done only when the recipient will receive an organ from a living donor. Cadaveric specimens cannot be tested using this technique because by the time the testing is complete, the organ will no longer be viable.

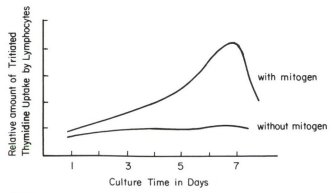

FIGURE 17-7
In the lymphocyte transformation procedure, the cells that are transformed with mitogen incorporate the radioactive DNA precursors into the cell. The amount of radiation observed in these cells reaches a peak at days 5 to 6 of the assay.

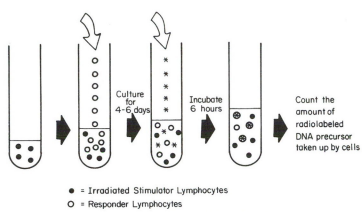

FIGURE 17-8
Irradiated stimulator lymphocytes are incubated with responder lymphocytes in cell culture for 4 to 6 days. After this incubation, radiolabeled DNA precursor, generally tritiated thymidine, is added to the culture and reincubated for an additional 6 hours. After the second incubation, the amount of radiation present in the cells is measured. If the stimulator lymphocytes and responder lymphocytes have different HLA antigens present on the cell surface, the amount of radiation present in the cells is increased.

● = Irradiated Stimulator Lymphocytes
O = Responder Lymphocytes
* = Radiolabeled DNA Precursor (Titiated Thymine)

Cytotoxicity

Cytotoxicity refers to the ability of a cell to kill a target cell. There are various mechanisms through which immune cells accomplish this. Cell-mediated killing may be MHC dependent (CD8+ cells) or MHC independent (NK activity). Cell-mediated cytotoxicity testing is extremely difficult to standardize and requires extensive controls. Antibody-mediated cytotoxicity is used as the classic test for determining HLA-A and HLA-B antigens (Fig. 17-9). This test is much easier and is widely used in histocompatibility laboratories.

CELL-MEDIATED CYTOTOXICITY

All cell-mediated cytotoxicity assays begin with separated mononuclear peripheral blood leukocytes, with cells removed from lymph nodes or spleen, or with cells isolated from bone marrow. For some assays, further separation to remove B cells or to isolate T-lymphocyte subsets may be desirable. Each of the assays described also requires the preparation of appropriate target cells, which may require prior sensitization.

Target cells must be selected based on the effector cell being analyzed. For instance, when testing for NK activity, the target cells must be sensitive to NK cell

killing. For monocyte function assays, target cells must be NK resistant but monocyte sensitive.[14] Some effector cells are effective only against MHC identical cells, and some kill cells that are infected by viruses. Tumor cells can also be used as targets. Most cell-mediated cytotoxicity assays are designed using appropriate target cells labeled with radioactive chromium (^{51}Cr). Test cells and labeled target cells are mixed together in microtiter wells with an excess of test cells. After incubation, the supernatant is harvested and counted to detect the release of radioisotope, which is proportional to the extent of cell killing. Obviously, it is essential that appropriate controls be used in these assays.

ANTIBODY-MEDIATED CYTOTOXICITY

These assays are used to determine the HLA-A and HLA-B phenotype of donor and recipient lymphocytes in preparation for organ transplantation.[15] Although HLA-C can also be detected using the same method, it is of limited clinical significance. The primary source of reagent antibody is the serum of multiparous women. During pregnancy, women are exposed to non-self MHC Class I molecules present on fetal red blood cells and respond by synthesizing antibody. The structure of MHC Class I molecules is such that immunization of

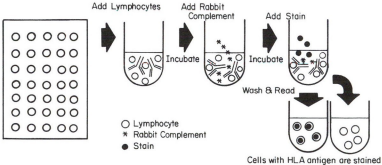

O Lymphocyte
* Rabbit Complement
● Stain

Cells with HLA antigen are stained
Cells without HLA ag are not stained

FIGURE 17-9
The microcytotoxicity test to detect MHC Class I molecules is done using a microtiter tray. Each well contains a specific antibody, and the purified lymphocytes are added to each well. Rabbit complement is added, and the tray is incubated to allow antigen, antibody, and complement to react. If the Class I antigen is present on the lymphocyte, antibody will react with the antigen and the complement cascade will cause the lysis of the lymphocyte. Eosin is added and will enter cells that have been lysed. The tray is washed free of all stain that is not bound. Each well is read microscopically for the presence of eosin-stained cells.

animals has been unsuccessful. The antiserum reagents are characterized and distributed in prepackaged microtiter plates, with each well containing 1 µL of antiserum (see Fig. 17-9). Reagent manufacturers include antisera against the most common HLA types in each tray, and special or extended trays with further specificities can also be purchased.

The test cells are peripheral blood lymphocytes that have been isolated using a density gradient. To remove contaminating monocytes, incubate the cells with metal filings. The monocytes will ingest the metal and can be removed with a magnet. When detecting HLA-DR and HLA-DQ, the test cells must be B cells because these HLA specificities are not present on resting T cells. The B-cell–enriched preparation can be achieved by passing the cell mixture through a nylon wool column or by using magnetic beads coated with monoclonal anti–B-cell antibodies.

In the assay, test cells are added to a microtiter well containing the reagent antiserum. After incubation, fresh rabbit complement is added and will bind to any cell coated with reagent antiserum. Cytolysis occurs and can be detected using a vital stain, such as eosin Y or trypan blue, and by examining the plate using phase microscopy. The stain enters dead cells and is excluded from living cells. A colored cell is positive, suggesting that it expresses the antigen defined by the reagent antiserum. A clear cell is living, and thus it excludes the stain, suggesting that it does not express the antigen.

Measurement of Immune Activation

Immune activation refers to the physiological events involved in the development of the immune response. The hematology laboratory first performs a white blood cell count and differential. Other assays performed in the clinical immunology laboratory measure and monitor immunoglobulin and complement levels. Cellular assays are performed when the patient develops conditions, for example, fungal infections, that suggest a cellular immune defect. The physical signs of immune activation include swollen lymph nodes, fever, and malaise. Enlarged lymph nodes may be removed to analyze the cell populations using flow cytometry. A polyclonal increase in T and B cells suggests immune activation rather than a malignant process. The presence of the HLA-DR antigen on T cells also indicates immune activation.

Cytokine is a generic term for the soluble mediators produced by immune cells. These molecules are usually in low concentration in blood, have a low molecular weight, and many have short half-lives, making them extremely difficult to detect and monitor. Sensitive techniques for measuring cytokines are contributing to the understanding of cell communication and interaction.

There are two approaches to cytokine measurement: direct measurement of patient cell production and serum measurement. Both are fraught with difficulties because of the problems cited earlier. In addition, direct measurement of cultured cell products has the potential of interference from other cytokines. Separated cells are placed in culture and provided with an appropriate stimulus. Culture supernatant is then removed and testing is done using radioimmunoassay or enzyme immunoassay.

The most common serum cytokine measurement is interleukin-2 (IL-2). IL-2 induces the proliferation and maturation of T cells. It is measured using standard noncompetitive enzyme immunoassay techniques with antibody specific for IL-2 bound by its Fc receptor to the solid phase. Patient serum is added to the antibody-coated solid phase. After incubation and washing, the labeled IL-2 antibody is added. After washing, substrate is added. Results are detected by color development using a spectrophotometer.

Neutrophil Function Assays

Neutrophils function as nonspecific phagocytic cells. Their action does not involve the MHC recognition nor immunologic memory. Patients with dysfunctional neutrophils present with recurring bacterial diseases. The most common disease involving defective neutrophils is chronic granulomatous disease (CGD), an X-linked disorder.

The screening assay for CGD is the nitroblue tetrazolium (NBT) test.[16] This test measures the respiratory burst of neutrophils. During the respiratory burst, neutrophils reduce the dye NBT to formazan, which appears as dark blue grains in the cell cytoplasm. The neutrophils of patients with CGD lack the ability to reduce NBT. Thus, the cells from patients with CGD will not have the blue granules after incubation with NBT. In normal control neutrophils, 95% exhibit blue granular cytoplasm after incubation with NBT. Patients who are X-linked carriers of the disease show positive granules in 30% to 80% of their neutrophils.

The Chediak-Higashi syndrome is diagnosed in the hematology laboratory based on its characteristic morphology. Neutrophils from patients with this syndrome exhibit defects in chemotaxis. Chemotaxis is measured by providing the cells with a stimulant such as N-formyl-L-methionyl-L-leucyl-phenylalanine (FMLP) and measuring the movement of cells under agarose for a prescribed time period. The FMLP is placed in one well cut in the agarose, and the neutrophils from patients or controls are placed in an adjacent well. The FMLP diffuses through the agarose and acts as a neutrophil stimulant. The test result is interpreted by comparing the migration of patient neutrophils with that of normal controls. Each laboratory must establish its own control range.

SUMMARY

Cellular immunity assessment remains an essential component of the clinical immunology laboratory. Quantitating cells is performed using monoclonal antibodies to identify the individual constituents, with flow cytometry as the measuring tool. These tests can now be performed on anticoagulated whole blood or on cells from bone marrow, lymph nodes, or other organs. Other assays are available for measuring cell function. Cellular immunity testing is also fundamental in preparing patients for organ transplantation.

Review Questions

1. In flow cytometry, cell size is measured by

    a. forward scatter
    b. side scatter
    c. red fluorescence
    d. green fluorescence

2. Helper T cells are defined by the presence of

    a. CD1
    b. CD4
    c. CD8
    d. CD19

3. B-cell monoclonality is determined by

    a. the presence of CD19 on the cell surface
    b. the ability to respond to pokeweed mitogen
    c. cell size and granularity
    d. the presence of a single light-chain type

4. The cell receptor for HIV is

    a. CD2
    b. CD3
    c. CD4
    d. CD5

5. In Ficoll-Hypaque separation, the lymphocyte layer also contains

    a. red cells
    b. granulocytes
    c. monocytes
    d. platelets

6. What is the classic method of determining HLA-Dw antigens?

    a. flow cytometry
    b. antibody-mediated cytotoxicity
    c. E-rosette formation
    d. mixed-lymphocyte culture

7. The nitroblue tetrazolium assay tests the functional ability of

    a. red cells
    b. granulocytes
    c. monocytes
    d. platelets

References

1. Cooper MD, Peterson RDA, South MA, Good RA: The functions of the thymus system and the bursa system in the chicken. J Exp Med 123:75–102, 1966
2. Roitt IM, Torrigiani G, Greaves MF, Brostoff J, Playfair JH: The cellular basis of immunological responses. Lancet 2:367–371, 1969
3. Kohler G, Milstein C: Continuous cultures of fused cells secreting antibody of predefined specificity. Nature 256:495–497, 1975
4. Barclay AN, Birkeland ML, et al: The Leucocyte Antigen Facts Book. London, Academic Press, 1993
5. Dyter JM: Identifying and enumerating human T and B lymphocytes. Prog Allergy 21:178–260, 1976
6. Foon KA, Rodd RF: Immunologic classification of leukemia and lymphoma. Blood 68:1–31, 1986
7. Stites DP: Clinical laboratory methods for detection of cellular immune function. In Stites DP, Stobo JD, Wells JV (eds): Basic and Clinical Immunology, 8th ed, p 286. Norwalk, CT, Appleton and Lange, 1994
8. CDC: Guidelines for the performance of CD4+ T-cell determinations in persons with human immunodeficiency virus infections. MMWR 41(RR-8):1–12, 1992
9. CDC: 1993 revised classification system for HIV infection and expanded surveillance case definition for AIDS among adolescents and adults. MMWR 41(RR-17):1–19, 1992
10. Boyum A: Separation of leukocytes from blood and bone marrow. Scand J Clin Lab Invest 21:97–114, 1968
11. Fletcher MA, Klimas N, Morgan R, Gjerset G: Lymphocyte proliferation. In Rose NR, DeMacario EC, Fahey JL, Friedman H, Penn GM (eds): Manual of Clinical Laboratory Immunology, 4th ed, p 213. Washington, DC, American Society for Microbiology, 1992
12. Palutke M, KuKuruga D, Tabaczka P: A flow cytometric method for measuring lymphocyte proliferation directly from tissue culture plates using Ki-67 and propidium iodide. J Immunol Meth 105:97–105, 1987
13. Hansen JA, Mickelson EM, Choo S, et al: Clinical bone marrow transplantation: Donor selection and recipient monitoring. In Rose NR, DeMacario EC, Fahey JL, Friedman H, Penn GM (eds): Manual of Clinical Laboratory Im-

munology, 4th ed, p 850. Washington, DC, American Society for Microbiology, 1992

14. Whiteside TL, Rinaldo CR, Herberman RB: Cytolytic cell functions. In Rose NR, DeMacario EC, Fahey JL, Friedman H, Penn GM (eds): Manual of Clinical Laboratory Immunology, 4th ed, p 220. Washington, DC, American Society for Microbiology, 1992

15. Milford EL: Immunologic testing for renal transplantation. In Rose NR, DeMacario EC, Fahey JL, Friedman H, Penn GM (eds): Manual of Clinical Laboratory Immunology, 4th ed, p 825. Washington, DC, American Society for Microbiology, 1992

16. Coates TD, Beyer LL, Baehner RL: Laboratory evaluation of neutropenia and neutrophil dysfunction. In Rose NR, DeMacario EC, Fahey JL, Friedman H, Penn GM (eds): Manual of Clinical Laboratory Immunology, 4th ed, p 409. Washington, DC, American Society for Microbiology, 1992

CHAPTER 18

Nucleic Acid Probes and Blotting Techniques

William C. Wagener

Objectives

Upon completion of the chapter, the reader will be able to:

1. Explain the biochemical principles underlying the use of nucleic acid probes
2. Define Southern blot, Northern blot, and Western blot, and differentiate between the procedures
3. State the relative importance of molecular techniques in clinical laboratory science
4. Understand and explain the basic principles of the polymerase chain reaction
5. Give specific examples of the clinical utility of molecular techniques in the laboratory

BACKGROUND

The late 19th and early 20th centuries are known as the golden age of bacteriology. During this time many infectious agents were first isolated and identified, specific culture media were defined, and the gram stain was developed. These events had great significance for medicine and the clinical sciences. Similarly, the 1980s were the age of molecular biology and biotechnology. Many procedures were developed to clone specific structural and regulatory genes and to sequence DNA. It is now possible to study mechanisms of gene regulation in both prokaryotic and eukaryotic cells, and to observe the effects of DNA mutations on the structure/function of specific proteins. The biotechnology boom has extended into modern medicine and laboratory science, especially in the area of infectious diseases. The tools of molecular biology allow the clinical laboratory to detect and diagnose several infectious agents with greater speed, sensitivity, and specificity. For example, *Mycobacterium tuberculosis* grows very slowly in vitro, thus delaying diagnosis and proper treatment. In addition, *Chlamydia*, *Borrelia burgdorferi*, and viruses require special equipment and procedures unavailable to most clinical laboratories. Molecular techniques can be used to confirm the identity of an isolated organism or to detect the presence of the organism in clinical specimens. In addition, molecular techniques have increased the ability to measure specific antibodies in patient serum. This chapter reviews the principles of these selected molecular techniques and highlights some specific applications.

PRINCIPLES

Nucleic Acid Probes

The nucleic acids present in eukaryotic and prokaryotic cells consist of both deoxyribonucleic acid (DNA) and ribonucleic acid (RNA). DNA is a double-stranded molecule consisting of a 2-deoxyribose-phosphate backbone to which the four nucleotide bases (guanine [G], cytosine [C], thymine [T], and adenine [A]) are attached (Fig. 18-1). The bases on one strand pair with a nucleotide on the complementary strand via hydrogen bonding. In DNA, adenine base pairs with thymine via two hydrogen bonds and cytosine pairs with guanine via three hydrogen bonds. It is the sequence of the bases along the DNA molecule that specifies the genetic code and thus the sequence of the amino acids that make up each protein molecule. RNA differs from DNA in that uracil (another base) replaces thymine; it is single stranded, and the sugar is ribose.

The two strands of DNA can be separated by a process called denaturation. Any physical or chemical process that disrupts the hydrogen bonding between the bases can cause denaturation. Once DNA is denatured,

the two complementary strands can reassociate, a process called reannealing. When two single-stranded DNA molecules reanneal, they do so according to the base-pair rules, and thus the original DNA molecule is recovered.

These processes of denaturation and reannealing are the basis of nucleic acid probe technology. A probe is a small segment of either RNA or single-stranded DNA. If a probe is added to a solution of denatured DNA, the probe will base pair, or hybridize, with target sequences of the DNA strand if there is sufficient homology between the base sequences of the target and probe. If the probe is labeled, then the DNA-probe duplex DNA can be detected. Traditionally, radioactive probes labeled with ^{32}P have been used. Today, however, other, nonradioactive labels are available for producing probes, such as chemiluminescence and biotin-avidin labels. Remember, however, that a probe may consist of either RNA or DNA to detect a target sequence of either RNA or DNA. Blotting methods that detect DNA sequences are called Southern blotting, while a similar method to detect RNA is called Northern blotting.

SOUTHERN BLOTS

In 1975 Southern perfected a method of transferring DNA fragments from agarose gels to nitrocellulose membranes.[1] The procedure became known as the Southern blot. This procedure makes it possible to detect a specific target sequence among the tremendous number of sequences of DNA in a mixture. The procedure is outlined in Figure 18-2. Basically, the DNA from a bacterial cell or other source is isolated in pure form. The DNA may then be treated with enzymes that digest DNA at specific nucleotide sequences. Such enzymes are called restriction endonucleases or restriction enzymes. There are many restriction enzymes and most exhibit amazing specificity in the nucleotide sequences at which they cut DNA. For example, the enzyme EcoR1 cuts DNA only at the sequences consisting of [P]GAATTC[OH]. The sequence makes up a palindrome, that is, a sequence that is the same when read in the opposite direction on the complementary strands.

The resulting digested DNA fragments of various lengths are then separated according to size (number of nucleotides) by agarose gel electrophoresis.[2] Because the DNA fragments are acidic, owing to the phosphate residues on the sugar phosphate backbone, the fragments migrate in an electric field. In a solid matrix, such as agarose, the fragments migrate at different rates determined by their size in base pairs. Thus, smaller fragments migrate faster than larger fragments. After the DNA in the gel is denatured by alkali, a nylon or nitrocellulose membrane is applied to the gel in an apparatus such as the one shown in Figure 18-2. The DNA fragments in the gel are transferred to the membrane via capillary action as the buffer solution flows through

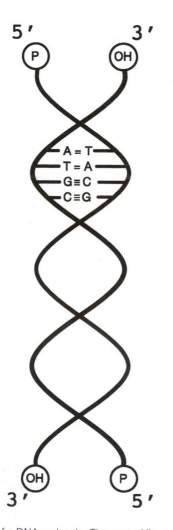

FIGURE 18-1

Representation of a DNA molecule. The curved lines are the deoxyribose-phosphate backbone of each complementary strand running in opposite directions from the phosphate (P) to the hydroxyl (OH) end. AT is adenine base-paired to thymine via two hydrogen bonds, and GC is guanine base-paired to cytosine via three hydrogen bonds. Hydrogen bonds between the two strands may be broken and the DNA denatured. The phosphate may be replaced with ^{32}P to produce a radioactively labeled probe.

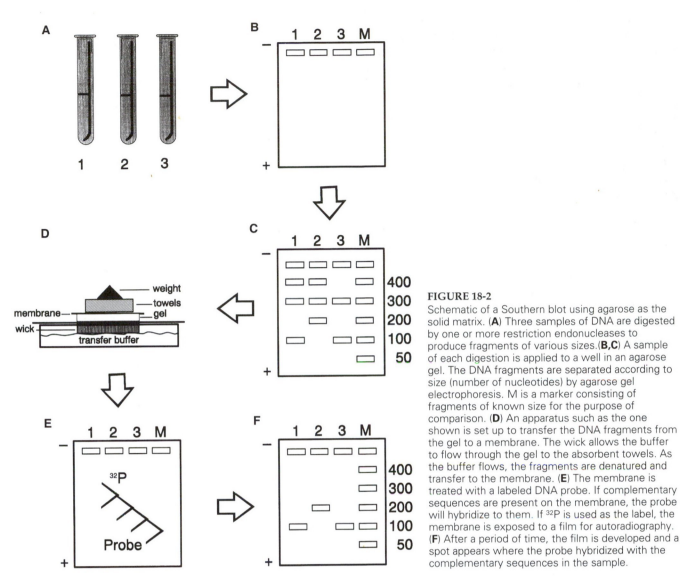

FIGURE 18-2

Schematic of a Southern blot using agarose as the solid matrix. (**A**) Three samples of DNA are digested by one or more restriction endonucleases to produce fragments of various sizes.(**B,C**) A sample of each digestion is applied to a well in an agarose gel. The DNA fragments are separated according to size (number of nucleotides) by agarose gel electrophoresis. M is a marker consisting of fragments of known size for the purpose of comparison. (**D**) An apparatus such as the one shown is set up to transfer the DNA fragments from the gel to a membrane. The wick allows the buffer to flow through the gel to the absorbent towels. As the buffer flows, the fragments are denatured and transfer to the membrane. (**E**) The membrane is treated with a labeled DNA probe. If complementary sequences are present on the membrane, the probe will hybridize to them. If ^{32}P is used as the label, the membrane is exposed to a film for autoradiography. (**F**) After a period of time, the film is developed and a spot appears where the probe hybridized with the complementary sequences in the sample.

the gel and membrane. As a consequence, the pattern of DNA fragments on the membrane is an exact replica of the pattern in the gel. After the membrane is neutralized, it is incubated with a labeled single-stranded DNA (or RNA) probe complementary to the sequences of interest. If the target DNA is on the membrane, the probe hybridizes to it via base pairing. By varying the temperature and/or the salt concentration during reannealing, the hybridization may be done under either high or low stringency. Stringency is a reflection of the extent of mismatch base pair allowed in the probe-target duplex. The presence of the duplex DNA is then determined by the label on the probe.

There are variations of the Southern blot that do not require gel electrophoresis, such as slot blots, dot blots, and in-situ hybridization.[2] The hybridization procedure may also be performed in a liquid phase instead of transferring DNA fragments to a membrane. In this case, the DNA-probe duplex may be "captured" on a solid matrix, such as a microtiter tray, and detected by one of several methods.

NORTHERN BLOTS

The RNA counterpart to the Southern blot is called the Northern blot. The technique is essentially the same as the Southern blot except that a nucleic acid probe is used to detect RNA target sequences. In some applications, detection of RNA is more sensitive because there are multiple copies of the genes encoding rRNA in the genome of prokaryotes and, therefore, more target sequences exist.

Immunoblots (Western Blots)

The Western blot is used to detect specific antibody. In this procedure proteins are isolated, denatured, and separated by sodium dodecyl sulfate polyacrylamide gel electrophoresis (SDS-PAGE).[2] SDS is a detergent that denatures proteins and imparts an overall negative charge to the denatured protein. PAGE separates proteins based on the molecular weight of the proteins. As with nucleic acids, the proteins in the gel can be transferred to a nylon, nitrocellulose, or polyvinylidene difluoride membrane. The membrane is incubated with patient serum, and if an antibody recognizes a protein, an immobilized complex is formed. The patient antibody in the complex is detected using a labeled reagent such as anti–human IgG conjugated with alkaline phosphatase. The actual label attached to the antibody reagent determines the mode of detection. The resulting bands on the membrane are compared with the position of bands generated from known positive and negative sera that were assayed on the same membrane. The interpretation of the test may be difficult, however, and requires an experienced technologist because of the subjective nature of the test. The Western blot is a very sensitive test to detect antibody and is presently the method of choice for detecting antibodies to the human immunodeficiency virus (HIV) (Fig. 18-3).[3,9]

Polymerase Chain Reaction

The polymerase chain reaction (PCR) was developed by Mullins[4] and is used to *amplify* a specific target sequence of DNA in a specimen. Amplification is needed because only one copy of the target sequence may be present among the millions of DNA sequences in a specimen. Thus, detection and isolation of the DNA is easier. PCR relies on the same general principles that an organism uses to replicate its DNA in vivo, although several reagents are required to replicate the target. The basic procedure is shown in Figure 18-4. First, there must be short pieces of DNA complementary to the sequences flanking each side of the target sequence. These short DNA sequences are called primers because the enzyme used to replicate DNA, DNA polymerase, requires such primer sequences. In the presence of DNA polymerase, the four nucleotide triphosphates (ATP, GTP, CTP, and TTP), and the proper salt concentration, the sequence of DNA between the primers will be copied or replicated. If this process is repeated, or cycled, many times, the target will be amplified many fold. It is important to note that the target DNA must be denatured before the primers can bind to the complementary sequences flanking the target. Because denaturation requires a high temperature, a special thermoresistant DNA polymerase, Taq polymerase, is used. There are three basic steps: first, the target DNA and primer DNA must be denatured by high temperature; next, the temperature is rapidly lowered to a temperature that allows the primers to anneal to the target DNA, and lastly, the temperature rises to a point at which the polymerase extends the primer. It is possible after 30 rounds of amplification to increase the target

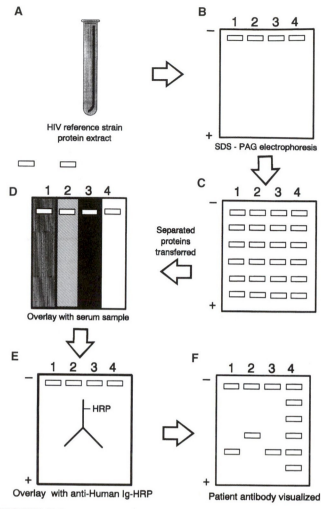

FIGURE 18-3

Immunoblotting (Western blot) using an HIV reference strain to identify specific antibody for complex HIV protein antigens. PAG = polyacrylamide gel; SDS = sodium dodecyl sulfate. (**A,B**) A protein extract of an HIV reference strain is prepared and samples are added to the wells of a PAG for SDS-PAGE. SDS denatures proteins and confers a large negative charge to each protein so that separation of individual proteins is based on size alone (molecular weight). (**C**) After electrophoresis, the proteins may be visualized by staining before transfer to a membrane. (**D**) After the proteins are transferred, individual patient serum samples are incubated on different lanes of the membrane (labeled 1 to 4). Each serum is separated and confined to one lane by a special apparatus to ensure there is no crossover between specimens. (**E**) After incubation and washing, an anti–human immunoglobulin is added to each lane. In this example, the antibody is labeled with horseradish peroxidase (HRP). (**F**) The membrane is washed to remove excess reagent and the substrate is added. If the sample contains antibody to HIV protein(s), they will bind to the protein on the membrane. The conjugated anti–human immunoglobulin will bind to this immune complex. The complex is detected by addition of the substrate, which results in a colorimetric change. In this example, patient lanes 1–3 have one antibody and lane 4 demonstrates the migration of all HIV proteins in the extract.

sequences about a billionfold. The target can then be identified by Southern blot, for instance, and isolated for further study. PCR is very sensitive. A single target DNA sequence in a clinical specimen can be amplified, thus making it possible to identify and confirm the presence of unique microbial DNA.

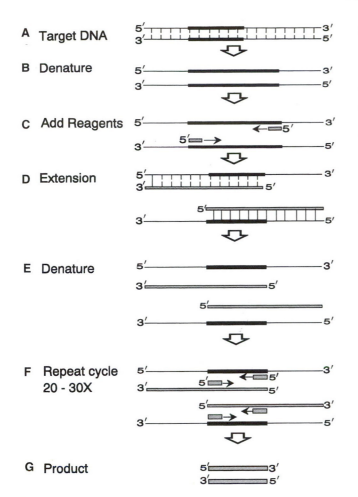

A Target DNA

B Denature

C Add Reagents

D Extension

E Denature

F Repeat cycle
20 - 30X

G Product

FIGURE 18-4
General scheme of amplifying DNA sequences using the polymerase chain reaction. (**A**) The target DNA sequence is indicated by bold lines. (**B**) The temperature is increased to denature the double-stranded target DNA. (**C**) The reagents for amplification are added, which include the four nucleotides, buffer, DNA polymerase, and primer DNA. Primer DNA is indicated by the smaller hatched fragments, which hybridize to complementary sequences flanking the target sequences. (**D**) The polymerase extends the primers to the ends of the template DNA. (**E–G**) The cycle is repeated by denaturing the products of the previous reaction, annealing of primers, and extension. After many cycles, the product consists of the target DNA sequences, which have been amplified many fold. The product DNA may be detected by Southern blot using the primer DNA sequences as a probe.

When microbial RNA is present, the procedure is modified. The organism's RNA is converted into DNA using the enzyme reverse transcriptase, the same enzyme found in retroviruses such as HIV. The resulting DNA is called complementary DNA (cDNA) to indicate the DNA was synthesized from RNA. cDNA may then be detected by amplification and DNA probes.

PCR is somewhat expensive and requires special instrumentation, such as a thermocycler which automatically increases and decreases the temperature throughout the amplification cycle. In addition, it is possible for amplified DNA to escape into the air and contaminate other specimens, thus producing false

positive results. The area for amplification must be physically separated from the area where the amplified DNA is manipulated. This problem can also be overcome by incorporating uracil instead of thymine into the nucleotide reaction mixture. In this manner, the amplified product contains uracil. For subsequent reactions that may have become contaminated with previously amplified DNA, adding an enzyme called uracil-N-glycosylase (UNG) to the reaction mixture destroys the contaminating uracil containing DNA, thus rendering it unsuitable to serve as a template.[5]

PCR as originally described is somewhat outdated because variations of the procedure have been developed. The techniques vary, but an interesting change is to amplify the signal rather than a specific DNA target. Such procedures include the ligase chain reaction (LCR), 3SR amplification, and QB replicase amplification (Table 18-1 on p. 196).[5] Advantages offered by these methods include shorter turnaround time, less expense, and room-temperature amplification, which eliminates the need for expensive instrumentation. Work is in progress to transfer one or more of these methods for use in the clinical laboratory.

CLINICAL APPLICATIONS

Nucleic Acid Probes

The use of nucleic acid probes in the diagnostic laboratory falls into two main categories: to confirm an organism isolated in culture and to identify an organism in a patient specimen. The organism can be isolated on solid medium or in broth culture, such as a blood culture bottle. Depending on the manufacturer, the target nucleic acid may be amplified before using DNA probes. Presently, probes are available commercially to identify *Mycobacterium* species, *Legionella* species, *Salmonella*, diarrheagenic *Escherichia coli* strains, *Shigella*, and *Campylobacter* species.[6–8] For *Mycobacterium* species, clinical isolates from either solid medium or broth cultures can be identified as *Mycobacterium tuberculosis* complex and *Mycobacterium avium* complex in as little as 2 hours, depending upon the manufacturer. The Accuprobe® Culture identification kit (Gen-Probe, San Diego, CA) uses DNA-rRNA hybridization to identify clinical *Mycobacterium* isolates. This is obviously an advantage over the traditional biochemical identification schemes, which require days to weeks to perform. All probes show good specificity.

In addition to probes for bacteria, commercially available probes for fungi may be used to identify *Cryptococcus neoformans*, *Coccidioides immitis*, *Histoplasma capsulatum*, and *Blastomyces dermatiditis*. To date, there

TABLE 18-1
Comparison of Nucleic Acid Amplification Procedures

METHOD	TARGET SEQUENCES	PRINCIPLES
PCR	DNA, cDNA from RNA	Amplification
		Thermocycling
LCR	DNA	DNA ligase used instead of polymerase
3SR	Primarily RNA	Room temperature
		Uses two polymerases
		Short turnaround time (15 min)
QB replicase	DNA	Signal is amplified, not DNA

Adapted from Thomas JG: Molecular diagnostics: The continuing saga. Presented at the Annual Meeting of the West Virginia State Society for Medical Technology, Huntington, WV, April 1995.

is not a commercially available DNA probe to identify *Candida albicans*.

The second application of DNA probe technology is to identify organisms directly in a patient specimen. Organisms for which probes are available have targeted those that traditionally require special culture media or the use of cell culture. Probes are particularly useful to identify the agents of sexually transmitted diseases, including *Neisseria gonorrhoeae*, *Chlamydia trachomatis*, and herpes simplex virus. Procedural details vary according to the manufacturer. The appropriate specimen is collected, usually from the urogenital area, and treated to kill the organism and to release the target DNA from the organism.

Probe technology is used extensively in the field of molecular genetics to study DNA rearrangements that lead to a variety of pathologic disorders and malignancies. For example, probes, in conjunction with PCR and DNA sequencing techniques, have been used to study the gene rearrangements in B cells in multiple myeloma,[9] T cells in chronic myelogenous leukemia,[10] and Philadelphia-chromosome–positive leukemic cells.[11]

Polymerase Chain Reaction

To date, a large number of important pathogens may be identified by PCR, including parasites, bacteria, and viruses. One procedure commercially available is the Amplicor® PCR Assay for Chlamydia (Roche Diagnostic Systems, Branchburg, NJ). This test uses PCR to amplify a target located on a plasmid, not in the genome, in all strains of *Chlamydia trachomatis*. About 10 copies of this plasmid are in the elementary bodies and reticulate bodies of the organism so that sensitivity is increased 10-fold immediately. In this assay biotinylated primers (biotin attached to primers) are used to amplify the target DNA sequences. After amplification, the amplified

product (amplicon) is added to microtiter wells coated with probes that are complementary to the target sequences. The capture of the amplified DNA is detected by adding an enzyme conjugate (antibody labeled with avidin-horseradish peroxidase). The amount of conjugate is detected by adding the substrate reagent (peroxide and tetramethylbenzidine) for color development. The test appears to be sensitive and specific; however, some clinical specimens cause a false negative test by inhibiting the biochemical amplification of the target DNA. In addition, because the target DNA is located on a plasmid, strains of the organism without the plasmid will not be detected. Another method marketed by Gen-Probe uses chemiluminescent labeled DNA probes to detect the rRNA of *C. trachomatis* in clinical specimens.[7]

Immunoblotting

The Western blot (WB) is a high complexity test performed in larger clinical laboratories. It is useful to identify one or more patient antibodies produced in response to a complex organism, such as HIV and *Borrelia burgdorferi*. In HIV infection, WB is used to confirm the presence of antibodies detected by the screening method, usually enzyme immunoassay.[3,9] The nature of the infection requires the maximum confidence related to the antibody specificity. Also, the pattern of antibody detection varies between infected individuals and during the course of the disease. In *B. burgdorferi* infection, WB has been used to confirm results from indirect immunofluorescence or enzyme immunoassays and to evaluate problem cases.[12,13] Care should be taken when interpreting results because false positive results can occur due to crossreactivity with *E. coli*, *M. tuberculosis*, *Legionella pneumophila*, *Coxiella burnetii*, and pathogenic *Treponema* species.[12,14]

Review Questions

1. The _____ blot is a technique used to detect specific microbial _____ in clinical specimens.

    a. Northern, DNA
    b. Southern, DNA
    c. Southern, RNA
    d. Western, protein

2. Immunoblot procedures are useful in sero-diagnosis because

    a. components of enzyme immunoassay (EIA) procedures may be incorporated into the test
    b. they are easier to interpret than EIA procedures
    c. the antibody response to a wide array of microbial antigens may be detected
    d. they are at least as sensitive as EIA procedures for all microbial antigens

3. In PCR, the amplified DNA product is called the

    a. replicon
    b. amplicon
    c. primer
    d. target

4. In order for DNA in a clinical specimen to be amplified, it must first be

    a. released from the microbial cell and denatured
    b. isolated in pure form
    c. digested with restriction endonucleases
    d. all of the above

5. Indicate the correct sequence of steps performed in a Western blot. The first step is "1."

    _5_ a. The label is detected.
    _1_ b. Isolated proteins are separated by SDS-PAGE.
    _3_ c. Patient antibody binds to specific protein.
    _2_ d. Proteins are transferred to a membrane.
    _4_ e. The conjugate is added.

6. PCR is used in the clinical laboratory to

    a. detect microbial proteins
    b. quantitate low concentrations of antibody in patient serum
    c. detect microbial DNA
    d. detect gene rearrangement in B-cell maturation

References

1. Southern EM: Detection of specific sequences among DNA fragments separated by gel electrophoresis. J Mol Biol 98:503–517, 1975
2. Sambrook J, Fritsch EF, Maniatis T: Molecular Cloning: A Laboratory Manual. Cold Spring Harbor, NY, Cold Spring Harbor Laboratory Press, 1989
3. Turgeon ML: Immunology and Serology in Laboratory Medicine. St. Louis, CV Mosby, 1990
4. Mullis K, Faloona F, Scharf S, et al: Specific enzymatic amplification of DNA in vitro: The polymerase chain reaction. Cold Spring Harbor Symp Quan Biol 51:263, 1986
5. Thomas JG: Molecular diagnostics: The continuing saga. Presented at the Annual Meeting of the West Virginia State Society for Medical Technology, Huntington, WV, April 1995
6. Ellner PD, Kiehn TE, Cammarata R, et al: Rapid detection and identification of pathogenic mycobacteria by combining radiometric and nucleic acid probe methods. J Clin Microbiol 26:1349–1352, 1988
7. Iwen PC, Blair TMH, Woods GL: Comparison of the Gen-Probe PACE 2 system, direct fluorescent-antibody and cell culture for detecting *Chlamydia trachomatis* in cervical specimens. Am J Clin Pathol 95:578–582, 1991
8. Pasculle AW, Vito GE, Krystofiak et al: Laboratory and clinical evaluation of a commercial DNA probe for detection of *Legionella* spp. J Clin Microbiol 27:2350–2358, 1989
9. Biggs DD, Kraj P, Goldman J, et al: Immunoglobulin gene sequence analysis to further assess B-cell origin of multiple myeloma. Clin Diagn Lab Immun 2:44, 1995
10. Jonas D, Lubbert M, Kawasaki ES et al: Clonal analysis of bcr-abl rearrangement in T lymphocytes from patients with chronic myelogenous leukemia. Blood 79:1017–1023, 1992
11. Aurer I, Butturini A, Gale RP: BCR-ABL rearrangements in children with Philadelphia chromosome-positive chronic myelogenous leukemia. Blood 78:2401–2410, 1991
12. Stevens CD: Clinical Immunology and Serology—A Laboratory Perspective. F.A. Davis, Philadelphia, 1996
13. Steere AC: Lyme disease. In Schaechter M, Medoff G, Eisenstein BI (eds): Mechanisms of Microbial Disease, 2nd ed. Baltimore, Williams and Wilkins, 1993
14. Schwan TG, Burgdorfer W, Rosa PA: Borrelia. In Murray PR, Baron EJ, Pfaller MA, et al (eds): Manual of Clinical Microbiology, 6th ed. American Society for Microbiology, Washington, DC, 1995

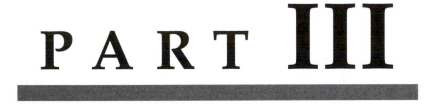

PART III

Clinical Immunology

Section A
Infectious Disease Serology

CHAPTER 19

Overview of Infectious Disease and Serology

Rosemarie Rumanek Romesburg

Objectives

Upon completion of the chapter, the reader will be able to:

1. Differentiate between infection and disease
2. Define colonize, pathogenicity, and virulence in relation to infectious diseases
3. List and describe the stages of an infectious disease
4. Define primary and secondary antibody response
5. Discuss significant titers of IgG and IgM in determining recent and past infections
6. Discuss the significance of a fourfold rise in antibody titer
7. List several characteristics used to classify viruses
8. Define capsid, envelope, capsomere, and peplomer
9. Name and describe the steps in viral replication
10. Discuss cytotoxic effects of viruses on host cells
11. Describe the properties of transformed cells
12. Discuss the role of interferon in response to viral infection

NATURAL COURSE OF INFECTIOUS DISEASE

Infection

Infectious diseases are caused by a variety of microorganisms, including bacteria, viruses, fungi, and parasites. Normal host defense mechanisms are designed to combat continual exposure to microorganisms. However, when the host defenses are no longer adequate to resist, disease occurs. Disease is characterized by changes in the host that interfere with normal function. Although infection and disease are sometimes used interchangeably, they are significantly different. Infection refers to the establishment and multiplication of an organism within or on the body. If the infection disturbs the health of the host producing signs and symptoms, it is called disease.

The presence of microorganisms on body surfaces is insufficient to cause an infection. They must gain access to the body and interact with the host. This access may occur in a variety of ways, including through ingestion, inhalation, close contact, arthropods, cuts and bites, and fomites or inanimate objects contaminated with the infectious agent. After gaining access, the microorganisms must attach or adhere to a host surface and then colonize, survive, and multiply long enough to produce sufficient numbers. At this point most microorganisms produce disease either by invading host tissues or by producing toxins that cause host damage.

The ability of an organism to cause disease is called pathogenicity. Some organisms readily cause illness in otherwise healthy hosts, while others can cause disease only in hosts already compromised by some other condition. The degree of pathogenicity (virulence) varies significantly, with some organisms causing serious illness in a normally healthy host and others causing relatively mild illnesses.

Stages of Disease

Most infectious diseases follow a standard course and progress through a series of stages irrespective of the administration of treatment.[1,2,3]

INCUBATION PERIOD

The incubation period is the time between the initiation of infection and the appearance of signs and symptoms, and varies depending on the pathogen involved. This is the time required by the infectious agent to establish itself, to overcome the host defenses, and to multiply in sufficient numbers to have an impact on the host. Factors affecting the length of time in the incubation period include the virulent properties of the organism, the number of organisms infecting the host, and the ability of the host to respond to the infecting organisms. The incubation period ranges from a few days to several weeks or months, depending upon the infectious agent, but averages 1 to 2 weeks.

PRODROMAL PHASE

The prodromal phase of a disease is the time when nonspecific symptoms, such as general malaise or headache, appear. This usually occurs 1 to 2 days preceding the acute illness and is not present in all diseases. Some diseases begin very abruptly with little or no prior warning.

ACUTE PHASE

During the acute phase of illness, the most severe signs and symptoms appear. The symptoms may be very acute, appearing suddenly, or they may develop over a period of several days. Common symptoms during the acute phase include fever, chills, muscle pain, sore throat, vomiting, and diarrhea. Survival depends upon the extent and nature of the damage to the host, the host's defense mechanisms, and treatment.[3]

CONVALESCENT PHASE

The final phase in the course of the disease process is recovery or convalescence. In this phase symptoms are no longer apparent, but in some diseases patients are still infectious. Antibodies are at peak levels, with protective antibodies contributing significantly to the recovery and inactivation of the organisms. Long-lasting immunity develops during the convalescent phase. However, if antibiotic therapy is administered promptly, thus eliminating the organism early in the course of disease, antibody levels may be lowered.[3]

SEROLOGIC SUPPORT OF DIAGNOSIS

Primary and Secondary Antibody Responses

When a host comes into contact with antigens of an infectious agent for the first time, a primary immune response is elicited. Initially IgM antibodies appear in 1 to 2 weeks, peak in 3 to 6 weeks, and decline to undetectable levels over the following few months. IgG and sometimes IgA antibodies begin to appear as IgM antibodies reach their peak, and IgG reaches maximum levels in about 4 to 12 weeks. The titer of IgG antibodies is greater than that of IgM and remains elevated for months or years.[2,4] Repeat exposure to the same infectious agent produces a secondary or anamnestic immune response. In this response, IgG antibodies rapidly reach higher levels than previously and remain elevated for long periods of time. IgM antibodies are less significant in secondary responses.

Significance of Antibody Class

In serologic testing for a specific antibody, the concentration or titer of total antibody or class-specific antibody can be measured. If a single specimen is used to determine a current infection, both an IgM and IgG assay should be performed. If both assays are negative, no infection exits. If only IgM is detected or both IgG and IgM are detected, the infection is recent. Appearance of only IgG indicates a past infection.[5]

It is important to distinguish between IgG and IgM titers in newborn serum. Significant levels of total IgM indicates infection in utero; fetuses are exposed to microorganisms and respond by producing antibodies. The source of IgM antibody is solely from the fetus because IgM does not cross the placenta. IgG in newborn serum reflects placental transport of maternal IgG or fetal production.[4]

Acute and Convalescent Titers

Serologic evidence of an infectious disease requires a fourfold rise in antibody titer between acute phase and convalescent phase serum. Serum should be collected within 1 week of the onset of symptoms (acute phase) and again 2 weeks later (convalescent phase). The titer of IgG is usually undetectable or low in the acute phase serum, but rises significantly in the convalescent phase. Both sera should be tested simultaneously to avoid errors caused by inherent day-to-day variability in serological testing. Elevated IgG titers in a single serum specimen may be considered diagnostic when the infection is rare or the disease has a prolonged incubation period.

VIRAL INFECTIONS

Classification of Viruses

Viruses are obligate intracellular parasites that can infect animals, plants, insects, or bacteria. Those animal viruses infecting humans range in size from 25 to 30 nm to 225 to 300 nm. In viruses, the nucleic acid (either RNA or DNA) is surrounded by a capsid (protein coat); an envelope may enclose the nucleic acid–capsid structure. Capsids are composed of identical protein subunits, capsomeres, geometrically arranged to form a helical, icosahedral (20-sided), or complex symmetry. The lipid bilayer of the envelope contains surface spikes (peplomers) composed of compound proteins such as glycoproteins, which serve as antigenic determinants of the envelope.[6,7] The entire virus particle is called a virion.

Viruses are classified into families based upon various characteristics, including the type of nucleic acid, capsid symmetry, number of capsomeres, presence or absence of an envelope, and size.

Steps in Viral Infection

Viruses can be transmitted by direct or indirect contact, inoculation by arthropods, or from parent to offspring. Viruses have an affinity for certain types of tissues, where they replicate in specific cells. Some animal viruses are species specific, while others infect a variety of different species. After entering the host, viruses replicate inside host cells. A typical replication cycle occurs in a stepwise process that includes the following phases: (1) attachment, (2) penetration, (3) uncoating, (4) biosynthesis, and (5) maturation and release. Although this is a typical cycle, variations occur, depending on the type of viral nucleic acid and the viral group.[8]

Attachment, the first step in infection, occurs when a surface site on the virion binds to a receptor site on the host cell. Attachment of the virion is sometimes reversible. For infection to occur, penetration of the virus into the host cell must follow. This process may involve several mechanisms: (1) fusion of the viral envelope with the host cell membrane, (2) direct penetration of the membrane, (3) interaction with receptor sites on the cell membrane, or (4) phagocytosis.[7,8]

Next, the viral nucleic acid must be uncoated, releasing it from the surrounding envelope or capsid. Uncoating occurs at the cell surface or in the host cell. Generally, this is an enzymatic process that uses preexisting lysosomal enzymes or involves synthesis of new enzymes. Following uncoating, biosynthesis of nucleic acid and viral proteins is necessary. Synthesis of viral components occurs in either the nucleus or the cytoplasm of the host cell, depending on the type of viral nucleic acid and the viral group. In RNA viruses, such as the rubella virus, synthesis occurs in the cytoplasm. In most DNA viruses, however, the viral nucleic acid is replicated in the host cell nucleus, whereas the viral protein is synthesized in the cytoplasm. In the final step of viral replication, maturation or assembly of the viral particles occurs. The mature particles are then released by budding through the cell membrane or by cell lysis.[7,8]

Effects of Viral Infection

CYTOTOXIC EFFECTS

Once a host cell is infected, viruses may cause a variety of changes, called cytopathic effects (CPE), or even cell death. If viruses are inoculated into cell cultures in the laboratory, CPE can be observed and used as a means for viral identification. Viral infection may be harmful to host cells in several ways.[7] Viruses are able to divert the host's synthetic processes, thereby stopping the production of important cellular components. Infection may also cause the release of enzymes from cellular lysosomes, resulting in host-cell lysis. Changes in antigenic determinants on the host cell surface caused by viral infection may subsequently induce humoral and cell-mediated immunity in the host.

DIAGNOSTIC MORPHOLOGIC CHANGES

Certain morphologic changes that occur in the host cell in response to viral infection are important markers in viral identification. As viruses replicate, viral and cellular components, such as nucleic acids and proteins not yet assembled into viruses, may accumulate in the form of inclusion bodies. Detection of certain inclusion bodies, such as Negri bodies in rabies infection, is diagnostic. Certain enveloped viruses form syncytia, or giant cells, by causing fusion of several adjacent infected cells. These giant cells are multinucleated.

TRANSFORMED CELLS

In addition to cytotoxic effects, chromosomal changes may occur as a result of infection with certain viruses.[7] These changes may include induction of tumors, called transformation. Tumors may be induced by either RNA or DNA viruses. Through the process of transformation, tumor cells acquire certain unique properties.

Viral genetic material integrates into the host cell DNA and subsequently replicates with the host chromosome. Chromosomes of transformed cells tend to be fragmented and are present in abnormal numbers. Transformed cells lose contact inhibition, a property of normal cells. Contact inhibition signals cells to stop dividing when they come into contact with other cells. Without contact inhibition, tumor cells divide uncontrolled and form a mass. Transformed cells appear rounder than normal cells.

Changes in the permeability and chemical composition of the host cell membrane may also occur in transformed cells. The ability of transformed cells to agglutinate with lectins is increased because of an alteration of their binding sites. Many tumor cells develop antigens on their surface, which may be specified by either the virus or the host cell. Some of the virus-specific antigens produced are referred to as tumor-specific transplantation antigens (TSTAs).

ROLE OF INTERFERON

Some cells produce a protein in response to viral infection shortly after the virus enters the cell. This protein, called interferon, is encoded by the host cell DNA and is important in host defense. Interferon is a group of chemical mediators with antiviral, immune modulatory, and antiproliferative effects. Interferons are low molecular weight glycoproteins synthesized in response to viral infection, immune stimulation, fever, and bacteria.[5] There are three types of interferon: alpha interferon, made by leukocytes, beta interferon, made by fibroblasts, and gamma interferon, made by T cells. A few hours after infection, cells release interferon, which binds to receptors on nearby uninfected cells. Once interferon binds to a cell, it causes the cell to make antiviral protein. This protein interferes with translation of viral mRNA but has no effect on host mRNA. Interferon is relatively species specific but is not virus specific.

Interferon can be made in laboratory cultures of white blood cells and fibroblasts, and in bacteria by re-combinant DNA techniques. Alpha interferon has been approved by the Food and Drug Administration for treatment of venereal warts, Kaposi sarcoma in patients infected with HIV, and in chronic hepatitis caused by hepatitis B virus and hepatitis C virus. Interferon is ineffective in acute viral infections.[5] It appears to delay the onset of symptoms of influenza, but is not effective in treating the disease.[1] Although interferon inhibits rhinoviruses (cold viruses), it causes irritation and nasal bleeding.[1]

Interferon has been shown to reduce metastasis in bone cancer following surgery and radiation treatment used to remove and destroy as much of the cancerous tissue as possible. Interferon has proven to be effective in treating hairy cell leukemia and somewhat effective in treating melanoma, but shows no immediate promise for lung, breast, or colon cancer.

TREATMENT OF VIRAL INFECTIONS

Viral infections are most successfully controlled through the administration of vaccines to prevent infection. Because vaccines are not available for most viral infections, chemotherapeutic agents have been used and have limited success. Because a virus uses the host cell metabolic systems and enzymes to perform its own metabolic functions, an antiviral agent that inhibits viral activity will interfere with the host's cellular function. Consequently, antiviral agents are toxic to human cells. Antiviral drugs currently licensed for use act either by inhibiting attachment of the virus to the host cell or by inhibiting viral replication within the host.

Review Questions

1. The establishment and multiplication of an organism within or on the body is called

   a. adherence
   b. disease
   c. infection
   d. pathogenicity

2. The ability of an organism to cause disease is called

   a. colonization
   b. communicability
   c. pathogenicity
   d. virulence

3. The time during a disease process when the symptoms are nonspecific is the

   a. acute phase
   b. convalescent phase
   c. incubation period
   d. prodromal phase

4. A glycoprotein with antiviral properties produced by the host cell in response to a viral infection is a(n)

   a. inclusion body
   b. interferon
   c. lysosome
   d. tumor-specific transplantation antigen

5. In a viral replication cycle, the step following penetration is

   a. biosynthesis
   b. maturation
   c. replication of viral particles
   c. uncoating

6. Which of the following is true regarding viruses?

   a. Viruses contain both DNA and RNA.
   b. Viral capsids are composed of identical protein subunits.
   c. Viral envelopes contain surface spikes called capsomeres.
   d. Animal viruses infecting humans range in size from 300 to 900 nm.

7. The presence of IgM specific antibody could signify

   a. permanent immunity to the infectious agent
   b. recovery
   c. in utero infection
   d. immunologic memory

8. Which pair of titers (acute; convalescent) suggests a recent bacterial infection?

   a. 10; 20
   b. 40; 320
   c. 400; 800
   d. 1000; 2000

References

1. Black JG: Microbiology Principles and Applications, 2nd ed., Englewood Cliffs, NJ, Prentice Hall, 1993
2. Larson HS: Host-parasite interaction. In Mahon CR, Manuselis G (eds): Textbook of Diagnostic Microbiology, pp 214–233. Philadelphia, WB Saunders, 1995
3. Morello J, Miler HE, Wilson ME, Grained PA: Microbiology in Patient Care, 5th ed. Dubuque, IA, WC Brown Publishers, 1994
4. Marcon MJ: Serologic diagnosis of infectious diseases. In Mahon CR, Manuselis G (eds): Textbook of Diagnostic Microbiology. Philadelphia, WB Saunders, 1995
5. Baron EJ, Chang RS, Howard DH, Miller JN, Turner J: Medical Microbiology: A Short Course. New York, Wiley-Liss, 1994
6. Smith T: Laboratory diagnosis of viral infections. In Howard BJ (ed): Clinical and Pathogenic Microbiology, 2nd ed. St. Louis, MO, Mosby Year Book, Inc., 1994
7. Tortora GJ, Funke BR, Case CL: Microbiology: An Introduction. Menlo Park, CA, Benjamin/Cummings, 1995
8. Chicory L, Myrvik QN: Pathways and classes of virus replication. In Kucera LS, Myrvik QN (eds): Fundamentals of Medical Virology, 2nd ed, p 27. Philadelphia, Lea & Febiger, 1985

CHAPTER 20

Streptococcal Infection and Serology

Ann C. Albers

Objectives

Upon completion of the chapter, the reader will be able to:

1. Explain the role of *Streptococcus pyogenes* and its components in the development of rheumatic fever (RF), rheumatic heart disease (RHD), and acute glomerulonephritis (AGN)
2. Describe the importance of immunologic procedures in the diagnosis of RF, RHD, and AGN
3. Discuss the relationship of an increased anti-streptolysin O (ASO) titer with the antecedent streptococcal infection
4. Differentiate between positive and negative ASO results
6. Explain the relationship between a positive ASO and a negative anti–hyaluronidase test (AHT)
7. Outline the procedure for the ASO, AHT, anti–DNase B, and the Streptozyme® tests
8. Describe the basic methods employed for diagnosis of antecedent streptococcal infections
9. Identify significant test results
10. Explain reasons for false positive results

ORGANISM

All members of the genus *Streptococcus* are gram-positive cocci. Division occurs in only one plane, resulting in cocci in pairs or chains. First described by Pasteur, these catalase-negative, facultative anaerobes comprise a heterogeneous group of homofermentative bacteria whose principal fermentation product is lactic acid.[1]

Streptococcus pyogenes, group A β-hemolytic streptococci, is a major pathogen of this genus. The organism is found only in humans, and person-to-person spread is usually by upper respiratory secretions or by direct contact. Group A streptococci constitute the principal bacterial cause of oropharyngitis and are involved in many other suppurative infections, including pyoderma, puerperal sepsis, and acute endocarditis. These organisms are also responsible for the toxigenic condition scarlet fever, and for two nonsuppurative conditions (i.e., rheumatic fever and acute poststreptococcal glomerulonephritis). These conditions are considered nonsuppurative because the affected organs do not have the purulent inflammatory response associated with infection; rather, the response in the affected organs is caused by the antibodies elicited by the infection.

The serogroups of streptococci are determined by the C carbohydrate of the cell wall. All group A streptococci are antigenically identical for this carbohydrate.

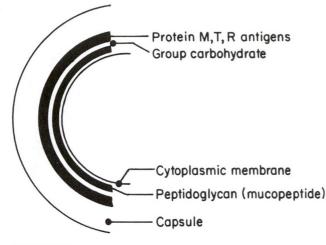

FIGURE 20-1
Layers of the cell wall and capsule of group A streptococcus.

Group carbohydrates are not known to be associated with any particular disorders.

Serotypes of group A are determined by the proteins in the cell wall (M, T, and R; Fig. 20-1). M antigens are significant in disease association; they are important in adherence of the bacterial cell to the host cells, they allow the bacteria to evade engulfment by phagocytic cells, and antibodies to them are protective.[2] There are at least 80 antigenically distinct M serotypes.[3] Usually, different serotypes of group A are involved in skin infections than those involved in upper respiratory tract infections. These two types of infections do not usually occur simultaneously in the same person. Although serogrouping of streptococci is a routine procedure for many clinical microbiology labs, serotyping is generally limited to a few research labs. The serotypes that are frequently associated with glomerulonephritis[2,13,14] are referred to as nephritogenic serotypes and those that have a high rate of association with rheumatic fever are referred to as rheumatogenic serotypes.[1,3,5,6,18,19,24]

POSTSTREPTOCOCCAL SEQUELAE

Infection with group A β-hemolytic streptococci may be followed by two separate sequelae, rheumatic fever (RF) and acute poststreptococcal glomerulonephritis (APSGN). Rheumatic fever follows streptococcal infection of the throat, and glomerulonephritis follows either streptococcal infection of the throat or streptococcal pyoderma. Diagnosis of either syndrome requires evidence of antecedent group A streptococcal infection. Most patients no longer have streptococcal infection when they present with RF or acute glomerulonephritis (AGN), so evidence of such infections is obtained by serologic assays. The tests most frequently employed—antistreptolysin O (ASO), Streptozyme®, anti-hyaluronidase (AHT), and anti-deoxyribonuclease B (anti–DNase B)—all measure the presence of antibodies to enzymes produced by the organisms during acute infection.

Rheumatic Fever

Rheumatic fever, which is characterized by carditis, chorea, and/or erythema marginatum, follows about 2% to 3% of untreated cases of streptococcal pharyngitis.[4,5] Patients who are treated with antibiotics but who still have organisms recovered from the throat ≥3 weeks after acute infection have a similar RF attack rate.[6] Rheumatic fever usually occurs 3 to 4 weeks after group A streptococcal infection in the throat but does not follow skin infection. The syndrome is related to production of antibodies to the streptococci; RF apparently does not develop in patients who fail to produce antibodies to the organisms.[6,7] Because the cholesterol in the skin binds streptolysin O, it is not immunogenic in skin infections.

Although RF has been observed in many age groups, the first attack is most common in the 5 to 15 year age group. Both sexes are equally affected. Carditis occurs at the same rate in both sexes; however, chorea is observed in girls two to three times more frequently than in boys. Also, chorea may occur months after the antecedent streptococcal infection, so the antibody titers may have returned to normal before chorea appears. The course of the disease varies, but in most cases the signs subside within a few weeks, 90% have subsided within 3 months, and <5% have signs persisting for longer than 6 months. Prior to the antibiotic era, symptoms of RF recurred once or more in more than 50% of patients, increasing the possibility of permanent valvular damage.

The process that leads from streptococcal infection in the oropharynx to rheumatic fever is not understood. This is a nonsuppurative inflammatory process involving connective tissue and resulting in injury to the heart, joints, and central nervous system. Rheumatic inflammation of the joints (rheumatic polyarthritis) or brain (Sydenham's chorea) rarely results in permanent damage. Rheumatic carditis, however, may become chronic and progressively debilitating. It may involve the pericardium, myocardium, and/or endocardium; however, it is the inflammation of the endocardium of the mitral valve that accounts for most of the morbidity and mortality of this disease. The inflammation of the mitral valve continues long after clinical evidence of carditis has disappeared, resulting in progressive scarring and malfunction, with end-stage mitral stenosis.[8]

There are several theories regarding the pathogenesis of rheumatic fever. The most popular is that the streptococcal infection induces an autoimmune response in the host. The group A streptococci are known to share antigenic determinants with some host cells, tissues, and organs.[9–11] The immune response that is directed against the organisms will crossreact with the host immunodeterminants; thus, these antibodies induced by group A streptococci are also autoantibodies to heart tissue. Patients with acute rheumatic fever have about four times as much of this heart-reactive antibody as patients convalescing from uncomplicated streptococcal infections or acute glomerulonephritis.[12]

Diagnosis of rheumatic fever is by the revised Jones criteria, which require supporting evidence of preceding streptococcal infection plus a combination of major manifestations (i.e., carditis, polyarthritis, chorea, erythema marginatum, subcutaneous nodules) and minor manifestations (i.e., previous rheumatic fever or rheumatic heart disease, arthralgia, fever, increased erythrocyte sedimentation rate, increased C-reactive protein, leukocytosis, and electrocardiographic changes).[13]

Acute Glomerulonephritis

Acute glomerulonephritis, like RF, is a nonsuppurative sequel to group A streptococcal infection. It occurs in quite varied attack rates ranging from 0.03% to 18%.[14] The disease occurs primarily in childhood and presents with proteinuria, hematuria, hypertension, impaired renal function, and edema, especially about the face and legs. It is thought that this syndrome, like RF, is immunologically mediated. Several theories have been proposed to explain the disease, but the one most commonly accepted is that the circulating antigen-antibody complexes are deposited in the glomerular basement membrane, where they activate complement, with damage to the glomeruli resulting from complement-mediated release of lysosomal content from white blood cells. There is an aggregation of platelets and a buildup of fibrin and fibrinogen. These, in turn, cause capillary obstruction, which impairs renal function.

Acute glomerulonephritis occurs approximately 10 days after streptococcal infection of the throat, or 18 to 21 days after skin infection.[15] It occurs twice as often in males as in females. Only a few specific nephritogenic M serotypes are responsible for acute poststreptococcal glomerulonephritis.

LABORATORY ASSAYS

The most reliable laboratory finding to support an antecedent streptococcal infection is isolation of the organism; however, many patients no longer have the organisms when either of the nonsuppurative poststreptococcal sequelae develop. Serologic evidence is then the only means to demonstrate the antecedent infection. The ASO test is positive in 80% of patients with

RF but is rarely positive in patients with AGN secondary to streptococcal pyoderma. The AHT test is positive in a smaller percentage of RF patients but is also positive in most patients with AGN. The anti-DNase B test is perhaps the most reliable of these three; moreover, it is positive for a longer period of time. It is strongly recommended that a combination of tests be performed for laboratory identification of an antecedent streptococcal infection. The Streptozyme test is a screening test and gives both false negatives and false positives compared with each of the other three assays. The relative reliability of these tests is described in Table 20-1.

ASO Neutralization Test

Streptolysin O is produced by most strains of β-hemolytic group A streptococci and by a few strains of groups C and G. It is responsible, together with streptolysin S, for the hemolysis observed on blood agar. The antibodies to streptolysin O neutralize its hemolytic activity. An increased titer of ASO indicates a recent infection with group A streptococci. Infection with groups C and G are very rare compared with group A infections, and few strains of these two groups produce streptolysin O. Thus, it is very rare that the increased ASO will be caused by antecedent infection with groups C or G; however, it is possible.

In patients with culture-documented streptococcal infection of the upper respiratory tract, the ASO titer begins to rise after 1 week and peaks at 3 to 6 weeks after infection.[2,16,17] Thus, by the time RF develops, the ASO titer may be declining, particularly in those patients who do not develop any signs of RF for months after the antecedent group A streptococcal infection. In 75% to 80% of patients with RF, there will be an increase in ASO titer; consequently, the diagnosis of RF cannot be excluded on the basis of a low ASO titer.[17] Patients with pyoderma and its sequela, acute glomerulonephritis, are less likely to have an increased ASO titer. Streptolysin O is produced by group A streptococci in pyoderma as well as in pharyngitis, but the cholesterol in the skin binds to the enzyme, thus preventing it from becoming an effective immunogen.

TABLE 20-1
Relative Reliability of Serologic Tests for Antecedent Group A Streptococcal Infections

TEST	RF	AGN
ASO	+++	0
AHT	++	++
Anti–DNase B	++++	++++
Streptozyme	+	+

RF, rheumatic fever; AGN, acute glomerulonephritis.

PRINCIPLES

This assay is an enzyme-inhibition (neutralization) reaction. In a patient who has had a recent group A streptococcal infection, the antistreptolysin O antibodies neutralize the streptolysin O reagent, thus preventing it from hemolyzing human group O red blood cells.

PROCEDURE

Dilutions of heat-inactivated patient serum and ASO control are prepared in buffer. Streptolysin O reagent is added to the control and patient serum dilutions. After a short room-temperature incubation, 5% group O human red blood cell suspension is added, followed by an incubation at 37°C. Tubes are centrifuged and read for hemolysis.

RESULTS

Tubes are read for hemolysis. Streptolysin O reagent hemolyzes human group O cells; lack of hemolysis is caused by neutralization of the streptolysin O reagent by the antibodies in the patient serum. The titer is the unit of the last tube (i.e., the highest dilution) showing total absence of hemolysis. The reciprocal of the original serum dilution (not the final dilution) in each tube is equal to the Todd units or the international units; these two units are the same.

INTERPRETATION

A fourfold increase in titer between acute and convalescent sera is evidence of a recent group A streptococcal infection. It is recommended that this test be performed on paired sera because a wide range of normal values has been reported. Streptococcal infections are fairly common; thus, normal individuals have low titers. The committee for revising the Jones criteria for diagnosis of RF recommended that single titers of at least 250 units in adults and 333 in children over 5 years of age be considered evidence of a recent streptococcal infection.[13] The titer of the ASO is unrelated to the clinical severity of RF.[17] There may be false positive titers associated with liver disease, with the growth of bacteria in the serum specimen, or caused by oxidation of the streptolysin O reagent.[16]

ASO Rapid Latex Agglutination

PRINCIPLES

Polystyrene latex particles coated with streptolysin O antigen will agglutinate with antibody to streptolysin O (ASO). This is a screening test and, if positive, can be performed as a semiquantitative procedure as well.

PROCEDURE

Dilutions of patient serum and positive and negative serum controls are mixed with the latex reagent on a glass serum slide. The slide is rotated for 3 minutes.

RESULTS

Agglutination is positive and no agglutination is negative.

INTERPRETATION

Positive results indicate ≥200 U/mL of ASO. In the semiquantitative procedure, the results are reported as the reciprocal of the highest dilution of serum to produce visible agglutination.

Streptozyme

Streptozyme® is a screening test marketed by Wampole (Wampole Laboratories, Cranbury, NJ) for detection of antibodies to five streptococcal enzymes: DNase B, hyaluronidase, NADase, streptokinase, and streptolysin O. The slide test is a passive hemagglutination assay that employs sheep erythrocytes coated with the streptococcal enzymes. The reagent is mixed with 1:100 dilution of patient serum or plasma (whole blood may also be used). If antibodies to any of these enzymes are present, agglutination is observed. If the test is positive, the patient serum can be further diluted to determine the Streptozyme titer (STZ titer). The titer is the reciprocal of the highest dilution showing agglutination and is expressed as STZ units.

Early evaluations of this test kit found good agreement with ASO, anti-hyaluronidase, and anti–streptokinase,[21] and with ASO and anti–DNase.[22] However, more extensive evaluation demonstrated that it is not as reliable when compared with ASO and anti–DNase B together to confirm an antecedent streptococcal infection. Golubjatnikov et al. found both false positive and false negative results when compared with ASO and anti–DNase assays.[23] They also reported that agreement rates appear to be age dependent, and as the patient population becomes older, Streptozyme will fail to detect up to 25% of elevated anti–DNase B titers.

Anti-Hyaluronidase Test

The enzyme hyaluronidase is produced by group A β-hemolytic streptococci, and antibodies to it, anti-hyaluronidase, are found in the blood of patients with recent streptococcal infections. The number of patients developing antibodies to this enzyme is somewhat lower than the number developing antibodies to streptolysin O; however, antibodies to hyaluronidase are produced by patients with either throat or skin infections, whereas ASO is produced only following throat infections.

PRINCIPLES

This test is a neutralization assay in which the antibodies to the enzyme are allowed to neutralize it, thus preventing the subsequent enzymatic breakdown of the substrate, potassium hyaluronate.

PROCEDURE

Serial dilutions of patient serum are prepared and the enzyme, hyaluronidase, is added to each tube. If the patient serum contains anti-hyaluronidase antibodies, the hyaluronidase will be inactivated. After a short incubation at 37°C, the tubes are cooled and substrate, potassium hyaluronate, is added to each tube. The tubes are reincubated at 37°C and cooled in the refrigerator. To each tube is added 2N acetic acid. If the patient has no antibodies to inactivate the hyaluronidase, hyaluronate will be hydrolyzed and there will be turbidity after the acid is added. In tubes where the enzyme was inactivated (neutralized) by patient anti-hyaluronidase antibodies, a mucin clot forms because the acid reacts with the potassium hyaluronate. The potassium hyaluronate is not destroyed if the hyaluronidase has been inactivated by antibodies, and potassium hyaluronate is therefore available to react with the acid, forming a mucin clot.

RESULTS

The titer is the reciprocal of the highest dilution with definite clot formation. Threads are not considered clot formation.

INTERPRETATION

If both acute and convalescent sera are tested, a fourfold rise in titer is considered evidence of streptococcal infection. If a single convalescent serum is tested, it is considered significant if the titer is >256. Reproducibility of this test is not as good as that of the ASO test and the anti–DNase B test; however, it is superior to ASO in demonstrating an antecedent streptococcal infection in patients presenting with skin-related acute glomerulonephritis.[16]

Anti–Deoxyribonuclease B Test

Streptococcus pyogenes strains are known to produce four DNases, A, B, C, and D.[18] DNase B is produced by nearly all strains of group A streptococci and by some strains of groups C and G. Group B streptococci produce three known DNases that are antigenically distinct from those produced by group A strains. Antibodies to DNase B are produced later than ASO, peaking at 4 to 6 weeks after infection and remaining in the serum for several months.[16] Anti-DNase antibodies are produced by organisms in the throat as well as those of the skin. Thus, anti–DNase B is a more reliable marker of antecedent streptococcal infection than is ASO, particularly in those patients whose symptoms (usually carditis or chorea) of RF are not observed for several months. This test is thought by many to be the single most reliable test to demonstrate antecedent group A streptococcal infection.

PRINCIPLES

The anti–DNase B test is also a neutralization test. Antibodies in the patient's serum will prevent the enzyme, DNase B (streptodornase), from depolymerizing DNA.

PROCEDURE

Inactivated patient sera and control serum are diluted in buffer and incubated at 37°C with the enzyme DNase B to allow the antibodies, if present, to inactivate (neutralize) the enzyme. The substrate (DNA–methyl green complex) is added to each tube. After overnight incubation at 37°C, the tubes are observed for color. Methyl green is green when combined with DNA. When DNase B hydrolyzes DNA, the methyl green is concomitantly reduced and becomes colorless.[19]

RESULTS

Color in each tube is graded from 0 (no color) to 4+ (green). The titer is the reciprocal of the highest dilution with at least a 3+ reaction.

INTERPRETATION

This test should be performed on paired acute and convalescent sera. A fourfold rise is considered indicative of a recent group A streptococcal infection. Interpretation of results of a single serum specimen depends on the age of the patient. Normal preschoolers have a titer of <120; everyone else has a titer of <1360.[20]

Case Study

On July 11, a 20-year-old female patient developed oropharyngitis. The physician prescribed 10 days of penicillin. She recovered in 3 days and discontinued taking the penicillin. On July 25 she again became ill with fever, transient generalized macular rash, and a swollen, painful left knee. She was admitted to the hospital on July 28, with the following signs and symptoms: temperature 37.7°C, pulse 100 beats/min, ECG normal, ESR 120 mm/h, and ASO titer 700 TU, and her left knee was still swollen and painful. The throat swab revealed no hemolytic streptococci. She was given penicillin and aspirin every 6 hours. By August 4 the fever was normal and the left knee had improved. On August 7 the ASO was 500 TU and the ESR 96 mm/h. By August 11 the patient was well except for a small residual left knee effusion. The patient was fully recovered with a normal ECG by September 24, at which time prophylactic penicillin was started.

Case Study Questions

1. What is the probable diagnosis? Which laboratory tests were necessary to confirm this diagnosis?

2. How could the patient have prevented this disease from developing?

3. Why was the patient put on prophylactic penicillin?

4. Will the disease recur?

References

1. Deibel RH, Seeley HW: Streptococceae. In Buchanan RE, Gibbons NE (eds): Bergey's Manual of Determinative Bacteriology, 8th ed, p 490. Baltimore, Williams & Wilkins, 1974

2. Wannamaker LW, Ayoub EM: Antibody titers in acute rheumatic fever. Circulation 21:598, 1960

3. Howard BJ, Ducate MJ: Streptococci. In Howard BJ (ed): Clinical and Pathogenic Microbiology, p 245. St Louis, CV Mosby, 1987

4. Denny FW Jr, Wannamaker LW, Brink WR, et al: Prevention of rheumatic fever: Treatment of the preceding streptococcic infection. JAMA 143:151–153, 1950

5. Wannamaker LW, Rammelkamp CH Jr, Denny FW, et al: Prophylaxis of acute rheumatic fever by treatment of the preceding streptococcal infection with various amounts of depot penicillin. Am J Med 10:673–695, 1951

6. Stollerman GH: Rheumatic Fever and Streptococcal Infection, p 63. Orlando, Grune & Stratton, 1975

7. Markowitz M: Rheumatic Fever, p 1. Philadelphia, WB Saunders, 1972

8. Paterson PY: The enigma of rheumatic fever. In Youmans GY, Paterson PY, Sommers HM (eds): The Biological and Clinical Basis of Infectious Diseases, 3rd ed, p 195. Philadelphia, WB Saunders, 1985

9. Kaplan MH, Svec KH: Immunologic relation of streptococcal and tissue antigens. J Exp Med 119:651, 1964

10. Zabriskie JB, Freimer EH: An immunological relationship between the group A streptococcus and mammalian muscle. J Exp Med 124:661, 1966

11. Husby G, van de Rijn I, Zabriskie JB, et al: Antibodies reacting with cytoplasm of subthalamic and caudate nuclei neurons in chorea and acute rheumatic fever. J Exp Med 144:1094, 1976

12. Zabriskie JB, Hsu KC, Seegal BC: Heart-reactive antibody associated with rheumatic fever: Characterization and diagnostic significance. Clin Exp Immunol 7:147, 1970

13. Committee to Revise Jones Criteria, Stollerman GH (chair): Jones criteria (revised) for guidance in the diagnosis of rheumatic fever. Circulation 32:664, 1965

14. Freeman BA: Burrows Textbook of Microbiology, p 401. Philadelphia, WB Saunders, 1985

15. Facklam RR, Washington II JA: Streptococci and related catalase-negative gram-positive cocci. In Lennette EH, Balows A, Hausler WJ Jr, et al (eds): Manual of Clinical Microbiology, 4th ed, p 154. Washington, DC, American Society for Microbiology, 1985

16. Escobar MR: Hemolytic assays: Complement fixation and antistreptolysin O. In Balows A, Hausler WJ Jr, Herrmann KL, et al (eds): Manual of Clinical Microbiology, 5th ed, p 73. Washington, DC, American Society for Microbiology, 1991

17. Davis E: Acute rheumatic fever. Practitioner 213:159, 1974

18. Slechta TF, Gray ED: Isolation of streptococcal nuclease by batch adsorption. J Clin Microbiol 2:528, 1975

19. Klein GC, Baker CN, Addison BV, et al: Micro test for streptococcal antideoxyribonuclease B. Appl Microbiol 18:204, 1969

20. Peacock JE, Tomar RH: Manual of Laboratory Immunology, p 50. Philadelphia, Lea & Febiger, 1980

21. Janeff J, Janeff D, Taranta A, et al: A screening test for streptococcal antibodies. Lab Med 2:38, 1971

22. Klein GC, Jones WL: Comparison of the streptozyme test with the antistreptolysin O, antideoxyribonuclease B, and antihyaluronidase tests. Appl Microbiol 21:257, 1971

23. Golubjatnikov R, Koehler JE, Buccowich J: Comparative study of antistreptolysin O, antideoxyribonuclease B and multi-enzyme tests in streptococcal infections. Health Lab Sci 14:284, 1977

24. Cosh JA, Lever JV: Rheumatic Diseases and the Heart, p 11. London, Springer-Verlag, 1988

CHAPTER 21

Syphilis

Ann Marie McNamara

Objectives

Upon completion of the chapter, the reader will be able to:

1. State the treponemes that infect humans, the syndromes and infections they cause, and the epidemiological differences
2. Describe the four stages of syphilis and congenital syphilis
3. Identify appropriate therapy for syphilis and congentital syphilis
4. Describe three types of direct detection tests for syphilis and in what stage of syphilis they are useful for diagnosis
5. Describe the serological diagnosis of syphilis, indicating the differences between nontreponemal and treponemal tests, and name the stages of syphilis for which serological tests are most useful

SYPHILIS

Treponema pallidum

The etiologic agent of syphilis is the bacterium *Treponema pallidum*, subspecies *pallidum*. This aerobic bacterium is a member of the order Spirochaetales, the family Treponemataceae, and the genus *Treponema*. These spirochetes are long, thin, spiral-shaped, unicellular organisms that are 5 to 15 μm long and 0.09 to 0.18 μm wide (Fig. 21-1).[1] These bacteria are loosely coiled, with 6 to 24 coils (average 14). Spirochetes are unique among bacteria in that their characteristic corkscrew motility is produced by internal periplasmic flagella located between the outer membrane and the periplasmic cylinder (body) of the spirochete.[2]

Two species of the genus *Treponema* infect humans: *T. pallidum* and *T. carateum*, the causative agent of pinta. *T. pallidum* is further divided into three subspecies: *T. pallidum*, subspecies *pallidum*, the causative agent of syphilis; *T. pallidum*, subspecies *pertenue*, the causative agent of yaws; and *T. pallidum*, subspecies *endemium*, the causative agent of nonvenereal endemic syphilis or bejel.[3] Unless noted otherwise, *T. pallidum* refers to subspecies *pallidum* throughout the remainder of this chapter. A third species of the genus is *T. paraluis-cuniculi*, the causative agent of rabbit syphilis. All treponemas infecting humans are identical sero-

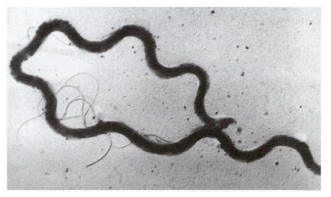

FIGURE 21-1
Electron micrograph of *Treponema pallidum*. (Courtesy of CDC Slide Archives.)

213

logically, sharing similar surface macromolecules and antigens. The three other treponemal diseases (yaws, pinta, and endemic syphilis) are distinguished from syphilis based on their geographic localization and clinical disease syndromes because the treponemas causing them are morphologically and serologically indistinguishable using current diagnostic methods. Evidence suggests that these three pathogenic treponemes are variants of a single prototype organism whose different clinical syndromes developed in response to host or environmental influences.[3]

In addition to the pathogenic treponemas, a number of nonpathogenic treponemas have been isolated from the human body, particularly from the oral cavity. *Treponema denticola* is an example of a nonpathogenic treponemas. Nonpathogenic and pathogenic treponemas can be distinguished by the failure of pathogenic treponemas to reproduce in standard laboratory conditions. However, pathogenic treponemas are capable of surviving and retaining their mobility in enriched and chemically defined media for up to 7 days at 25°C and up to 48 hours at 37°C.[1] Intratesticular passage of treponemas in rabbits is necessary to maintain a source of treponemas for laboratory studies. This makes research into the biology and pathogenesis of treponemas difficult.

Little is known about the interaction between *T. pallidum* and the human host. There is evidence that the complex symptomatology of syphilis is influenced by both humoral and cell-mediated immune responses. The body produces antitreponemal and anticardiolipin antibodies, initiates an inflammatory response (involving lymphocytes, plasma cells, and macrophages), forms immune complexes, walls off the organism in lesions, and enters a latency (remission) stage of the disease.[3]

Clinical Features

EPIDEMIOLOGY

Cases of syphilis are on the increase, despite effective therapies. In the United States, 112,581 cases were reported in 1992, including 33,973 cases of primary and secondary syphilis and 3850 cases of congenital syphilis.[4] Syphilis is transmitted by four main routes: sexual contact, transfusion of fresh human blood, direct inoculation, and through the placenta (congenital syphilis). The most common route of acquiring syphilis is through sexual intercourse. Most cases occur in the sexually active age group (15 to 30 years old), nonwhites, and homosexual men. Transmission can occur through the act of sexual intercourse itself, kissing, or touching active lesions.

Transmission of syphilis through blood transfusions or blood products is rare in the United States. This is because of the low incidence of syphilis in the United States, combined with the fact that under current blood bank storage conditions, *T. pallidum* cannot survive longer than 24 to 48 hours (at 4°C).[5]

DISEASE STAGES

Incubation Period

Treponema pallidum enters the human body through abrasions in the skin or by penetrating intact mucous membranes. Once inside the human host, the bacterium begins to multiply. Within hours it enters the lymphatics and/or the bloodstream and is disseminated to the various organs of the body.[1] This stage occurs from 0 to 33 hours postinfection and lasts from 9 to 90 days (average, 3 weeks; Fig. 21-2).[6] During the incubation period there are no clinical symptoms of the disease and all serologic tests are negative. Negative skin tests and depressed mitogenic responses indicate that T-cell immunity is impaired.

Primary Syphilis

The primary stage of syphilis begins with the appearance of the initial lesion called a *chancre*. The chancre is usually a firm, eroded, painless papule with raised, indurated margins that progresses to a clean-based, nonbleeding, painless ulcer.[1] Generally, chancres appear at the site of inoculation after a 2- to 3-week incubation period. They are commonly found in the genital and perianal regions or extragenitally on the lips, tongue, nipples, tonsils, and fingers. Often they are single lesions, although multiple lesions can occur. Within a week of the appearance of the chancre, regional lymph nodes become enlarged (although painless). These enlarged lymph nodes are termed *satellite bulboes*. The chancre heals spontaneously within 3 to 6 weeks; however, the lymphadenopathy persists.[1] The patient usually enters an asymptomatic period following the healing of the chancre, although some patients begin to develop symptoms of secondary syphilis during the primary stage.

In the early primary stage, patients are seronegative, as humoral antibodies generally begin to develop from 1 to 4 weeks after the appearance of the chancre. Darkfield microscopy examination of the lesion fluids for the presence of spirochetes can confirm the diagnosis prior to the development of antibodies. If nontreponemal screening tests are negative but the patient presents with a lesion characteristic of syphilis, the nontreponemal screening test should be repeated after 1 week, 1 month, and 3 months before ruling out a diagnosis of syphilis.[7] Cellular immunity remains depressed at this stage.

Secondary Syphilis

Secondary syphilis marks the disseminated stage of the disease. This stage is characterized by skin rashes

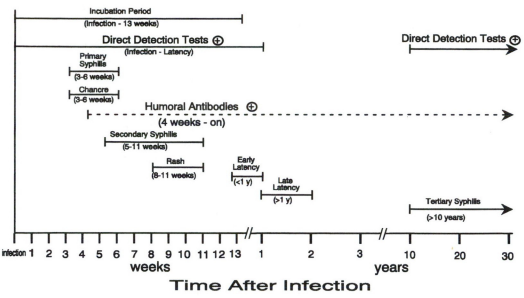

FIGURE 21-2
A timeline showing the progression of syphilis. The times are approximate. Consult the text for further details.

and the demonstration of large numbers of treponemas throughout the body. Almost any type of skin rash (except vascular rashes) can be seen in secondary syphilis, with the rash being quite marked on the palms and soles, and rarely on the face. The patient also presents with low-grade fever, malaise, pharyngitis, laryngitis, weight loss, arthralgia, and generalized painless lymphadenopathy.[1] Highly infectious lesions called *mucous patches* develop on the mucous membranes. These erosions are silver-gray in color, with a red periphery, and contain numerous spirochetes. Because of the large numbers of spirochetes in the blood stream, these bacteria are disseminated to the organs of the body, including the central nervous system. At this stage of syphilis, all serologic tests are positive and T-cell responses become normal. The diagnosis of secondary syphilis should also be considered when a prozone phenomenon (a false negative test in persons with high titers) results in a negative nontreponemal test result.

Latency

Latent syphilis is a stage of acquired or congenital syphilis without signs and symptoms of the disease, but with positive nontreponemal and treponemal antibody tests. Latency is divided into two stages: early latency (<1 year after initial infection) and late latency (>1 year after infection). In at least 25% of untreated syphilis cases, signs and symptoms of relapses into secondary syphilis occur during early latency.[5] A patient is considered to have early latent syphilis if there is a history of lesions consistent with untreated primary or secondary syphilis or if the patient has had a nonreactive, nontreponemal reagin

test within the last year.[5] During late latent syphilis, the patient becomes more resistant to reinfection and to relapses.[1]

Spirochetemia is reduced during latency, although the patient remains infectious. When lesions are present, syphilis may still be transmitted by sexual contact; otherwise, blood transfusions and congenital transfer are the main routes of transmission during latency. Serologic tests are reactive during the latency stage and are the only means of diagnosing latent syphilis when clinical symptoms are absent.

Tertiary Syphilis

Tertiary syphilis is a slowly progressive inflammatory disease that can produce clinical illness 2 to 40 years after initial infection. This stage has been called *gummatous syphilis, neurosyphilis,* or *cardiovascular syphilis.*[1] Gummas are lesions of syphilis that resemble tuberculosis and may occur in the skin, bones, mucosa, muscles, and organs of the body.[8] These lesions are believed to be the result of delayed hypersensitivity reactions and contain few treponemas. Penicillin rapidly resolves gummatous lesions.[1] Cardiac anomalies contribute to the morbidity and mortality in tertiary syphilitic patients. Most commonly, syphilitic aortitis, aortic valve insufficiency, and thoracic aneurysm and rupture occur.[8] Central nervous system (CNS) involvement results from the multiplication of treponemas in CNS lesions. Neurosyphilis may present in asymptomatic or symptomatic stages and often causes blindness and/or insanity. The symptomatic phase may present with symptoms of endarteritis obliterans, general paresis, or tabes dorsalis.[1] Neurosyphilis generally ocurs in tertiary syphilis cases, rarely in primary and secondary[9] syphilis, and often in patients with human immunodeficiency virus (HIV) infections.[10] Nontreponemal reagin tests are less sensitive than treponemal tests for detecting tertiary syphilis. Neurosyphilis can be confirmed by a positive Venereal Disease Research Laboratory–cerebrospinal fluid (VDRL–CSF) test (described later).

Congenital Syphilis

Transfer of *T. pallidum* across the placenta can occur in any untreated mother in any stage of syphilis. Generally, the severity of congenital infection correlates with the clinical stage of the mother, with the most severe cases occurring when the mother has early primary or secondary syphilis. Clinical outcome may be late abortion, stillbirth, neonatal death, neonatal disease, or latent infection.[1] Treatment of the mother during the first 4 months of pregnancy almost always prevents congenital syphilis.[1] Signs of early congenital syphilis include rhinitis (snuffles) and a diffuse maculopapular desquamatous rash, particularly about the mouth and on the palms and soles. The child may also have hemolytic anemia, jaundice, hepatosplenomegaly, and bone involvement.[1] Signs of late syphilis, after 1 year of age, include corneal involvement, deafness, and abnormal bone and tooth development.[1] Treponemas are present in almost every tissue of the infant. A definitive diagnosis may be made by direct detection of *T. pallidum* in the umbilical cord, placenta, skin lesions, or nasal discharge. A presumptive diagnosis is defined by any infant with a reactive treponemal test.[11]

DIAGNOSIS

The diagnosis of syphilis is based on recognition of the clinical signs and symptoms in the various disease stages of syphilis, direct examination of fluid from syphilitic lesions for spirochetes, and syphilis serologic testing. The most important of these three is syphilis serology, because of the transient and sometimes nonspecific symptoms of the disease, and the lack of well-trained darkfield microscopists who must be able to distinguish between pathogenic and nonpathogenic spirochetes in patient samples.

TREATMENT

The treatment of choice for all stages of syphilis (early syphilis, secondary syphilis, tertiary syphilis, neurosyphilis, congenital syphilis, syphilis during pregnancy) is penicillin. For penicillin-allergic patients, alternative drugs of choice are tetracycline or doxycycline.[12]

DIRECT DETECTION

A definitive diagnosis of syphilis is made by direct microscopic identification of *T. pallidum* in lesion material, lymph node aspirates, biopsy tissue (primary and occasionally secondary syphilis), cerebrospinal fluid (neurosyphilis), or umbilical cord, placenta, nasal discharge, or skin lesions (congenital syphilis, especially early congenital syphilis). In latent-stage syphilis, direct detection tests are negative because treponeme-containing lesions are absent. Treponemas may be directly detected using darkfield microscopy, a direct fluorescent antibody test,[12,13] or by the polymerase chain reaction.[13,14]

Syphilis has traditionally been diagnosed by examining serous exudates from primary and secondary syphilitic lesions by darkfield microscopy for the presence of *T. pallidum*. Distinguishing *T. pallidum* by its characteristic morphology and motility from other nonpathogenic human commensal treponemas is exceedingly difficult, requiring a trained microscopist and resulting in a sensitivity of approximately 75%.[15]

Newer direct fluorescent antibody tests (DFA-TP) have been developed and have been determined to be as sensitive and specific as darkfield microscopy. In these tests serous lesion exudate (antigen) is collected on a microscope slide, fixed in acetone, and overlaid with either absorbed fluorescein-labeled polyvalent rabbit antitreponemal antiserum (antibody)[16] or *T. pallidum*–specific monoclonal antibodies (antibody).[17] When Evans blue stain is used as a counterstain, treponemas fluoresce green in a red background in a reactive test.

The polymerase chain reaction (PCR) is under investigation and considered experimental for this application. Most tests are based on detecting treponemal DNA, which codes for surface antigens. PCR could be valuable in diagnosing those disease states in which the direct examination of serologic detection is negative or difficult to interpret, such as congenital syphilis, neurosyphilis, and early primary syphilis, and for distinguishing new infections from old infections.[11]

SEROLOGIC DIAGNOSIS

General Principles

Infection of humans by *T. pallidum* leads to the production of two major types of antibodies: nonspecific (reagin) antibodies and specific treponemal antibodies. Nonspecific antibodies are measured in "nontreponemal" screening tests for syphilis, whereas specific treponemal antibodies are measured in "treponemal" confirmatory tests for syphilis.

The nontreponemal tests for syphilis detect the presence of nonspecific antibodies directed against lipid antigens of the treponemas' outer membrane, or against lipid antigens produced by interaction of the treponema and the human host. Because these lipid antigens are present in other diseases (systemic lupus erythematosus, autoimmune diseases, pregnancy, some chronic infections of the elderly, and drug addicts) and in normal tissue, the antibodies they elicit are not specific for syphilis and the tests that detect them are useful only as screening tests for the disease. The antigen for the nontreponemal tests is a cardiolipin-lecithin-cholesterol antigen. The antibody that reacts with this antigen has been termed reagin. Reagins are immunoglobulins of the IgG and IgM classes.

Although nontreponemal tests are inexpensive, rapid, and easy to perform, they may be insensitive in detecting primary, latent, and tertiary infections (Table 21-1). They may be particularly insensitive in early primary syphilis before reagin antibodies have had a chance to form. Because reagins are nonspecific, false positive tests may occur. The proportion of falsely reactive nontreponemal tests has been estimated at 3% to 40%,[9] depending on the type of test used and the incidence of syphilis in the test population studied. For this reason, all positive nontreponemal tests for syphilis are confirmed by a treponemal test in which patient sera are tested for antibodies developed specifically against *T. pallidum*. Nontreponemal tests are also useful in monitoring the effectiveness of therapy, in determining reinfection in patients with a history of syphilis, and in the diagnosis of congenital syphilis.

Treponemal confirmatory tests determine the presence of specific antitreponemal antibodies in the patient's serum. The antigens used in these tests are the nonpathogenic *T. phagedenis* biotype Reiter treponeme (to remove crossreacting antibodies to nonpathogenic treponemas) and *T. pallidum* antigens (to detect antibodies specific for *T. pallidum*). Treponemal tests are most useful in confirming latent and tertiary disease states (see Table 21-1) and, once positive, remain reactive for the life of the patient. Because all pathogenic treponemas show crossreactions in these tests, the different treponemal diseases (syphilis, bejel, yaws, and pinta) cannot be distinguished by serologic means alone but must rely on appearance and location of the lesion, the mode of transmission, the age of the patient, geographic location, and positive serologic tests. The treponemal tests may be divided into four categories: the *Treponema pallidum* immobilization test, fluorescent antibody tests, hemagglutination tests, and enzyme-linked immunoassays.

Nontreponemal Screening Tests

VDRL SLIDE TEST

The standard nontreponemal test is the Venereal Disease Research Laboratory (VDRL) slide test. The principle of this test is to examine microscopically patients' heat-treated sera (source of reagin antibodies) for the ability to flocculate (to form antigen-antibody complexes in suspension) with an antigen containing 0.03% cardiolipin, 0.9% cholesterol, and 0.21% lecithin (VDRL antigen).[18] This test may be either qualitative or quantitative, and each step in the testing has been meticulously described and must be strictly adhered to.[18] Results are reported as nonreactive (no clumping), weakly reactive (small clumps), or reactive (medium or large clumps). Because prozone reactions occur in which undiluted serum gives partial or complete inhi-

TABLE 21-1
*Percentage of Patients Reactive in Serologic Tests for Syphilis**

| TEST | STAGES OF SYPHILIS | | | | |
	Primary	Secondary	Latent	Tertiary	Congenital
VDRL	70–80	100	75–90	62–75	88
RPR	~80	100	75–90	~75	100
USR	72–88	100	88–100		
RST	77–86	100	88–100		
FTA-ABS	85–92	100	97	97–100	100
MHA-TP	65–78	100	98–99	94–98	100
TPI	57	99	97	92	NA
ELISA†	82–100	100	72–100	83–100	NA

*Percent rounded to nearest whole number. Compiled from reference list sources.
†Bio-Enzabead ELISA, Organon Teknika Corp. Lower percentages reflect test results read visually versus the use of a spectrophotometer.

bition of reactivity and corresponding diluted serum is reactive, weakly reactive results in the qualitative VDRL test should be followed by a quantitative VDRL test to rule out this phenomenon. The VDRL test generally becomes positive 1 to 3 weeks after the appearance of the chancre. The antibody titer then increases during the secondary stage and begins to fall during latency. Although largely replaced by newer nontreponemal tests for syphilis, the VDRL–cerebrospinal fluid (VDRL–CSF) test is the only test used to diagnose neurosyphilis.

The nontreponemal tests that follow are all modifications of the VDRL test. The main modification has been the addition of choline chloride and ethylenediamine tetracetic acid (EDTA) to the VDRL antigen. These two chemicals allow non–heat-inactivated serum to be used in place of the heat-inactivated serum and stabilize the antigen, respectively. Another modification of these tests is the use of compounds to increase the visibility of the flocculation reaction. The ability to perform these tests on disposable microscope slides or paper cards makes them simpler and less expensive to perform than the standard VDRL test.

All reactive qualitative nontreponemal tests should be followed by a quantitative nontreponemal test of the same type because differences in the titers may be obtained using each of these various tests. A rise in titer in a quantitative nontreponemal test may indicate recent infection or reinfection. Quantitative nontreponemal tests are also useful in monitoring the antibody titer in congenital syphilis. Newborns are monitored with quantitative nontreponemal tests for the first 6 months of life. A rise in antibody titer is diagnostic; however, an infant who was not infected in utero should show a decrease in antibody titer after 3 months because maternal antibody levels decrease. An important use of quantitative nontreponemal tests is in monitoring the effectiveness of therapy. Brown et al.[19] showed that there is at least a fourfold decrease in titer by 3 months after appropriate treatment for primary and secondary syphilis. Antibody titers may decline until no serologic reaction is detectable; however, low titers may persist when the patient is in the latent stage.[20]

UNHEATED SERUM REAGIN TEST

The unheated serum reagin test (USR) is a microscopic flocculation test that uses the choline chloride–EDTA-modified VDRL antigen.[21] This test is primarily used as a screening test or for monitoring the efficacy of treatment. The principle is that unheated serum (a qualitative test) or unheated serum dilutions (a quantitative test) are mixed with the modified VDRL antigen suspension on glass slides. The slides are then rotated mechanically and read microscopically for flocculation. Results are read as nonreactive, weakly reactive, or re-

active, as in the VDRL test. All reactive qualitative USR tests should be followed by a quantitative USR test.

RAPID PLASMA REAGIN CARD TEST

The rapid plasma reagin card test (RPR) is a macroscopic flocculation test that uses the modified VDRL antigen and charcoal particles to aid in visualizing the flocculation reaction with the naked eye. These modifications allow the use of non–heat-treated serum and eliminate the use of a microscope, resulting in a fast, easy-to-read nontreponemal test. Performing the test on cardboard with designated test circles makes the test disposable for screening large numbers of samples. There are two different formats for RPR card testing, the RPR teardrop card test and the RPR circle card test. The RPR teardrop card test was designed as a screening test for field use. Fingerstick blood plasma is mixed with a modified VDRL antigen suspension containing charcoal particles on a disposable card within a teardrop-shaped circle. The card is rocked by hand, and the results are read as reactive (flocculation) or nonreactive (no flocculation). This test is only qualitative.[22] The RPR circle test, however, can be read as a qualitative or a quantitative test for both screening and diagnostic purposes, respectively.[23] In contrast to the RPR teardrop card test, the RPR circle card test uses patient serum and is rotated on a mechanical rotator. Results are read as reactive or nonreactive.

REAGIN SCREEN TEST

The reagin screen test (RST) is another macroscopic flocculation test that can be read qualitatively and quantitatively for the screening and diagnosis of syphilis.[24] This test uses the modified VDRL antigen with added Sudan Black B, a lipid-soluble diazo dye, for visualization of the flocculation reaction. Results are read as reactive (flocculation) or nonreactive (no flocculation). This test is no longer available in the U.S. market.

Confirmatory Treponemal Tests

TREPONEMA PALLIDUM IMMOBILIZATION TEST

The *Treponema pallidum* immobilization (TPI) test was once the standard test against which all treponemal tests were compared. This test has since been replaced by newer confirmatory tests that are more sensitive, less difficult to perform, and less expensive. The TPI test was the first serologic treponemal test, developed in 1949 by Nelson and Mayer.[25] The purpose of this test was to measure the ability of antibody and complement to immobilize a suspension of live treponemes as visualized under darkfield microscopy.

Live, motile *T. pallidum* from a testicular lesion in a rabbit is mixed with patient sera and guinea pig complement. The mixture is incubated in an atmosphere of 5% carbon dioxide and 95% nitrogen. An aliquot is then examined under a darkfield microscope for immobilization of the *T. pallidum* present. If 50% or more treponemes are immobilized, the test is positive. Less than 20% immobilization constitutes a negative test, and the range between 20% and 50% immobilization represents a "doubtful" result. Antibiotics in the patient sera will also immobilize the treponemes present, resulting in a false positive test. Interpretation of the TPI test must also take into account the patient's stage of syphilis, because reactivity to the TPI test develops slowly and the sensitivity of the TPI test in the primary stage is approximately 50% (see Table 21-1).

FLUORESCENT TREPONEMAL ANTIBODY ABSORPTION TEST

Treponema pallidum may be detected in a fluorescent treponemal antibody absorption test (FTA-ABS). In this indirect fluorescent antibody test, dried Nichols strain *T. pallidum* grown in rabbit testes is used as the antigen. This material is smeared onto glass slides, air dried, and acetone fixed. Heat-inactivated patient serum (antibody) is then mixed with "sorbent," a culture of Reiter treponemas that removes antibodies to group antigens common to *T. pallidum* and the nonpathogenic treponemas. This step makes the test more specific in detecting *T. pallidum* antibodies. Absorbed patient serum is then added to the antigen smears, and fluorescein–isothiocyanate-labeled antihuman gamma globulin is added.

If antitreponemal antibody is present in the patient's serum, green fluorescent treponemas are visible under the fluorescence microscope. Positive reactions are graded from 1+ to 4+ by comparing them with appropriate 1+ to 4+ control sera. Nonreactive tests lack fluorescent treponemas. A modification of the FTA-ABS test for use with epi-illumination fluorescence microscopes is the fluorescent treponemal antibody absorption doublestaining test (FTA-ABS-DS). This procedure uses a rhodamine-labeled, class-specific, anti–human IgG primary stain and the fluorescein-labeled antitreponemal globulin as a counterstain. In this test treponemas exhibit specific red fluorescence. Farshy et al. have shown that the FTA-ABS-DS test gives results comparable with the FTA-ABS test, with the added advantage of being easier to read, especially with borderline reactive sera.[26]

For the diagnosis of congenital syphilis, an FTA-ABS test that detects IgM antibodies (FTA-ABS-IgM) has been developed. This test may be used as a confirmatory test for congenital syphilis but should not be used as a screening test, because the false positive rate of the test is 10% and the false negative rate is ≥35%.[27]

Fluorescent antibody tests are the most widely used confirmatory treponemal tests for syphilis. This is because of their advantages over darkfield microscopy and their sensitivity in detecting syphilis, particularly in the early stage of the disease (see Table 21-1).

HEMAGGLUTINATION ASSAYS: MHA-TP, HATTS, AND TPHA

Three hemagglutination assays for the detection of antibodies to syphilis are currently available: the microhemagglutination assay for antibodies to *T. pallidum* (MHA-TP), the hemagglutination treponemal test for syphilis (HATTS), and the *T. pallidum* hemagglutination assay (TPHA). Each is produced by a different manufacturer and differs in the types of erythrocytes employed in these passive (indirect) hemagglutination assays. The MHA-TP uses tanned formalin-fixed sheep erythrocytes, whereas the HATTS and TPA use gluteraldehyde-stabilized turkey erythrocytes. The sensitivity and specificity of these tests are virtually identical, and the choice of one as a confirmatory test depends on the preference of the user.

All these tests, however, give comparable test results to the FTA-ABS test in all stages of syphilis except the primary stage. In the primary stage, the FTA-ABS or nontreponemal tests are better choices (see Table 21-1). Each of these hemagglutination assays is performed by mixing erythrocytes sensitized with an ultrasonicate of *T. pallidum* with absorbed patient serum in either microtiter plate wells or in test tubes. Unsensitized cells in a second well or tube act as a control. The tests are incubated at room temperature, and agglutination of the sensitized cells constitutes a positive test. The unsensitized control cells and negative test results fail to agglutinate, forming a button of erythrocytes in the well or test tube bottom.

ENZYME-LINKED IMMUNOSORBENT ASSAY (ELISA)

ELISA tests have recently been developed for the diagnosis of syphilis. The Bio-Enza Bead (Organon Teknika Corp.) test kit uses Nichols-strain *T. pallidum* antigen fixed to metal beads. Patient serum provides the antibody source, and the detection system is horseradish peroxidase–conjugated anti–human IgG (second antibody) and 2,2′-azinodi(3-ethyl-2,3 dihydro-6-benzthiazoline-sulfonate), the enzyme substrate. Results are read visually[28] or on a spectrophotometer at a wavelength of 690 nm for green color development.[29] Results obtained in this ELISA test were found to be comparable with those obtained in the FTA-ABS test (see Table 21-1).[28–30]

Similar antibody capture ELISA tests in microtiter-well format assays have been developed for patient

IgG, the CAPTIA Syph-G assay (Centocor),[31] and for IgM, the CAPTIA Syph-M assay (Centocor).[32] These tests are currently confirmatory tests for syphilis and congenital syphilis (CAPTIA Syph-M); however, the CAPTIA Syph-G and similar ELISA tests have been demonstrated to detect syphilis in low-risk populations as well as or better than the RPR test and may soon be accepted as replacements for nontreponemal screening tests.[31] The major advantage of ELISA tests over immunofluorescent and hemagglutination tests for syphilis is their ability to be read spectrophotometrically, which eliminates the subjective judgments of visual methods. In addition, ELISA methodology makes screening large numbers of sera possible in sexually transmitted disease clinics and public health departments.

SUMMARY

Syphilis is caused by the bacterium *Treponema pallidum*, subspecies *pallidum*. Following an incubation period, the disease presents as three clinical stages in the adult (primary, secondary, or tertiary syphilis) or via transplacental transmission as congenital syphilis in the neonate. Each stage can be diagnosed by appropriate use of direct detection techniques or serologic testing. Two major antigens elicit the production of antibodies in syphilis: lipid antigens and specific treponemal antigens. Lipid antigens elicit the production of nonspecific, reagin antibodies detected by nonspecific nontreponemal tests for syphilis. Because these lipid antigens are present in some normal tissue and in disease states other than syphilis, nontreponemal tests may give false positive results and therefore are used only as screening tests for syphilis. Patient sera giving positive reagin tests or patients whose sera give negative reagin test results but who have signs and symptoms of syphilis are further evaluated using treponemal tests for syphilis. Treponemal tests are confirmatory and highly specific tests for syphilis because they detect antigens produced by *T. pallidum*.

Case Studies

1. A 23-year-old white male presented to a sexually transmitted disease clinic with symptoms of low-grade fever, malaise, weight loss, arthralgia, painless lymphadenopathy, and a skin rash. Blood work showed a positive rapid plasma reagin card test.

What subsequent testing should be performed?

2. A pregnant female contracts syphilis in her second month of pregnancy and is treated with penicillin. At 9 months, she delivers an apparently healthy baby. When her child is 3 months of age, the baby presents with hepatosplenomegaly, cutaneous lesions, and snuffles.

How is a diagnosis of congenital syphilis made?

Bibliography

1. Tramont EC: *Treponema pallidum* (syphilis). In Mandell GE, Douglas RG Jr, Bennett JE (eds): Principles and Practices of Infectious Diseases, 3rd ed, p 1794. 1990
2. Johnson, RC: Spirochetes. In Howard B, Klaas J, Rubin S, et al (eds): Pathogenic Microbiology, p 503. 1986
3. Baseman JB: The biology of *Treponema pallidum* and syphilis. Clin Microbiol Newslett 5:157, 1983
4. Centers for Disease Control and Prevention: Summary of Notifiable Diseases, United States 1992. Weekly Rep 41(55):9
5. Fiumara NJ, Finegold S: The surgical diagnosis: Ruling out VD, Part 2. Syphilis. Infect Surg 3:359, 1984
6. Wilcox RR, Guthe T: *Treponema pallidum*. A bibliographic review of the morphology, culture, and survival of *T. pallidum* and associated organisms. Bull WHO 35:1, 1966
7. U.S. Department of Health Education and Welfare: Criteria and techniques for the diagnosis of early syphilis. Atlanta, Centers for Disease Control, 1980
8. Larsen SA, Beck-Sague CM: Syphilis. In Balows A, Hausler WJ Jr, Lennette EH (eds): The Laboratory Diagnosis of Infectious Diseases: Principles and Practice. New York, Springer-Verlag, 1988
9. Hook EW III, Marra CM: Acquired syphilis in adults. N Engl J Med 326:1060–1069
10. Marra CM: Syphilis and human immunodeficiency virus infection. Semin Neurol 12:43–50, 1992
11. Larsen SA, Steiner BM, Rudolph AH: Laboratory diagnosis and interpretation of tests for syphilis. Clin Microbiol Rev 8:1–21, 1995
12. Larsen SA, Hunter EF, Kraus SJ (eds): A Manual of Tests for Syphilis, 8th ed. Washington, DC, American Public Health Association, 1990
13. Jethwa HS, Schmitz JL, Dallabetta G, et al: Comparison of molecular and microscopic techniques for detection of *Treponema pallidum* in genital ulcers. J Clin Microbiol 33:180–183, 1995
14. Daniels KD, Ferneyhough HS: Specific direct fluorescent antibody detection of *Treponema pallidum*. Health Lab Sci 14:164, 1977
15. Jue R, et al: Comparison of fluorescent and conventional darkfield methods for the detection of *Treponema pallidum* in syphilitic lesions. Am J Clin Pathol 47:809, 1967
16. Hook EW III, Roddy RE, Lukehart SA, et al: Detection of *Treponema pallidum* in lesion exudate with a pathogen specific monoclonal antibody. J Clin Microbiol 22:241, 1985
17. Sanchez PJ, Wendel GD, Gimprel E, et al: Evaluation of molecular methodologies and rabbit infectivity testing for the diagnosis of congenital syphilis and neonatal central nervous system invasion by *Treponema pallidum*. J Infect Dis 167:148–157, 1993

18. U.S. Department of Health Education and Welfare, National Communicable Disease Center, Venereal Disease Program: Manual of Tests for Syphilis. Atlanta, Centers for Disease Control, 1969

19. Brown ST, Zaidi A, Larsen SA, Reynolds GH: Serological response to syphilis treatment: A new analysis of old data. JAMA 2593:1296, 1985

20. Fiumara NJ: Serological response to treatment of 128 patients with late latent syphilis. Sex Transm Dis 6:243, 1979

21. Portnoy J, Bossak HN, Falcone VH, et al: Rapid reagin test with unheated serum and new improved antigen suspension. Public Health Rep 76:933, 1961

22. Portnoy J, Brewer JH, Harris A: Rapid plasma reagin test for syphilis. Public Health Rep 72:761, 1957

23. Falcone VH, Stout GW, Moore MBM: Evaluation of rapid plasma reagin (circle) card test. Public Health Rep 79:491, 1964

24. March RW, Stiles GE: The reagin screen test: A new reagin card test for syphilis. Sex Transm Dis 7:66, 1980

25. Nelson RA Jr, Mayer MM: Immobilization of *Treponema pallidum* in vitro by antibody produced by syphilitic infection. J Exp Med 89:369, 1949

26. Farshy CE, Kennedy EJ, Hunter EF, et al: Fluorescent treponemal antibody absorption double staining test evaluation. J Clin Microbiol 17:245, 1983

27. Kaufman RE, Olansky DC, Weisner PJ: The FTA-ABS (IgM) test for neonatal congenital syphilis: A critical review. J Am Venereal Dis Assoc 1:79, 1974

28. Stevens RW, Schmitt ME: Evaluation of an enzyme-linked immunosorbent assay for treponemal antibody. J Clin Microbiol 21:399, 1985

29. Moyer NP, Hudson JD, Hausler WJ: Evaluation of the Bio-EnzaBead Test for Syphilis. J Clin Microbiol 25:619, 1987

30. Larsen SA, Hamble EA, Cruce DD: Review of the standard tests for syphilis and evaluation of a new commercial ELISA, the Syphilis Bio-Enzabead test. J Clin Lab Anal 1:300, 1987

31. Silletti R: Comparison of CAPTIA syphilis G enzyme immunoassay with rapid plasma reagent test for detection of syphilis. J Clin Microbiol 33:11929–1831, 1995

32. Ijsselmuiden OE, et al: An IgM capture enzyme-linked immunosorbent assay to detect IgM antibodies to treponemas in patients with syphilis. Genitourin Med 65:79–83, 1989

CHAPTER 22

Borrelia burgdorferi
Infection and Serology

Rosemarie Rumanek Romesburg

Objectives

Upon completion of the chapter, the reader will be able to:

1. Describe the causative agent of Lyme disease
2. List the major antigenic components of *Borrelia burgdorferi*
3. Describe how Lyme disease is transmitted
4. Describe the stages of Lyme disease and the major symptoms in each stage
5. Discuss the appearance of IgG and IgM in the course of Lyme disease
6. Discuss the principles of the following tests used in the diagnosis of Lyme disease:
     Immunofluorescent assay
     Enzyme-linked immunosorbent assay
     Western immunoblot
7. Discuss methods of treatment, prevention, and control of Lyme disease

ORGANISM

Borrelia burgdorferi, the causative agent of Lyme borreliosis or Lyme disease, is a medium to loosely coiled, thin, flexible, actively motile spirochete. It is approximately 4 to 30 μm in length and 0.18 to 0.25 μm in diameter. The organism is best recognized by darkfield microscopy, but stains well with Giemsa, Wright, and silver impregnation methods. Cultivation is best accomplished in Barbour-Stoenner-Kelly (BSK) broth, a medium enriched with bovine serum albumin and heat-inactivated rabbit serum, at 34 to 35°C in a microaerophilic environment.[1]

Antigenic Structure

Two lipoproteins, Osp A and Osp B, are located below the surface of the organism. Although the role of Osp A and Osp B in the virulence of the organism has not been established, Osp A has been used as a vaccinogen against experimental disease in the mouse.[1] Extracellular virulence factors have not been identified.

Transmission

Lyme disease is the most common vector-borne disease in the United States, with the majority of cases occurring in Connecticut, Massachusetts, Minnesota, Pennsylvania, New Jersey, New York, Rhode Island, Wisconsin, and the northern part of California. Lyme disease is transmitted by the deer tick, *Ixodes*. The species of the vector varies with its geographic location. In the United States, *Ixodes scapularis* (formerly *I. dammini*) is found in the Northeast and Midwest, and *I. pacificus* is found in the West. *Ixodes racinus* and *I. persulcatus* are the vectors in Europe and Asia, respectively.[1]

Transmission occurs by the bite of a tick. Although the disease may be transmitted by a tick at any developmental stage, most often it occurs via a nymph. Tick saliva contaminated with *B. burgdorferi* is injected directly into the circulation or is deposited onto epidermal surfaces.

LIFE CYCLE OF *IXODES*

The life cycle of the *Ixodes* tick is 2 years. The first or larval stage must take a blood meal before developing into the nymph stage. Nymphs are only 1 to 2 mm in size and are active mostly during June and July.[3] Both larvae and nymphs feed on the white-footed mouse. Humans are an accidental host. Nymphs must also take a blood meal before developing into the adult stage. Adults feed only on large mammals, primarily the white-tailed deer. Because ticks require several days to become fully engorged, removal within 24 to 36 hours will prevent infection.[3]

LYME DISEASE

Lyme disease was first recognized in the United States in 1975 by Burgdorfer in Lyme and Old Lyme, Connecticut, with the occurrence of an outbreak of juvenile arthritis. By 1982 Dr. Burgdorfer isolated the organism from an *Ixodes* tick, and in 1984 the organism was named. Lyme disease is usually divided into the early and late stages; however, the stages may be difficult to determine and sometimes overlap occurs. Some cases show no symptoms during the early stage, and some never progress to the late stage.[3]

Early Stage

Within 2 to 32 days (usually 8 to 9 days) after exposure to an infected tick, 60% to 80% of patients develop a red papule at the site of the bite.[2] The papule, called erythema chronicum migrans, is usually about 5 cm in diameter in the early stages but may later expand to form an annular erythematous lesion resembling concentric rings, with a clear center, reaching 70 cm in diameter.[1,2] Erythema chronicum migrans may last for several months before clearing, which appears to involve phagocytosis of the organism by macrophages. The lesions may recur at the same or a distal site.[1] Spirochetes prefer solid tissue over blood or body fluids.[2]

Late Stage

The most common manifestation of the late stage is arthritis, with approximately 60% of the patients having at least one episode. Usually the large joints, especially the knees, shoulders, and elbows, are affected.[2] About 10% of patients with joint involvement develop a chronic condition leading to permanent damage; this is frequently associated with HLA-DR2 and HLA-DR4 alloantigens.[1] The arthritis may be mediated by the host immune system rather than by the organisms. Untreated patients may experience decreasingly severe attacks with the passage of time.

In untreated cases, 15% show neurologic abnormalities, such as aseptic meningitis, facial nerve palsy, encephalitis, cranial neuritis, and radiculoneuritis.[3] Carditis occurs in approximately 8% of cases. Neurologic abnormalities occur with greater frequency in Europe, where 40% of patients exhibit such symptoms.[1]

Chronic disseminated disease may manifest as a sclerotic or atrophic skin lesion, called acrodermatitis chronica atrophicans (ACA), or a lymphocytoma cutis with a predilection for earlobes in children and the nipple-areola region in adults.[1] Although ACA is well known in Europe, it is seldom seen in the United States.[1]

Antibody Response

According to most reports, the first detectable antibody in early Lyme disease is of the IgM class, and it is directed to 41 kDa protein corresponding to flagellin antigen.[5] The antibody is not specific for *B. burgdorferi* and is seen in healthy individuals and in those with other bacterial or viral infections. Antibodies against 25, 31, 34, 39, and 83 kDa antigen have been observed and are considered indicative of Lyme disease.[5,8] Antibodies persist for 3 years in patients with erythema chronicum migrans.[5]

The highest levels of borreliacidal antibody have been detected in patients with arthritis.[7] Lower levels have been detected in early disease and in patients with infections of long duration. Serum from Lyme disease patients can immobilize and kill *B. burgdorferi*. No borreliacidal activity has been demonstrated in potentially crossreactive serum.[7]

DIAGNOSIS

Physical Examination

Physical examination is paramount in diagnosing Lyme disease and includes establishing a history of prior tick bite or visiting a tick-infested area. Of special interest are clinical manifestations in the skin, nervous system, heart, and joints.

Isolation of Organism

Skin biopsies, lymph node aspirates, synovial fluid, cerebrospinal fluid (CSF), and blood are appropriate specimens. Culture in general yields a low rate of recovery and requires incubation of up to 12 weeks or more, although cultures of skin biopsies are positive in up to 85% of cases.[1]

Serologic Tests

Serological evidence of Lyme disease is accomplished primarily through the indirect immunofluorescence assay (IFA) and the enzyme-linked immunosorbent assay (ELISA) procedures. In IFA, killed *B. burgdorferi* is used as the antigen, while the ELISA employs an ultrasonic lysate of the organism. Demonstration of a fourfold increase in titer on paired sera taken at 6- to 8-week intervals confirms the diagnosis.[1] Because tests and reagents are not yet standardized for either methodology,[4] interlaboratory reliability is poor.[2] A third serologic test, the Western blot, is also available for use primarily as a confirmatory test. Serum, CSF, and other body fluids are acceptable specimens for all assays and should be refrigerated or frozen until assayed.[8]

IMMUNOFLUORESCENCE ASSAY

The IFA procedure is appropriate for low-volume testing because of its labor-intensive nature.

Procedure

This is a standard indirect immunofluorescence assay in which the antigen (substrate) is cultured *B. burgdorferi* that is acetone fixed on a microscope slide. Serial dilutions of patient serum, positive serum control, and negative serum control are placed onto the antigen. After incubation at 37°C for 30 minutes, the slide is washed and the conjugated anti–human immunoglobulin is applied. The slide is incubated and washed in the same manner; a coverslip is applied, and the slide is read using the oil immersion objective.[8]

Results and Interpretation

Titers of ≥128 for serum and ≥16 for CSF are considered positive. The titer is read as the reciprocal of the highest dilution of specimen in which 50% of the cells exhibit a definite fluorescence.[8] False negative test results are seen during the first few weeks of infection before sufficient free antibody is present or after treatment with antibiotics given in inappropriate doses, thereby preventing a sufficient immune response. Only 50% of cases are seropositive in early Lyme disease, while 71% to 100% of cases are reactive in late disease.[1] False positive results occur in patients with other spirochetal infections, such as syphilis and relapsing fever,[4] and in autoimmune diseases, AIDS, and occasionally in normal individuals.[1]

ENZYME-LINKED IMMUNOSORBENT ASSAY (ELISA)

ELISA is the assay of choice in laboratories doing high volume testing and is easily automated. Currently, the cell lysates used for the antigen are unpurified. Purified flagellin antigen is also available to evaluate some false positive results.

Procedure

Most commercially available kits are noncompetitive assays. Sonicated *B. burgdorferi* antigen is attached to the solid phase. Diluted patient serum, control sera, and calibrators are added. After incubation and washing, the enzyme labeled anti–human globulin (the conjugate) is added. After incubation and washing, substrate is added. The enzymatic reaction is stopped and the intensity of colored product is read. Some kits include a serum pretreatment step to minimize crossreactivity caused by antibodies against *E. coli* flagellar antigen.

Results and Interpretation

The absorbance of each well is read at the wavelength specified by the manufacturer. To validate the performance of the assay, the parameters specified by the manufacturer must be carefully applied. Likewise, to interpret the absorbance readings in the patient sample, appropriate calculations are performed according to the manufacturer's directions. One such calculation is to compare the absorbance of the patient sample to the absorbance of a low positive control serum. The low postive control serum contains the minimum concentration of antibody to indicate infection with *B. burgdorferi*. If the patient sample absorbance is significantly greater than the low positive control absorbance, antibody to *B. burgdorferi* is present. Factors contributing to false negative and false positive test results in the IFA procedure also apply to the ELISA procedure.

WESTERN BLOT

The Western blot is best used to confirm IFA and ELISA results because it is too time consuming, laborious, and difficult to interpret to be used as a primary test and requires special equipment.

Procedure

Antigen and standards are separated according to their molecular weights by electrophoresis on polyacrylamide gels. The separated bands of protein are electrotransferred to an inert membrane filter. After incubation with patient serum, the membrane is washed and allowed to react with an enzyme-labeled anti–human immunoglobulin. Antigen-antibody reactions are detected after adding the enzyme substrate and washing.[2,8]

Results and Interpretation

After evaluating the controls, the strips incubated with patient sera are compared with the strip showing the migration of the reference antigens based on their molecular weights. A strongly positive serum should react with several antigens. A negative test exhibits no reaction or a minimal reaction.[8]

Detection of the Organism

By detecting antigen directly, the shortcomings of measuring antibody are avoided. The shortcomings include false negative results early in the infection, decreased antibody response resulting from inappropriate treatment, and false positive results in endemic areas and from crossreactive antibodies. Although in the developmental stages, polymerase chain reaction (PCR) methods have been used to detect organisms in clinical specimens, providing direct evidence of current infection. A PCR performed on skin biopsy specimens was sensitive in detecting <10 spirochetes and was highly specific for *B. burgdorferi*. PCR has been used to confirm the diagnosis in 50% of untreated patients who were seronegative at the initial visit.[6]

TREATMENT

Oral medications such as doxycycline, amoxicillin plus probenicid, or cefurorime are useful in the treatment of early Lyme disease. Neurologic and disseminated disease is best treated using intravenous ceftriaxone, cefotaxime, or penicillin G. Doxycycline is contraindicated in children less than 9 years old and in pregnant women.[3]

PREVENTION AND CONTROL

Prevention and control of Lyme disease depends on the education of the general public and control of the arthropod vector and its reservoir host. Education of the general public should include information on preventing tick bites, inspecting and effectively removing ticks, recognizing the clinical manifestations of the disease, and strengthening awareness of endemic tick areas. A vaccine is being evaluated.[1]

Case Study

A 28-year-old woman had a fever of 104°F 1 week before her visit to the Mill Creek Clinic. Although it resolved spontaneously, headache and arthralgia followed. A maculopapular rash developed over her abdomen and the front of her arms and legs 3 days later. The head, neck, and throat were clear, and there was no adenopathy. There was no prior history of illness, drug use, sore throat, or rheumatoid arthritis, and no joint tenderness, cyanosis, edema, or clubbing. The range of joint motion was full and the nervous system was intact. She was allergic to codeine and tetracycline. Examination of the heart, lungs, and abdomen revealed no abnormalities other than the rash.

The blood count included 4800 leukocytes/μL and a hematocrit of 33%. The only abnormal liver function test was lactate dehydrogenase of 225 U/L (reference range 109–193 U/L). Tests for rheumatoid factor and anti-nuclear antibody and throat cultures for streptococci were negative. The Lyme disease antibody test gave an index of 1.16 (0.95 negative; 0.95 to 1.05 equivocal; 1.05 positive). The patient was immediately started on erythromycin 1.0 g daily by mouth and continued the medication while the tests were on order for 30 days. She gradually improved and has not relapsed. The Lyme antibody titer was 0.34 at the end of treatment.[10]

Case Study Questions

1. What symptoms related to Lyme disease did the patient exhibit prior to her visit to the clinic?

2. What symptoms developed later? Are any of these symptoms indicative of Lyme disease?

3. What is the significance of the negative throat culture and results for rheumatoid factor and ANA?

4. What test(s) are diagnostic for Lyme disease?

References

1. Baron EJ, Chang RS, Howard DH, Miller JN, Turner JA: Medical Microbiology: A Short Course. New York, Wiley-Liss, 1994

2. Mahon CR, Manuselis G (eds): Textbook of Diagnostic Microbiology. Philadelphia, WB Saunders, 1995

3. Howard BJ (ed): Clinical and Pathogenic Microbiology, 2nd ed, St. Louis, MO, Mosby Year Book Inc., 1994

4. Burgdorfer W, Schwan TG: Borrelia. In Lennette EH, Balows A, Hausler WJ Jr, et al (eds): Manual of Clinical Microbiology, 5th ed, p 560. Washington, DC, American Society for Microbiology, 1991

5. Aguero-Rosenfels ME, Nowakowski J, McKenna DF, Carbonaro CA, Wormser GP: Serodiagnosis in early Lyme disease. J Clin Microbiol 31:3090–3095, 1993

6. Schwartz I, Wormser GP, Schwartz JJ, Cooper D, Weissensee P, Gazumyan A, Zimmermann E, Goldberg NS, Bittker S, Campbell GL, Pavia CS: Diagnosis of early Lyme disease by polymerase chain reaction amplification and culture of skin biopsies from erythema migrans lesions. J Clin Microbiol 30:3082–3088, 1992

7. Callister SM, Schell RF, Lovrich SD: Lyme disease assay which detects killed *Borrelia burgdorferi*. J Clin Microbiol 29:1773–1776, 1991

8. Gill JS, Johnson RC: Immunologic methods for the diagnosis of infections by *Borrelia burgdorferi* (Lyme disease). In Rose NR, DeMacario EC, Fahey JL, et al (eds): Manual of Clinical Laboratory Immunology, 4th ed, p 452. Washington, DC, American Society for Microbiology, 1992

9. Szczepanski A, Benach JL: Lyme borreliosis: Host responses to *Borrelia burgdorferi*. Microbiol Rev 55:21–34, 1991

10. Paulk DA: Lyme disease case studies. WV Med J 88:102, 1992

CHAPTER 23

Rubella Virus Infection and Serology

Rosemarie Rumanek Romesburg

Objectives

Upon completion of the chapter, the reader will be able to:

1. Describe the size and composition of the rubella virus
2. Describe the symptoms and complications of acute rubella virus infection
3. List the major abnormalities associated with congenital rubella infection
4. Discuss the appearance of IgG and IgM antibodies in the course of acute disease and congenital infection
5. Discuss the principles of the following tests used in rubella antibody testing:
    Hemagglutination inhibition
    Passive hemagglutination
    Solid-phase immunoassays
    Sucrose density gradient ultrcentrifugation
6. List appropriate tests for diagnosing congenital infection and determining recent rubella infection and immune status
7. Discuss the rubella vaccine in terms of composition, recommended administration, and contraindications for use

VIRUS

Size and Composition

The rubella virus, composed of single-stranded RNA, is a member of the family Togaviridae.[1] It is a roughly spherical particle with a diameter between 60 and 70 nm.

The virion contains a dense core surrounded by a lipid bilayer covered with short, fine projections.[1,2] Only one serotype of rubella virus is known,[1,3] and it remains immunologically distinct from any other described group.[1]

Rubella virus contains three major structural proteins, two (E1 and E2) associated with the viral envelope and one capsid (C) protein associated with the viral RNA.[4] Several major and minor polypeptides have been identified in purified rubella virus.[5] Each of these polypeptides is immunologically active, but infectivity has not been associated with a distinct antigenic site.[1]

Isolation and Identification

Although the rubella virus may be propagated in a variety of primary cell cultures and cell lines,[6,7] rubella infections are routinely diagnosed through serologic methods that are less time consuming and cumbersome. Primary cell lines, especially monkey kidney, are superior for viral isolation, whereas continuous cell lines produce higher levels of virus and are generally better for antigen production.[7] Growth of the virus has not been reproduced in embryonated eggs, suckling mice, or adult rabbits.[5,6,8]

Antigenicity

The E1 envelope protein has hemagglutinating activity[4,7,9] and reacts with newborn chick, goose, and pigeon red blood cells at 4°C and 25°C, but not at 37°C.[10] Both the red blood cells and serum of individuals infected with rubella virus contain a nonspecific β–lipoprotein that can inhibit hemagglutination.[7] Both E1 and E2 have immunogenic domains that give rise to neutralizing antibodies.[4] The major complement-fixing activities are associated primarily with the envelope, although some activity is also associated with the nucleoprotein core.[7] Both the hemagglutinin and the complement-fixing antigens can be detected through serologic testing.

DISEASES

German Measles

Rubella, a mild, contagious illness characterized by an erythematous maculopapular rash, is observed primarily in children 5 to 14 years old and in young adults.[1,11] The disease, commonly called German or 3-day measles, may be asymptomatic or may involve a 1- to 5-day prodromal period of malaise, headache, cold symptoms, low-grade fever, and suboccipital lymphadenopathy.[11]

In children, the first sign of illness is the appearance of a rash.[11] However, in adolescents and adults the rash is preceded by the prodromal period, which occurs approximately 14 to 21 days after exposure to the virus. The rash appears first on the face, spreads downward,[7,11] and clears in a similar fashion within 1 to 5 days.[11] The rash is characterized by discrete pink-red lesions that may or may not coalesce. Lesions that coalesce form a uniform red blush that generally appears on the trunk and resembles the rash of mild scarlet fever.[11] The rash may also be confused with that induced by certain drugs. Therefore, rendering a diagnosis of rubella solely on clinical grounds is unreliable, especially during periods between epidemics.[1]

The portal of entry for rubella virus is the upper respiratory tract, perhaps through the lymphoid tissue, where it establishes intracellular reproduction in a susceptible host.[9] Within 9 to 11 days following the onset of infection, detectable levels of virus may be demonstrated in nasopharyngeal secretions, urine, the cervix, and feces.[9] Shedding of the virus is most prolonged and reaches the highest levels in pharyngeal secretions.[9]

Arthritis may be a complication of rubella infection in adolescents and young adults, involving the knees, ankles, or elbows. The arthritis may resemble the type observed in cases of rheumatic fever or rheumatoid arthritis.[9] Other complications may include transient arthralgias (15% to 52% of cases), encephalitis (1 in 6000 cases), and thrombocytopenic purpura.[1,11] The prognosis of rubella without complications is excellent because the disease is benign and self-limited.

Congenital Rubella

Although recognized by German authors in the mid-18th century as a clinical entity,[9] it was not until 1941 that Sir Norman Gregg discovered a causal relationship between maternal infection during pregnancy and congenital defects.[12] Maternal infection may result in spontaneous abortion, stillbirth, or infection of the fetus.[12] Infection of the placenta may occur without fetal involvement.[9] Fetal infection during the first trimester of pregnancy and, to a lesser extent, the second trimester, may result in congenital defects. As many as 85% of infants infected during the first 8 weeks of gestation have detectable defects by 4 years of age.[9] The classical abnormalities associated with the rubella syndrome include congenital heart disease, cataracts, and neurosensory deafness.[13,14] After 20 to 24 weeks of gestation, congenital abnormalities are rare. Defects may not be apparent until late childhood, with the most common manifestations being ocular defects and deafness.[15,16]

Infants born with the rubella syndrome usually have a low birthweight. Other symptoms, such as thrombocytopenia, hepatitis, long-bone lesions, retinitis, encephalitis, interstitial pneumonitis, psychiatric disorders, thyroid disorders, and diabetes mellitus, may also be present in a variety of combinations.[1,11] The virus can be isolated readily from the throat and less

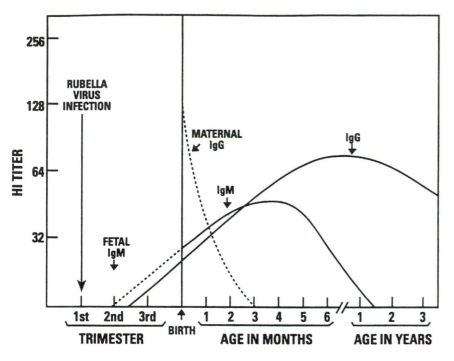

FIGURE 23-1

Antibody responses in an infant congenitally infected with rubella virus. (From Chernesky MA, Mahony JB: Rubella virus. In Murray PR, Baron EJ, Pfaller MA, Tenover FC, Yolken RH (eds): Manual of Clinical Microbiology, 6th ed, p 970. Washington, DC, American Society of Microbiology, 1995, with permission.)

frequently from the feces and urine,[17] and may persist up to a year in infected infants.[11]

Immunologic Response

Antibodies to rubella virus appear as the rash fades, with both IgG and IgM reaching detectable levels at this time.[1,7] Antibodies to IgG persist throughout life, whereas antibodies to IgM usually decline after 4 to 5 weeks.[1,7] Fetal infection is usually accompanied by early placental transfer of maternal IgG. In addition, substantial levels of fetal IgM are produced by midgestation (Fig. 23-1).[9] Because levels of IgM are generally increased at birth in infected infants, screening for congenital infection may be accomplished by quantitating IgM.

Although reinfection with the virus can occur, it is almost always asymptomatic and can be detected by a rise in IgG antibodies.[1,7,18] Viremia has been detected in volunteers with low rubella titers after experimental challenge with rubella vaccine.[19] This demonstrates that viremia can indeed occur after reinfection. Although studies have shown that rubella vaccine virus can cross the placenta and infect the fetus during early stages of development, the risk of congenital malformations appears to be low to nonexistent.[20]

LABORATORY TESTING

Reliable serologic techniques to detect rubella antibodies provide the methods of choice to (1) determine immunity to rubella, (2) diagnose congenital rubella, and (3)

diagnose acute rubella infection.[1,3] Methods currently available include passive hemagglutination (PHA), hemagglutination inhibition (HI), radial hemolysis, latex agglutination, enzyme-linked immunosorbent assay (ELISA), neutralization, mixed hemadsorption, complement fixation (CF), and time-resolved fluoroimmunoassay. Of these methods, PHA and CF do not show peak titers until later in the disease (Fig. 23-2 on p. 232). More than 95% of rubella antibody testing in the United States is being performed with commercially prepared test kits that have been evaluated and monitored by the Centers for Disease Control and Prevention.[1]

CLINICAL INDICATIONS

Determining Recent Infection

SERA AVAILABLE AT ONSET OF SYMPTOMS

A rapid and accurate serologic diagnosis is needed to investigate a pregnant patient who was exposed to the rubella virus. If signs and symptoms develop, two serum specimens should be collected. An acute-phase serum is obtained at the onset of symptoms and a convalescent serum is obtained 5 to 7 days later. Both specimens should be tested in parallel on the same day using the same test and appropriate controls.[1,3] Otherwise, changes in titer may merely reflect variation in testing rather than true antibody levels.[7] A fourfold or greater rise in antibody titer together with clinical symptoms is diagnostic of a recent rubella infection.[1,3] The HI antibodies reach peak titers in 10 to 20 days,

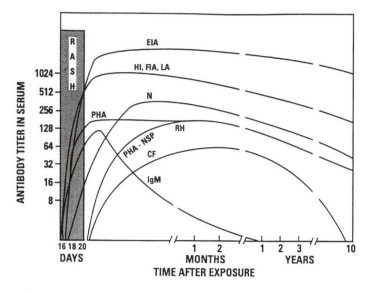

FIGURE 23-2

Antibody response after rubella virus infection. (From Chernesky MA, Mahony JB: Rubella virus. In Murray PR, Baron EJ, Pfaller MA, Tenover FC, Yolken RH (eds): Manual of Clinical Microbiology, 6th ed, p 969. Washington, DC, American Society of Microbiology, 1995, with permission.)

whereas CF antibodies appear approximately a week later, do not reach as high a level, and decline more rapidly.[1] The CF test may be useful in cases where the acute-phase serum was collected too late to show a rise in HI titer.[3]

SERA NOT AVAILABLE AT ONSET OF SYMPTOMS

Testing for specific IgM antibody in serum collected several days after the onset of symptoms may aid in retrospectively establishing a diagnosis of rubella.[1,3] In this case, all serologic tests will show a titer. However, titers of IgM antibody wane rapidly and may disappear within 4 weeks. Therefore, a negative result does not exclude the possibility of a recent rubella infection.

Diagnosing Congenital Infection

Although congenital infection may be confirmed by isolating the virus from throat washings, urine, and other body fluids, isolation may require repeated attempts.[1] Therefore, serologic testing is the recommended method. Testing for the presence of specific IgM antibody is indicated for any neonate of low birthweight who also presents with any of the symptoms associated with congenital rubella.[3,19] The demonstration of IgM antibody in the infant is diagnostic of congenital infection because these antibodies do not cross the placenta.[1,3]

Specific rubella IgG antibodies may be produced by the infant in utero. However, because maternal IgG crosses the placenta, it is difficult to differentiate between passively transferred antibody and specific antibody produced by the infant.[7] Persistence of specific rubella IgG antibody beyond 6 to 12 months of age in-

dicates that the antibody is being produced by the infant and is therefore retrospective evidence of congenital infection.

Determining Immune Status

The most widely used tests for determining rubella immunity status are the latex agglutination, HI, PHA, ELISA, and indirect immunofluorescence methods.[21] Detectable levels of antibody are indicative of past infection with the rubella virus. Individuals with detectable antibody levels are considered immune.

HEMAGGLUTINATION INHIBITION TEST

A hemagglutination inhibition (HI) test for the detection of rubella antibody was first described in 1967.[10] A standardized reference HI procedure was developed in 1970 and has been adopted by the National Committee for Clinical Laboratory Standards and the World Health Organization as the reference method.[1] Serologic tests for rubella should be compared with the HI test for accuracy before being employed for diagnostic purposes. Both IgM and IgG antibodies can be detected using the HI test.[21]

Principles

Rubella virus has the ability to agglutinate chick erythrocytes. When patient serum containing rubella antibody is incubated with rubella antigen, binding occurs. To determine whether binding has occurred, chick erythrocytes are added. Any unbound rubella antigen present is free to agglutinate the chick erythrocytes.

Procedure

ANTIGEN PREPARATION

Rubella antigen is prepared in BHK-21 or Vero cell cultures, and may be purchased commercially.[7]

ERYTHROCYTES

Erythrocytes (indicator cells) used in the test proper and antigen titration procedure are obtained from 1- to 3-day-old unfed baby chicks.[1,7,10] These cells may be stored for up to 2 weeks in Alsever's solution without loss of sensitivity.[1,7] Indicator cells are 0.25% suspensions. The cells used to adsorb patient sera for natural agglutinins are 50% suspensions.

ANTIGEN TITRATION

To determine the proper dosage of antigen, titration is necessary. Rubella antigens ranging in titer from 4 to 1024 are satisfactory for use. An excess amount of antigen will result in low antibody titers, whereas an insufficient amount gives rise to falsely elevated titers.[7]

Titration is performed by preparing serial twofold dilutions of test antigen in V-type microtiter plates and incubating at 4°C with indicator cells. Plates are read for agglutination. The highest dilution producing complete agglutination is called 1 HA unit. The reciprocal of the highest dilution producing complete agglutination is the titer of the antigen. The dilution of antigen to be used for the HI test must contain 4 HA units and is therefore a fourfold dilution lower.

REMOVAL OF NONSPECIFIC INHIBITORS

Before the HI test is performed, nonspecific β-lipoprotein inhibitors and nonspecific agglutinins must be removed.[3,5,19] This is accomplished by incubating all sera and controls with heparin-$MnCl_2$ or dextran sulfate-$CaCl_2$ to remove the nonspecific inhibitors[9] and by incubating all sera with a 50% suspension of chick erythrocytes to adsorb natural agglutinins.[1,3,7]

HI TEST

The HI test involves preparing serial twofold dilutions of treated serum and incubating at 4°C with antigen (4 HA). Plates are then incubated with indicator cells and read after 15 to 20 minutes at room temperature.

ANTIGEN BACKTITRATION

To ensure that the antigen dilution used in the HI test is correct, an antigen backtitration is performed simultaneously with the HI test. Serial twofold dilutions of the antigen representing 4, 2, 1, and 0.5 HA units are prepared.

Interpretation

The test is valid, providing the antigen backtitration confirms that the correct antigen dilution was used and controls show that nonspecific inhibitors and agglutinins were removed. The endpoint is read as the highest dilution of serum that completely inhibits hemagglutination.

Recent rubella infections are demonstrated by a fourfold or greater rise in titer between acute and convalescent (paired) sera. Interpretations of the HI antibody titer on single specimens do not present diagnostic information. High titers (≥512) may be observed in immune individuals with no recent rubella infection.[5] HI titers ≥8 indicate immunity to rubella disease.

PASSIVE HEMAGGLUTINATION

Principles

In the passive hemagglutination (PHA) test, stabilized human red blood cells are coated with soluble rubella virus antigen. These sensitized erythrocytes agglutinate in the presence of specific rubella antibody.[1,3,7,22]

Procedure

Patient and control sera are diluted in phosphate buffered saline (PBS), mixed with antigen-coated red blood cells, and incubated at room temperature for 2 hours to allow the cells to settle.[1]

Results and Interpretation

The plates are read for the presence or absence of agglutination. A button of erythrocytes forming at the bottom of the V-shaped well in the microtiter plate indicates a negative reaction (absence of antibody or susceptibility to rubella infection). Agglutination or a dispersal of erythrocytes indicates a positive reaction (presence of antibody or immunity to rubella).[1,3,7]

Advantages

An advantage of the PHA test is that sera do not require treatment for removal of nonspecific reactants prior to testing. The test can be performed rapidly and correlates well with HI test results in over 98% of cases.[1] The PHA test is most useful in detecting rubella immunity status and is sensitive to IgG antibodies.[21]

SOLID PHASE IMMUNOASSAYS (SPIA)

SPIA are heterogeneous labeled assays that are useful to detect and quantitate both IgG and IgM rubella antibodies, depending on the antiglobulin conjugate used.[21,23,24] Most commercially available kits are enzyme immunoassays; however, radioimmunoassays have been developed.[25]

Antigen Capture Assays

Immunoassays that employ rubella virus antigen adsorbed to a solid phase (plate or beads) are known as sandwich assays to detect antigen or antigen capture assays. After incubation with patient serum, rubella-specific antibody binds to the antigen on the solid phase. Rubella-specific antibody is subsequently detected by incubation with anti–human globulin that are enzyme labeled[23,26] or radiolabeled.[25] Enzyme-labeled assays using synthetic peptides[4] and purified forms of recombinant rubella virus E1 protein[27] rather than whole rubella virus antigen have recently been developed.

The antigen capture assay is effective for detection of IgG antibody, but false positive and false negative reactions may be encountered when assaying for IgM. False positive reactions may appear with IgM rheumatoid factor (IgM-RF) and specific IgG.[28] Immune IgG binds to the antigen and IgM-RF binds to the IgG. The IgM-RF will then bind to the labeled anti–human globulin, causing a false positive result.[29] High-titered IgG may cause false negative results by competing with the IgM antibody for the antigen coated on the solid phase.[29,30] These can be minimized by pretreatment of the serum to remove the IgG or the IgM-RF, or by using one of the antibody capture assays described later.[29]

Antibody Capture Assays

Sandwich assays to detect antibody or antibody capture assays use a solid phase coated with anti–human IgM globulin.[30–32] After incubation with patient serum, patient IgM antibodies bind to the anti–human IgM globulin on the solid phase. Specific rubella antibodies are then detected by incubation with rubella antigen, followed by another incubation with enzyme-labeled or radiolabeled rubella antibody (rubella conjugate).

Interpretation

No standard method of reporting results of enzyme immunoassay tests exists. Therefore, results must be interpreted according to the instructions in the specific test employed.[21]

SUCROSE DENSITY GRADIENT ULTRACENTRIFUGATION

Specific IgM antibodies to rubella can be detected by physical separation of IgG and IgM in serum using sucrose density gradient ultracentrifugation.[34] Patient serum is sedimented through a sucrose density gradient to fractionate serum, thus separating the IgM and IgG antibodies. The antibody-rich fractions are then tested for specific rubella antibodies using HI or a solid phase immunoassay. Because IgM antibodies do not cross the placenta, detection of these antibodies in infant sera is evidence of congenital infection.

RUBELLA VACCINATION

Vaccines

Three strains of a live, attenuated rubella vaccine were developed and licensed in 1969. Each of these vaccines has been proven safe, with low rates of fever, rash, arthritis, and lymphadenopathy as side effects in recipients. However, arthralgia has been reported to be as high as 40% in female vaccinees.[18] In January 1979, the RA 27/3 vaccine strain (rubella abortus, 27th specimen, third explant, grown in human diploid fibroblast culture) became the product generally available in the United States.[18]

Vaccine Distribution

The rubella immunization program was instituted after a worldwide rubella epidemic that occurred from 1962 to 1965. Beginning in 1969, federal support was given to the immunization program, and within 3 years more than 45 million doses were administered to nonpubescent children.[18] Within this time the incidence of rubella in the general population declined greatly (Fig. 23-3).[35] However, because 10% to 15% of adults in the continental United States have no detectable levels of rubella antibody, the potential for outbreaks of the disease still exists.[21]

Reinfection

Subclinical reinfection has been detected in persons with natural or vaccine-induced immunity after challenge with wild-type rubella virus. Reinfection is demonstrated by at least a fourfold rise in pre-existing antibody titer and is more likely to occur in previously immunized persons with low levels of antibody.[11] Although rubella vaccine viruses can cross the placenta and infect the fetus, no congenital rubella syndrome defects have been observed.[36] None of the three rubella vaccine strains have proven to be teratogenic.

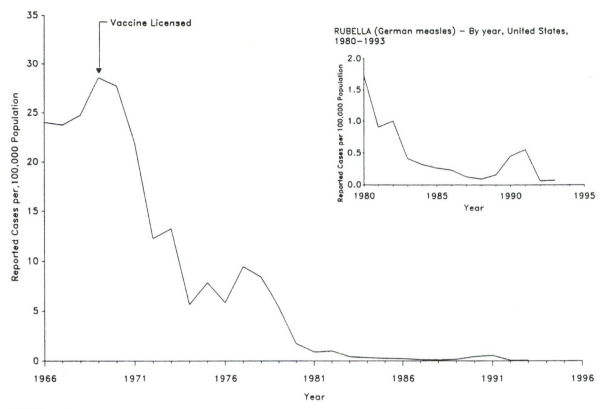

FIGURE 23-3
Incidence of rubella infection in the United States from 1966 to 1992. (From Centers for Disease Control and Prevention. Morbidity and Mortality Weekly Report, Summary of Notifiable Diseases, United States, 1993. Surveill Summ 42:50, 1994, with permission.)

Vaccination Practices

Immunization should be administered after 12 months of age or, if given in combination with the measles and mumps vaccines (MMR), not until 15 months of age. If the rubella vaccine is given before age 12 months, maternal antibodies present in the infant may interfere with immunization.[37] Vaccine should be administered to children and adults who are negative for rubella antibody or who have no history of immunization. No adverse reactions have occurred in individuals receiving the vaccine following previous immunization.

Contraindications

A potential risk to the fetus of acquiring congenital rubella syndrome following vaccination cannot be totally eliminated. Therefore, pregnancy remains a contraindication to rubella vaccination.[36] In addition, women of childbearing age should prevent pregnancy for 3 months after vaccination.[18] However, rubella vaccination of a pregnant woman should not ordinarily be a reason to consider abortion because the risk of congenital rubella syndrome is extremely low.[36] Additionally, rubella vaccination is not recommended for persons with impaired immunity, persons receiving radiation treatments, or persons being treated with corticosteroids, alkylating drugs, or antimetabolites.[37]

Case Study

The mother, a 24-year-old gravida 2 para 1 woman, received rubella vaccine 6 years ago. The vaccine was administered 5 days postpartum after she was identified as nonimmune to rubella during her first pregnancy. A rubella titer was not measured following vaccine administration. The mother had a rash lasting 1 day at 4 weeks of gestation during her second pregnancy. At that time she had rubella IgG antibody with a hemagglutination inhibition (HI) titer of 512 but no rubella IgM antibody. A second rubella serology was not obtained. A female infant was delivered at 37 weeks of gestation with a birth weight of 2.3 kg, a head circumference of 31.5 cm (10th percentile), and a length of 47.5 cm (50th percentile). The infant's rubella IgM antibody titer was positive and the mother's rubella IgG hemagglutination inhibition titer was 1054 postpartum. The baby was seronegative for toxoplasmosis. The infant had IgG and IgM antibodies to rubella at 11 months of age.

At 7 months of age, the baby showed moderate bilateral hearing loss and at 9 months of age developed a cataract of the right eye. Echocardiography revealed mild acceleration in velocity of flow in the main pulmonary artery, with no evidence of valve or branch stenosis. Examination at 21 months of age revealed mild developmental delay, moderate to severe bilateral sensorineural hearing loss, and no vision in the right eye.[38]

Case Study Questions

1. What does a rubella IgG titer of 512 indicate?

2. What is the significance of a second rubella serology done on the mother during her second pregnancy?

3. What did the infant's IgM titer indicate? What did the IgG titer indicate?

4. What symptoms exhibited by the baby were characteristic of congenital rubella?

References

1. Chernesky MA, Mahony HB: Rubella virus. In Lennette EH, Balows A, Hausler WJ Jr, et al (eds): Manual of Clinical Microbiology, 5th ed, p 918. Washington, DC, American Society for Microbiology, 1991

2. Alford CA Jr, Neva FA, Weller TH: Virologic and serological studies on human products of conception after maternal rubella. N Engl J Med 271:1275, 1964

3. Mahony JB, Cernesky MA: Rubella virus. In Rose NR, Friedman H, Fahey JL (eds): Manual of Clinical Laboratory Immunology, 4th ed, p 600. Washington, DC, American Society for Microbiology, 1992

4. Mitchell LA, Zhang T, Ho M, Décarie D, Tingle AJ, Zreiln M, Lacroix M: Characterization of rubella virus-specific antibody responses by using a new synthetic peptide-based enzyme-linked immunosorbent assay. J Clin Microbiol 30:1841–1847, 1992

5. Oker-Blom C, Kalkkinen N, Kaariainen L, et al: Rubella virus contains one capsid protein and three envelope glycoproteins, E12, E2a, and E2b. J Virol 46:964, 1983

6. Parkman PD, Buescher EL, Artenstein MS: Recovery of rubella virus from army recruits (27750). Proc Soc Exp Biol Med 111:225, 1962

7. Herrmann KL: Rubella virus. In Lennette EH, Schmidt NJ (eds): Diagnostic Proceedings for Viral, Rickettsial, and Chlamydial Infections, 5th ed, p 725. Washington, DC, American Public Health Association, 1979

8. Weller TH, Neva FA: Propagation in tissue culture of cytopathic agents from patients with rubella-like illness (27749). Proc Soc Exp Biol Med 3:215, 1962

9. Alford CA Jr, Griffiths PD: Rubella. In Remington JS, Klein JO (eds): Infectious Diseases of the Fetus and Newborn Infant, 2nd ed, p 69. Philadelphia, WB Saunders, 1983

10. Stewart GL, Parkman PD, Hopps HE, et al: Rubella-virus hemagglutination-inhibition test. N Engl J Med 276:554, 1967

11. Krugman S, Katz SL (eds): Infectious Diseases of Children, 7th ed, p 315. St. Louis, CV Mosby, 1981

12. Wesselhoeft C: Rubella (German measles). N Engl J Med 236:978, 1947

13. Cooper LZ, Ziring PA, Ockerse AB, et al: Rubella: Clinical manifestations and management. Am J Dis Child 118:18, 1969

14. Dudgeon JA: Congenital rubella: Pathogenesis and immunology. Am J Dis Child 118:35, 1969

15. Forrest JM, Menser MA: Congenital rubella in schoolchildren and adolescents. Arch Dis Child 45:63, 1970

16. Peckham CS: Clinical and laboratory study of children exposed in utero to maternal rubella. Arch Dis Child 47:571, 1972

17. Phillips AC, Melnick JL, Yow MD, et al: Persistence of virus in infants with congenital rubella and in normal infants with a history of maternal rubella. JAMA 193:1027, 1965

18. Preblud SR, Serdula MK, Frank JA, et al: Rubella vaccination in the United States: A ten-year review. Epidemiol Rev 2:171, 1980

19. O'Shea S, Best JM, Banatvala JE: Viremia, virus excretion, and antibody responses after challenge in volunteers with low levels of antibody to rubella virus. J Infect Dis 148:639, 1983

20. Modlin JF, Herrmann KL, Brandling-Bennett AD, et al: Risk of congenital abnormality after inadvertent rubella vaccination of pregnant women. N Engl J Med 294:972, 1976

21. Herrmann KL: Rubella. In Lennette EH (ed): Laboratory Diagnosis of Viral Infections, p 481. New York, Marcel Dekker, 1985

22. Safford JW Jr, Whittington R: A passive hemagglutination assay for detecting rubella antibody [abstr]. Fed Proc 35:813, 1976

23. Gravell M, Dorsett PH, Gutenson O, et al: Detection of antibody to rubella virus by enzyme-linked immunosorbent assay. J Infect Dis 136:S300, 1977

24. Voller A, Bidwell DE: A simple method for detecting antibodies to rubella. Br J Exp Pathol 56:338, 1975

25. Meurman OH, Viljanen MK, Granfors K: Solid-phase radioimmunoassay of rubella virus immunoglobulin M antibodies: Comparison with density gradient centrifugation test. J Clin Microbiol 5:257, 1977

26. Chernesky MA, Wymann L, Mahony JB, et al: Clinical evaluation of the sensitivity and specificity of a commercially available enzyme immunoassay for detection of rubella virus-specific immunoglobulin M. J Clin Microbiol 20:400, 1984

27. Lindquist C, Schmidt M, Heinola J, et al: J Clin Microbiol 32: 2192–2196, 1994

28. Champsaur H, Dussaix E, Taurmier P: Hemagglutination inhibition, single radial hemolysis, and ELISA tests for the detection of IgG and IgM to rubella virus. J Med Virol 5:273, 1980

29. Voller A, Bidwell D: Enzyme-linked immunosorbent assay. In Rose NR, Freedman H, Fahey JL (eds): Manual of

Clinical Laboratory Immunology, 3rd ed, p 99. Washington, DC, American Society for Microbiology, 1986

30. Bonfanti C, Meurman O, Halonen P: Detection of specific immunoglobulin M antibody to rubella virus by use of an enzyme-labelled antigen. J Clin Microbiol 21:963, 1985

31. Vejtorp M: Solid phase anti-IgM ELISA for detection of rubella specific IgM antibodies. Acta Pathol Microbiol Scand Sect B 89:123, 1981

32. Enders G, Knotek F: Detection of IgM antibodies against rubella virus: Comparison of two indirect ELISAs and an anti-IgM capture immunoassay. J Med Virol 19:377, 1986

33. Ankerst J, Christensen P, Kjellen L, et al: A routine diagnostic test for IgA and IgM antibodies to rubella virus: Adsorption of IgG with *Staphylococcus aureus*. J Infect Dis 130:268, 1974

34. Vesikari T, Vaheri A: Rubella: A method for rapid diagnosis of a recent infection by demonstration of the IgM antibodies. Br Med J 1:221, 1968

35. Centers for Disease Control: Summary of Notifiable Diseases, United States, 1986. Surveill Summ 35:35, 1986

36. Centers for Disease Control: Rubella vaccination during pregnancy—United States, 1971–1986. Surveill Summ 36:457, 1987

37. Alexander ER: Rubella. In Fulginiti VA (ed): Immunization in Clinical Practice, p 103. Philadelphia, JB Lippincott, 1982

38. Robinson J, Lemay M, Vaudry W. Congenital rubella after anticipated maternal immunity: Two cases and a review of the literature. Pediatr Infect Dis J 13:812–815, 1994

CHAPTER 24

Epstein-Barr Virus Infection and Serology

Dorothy J. Fike

EPSTEIN-BARR VIRUS

DISEASES
  Burkitt's Lymphoma and Nasopharyngeal Carcinoma
  Infectious Mononucleosis

LABORATORY TESTS
  Heterophile Antibodies
  EBV-Specific Tests

OTHER CHANGES
  Lymphocytosis
  Liver Function

Objectives

Upon completion of the chapter, the reader will be able to:

1. Describe the Epstein-Barr virus
2. Discuss the diseases caused by Epstein-Barr virus
3. Discuss the tests used to detect heterophile antibody
4. Discuss specific tests used to detect antibodies to the Epstein-Barr virus
5. Given laboratory results, suggest the most likely disease and whether the infection was recent, remote, or reactivated

EPSTEIN-BARR VIRUS

The Epstein-Barr virus (EBV) is a DNA virus that belongs to the herpesvirus group. EBV is widely distributed throughout the world, with 80% to 90% of all adults demonstrating previous infection.[1] Transmission of the virus appears to be almost exclusively through saliva, which explains its nickname, the "kissing disease." The virus is excreted orally by both symptomatic and asymptomatic individuals, and can be isolated from the saliva of 10% to 20% of healthy adults.[2] Primary infection, with or without disease, will induce production of neutralizing antibodies, usually resulting in lifelong immunity; however, the individual remains infected with the virus and is thus a carrier for life. Epstein-Barr virus can survive for years in peripheral blood lymphocytes without any disease but may become reactivated at any time.[2,3]

Like all herpesviruses, the double-stranded DNA-enveloped EBV has the characteristic icosahedral nucleocapsid, with 162 capsomeres surrounded by a 120 nm envelope. The virus can be isolated from both lymphoid tissues and epithelial tissues of the nasopharynx.[4] EBV binds to CD21 (CR2) found on B cells and enters the cytoplasm. EBV produces disease by transforming B lymphocytes, which then become self-perpetuating. Their multiplication is arrested by two mechanisms. One is a cellular immune response capable of eliminating the infected cells; the other is neutralizing antibodies that prevent the spread of virus to other B lymphocytes. The reactive (atypical) lymphocytes that are characteristic of infectious mononucleosis (IM) are mostly suppressor-cytotoxic lymphocytes that recognize and kill EBV-infected B lymphocytes.[5]

The presentation and course of disease varies with the age at which the primary infection occurs. If the disease occurs in early childhood, it is usually asymptomatic and is rarely associated with classical infectious mononucleosis. In areas of the world where there is poor hygiene and crowded conditions, infection usually occurs early in childhood. When primary infection does not occur until early adolescence or adulthood, 50% to 75% of individuals will be symptomatic, usually presenting as infectious mononucleosis. The infection is persistent and disease can be reactivated by immunosuppression.[3,6]

Isolation of EBV is time consuming and not practical for diagnostic purposes; therefore, serology is the basis for laboratory diagnosis of infection and disease. Two kinds of antibodies are used to diagnose infection and disease from EBV: the heterophile antibodies, which rise and fall rapidly, and the virus-specific antibodies, which persist for the duration of the infection and for the life of the patient.

DISEASES

There are many subclinical cases of EBV infections, and five diseases are known to be associated with the virus.[1] The most important disease, in terms of the number of symptomatic individuals, is infectious mononucleosis (IM). The other four diseases affect fewer people, but are more serious because they are human tumors: Burkitt's lymphoma, nasopharyngeal carcinoma, B-cell lymphomas in immunosuppressed individuals, and some cases of Hodgkin's disease. The last two tumors are very rare.

Burkitt's Lymphoma and Nasopharyngeal Carcinoma

A malignant neoplasm of B lymphocytes, Burkitt's lymphoma (BL) is found primarily among children in a restricted area of Africa and New Guinea. Although BL has a higher incidence in these areas, it is observed sporadically throughout the world. In the rest of the world, however, EBV-associated lymphoma is found primarily in immunocompromised adults. The clusters of this malignancy in two restricted areas prompted a search for viral etiology. This search culminated with the 1964 discovery of EBV, which bears the names of the researchers who first isolated it from BL tumor cells.[7]

Although the association of EBV with BL is strong, EBV DNA has not been detected in BL tumor cell DNA grown in situ. However, there is immunologic evidence for the presence of virus-specific antigens on the tumor cell surface, and all BL patients have elevated antibody titers against viral capsid antigens. Tumor cells grown in vitro produce the virus.[1]

Epstein-Barr virus has been consistently associated with a rare form of squamous cell carcinoma of the nasopharynx; the highest incidence is observed among southern Chinese. Unlike BL, nasopharyngeal tumor cells do contain EBV DNA.[1] Neither BL nor nasopharyngeal carcinoma is thought to be a primary infection. Environmental and genetic factors appear to affect the development of these two human malignancies.[1]

Infectious Mononucleosis

A disease of the reticuloendothelial system, IM has a broad spectrum of clinical presentations, ranging from asymptomatic to severe, although it is rarely life threatening. Heterophile-positive IM is caused by EBV; heterophile-negative IM may be induced by EBV and other agents, including cytomegalovirus, adenovirus, and *Toxoplasma gondii*.[3]

The incubation period has been estimated to be 4 to 7 weeks. The patient is probably infectious before illness, and based on studies of saliva of IM patients, infectivity continues for several weeks or months. The onset of the disease may be acute or insidious, and is characterized by fever, sore throat, and lymphadenopathy. Hepatosplenomegaly, lymphocytosis with many reactive lymphocytes, and enlarged cervical lymph nodes are common. The patient may develop a skin rash, and there may be conjunctivitis and central nervous system damage. The white blood cell count increases; there is a decrease in polymorphonuclear granulocytic cells and a marked increase in monocytes and reactive lymphocytes. The acute disease usually lasts about 2 weeks and is followed by a lengthy convalescence. The patients usually develop transient IgM heterophile antibodies, have an abnormal white cell picture, and have abnormal liver function tests.[5,8]

Socioeconomic conditions affect the incidence of IM. In underdeveloped countries, most children are infected by their third birthday. In developed countries infection is frequently delayed until early adulthood, with approximately 50% of students entering college in the United States not yet infected. By age 30 the prevalence of EBV antibodies approaches 100%, regardless of socioeconomic status.[3,9]

Generally IM infections resolve within 4 to 6 weeks, although complications do arise. Chronic illness subsequent to IM occurs has been reported. This long-term illness is characterized by lymphadenopathy, fever, headache, pharyngitis, and persistent fatigue. Although some patients with this chronic form of IM are immunocompromised, not all are so affected. It appears that there is also a chronic mononucleosis illness that is unrelated to EBV infection.[10,11] Other complications can involve any organ system, with more serious complications found in immunocompromised individuals (i.e., in AIDS and post-transplantation). In these patients polyclonal B cells can divide very rapidly and death can result.[1]

LABORATORY TESTS

Serologic evidence for infectious mononucleosis is obtained through examination of patient blood for heterophile or EBV-specific antibodies.[3] The Paul-Bunnell and Davidsohn differential tests detect heterophile antibodies and are almost specific for the disease with few false positives. Commercially available rapid tests, however, have a higher rate of false positives. Some patients, especially children, fail to develop classical heterophile antibodies; therefore, EBV-specific tests must be performed for laboratory diagnosis. Heterophile antibodies are transient and decrease after the initial infection, whereas some EBV-specific antibodies persist for the life of the patient.[3,5,6,12]

Heterophile Antibodies

Heterophile antibodies react with antigens found in species unrelated to the antigen that stimulated their formation. There are many heterophile antibodies: sheep erythrocyte antibodies in IM, the nonimmune antibodies to the ABO blood group, and nontreponemal antibodies (reagin) in syphilis. Heterophile antibodies, produced in response to the EBV-specific cell surface antigens during IM, react with erythrocyte surface antigens from several species (e.g., sheep, beef, ox, and horse). Other heterophile antibodies can also react with erythrocytes. For example, the serum sickness antibody produced in response to heterologous serum can also react with sheep, beef, and horse erythrocytes. The first heterophile antibody to be described, Forssman antibody, is formed in response to certain bacteria and reacts with sheep and horse erythrocytes, but not with beef erythrocyte antigens.

PAUL-BUNNELL PRESUMPTIVE TEST

Principles

Heterophile antibodies appear in the serum of 85% to 90% of young adults and adolescents who are in the acute phase of classical IM. Such antibodies usually reach significant levels by the end of the first week of illness and peak at 2 to 3 weeks.[12] These heterophile antibodies react with erythrocytes of several species, including sheep. Young children are usually seronegative unless they develop the classical disease. Infectious mononucleosis heterophile antibodies are of the IgM class and represent an early response.

Procedure

The Paul-Bunnell presumptive test employs a serial dilution of heat-inactivated patient serum mixed with a standard concentration of sheep erythrocytes. The dilutions of inactivated patient serum are twofold, beginning with a 1:5 dilution. Subsequent to preparing serum dilutions, a 2% sheep erythrocyte suspension is added, resulting in twofold dilutions, beginning with 1:7 dilution concentration. After room temperature incubation, the tubes are read for visible agglutination.

Results

The titer is the reciprocal of the highest dilution of serum showing visible agglutination of the erythrocytes. A titer of 28 or less (agglutination in four tubes or less) is normal, whereas a titer of ≥56 indicates the presence of a significant level of heterophile antibody.

Interpretation

The Paul-Bunnell is a screening test to detect heterophile antibodies, which are not necessarily specific for IM. If it is negative, no further testing is needed. If it is positive, it indicates the presence of heterophile antibodies, which are found in IM, serum sickness, and several rheumatic diseases. The false positive rate is approximately 3% and is caused by individuals who maintain persistent, albeit low, heterophile antibodies long after their illness. The false negative rate is 10% to 15% and is more common among children; these patients' sera should be tested for EBV-specific antibodies.[12]

DAVIDSOHN DIFFERENTIAL TEST

Principles

The Davidsohn differential test[14,15] assumes the presence of heterophile antibodies at a titer of at least 56, as measured in the Paul-Bunnell test. Heterophile antibodies of IM are adsorbed by beef erythrocytes (Fig. 24-1) and are adsorbed weakly, if at all, by guinea pig kidney cells. The converse is true of Forssman heterophile antibodies, whereas the heterophile antibodies of serum sickness are adsorbed by both the guinea pig and bovine erythrocyte antigens (Table 24-1). Therefore, by comparing the sheep erythrocyte reaction with the antibodies remaining in the serum after adsorption with guinea pig and bovine antigens, it is possible to differentiate between these three heterophile antibodies.

Procedure

Patient serum is added to a suspension of guinea pig kidney antigen and to a second suspension of bovine erythrocyte antigen. After mixing and a short incubation period at room temperature, the suspensions are centrifuged. The supernatants are saved for the test, and the guinea pig and bovine antigens are discarded. Each supernatant is a 1:5 serum dilution. Each is serially diluted twofold up to one dilution greater than the titer of the positive Paul-Bunnell test. When the 2% sheep erythrocyte suspension is added, the resultant dilutions begin with 1:7. After room temperature incubation, the tubes are read for visible agglutination.

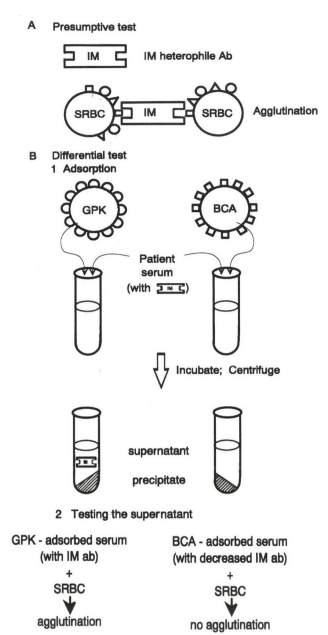

FIGURE 24-1
(**A**) In Paul-Bunnell test for infectious mononucleosis (IM), heterophile antibodies react with the antigens located on sheep red blood cells (SRBC) and cause visible agglutination. (**B**) In the Davidsohn differential test, the IM heterophile antibody does not react with the guinea pig kidney (GPK) antigen. After centrifuging, the supernate contains the IM heterophile antibody. Visible agglutination is observed after the addition of SRBC. The IM heterophile antibody reacts with the bovine cell antigens (BCA) and is adsorbed. After centrifuging, the supernate does not contain the IM heterophile antibody. No agglutination is observed after the addition of SRBC.

Results

The titer is the reciprocal of the highest dilution showing visible agglutination.

Interpretation

The titer in the Paul-Bunnell test is known and is ≥56. In infectious mononucleosis, the guinea pig kidney antigen adsorption reduces the Paul-Bunnell titer by no

TABLE 24-1
Davidsohn Differential Test Adsorption Patterns

HETEROPHILE ANTIBODY	ANTIBODY ADSORBED BY	
	Guinea Pig Kidney Cells	*Beef Erythrocytes*
Infectious mononucleosis	No	Yes
Serum sickness	Yes	Yes
Forssman	Yes	No

more than three tubes (sixfold or less reduction in titer), and the bovine erythrocyte antigen adsorption reduces the Paul-Bunnell titer by four tubes or more (at least an eightfold reduction in titer is required). In serum sickness, both adsorptions reduce the titer by at least eightfold. Forssman antibodies have an eightfold or greater reduction in the titer using the guinea pig kidney adsorbed serum, and the titer of beef erythrocyte adsorbed serum is the same as the Paul-Bunnell titer (Table 24-2).

RAPID TESTS

Slide Red Cell Tests

PRINCIPLES. A number of rapid slide tests are commercially available. One test is a differential test that employs differential agglutination by patient serum of horse erythrocytes[14,15] after the serum has been adsorbed with fine suspensions of guinea pig kidney antigen and beef erythrocyte antigens. The majority of the other commercially available kits do not use differential agglutination but directly add patient serum to the horse erythrocytes. Rapid latex tests are also available in which bovine erythrocyte antigens are on the latex particles.

PROCEDURE. There are a number of variations in each of the commercially available kits in which horse erythrocytes are added to unadsorbed patient serum. Read the manufacturers' procedure for the specifics of each

TABLE 24-2
Interpretation of Davidsohn Differential Test Adsorption Patterns

DISEASE	DECREASE IN PAUL-BUNNELL TITER AFTER ADSORPTION WITH	
	Guinea Pig Kidney Cells	*Beef Erythrocytes*
Infectious mononucleosis	≤ Sixfold	≥ Eightfold
Serum sickness	≥ Eightfold	≥ Eightfold
Forssman	≥ Eightfold	No change

procedure. The differential slide test is performed using serum or plasma samples (which do not have to be inactivated). The slide is divided into two sections and the serum is mixed separately with guinea pig kidney antigen and beef erythrocyte antigen; subsequently, each mixture is mixed with horse red blood cells. All tests should be run in parallel with known positive and negative serum controls.

RESULTS. All slide tests are read for agglutination.

INTERPRETATION. Slide tests (horse erythrocyte and latex) without a differential component are positive if any agglutination is present on the slide and negative if there is no agglutination. Differential test interpretation is positive if agglutination with the guinea pig antigen-adsorbed serum is observed but no agglutination with the beef erythrocyte antigen-adsorbed serum is observed. The test is negative if neither side has any agglutination or if both sides demonstrate agglutination. The sensitivity and specificity of the slide tests depend on the manufacturer; the horse cell agglutination procedure is the most sensitive (95% positive in serologically proven IM), but bovine cells are more specific.[16]

Membrane-Based Enzyme Immunoassay

PRINCIPLES. A newer rapid test incorporates ox erythrocyte antigens onto a membrane in a self-contained cassette. The patient serum is added to the appropriate spot along with the reagent enzyme-labeled globulin. The serum and reagent antibody diffuse along the membrane to the antigen, where color development occurs if IM heterophile antibodies are present. There is also an internal control area on the slide. Positive and negative serum controls should also be performed (Fig. 24-2).

RESULTS. The test is read for color development.

INTERPRETATION. The internal control area of the cassette should always show color development for valid results. The presence of color in the test area indicates the presence of IM heterophile antibodies. The absence of color is a negative test. This test is a qualitative test and correlates well with horse erythrocyte agglutination titers.

ENZYME-LINKED IMMUNOSORBENT ASSAY (ELISA)

In ELISA purified antigen from bovine erythrocyte stroma is attached to the solid phase.[16] After incubation with patient serum, the heterophile antibody will bind to the bovine antigen. The test employs a detector antibody reagent that is specific for the μ heavy chain, is labeled with alkaline phosphatases, and detects the captured heterophile antibody. The quantitative results correlate well with horse erythrocyte agglutination titers.

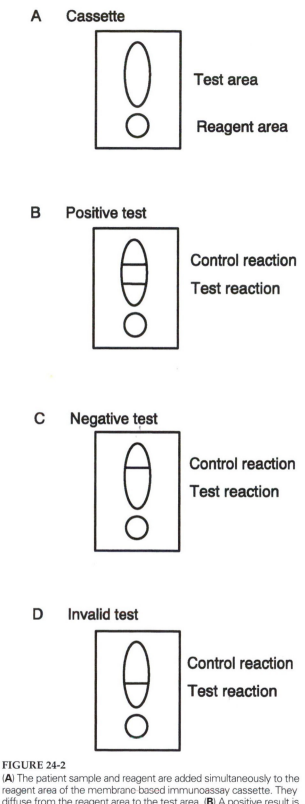

FIGURE 24-2
(**A**) The patient sample and reagent are added simultaneously to the reagent area of the membrane-based immunoassay cassette. They diffuse from the reagent area to the test area. (**B**) A positive result is indicated by two lines in the test area. IM antibodies binding to membrane-bound ox red cell antigen react with the enzyme antibody to form a line in the test result area. If the test system is reacting properly, a second line will form in the control area. (**C**) If no IM antibody is present, no line will be formed in the test area. A line will still form in the control area if the reagents are working properly. (**D**) Even though a line formed in the test area, there is no line in the control area. This indicates that there is an error in the testing procedure and the results are invalid.

EBV-Specific Tests

Enzyme immunoassays (EIA) and indirect immunofluorescence assays are available to detect EBV-specific antibodies. Many consider EIA to be more practical for use in routine clinical laboratories. Two groups of antigens produced during the lytic phase of infection are the early antigen (EA) and viral capsid antigen (VCA); antibodies to these two antigens may be found early in the disease (Fig. 24-3).[3,6,12] A third antigen, Epstein-Barr nuclear antigen (EBNA), causes antibody production later in the disease (Table 24-3).

IMMUNOFLUORESCENCE TESTS

Principles

The indirect immunofluorescence test is a sandwich technique in which the antigen (EBV-infected lymphoblastoid cells) is fixed to the slide, allowed to react with patient serum, and subsequently layered with fluorescein-conjugated anti–human IgG or IgM. Four antibodies are detected using class-specific antisera: VCA-IgM, VCA-IgG, EA-IgG, and EBNA-IgG.[2,17]

Results

The slides are read with a fluorescence microscope. The titer is the reciprocal of the highest dilution showing specific fluorescence.

Interpretation

Most often VCA antibodies are measured. In those older than 4 years, titers of anti-VCA peak 3 to 4 weeks following infection; the IgM becomes undetectable in the circulation by 12 weeks after infection, and the IgG titer

decreases but persists for life. Because IgG anti-VCA persists indefinitely, it is the most sensitive indicator of EBV infection. Although high levels of IgG anti-VCA are observed in acute infections, they are not specific for recent infections; increased levels are detected in a variety of other conditions, including immunodeficiency, malignancy, arthritis, systemic lupus erythematosus, and acquired immunodeficiency syndrome (AIDS). IgM anti-VCA is detectable in 97% of patients during the acute phase of IM and is therefore a reliable marker of acute or recent infection.[3,6,12]

Antibody to EBV early antigen (anti-EA) is produced concomitantly with IgM anti-VCA and persists for 8 to 12 weeks. Anti-EA is usually associated with recent infections; after the acute phase of infection, anti-EA disappears but reappears as the patient ages.

Antibody to the nuclear antigen (anti-EBNA) appears as early as 1 month after infection, but more commonly 2 to 3 months later, and persists indefinitely. The presence of anti-EBNA indicates that EBV infection has occurred and that it is not recent. Thus the presence of anti-VCA IgG or IgM in the absence of anti-EBNA supports a recent infection and the diagnosis of IM. Other patterns of reactivity indicate either previous infections or reactivation (Table 24-3). Table 24-4 indicates the pattern of antibodies present in other EBV diseases.

ENZYME IMMUNOASSAYS

Principles

The enzyme immunoassay procedures are sandwich assays in which the antigen is fixed onto a well in a microtiter plate. Patient serum is added to the well and in-

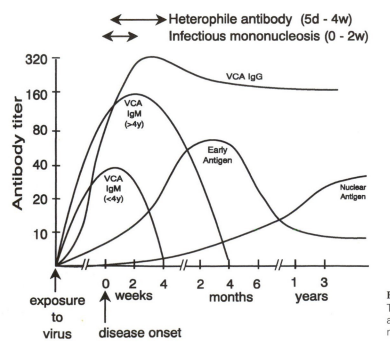

FIGURE 24-3
This schematic shows the development of different antibodies during the course of infectious mononucleosis following a primary EBV infection.

TABLE 24-3
EBV-Specific Serology in Infectious Mononucleosis

	ANTIBODIES			
	VCA (IgM)	VCA (IgG)	EA	EBNA
Acute primary infection	+	+	+	−
Recent primary infection	+/−	+	+/−	+
Remote primary infection	−	+	−	+
Reactivation	−	+	+	+

cubated. After washing, an enzyme-conjugated anti–human IgG or IgM is added.

Results

The microtiter plates are read spectrophotometrically. The amount of color produced is proportional to the amount of antibody present in the patient serum.

Interpretation

The interpretation for this type of procedure is the same as that of the immunofluorescence tests.

OTHER CHANGES

Lymphocytosis

When acute IM develops, there may be leukopenia caused by decreased granulocytes; however, usually there will be leukocytosis by the second or third week of illness. The white blood cell (WBC) count rises to 10 to $20 \times 10^9/L$, with >50% mononuclear cells with >10% reactive lymphocytes. In most cases, there are 60% to 80% mononuclear cells with >25% reactive lymphocytes. The peripheral blood picture remains abnormal for at least 2 weeks and may persist for months.[18]

When a patient becomes infected with EBV, the initial site of infection is lymphocytes in lymphoid tissue of the oropharynx. The host immune response may limit the virus to this site, or the virus may spread to the rest of the body. If spreading does not occur, clinical IM does not develop. Spreading may occur by viremia or circulation of the infected B lymphocytes. The infected B lymphocytes proliferate and invade many organs of the body. The polyclonal activation of EBV-infected B lymphocytes stimulates the production of many different antibodies (such as heterophile, cold agglutinins, anti-VCA, anti-EA, and anti-EBNA). The virally infected B lymphocytes stimulate the proliferation of T lymphocytes, which are essential in the recovery from IM. The lymph nodes and spleen become enlarged as the number of white cells increase in those organs; most frequently, cervical lymph nodes are involved, although generalized lymphadenopathy is often observed. Splenomegaly occurs in 50% to 60% of patients.[1,5]

During the incubation period, some infected B lymphocytes are transformed, resulting in a proliferation of B lymphocytes; however, some infected cells lyse, releasing viral antigens. These antigens stimulate the production of antibodies to membrane antigens, VCA, and EA that can be identified in the laboratory. The EBNA appears to be derived from transformed cells, not lytic cells; thus, these antibodies are not detected until convalescence.

Liver Function

Clinically apparent jaundice is observed in 5% to 10% of patients with IM and 10% to 25% have mild hepatomegaly. Abnormal liver function tests are observed in most patients. Liver enzymes, such as aspartate aminotransferase and alanine aminotransferase,

TABLE 24-4
Specific Antibody Responses in EBV-Related Diseases

	ANTIBODY				
	Heterophile	VCA (IgM)	VCA (IgG)	EA	EBNA
IM (acute or recent primary infection)	+	+	+	+/−	−
Burkitt's lymphoma	−	−	+	+	−
Nasopharyngeal Carcinoma	−	−	+	+*	+*

Both IgG and IgA antibodies are produced, although IgA has the higher concentration.

rise during the second and third weeks of the disease. Hyperbilirubinemia is also present in most patients. The increased lactate dehydrogenase level in IM is probably derived from the white blood cells and not from the liver.[5]

Case Study

DD, an 18-year-old female, went to her physician because she felt tired all the time. The physician ordered a screening test for infectious mononucleosis. The results of that test were negative. The screening test was repeated 2 weeks later, with the same results as the first test. The physician then ordered the following specific antibody tests to be done with the following results: VCA-IgM positive, VCA-IgG positive, EA-IgG positive, and EBNA-IgG negative.

Case Study Questions

1. What do the results of the specific antibody tests indicate?

2. Why were the results of the screening tests negative?

3. Why is the EBNA-IgG test negative when other test results are positive?

References

1. Coltran RS, Kumar V, Robbins SL (eds): Robbins Pathologic Basis of Disease, 5th ed, p 287. Philadelphia, WB Saunders, 1994
2. Henle G, Henle W: Immunofluorescence in cells derived from Burkitt's lymphoma. J Bacteriol 91:1248, 1966
3. Sumaya CV, Jenson HB: Epstein-Barr virus. In Rose NR, DeMacario EC, Fahey JL, Friedman H, Penn GM: Manual of Clinical Laboratory Immunology, 4th ed, p 568. Washington, DC, American Society for Microbiology, 1992
4. Lennette ET: Epstein-Barr virus. In Lennette ET, Balows A, Hausler WJ Jr (eds): Manual of Clinical Microbiology, 4th ed, p 728. Washington, DC, American Society for Microbiology, 1985
5. Coltran RS, Kumar V, Robbins SL (eds): Robbins Pathologic Basis of Disease, 5th ed, p 347. Philadelphia, WB Saunders, 1994
6. Ray CG, Minnich LL: Viruses, Rickettsia and Chlamydia. In Henry JB (ed): Clinical Diagnosis and Management by Laboratory Methods, 18th ed, p 1234. Philadelphia, WB Saunders, 1991
7. Epstein MA, Barr YM, Achong BG: Virus particles in cultured lymphoblasts from Burkitt's lymphoma. Lancet 1:702, 1964
8. Henle G, Henle W, Diehl V: Relation of Burkitt's tumor-associated herpes-type virus to infectious mononucleosis. Proc Natl Acad Sci USA 59:94, 1968
9. Niederman JC, Evans AS, Subrahmanya MS, et al: Prevalence, incidence and persistence of EB virus antibody in young adults. N Engl J Med 282:361, 1970
10. Isaacs R: Chronic infectious mononucleosis. Blood 3:858, 1984
11. Merlin TL: Chronic mononucleosis: Pitfalls in the laboratory diagnosis. Hum Pathol 17:2, 1986
12. Davey FR, Nelson DA: Leukocyte disorders. In Henry JB (ed): Clinical Diagnosis and Management by Laboratory Methods, p 686. Philadelphia, WB Saunders, 1991
13. Paul JR, Bunnell WW: The presence of heterophile antibodies in infectious mononucleosis. Am J Med Sci 183:90, 1932
14. Lee CL, Davidsohn I, Panczyszyn O: Horse agglutinins in infectious mononucleosis, II. The spot test. Am J Clin Pathol 49:12, 1968
15. Lee CL, Davidsohn I, Slaby R: Horse agglutinins in infectious mononucleosis. Am J Clin Pathol 49:3, 1968
16. Andiman WA: Antibody Responses to Epstein-Barr Virus. In Rose NR, Friedman H, Fahey JL (eds): Manual of Clinical Laboratory Immunology, 3rd ed, p 509. Washington, DC, American Society for Microbiology, 1986
17. Henle W, Henle G, Horowitz CA: Epstein-Barr virus-specific diagnostic tests in infectious mononucleosis. Hum Pathol 5:551, 1974
18. Niederman JC: Infectious mononucleosis at the Yale-New Haven Medical Center 1946–1955. Yale J Biol Med 28:629, 1956
19. Fleisher GR: Epidemiology and pathogenesis. In Schlossberg D (ed): Infectious Mononucleosis, Praeger Monographs in Infectious Disease, Vol 1, p 27. New York, Praeger, 1983

CHAPTER 25

Viral Hepatitis

Ann Marie McNamara

Objectives

Upon completion of the chapter, the reader will be able to:

1. Describe the pertinent characteristics of the five hepatitis viruses
2. Compare and contrast the epidemiology and clinical manifestations of the five hepatitis diseases
3. Describe the antigen and antibody responses for diagnosing acute and chronic stages of the five viral hepatitis diseases

Viral hepatitis refers to liver disease caused by five hepatotrophic viruses: hepatitis A (HAV), hepatitis B (HBV), hepatitis C (HCV), delta hepatitis (HDV), and hepatitis E (HEV). The reader should be aware, however, that hepatitis simply means an inflammation of the liver and is a clinical manifestation of liver disease caused by a variety of bacteria, viruses, fungi, parasites, toxins, autoimmune diseases, radiation, neoplasms, and drugs.[1-3] This chapter describes current laboratory methods for diagnosing the five viral hepatitis infections and discusses pertinent characteristics of these viruses, including their physical characteristics, epidemiology, clinical manifestations, and patterns of antibody and antigen response to infection.

HEPATITIS TESTING

General Principles

Detection of specific hepatitis antigens and antibodies from patient serum determines the responsible viral agent, the immune status of the host, and the clinical stage of the infection. Radioimmunoassay (RIA) and enzyme-linked immunosorbent assays (ELISA) are the most widely used diagnostic test methods. ELISA tests are usually preferred because no radioactive materials are involved, reagents are commercially available, and test kits have a long shelf life.[4] ELISA tests are about as sensitive as RIA, but their specificity is lower.[2] Because false positive results occur in both test formats, only repeatedly reactive specimens should be reported as positive tests. The advantages of RIA are that it is more specific than ELISA and commercial reagents are available. RIA tests have distinct disadvantages in that radioactive materials are involved, expensive equipment is required, and test kits have a short shelf life.[4]

Test methods for detecting hepatitis antigens and antibodies can be grouped into three successive "generations" of tests. Each subsequent generation shows improved test sensitivity when compared with the previous generation. Agar gel diffusion (Ouchterlony double diffusion) is the first-generation test, followed by three second-generation tests: counterimmunoelectrophoresis, complement fixation, and reverse passive latex agglutination.[4] All these test formats are outdated and will not be presented here. Third-generation tests include RIA, ELISA, and passive and reverse-passive hemagglutination. Because the hemagglutination tests are less sensitive than the RIA and ELISA, they are rarely used in clinical laboratories. Detection of specific antigens and antibodies for diagnosing the hepatitis viruses will be discussed under the sections appropriate to each virus.

Direct detection of hepatitis virus antigens and particles in patient specimens (liver biopsies, serum, or stools, where appropriate) is accomplished by electron microscopy and immunofluorescence or immunoperoxidase staining.[2] New polymerase chain reaction techniques can detect specific DNA or RNA genomic sequences from hepatitis viruses. Generally, these techniques are limited to research because diagnosis can generally be made serologically.

Radioimmunoassay

Radioimmunoassay (RIA) tests are of two formats: noncompetitive, solid-phase radioimmunoassay (sandwich technique) or competitive binding assays. Solid-phase radioimmunoassays to detect hepatitis antigens are performed by incubating patient sera or plasma (antigen source) with hepatitis antibodies adsorbed to a solid-phase support (plastic tubes or beads).[2] ^{125}I-labeled antibody is then added and allowed to incubate. If antigen is present in the patient sample, an antibody-antigen–labeled antibody sandwich forms. After washing away excess labeled antibody, the bound radioactive label is counted in a gamma counter. The counts per minute (CPM) recovered is proportional to the concentration of antibody in the sample. The CPM

of the patient's sample is compared with a positive cutoff value calculated by a mathematical manipulation of the negative control. Samples with a CPM higher than the cutoff value are considered reactive. This assay can be modified to detect hepatitis antibodies by adsorbing antigen to the solid support and adding labeled antigen or labeled anti–human globulin reagent.

Competitive binding assays to detect viral antigens are performed by incubating patient sera or plasma (antigen source) with radioactively labeled hepatitis antigen.[2] These antigens then compete for binding sites on plastic beads coated with hepatitis antibody. The amount of labeled antigen detected is inversely proportional to the amount of antigen present in the patient sample. Therefore, a reactive test result occurs when the CPM of the patient sample are less than those of the negative control.

Because false positive reactions can occur, all reactive test results must be repeated. Some causes for false positive tests include inadequate washing steps and cross contamination of the counting tubes or beads with radioactivity in nonreactive samples caused by faulty technique or contaminated pipette tips.

A confirmatory test is available to rule out false positive tests for hepatitis B surface antigen (HB$_s$Ag). This is a specific antibody neutralization test in which human antibody to hepatitis B surface antigen is incubated with the patient's sample before testing. If HB$_s$Ag is present in the patient's sample, it will combine with the added antibody and be unavailable to react in the RIA test. The sample is considered positive if the neutralized sample shows a reduction in CPM of at least 50% compared with a concomitantly run non-neutralized sample.[4]

Enzyme-Linked Immunosorbent Assay

ELISA tests can be used to detect hepatitis antigens or antibodies in both noncompetitive, solid-phase and competitive binding assays.[4] The principle of these assays is the same as that of the corresponding RIA, except that an enzyme label replaces the radioactive label. Addition of an appropriate chromogenic substrate for the enzyme produces a color change that is measured in a spectrophotometer. Reactive samples are determined by comparing the absorbance of the patient's sample with that of a cutoff value for the negative control. Confirmatory antibody neutralization tests are also available in ELISA format to confirm HB$_s$Ag.

False positive tests occur with ELISA testing, and all reactive results must be confirmed by retesting or by neutralization. Common sources of false positive ELISA results are inadequate washing, cross contamination of nonreactive sera with positive sera retained on the pipetting device, contaminating the o-phenylenediamine

(OPD) solution with oxidizing agents, contamination of the acid stopping reagent, or contamination of the reaction tray well rim with conjugate or specimen (AUSAB EIA package insert, Abbott Laboratories, North Chicago, IL).

HEPATITIS A

Hepatitis A Virus

Hepatitis A virus (HAV) is a member of the Picornaviridae family of viruses.[5] It is composed of a single serotype, classified as enterovirus type 72.[2] This virus was first isolated from the stool of acutely ill patients by Feinstone et al.[6] in 1973. Electron microscopy (Fig. 25-1) reveals a virion with a mean diameter of 27 nm, icosahedral in shape, and without an envelope.[5] It is both acid stable and ether resistant.[4] Although present in the stool of acutely ill patients, HAV is not detectable in serum. The hosts of the virus are limited to humans, marmosets, chimpanzees, and owl monkeys.[2,4] It has recently been grown in cell culture.[7]

Epidemiology

HAV infections occur worldwide, in both epidemic and endemic forms.[2] In industrialized nations, where standards of living are high, infection is generally seen in adults <50 years old.[1] In developing countries, where hygiene is poor, children are most commonly affected.[3] Transmission has been shown to occur most often by the fecal-oral route, although rare parenteral transmission has been documented after transfusion of blood products.[4] Epidemics generally occur from fecal contamination of a single source of food, water, or milk.[2]

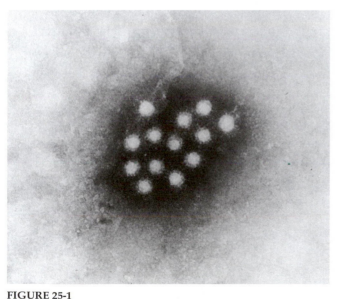

FIGURE 25-1
Electron micrograph of hepatitis A virus. (Courtesy of CDC Archives.)

Hospital outbreaks are rare.[4] Person-to-person spread is responsible in outbreaks linked to daycare centers, mental institutions, and military recruits.[4]

Clinical Manifestations

Hepatitis A infections may be asymptomatic or symptomatic. Symptomatic infections may include a period of jaundice (icteric stage) or not (anicteric). The incubation period of the disease is usually 10 to 50 days,[1] after which clinical illness develops abruptly in symptomatic cases. Clinical findings include fever, anorexia, vomiting, fatigue, and malaise.[1,3] Serum transaminase levels (especially alanine aminotransferase) are elevated and peak before the onset of jaundice. Right upper quadrant pain, dark urine, and pale stools mark the beginning of jaundice. This icteric stage lasts for a few days to a few weeks.[2] Other clinical findings include hyperbilirubinemia and decreased albumin levels.[1] Recovery is generally in 2 to 4 weeks, and the mortality rate is approximately 0.1%.[1] Rarely does chronic disease occur. Patients should be placed on enteric precautions, however, as they are considered infectious for approximately 2 weeks following the onset of jaundice.[3] Treatment is based on alleviating the patient's symptoms, because no antiviral drugs are known to be effective. Household contacts should receive immune serum globulin prophylaxis. A new HAV vaccine was licensed in 1995 and is prepared from inactivated virus grown in tissue culture.[8] It is recommended for healthcare workers, travelers to endemic areas, drug abusers, and children in communities with periodic HAV outbreaks.[8]

Laboratory Diagnosis

Figure 25-2 and Table 25-1 show the antibody and antigen markers present in hepatitis A infection. Fecal hepatitis A antigen (HAV-Ag) can be detected by immune electron microscopy, RIA antigen assays, and ELISA antigen assays. These tests are generally not performed, however, because antigen levels are usually declining as symptoms develop. Instead, RIA and ELISA tests are used to detect the presence of specific HAV antibodies in the patient's serum. Patient blood is collected as soon as exposure is known or at the onset of symptoms, again at 3 or 4 weeks after symptoms appear, and 2 to 3 months after the illness. A fourfold rise in antibody titer to IgM and total (IgG and IgM) antibodies is considered diagnostic. IgM anti-HAV antibody is present at the onset of symptoms and reaches a maximum titer in 1 to 3 weeks. Anti-HAV total antibodies are present at the onset of symptoms and can remain elevated for years. Patterns of antibody response can be interpreted as follows: both total anti-HAV and IgM anti-HAV signify acute or convalescent infection; total anti-HAV indicates

Antibody Response in Hepatitis A

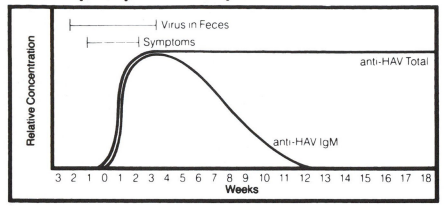

FIGURE 25-2

Antigen and antibody response in hepatitis A infection. (Reproduced with permission from Abbott Laboratories, ©1988 Abbott Laboratories.)

only prior infection, with the patient now immune; and neither antibody present indicates the absence of infection or the incubation phase of the disease.

HEPATITIS B

Hepatitis B Virus

Hepatitis B virus (HBV) is a small, enveloped, double-stranded DNA virus belonging to the Hepadnaviridae family[2] (Fig. 25-3). HBV exists in the serum of HBV-infected individuals in three morphologic forms: the infectious 42-nm spherical Dane particle, and two 22 nm diameter particles existing as spheres or filaments (50 to >200 nm in length).[5] These latter two forms are considered to be incomplete viral coat proteins, consisting of hepatitis B surface antigen (HB_sAg).[4] Because these particles are incomplete virions, they are not considered infectious.

The infectious Dane particle is a complete HBV virion and exhibits a more complicated structure than the smaller HB_sAg particles. The Dane particle consists of a 22-nm nucleocapsid surrounded by a lipid-protein-carbohydrate envelope containing HB_sAg.[5] HB_sAg was first described in 1964 in the serum of an Australian aborigine and has been previously termed the Australian antigen.[5] HB_sAg is a marker of viral replication in liver hepatocytes. The HB_sAg consists of several types of antigenic determinants, including a group-specific determinant *a* and two pairs of mutually exclusive, type-specific determinants located on two independent genetic alleles, the *d* or *v* and *w* or *r* pairs.[5] By combining the group-specific determinant, *a*, with one of each of the two type-specific pairs (i.e., *avw*), 10 different strains of HBV have been identified.[3] Strain determinations are not routinely performed in the clinical laboratory but may be useful in epidemiologic studies. Antibodies to HB_sAg (anti-HB_s) in a patient's serum indicate

---

TABLE 25-1
Viral Hepatitis Diagnostic Markers and their Significance in Infection*

MARKER[†]	INTERPRETATION
IgM anti-HAV	Diagnoses a recent acute HAV infection; tests for IgM antibodies
Total anti-HAV	Indicates past infection and immunity to HAV; tests for IgM and IgG antibodies
HB_sAg	Indicates acute HBV infection when present with IgM anti-HB_c; persistence beyond 6 months signals chronic infection
IgM anti-HB_c	Indicates recent acute HBV infection when present with HB_sAg
HB_eAg	Marker of HBV infectivity in either acute or chronic infections; indicates progression of disease to chronic liver infection is likely
Anti-HB_e	Indicates a more benign clinical HBV course
Anti-HB_s	Signifies recovery from HBV infection, natural immunity, or immunity after vaccination
Anti-HCV	Acute or chronic HCV disease
IgM anti-HDV	Acute HDV superinfection
Total anti-HDV	Chronic HDV superinfection; tests for IgM and IgG antibodies

*Table adapted from references 11, 13, and 17.
[†]See text for meaning of abbreviations.

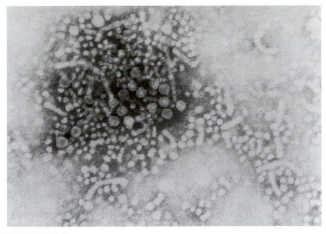

FIGURE 25-3
Electron micrograph of hepatitis B virus. (Courtesy of CDC Archives.)

past infection and subsequent immunity of the patient to HBV (Fig. 25-4).

If the envelope of the Dane particle is removed using detergents, the nucleocapsid remains. This nucleocapsid contains the viral DNA, viral polymerase, and hepatitis B core antigen (HB$_c$Ag). HB$_c$Ag can be detected in liver hepatocytes, but more often serologic diagnosis is determined by the presence of antibodies to HB$_c$Ag (anti-HB$_c$). Anti-HB$_c$ levels are always interpreted relative to finding HB$_s$Ag or anti-HB$_s$ in the patient's serum and signify either chronic infection or patient immunity (Figs. 25-4 and 25-5 on p. 252).

An antigen found in some HB$_s$Ag-positive sera, either bound to immunoglobulins or free in solution, has been correlated with viral infectivity. This is the HB$_e$Ag antigen, and it is associated with viral replication in the liver (see Figs. 25-4 and 25-5).[5] Antibodies to anti-HB$_e$Ag (anti-HB$_e$) usually occur when the patient is recovering from active infection (see Fig. 25-4).

Epidemiology

HBV infections were originally called serum hepatitis, as opposed to HAV fecal-oral–transmitted infectious hepatitis. Serum hepatitis is now a misnomer, because

hepatitis C (HCV) and hepatitis delta virus (HDV) are also transmitted by blood and blood products.

HBV can be recovered from the blood and body fluids of infected persons. Infected body fluids include semen, saliva, breast milk, tears, cerebrospinal and ascitic fluids, and urine.[3,4] Transmission occurs either through a parenteral route or through contact of mucous membranes or open wounds with infected body fluids. Parenteral transmission can occur through the use of infected blood or blood products, hemodialysis, intravenous drug use, accidental needle sticks, tattooing, acupuncture, ear piercing, or arthropod-borne vectors.[3,4] Blood banks routinely screen blood and blood products for HB$_s$Ag, and infected units are destroyed. Transmission through contact with contaminated body secretions occurs in institutionalized mentally retarded children, sexual partners of infected persons, household contacts, and infants of infected mothers.[3,4] Infections occur worldwide; high-risk groups have been defined as intravenous drug users, homosexual men, hemodialysis patients, and medical and dental personnel. Reservoirs of HBV are chronic carriers of HBV infection.

Clinical Manifestations

Approximately 300,000 new cases of HBV infection occur annually in the United States.[9] Clinical symptoms and signs are similar to those found in HAV infections; however, HBV infections tend to have more arthralgia, a more abrupt onset of symptoms, a longer clinical course, and a slower resolution.[1] The infection has an incubation period of 50 to 180 days (mean of 75)[1] and may present as asymptomatic infection, either icteric or nonicteric symptomatic infection, or fulminant hepatitis. Chronic infections can be persistent or active infections. All chronic cases are HB$_s$Ag positive. Chronic persistent infections are usually benign, but chronic active infections manifest severe liver necrosis and may develop primary hepatocellular carcinoma.[4] All chronic carriers continue to shed active virus.

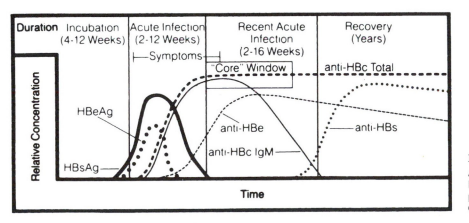

FIGURE 25-4

Antigen and antibody response in acute hepatitis B infection. (Reproduced with permission from Abbott Laboratories, ©1988 Abbott Laboratories.)

No Seroconversion

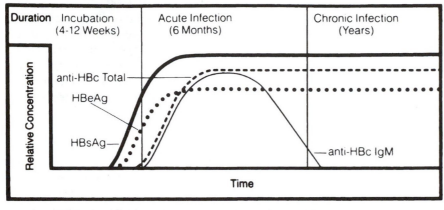

FIGURE 25-5

Antigen and antibody response in chronic hepatitis B infection. (Reproduced with permission from Abbott Laboratories, ©1988 Abbott Laboratories.)

Although no antiviral drug is known to be effective against HBV, effective vaccines exist and should be used to immunize high-risk persons. The vaccine consists of purified, formalin-fixed HB_sAg from the sera of HBV carriers[3] or recombinant HB_sAg, and it evokes a protective immune response to HBV when administered. Both commercially available immune serum globulin (ISG) and high-titer anti-HB_s HBV immune serum globulin (HBIG) are used prophylactically following exposure to HBV-contaminated blood and body fluids. ISG and HBIG provide passive immunity to HBV, and recipients should also receive an HBV vaccine for active immunity.[8] HBV vaccine is recommended for all children as a childhood vaccine, health-care workers, patients on hemodialysis, IV drug users, household contacts of cases, persons with multiple sexual partners, and travelers to endemic areas.[8]

Laboratory Diagnosis

The serologic diagnosis of HBV infections is more complicated than that for HAV infections. Both HBV antibody and antigen markers (Table 25-1; Figs. 25-4 and 25-5) can be demonstrated in samples using RIA and ELISA techniques. For simplification, the pattern of HBV antigen and antibody response will be divided into responses seen in acute and chronic HBV disease. In acute HBV hepatitis (Fig. 25-4), HB_sAg appears during the incubation period of the infection and is the first detectable serologic marker. HB_eAg develops next and is indicative of the infectivity of the patient. Development of anti-HB_e is the first serologic sign of clinical recovery and decreased patient infectivity. Anti-HB_c is the first antibody to appear in the serum. Anti-HB_c development begins during acute illness and remains high for years. Its presence suggests that the patient is in the later stages of the disease or is immune. This antibody is also a marker

of the "core window" period in which neither HB_sAg nor anti-HB_s is found in patient sera. Anti-HB_c is initially IgM and then is replaced by IgG antibodies measured by total anti-HB_c. Development of anti-HB_s occurs months to years after infection during the patient's recovery period. The presence of anti-HB_s signals the late stages of disease and the development of immunity.

In chronic HBV infections (Fig. 25-5), persistent HB_sAg in the serum is the characteristic diagnostic marker. Chronic carriers of HB_sAg have repeatedly demonstrable titers of HB_sAg for 6 months to several years after initial infection. Anti-HB_c and HB_eAg are also present in high titers in chronic hepatitis. A decrease in HB_eAg and a rise in anti-HB_e indicate chronic persistent hepatitis. If no seroconversion to anti-HB_e occurs and high HB_eAg titers persist, the person is highly infectious and is likely to develop serious liver disease.

The clinical stage of HBV infection and the immune status of the host are generally determined by screening for HB_sAg, anti-HB_s and anti-HB_c (both total and IgM), HB_eAg, and anti-HB_e.[4] In general, the presence of HB_sAg signifies HBV acute or chronic infection. Patients should then be repeatedly tested for the presence of both HB_sAg and anti-HB_s to detect the recovery stage of HBV illness, when HB_sAg decreases and anti-HB_s increases. If HB_sAg without anti-HB_s persists for more than 6 months, a chronic active or passive case of HBV can be diagnosed. Elevated liver enzymes indicate chronic disease, whereas normal enzyme levels suggest that the patient is a chronic carrier. When anti-HB_s is present in a sample, the patient is immune to HBV infection. Anti-HB_c indicates a chronic carrier state or late infection during the "core window" of acute infection. The presence of HB_eAg indicates infectivity of the patient and viral replication in the liver. Anti-HB_e occurs when the patient is in late disease or recovering.

HEPATITIS C

Hepatitis C Virus

Previously, viral hepatitis cases that could not be serologically defined as either hepatitis A or B were classified as non-A, non-B hepatitis (see the section Non–A–E Hepatitis). We now know that the majority of these cases can be attributed to HCV or HEV. HCV was first discovered in 1988 and is an enveloped, single-stranded RNA virus, approximately 38 to 50 nm in length.[11] It is related to both the pestivirus and flavivirus groups.[9] Comparing nucleotide sequences from HCV isolates suggests that at least five different classes of HCV exist.[10]

Epidemiology

It is estimated that 150,000 to 170,000 new cases of hepatitis C occur annually in the United States.[11] The major route of transmission is parenteral, either through transfusion of contaminated blood or blood products, inadvertent needle stick accidents in healthcare workers, or via intravenous drug use.[10] Sexual and perinatal transmissions are known to occur but are uncommon.[11]

Clinical Manifestations

HCV can result in either acute or chronic disease. The incubation period ranges from 2 to 26 weeks.[11] Most acute cases are asymptomatic or exhibit mild symptoms of hepatitis, such as nausea, anorexia, abdominal pain, fatigue, malaise, and jaundice.[10] Approximately 50% to 80% of cases become chronic, leading to cirrhosis of the liver in 20% to 25% of these cases.[8] Twenty percent of cirrhosis cases may progress to develop hepatocellular carcinoma.[9] The mortality rate is 1% to 2%.[8] For chronic cases of HCV with severe liver disease, interferon-alpha therapy may be prescribed.[8] Only approximately 50% of treated patients respond and relapses are common.[8] HCV vaccines are under development.

Laboratory Diagnosis

Antibodies to HCV appear in both acute and chronic cases of disease (see Table 25-1). Although an IgM-anti HCV assay has been developed, it does not consistently distinguish between acute and chronic disease states.[8] This is partially because of the fact that when HCV infections resolve spontaneously, antibodies to HCV are lost at the very slow rate of 0.6/100 patient years.[12] This means that anti-HCV levels in a patient's serum remain at high levels for years in most patients.[13] Distinguishing between acute and chronic HCV infection, therefore, depends not only on detecting HCV antibodies but also on a knowledge of the clinical history and previously positive anti-HCV serological tests (6 months' duration between positive tests denotes a change from acute to chronic infection).[8] Because false positive results occur with the anti-HCV ELISA screening tests currently on the market, recombinant antigen immunoblot assays were developed to distinguish between "true" and "false" anti-HCV reactions.[12] These immunoblot assays, RIBA HCV (Chiron, Emeryville, CA), and HCV Matrix (Abbott Laboratories, Abbott Park, IL), use four antigens selected from the core, NS3, and NS4 regions of HCV.[8] A serological sample is considered positive if antibodies to two or more HCV antigens are detected.[11] Nucleic acid probes and polymerase chain reaction techniques have been developed to detect HCV RNA in a patient's serum sample.[11,12] These assays are currently for research purposes only.

DELTA HEPATITIS

Hepatitis D Virus

Hepatitis delta virus (HDV) was first described by Rizzetto et al. in 1977.[14] Also called the delta antigen, this single-stranded RNA virus is spherical in shape, with a diameter of 36 nm.[15] It is a defective hepatotrophic virus in that it requires obligatory helper functions from HBV to ensure its replication and infectivity. One major helper function of HBV is to provide HDV with a protein coat of HB_sAg. This allows the formerly unenveloped, defective particle to function as an infectious agent.[16]

Epidemiology

HDV infection has been shown to occur worldwide. Transmission of HDV is linked to that of its HBV helper virus and occurs by parenteral and transmucosal routes of infection. High-risk populations of HB_sAg are also at risk for HDV infections: intravenous drug users, recipients of blood products, male homosexuals, and mentally retarded individuals.[15,16] Horizontal transmission occurs in households, and infections increase in non-hygienic, crowded living conditions.[16] Mosquitoes have been shown to be a vehicle for transmission of HDV in epidemics.[16]

Clinical Manifestations

HDV infection occurs as either acute or chronic infection in conjunction with concomitant HBV infection. Acute infection can occur in one of two forms: coinfection with acute HBV infection or superinfection of a chronic HBV infection. In cases of acute HDV-HBV coinfection, either both viruses are cleared rapidly or the patient progresses to fulminant hepatitis. There is a higher incidence of fulminant hepatitis and cases of relapse with HDV-HBV coinfection than when HBV is present alone.[16] More than 90% of cases of HDV superinfection of chronic HBV infection progress to chronic HDV infection.[16]

Chronic HDV infection has a poor prognosis for the patient. The severity of liver necrosis, inflammation, and clinical illness are all increased, and cirrhosis often occurs.[16] To date, there are no effective antiviral drugs or immunosuppressive agents for treatment of chronic infections. Vaccination against HBV also provides immunity to HDV because HDV is not infectious and cannot replicate without HBV helper functions.

Laboratory Diagnosis

Because HDV requires helper functions from HBV, only HB$_s$Ag-positive persons need to be tested for HDV infection. The first HDV marker to appear is HDV antigen (HDV-Ag). HDV-Ag is transient in serum (1 to 4 days) and appears prior to symptomatology and elevation of liver enzymes. For this reason, HDV-Ag is rarely detected, even though RIA, ELISA, and DNA probes exist for its detection. With the decline of HDV-Ag, IgM antibodies to HDV (IgM anti-HDV) appear (seroconversion), followed by low levels of IgG antibodies (IgG anti-HDV) in acute infection. The progression to high levels of IgG anti-HDV in HB$_s$Ag-positive individuals signals the switch to chronic HDV infection. Diagnosis of acute versus chronic HDV infection should be based on detection of IgM anti-HDV and total anti-HDV (IgM and IgG) in HB$_s$Ag-positive persons using commercially available RIA or ELISA kits.

HEPATITIS E

Hepatitis E Virus

Hepatitis E virus (HEV) is the agent of epidemic or enterically transmitted cases of hepatitis, formerly classified along with HCV as the non-A, non-B hepatitis enteric viral agents.[11] It is a small, non-enveloped, single-stranded RNA virus[11] belonging to the caliciviruses.[9]

Epidemiology

Hepatitis E is a disease of the underdeveloped areas of the world (Asia, Africa, and Mexico),[17] where there are poor sanitation, overcrowding, and unsafe water supplies.[17] All U.S. cases have been linked to recent travel to endemic areas.[11] HEV is transmitted by the fecal-oral route, either through poor personal hygiene or via fecally contaminated drinking water.[17] There have been no reports of secondary transmission.[11]

Clinical Manifestations

Hepatitis E disease is generally an acute, self-limiting disease with symptoms characteristic of hepatitis A: sudden onset of flulike symptoms, such as anorexia, malaise, nausea, and vomiting.[17] The incubation period lasts from 15 to 64 days, and symptoms are generally seen in adults.[9] Mortality is generally low (1% to 2% of cases) but increases to 10% to 20% in pregnant females.[9,17] No chronic cases have been documented. Prevention is achieved through practicing good sanitation in endemic areas.[17] A human vaccine is under development.[9]

Laboratory Diagnosis

In the United States, HEV infections are diagnosed by appropriate symptomology, history of recent travel to endemic areas, and exclusion of other serological hepatitis virus markers. Commercial anti-HEV serological tests exist outside the United States and molecular biology–based, HEV RNA assays have been developed for research purposes.[9]

NON–A-E HEPATITIS

Hepatitis cases that are viral in origin and cannot be attributed to the known five hepatitis viruses are classified as non–A-E hepatitis. It is estimated that 5% to 20% of hepatitis cases fall into this category.[11] Recent research suggests that non–A-E hepatitis may be caused by three new, flavivirus-like RNA viruses, designated GBV-A, GBV-B,[18] and GBV-C[19] (GB are the initials of the patient whose plasma was used for experimentation.) Although much remains to be learned from the study of these new viruses and the development of commercial serological tests to detect them, it is known that patients with non–A-E hepatitis may present with either acute or chronic illness. Serious sequelae of non–A-E hepatitis have been documented, such as liver failure, aplastic anemia, and fatal liver disease.[11]

SUMMARY

The term hepatitis viruses refers to five human hepatotrophic viruses: HAV, HBV, HCV, HDV, and HEV. These viruses have worldwide distribution and are transmitted by parenteral (HBV, HCV, HDV) or fecal-oral (HAV, HEV) routes of infection. Serologic tests to detect virus-specific antigens or antibodies determine the causative viral agent, the immune status of the host, and the clinical stage of infection. HDV is a defective hepatotrophic virus requiring helper functions from HBV to allow its replication and infectivity. Diagnosis of HDV infection is made by demonstrating HDV-specific antibodies in HB$_s$Ag-positive persons. Diagnosis of HEV is made through the serological exclusion of the other four hepatitis viruses.

Case Studies

Case 1

A 26-year-old white male presents to a free clinic with symptoms of anorexia, malaise, vomiting, abdominal pain, and mild jaundice. The patient is a known IV drug abuser. The physician orders liver function tests and an acute hepatitis serum panel. He discovers the following results:

    IgM anti-HAV = nonreactive
    HB$_s$Ag = reactive
    IgM anti-HB$_c$ = reactive
    anti-HCV = nonreactive

Case 1 Study Questions

1. What is the diagnosis?
2. What facts support the diagnosis? Explain the relationship of each fact to the diagnosis.

Case 2

The same white male patient who was previously diagnosed with acute hepatitis B presents to the clinic 7 months later for a follow-up exam. The physician orders liver function tests plus the following chronic hepatitis B serum panel:

    HB$_s$Ag = reactive
    HB$_e$Ag = reactive
    anti-HB$_e$ = reactive

Case 2 Study Questions

1. What is the diagnosis?
2. What additional tests may be run?

References

1. Fody EP, Johnson DF: The serologic diagnosis of viral hepatitis. J Med Technol 4:54, 1987
2. Hollinger FB, Melnick JL: Viral hepatitis. In Lennette EH (ed): Laboratory Diagnosis of Viral Infections, p 293. New York, Marcel Dekker, 1985
3. Tyrell DLJ, Gill MJ: Hepatitis. In Mandell LA, Ralph ED (eds): Essentials of Infectious Diseases, p 241. Boston, Blackwell Scientific, 1985
4. Rubin SJ: Hepatitis viruses. In Howard BJ, Klass J II, Rubin SJ, et al (eds): Clinical and Pathogenic Microbiology, p 817. St. Louis, CV Mosby, 1987
5. Ginsberg HS: Hepatitis viruses. In Davis BD, Dulbecco R, Eisen HN, et al (eds): Microbiology, p 1218. Philadelphia, Harper and Row, 1980
6. Feinstone SM, Kapikian AZ, Purcell RH: Hepatitis A: Detection by immune electron microscopy of a virus-like antigen associated with acute illness. Science 182:1026, 1973
7. Provost PJ, Giesa P, McAleer WJ, et al: Isolation of hepatitis A virus (in vitro) in cell culture directly from human specimens. Proc Soc Exp Biol Med 167:201, 1987
8. Kuhns M: Viral hepatitis: Treatment, prevention, and special precautions. Lab Med 26:786, 1995
9. Larsen JT, Larsen HS: Viral hepatitis: An overview. Clin Lab Sci 8:169, 1995
10. Larsen JT: Hepatitis C. Clin Lab Sci 8:273, 1995
11. Kuhns M: Viral hepatitis: Discovery, diagnostic tests, and new viruses. Lab Med 26:650, 1995
12. Faruki H: New developments in diagnostics for hepatitis B and C. Clin Lab Sci 8:174, 1995
13. Abbott Diagnostics: Hepatitis Sliderule. Abbott Park, IL, Abbott Diagnostics Educational Services, 1991
14. Rizzetto M, Canese MG, Arico S, et al: Immunofluorescence detection of a new antigen-antibody system associated to the hepatitis B virus in the liver and in the serum of HB$_s$Ag carriers. Gut 18:997, 1977
15. Bonino F, Smedile A, Verme G: Hepatitis delta virus infections. Adv Intern Med 32:345, 1987
16. Govindarajan S: Delta hepatitis: What have we learned in the last decade? Lab Mgt 26:36, 1988
17. Alter M, Goldschmidt R, Swartz J: Principles in Practice: Testing for Viral Hepatitis. Abbott Park, IL, Abbott Diagnostics Educational Services, 1994
18. Zuckerman AJ: The new GB hepatitis viruses. Lancet 345:1453, 1995
19. Simmons JN, Leary TP, Dawson GJ, et al: Isolation of novel virus-like sequences associated with human hepatitis. Nature Med 1:564, 1995

CHAPTER 26

Human Immunodeficiency Virus Infection and Serology

Ann Marie McNamara

Objectives

Upon completion of the chapter, the reader will be able to:

1. Describe the HIV virus, its structure, and its life cycle
2. Compare and contrast the epidemiology of HIV-1 and HIV-2 infections
3. Describe the clinical manifestations of AIDS and current therapy
4. Describe the laboratory diagnosis of HIV infections, including the appropriate use of screening and supplemental antibody tests
5. Describe several tests for directly detecting HIV viremia

The goal of this chapter is to show how immunologic methods can be used in the identification of human immunodeficiency virus (HIV), not to provide all the details of how HIV interferes with the body's immune response. Many articles have reviewed the effects of HIV on the immune system, and the interested reader is referred to this literature.[1–5]

HUMAN IMMUNODEFICIENCY VIRUS

The first case of AIDS was reported to the Centers for Disease Control and Prevention (CDC) in June 1981.[5] Since then this disease has reached epidemic proportions in the United States, with more than 66,000 cases reported in 1988[6] and 400,000 cases reported by 1993.[7] It has been estimated that the cumulative total number of worldwide cases was 10 to 12 million in 1993.[8] More than 80% of persons diagnosed as having the disease for 3 or more years have died.[9] To date, there is no cure.

The etiologic agent of the acquired immunodeficiency syndrome (AIDS) is a human retrovirus known as the human immunodeficiency virus (HIV). Retroviruses are RNA viruses that contain reverse transcriptase, an enzyme that makes DNA from the viral RNA. Two types of HIV have been found: HIV-1, the causative agent of AIDS in the United States and Europe, and HIV-2, associated with immunodeficiency and a less severe clinical syndrome seen in West Africa that is similar to AIDS.[10] The vast majority of U.S. cases are caused by HIV-1 infections. Approximately 50 cases of HIV-2 have been reported in the United States, and all were linked to recent travel to endemic areas. For this reason, HIV in this chapter shall refer to HIV-1 unless otherwise noted.

HIV, formerly known as lymphadenopathy-associated virus (LAV),[11] human T-cell lymphotrophic virus type III (HTLV-III),[12] or AIDS-related virus (ARV),[13] is closely related to a group of nontransforming, cytopathic retroviruses called lentiviruses. Lentiviruses cause chronic neurodegenerative and wasting diseases in animals, similar to the wasting disease and neurologic disorders produced by HIV in humans. Based on studies of crossreactions of viral proteins, HIV has been shown to be closely related to simian T-cell lymphotrophic virus type III (STLV-III). STLV-III causes a form of AIDS in African green monkeys, suggesting that HIV originated from a monkey virus prevalent in Africa that adapted to human hosts.

HIV Structure

The HIV virus particle, or virion, is approximately 100 nm in diameter. It consists of three parts: an outer envelope, a core shell of protein, and a cone-shaped inner core that contains the viral RNA (Fig. 26-1). Small viral surface proteins form a regular geometric structure that resembles a soccer ball in that it consists of pentagons and hexagons combined to form a spherical shape. These proteins are embedded in a lipid bilayer. At regular intervals in this surface structure, a large glycoprotein traverses the lipid bilayer membrane and pro-

trudes above the surface in a knoblike structure. This glycoprotein (gp) has two components: gp41 traverses the membrane, and gp120 extends beyond the surface as a knob. The names of these proteins are derived from their molecular weight (gp41 = glycoprotein of 41 kDa). The gp120 component is highly immunogenic (it provokes an immune response). The outer envelope also contains human leukocyte antigens. These antigens are derived from human cell membranes when new HIV virions bud from human cells during the process of virus particle formation.

Beneath the outer envelope lies a protein core composed of the viral proteins p24 and p17. Inside the protein core shell lies a cone-shaped central core containing the viral RNA and reverse transcriptase. The reverse transcriptase is unique to retroviruses and allows the viral RNA to be transcribed into DNA for incorporation into the infected human host cells' genome.

HIV Genome

Complete nucleotide sequences of the HIV-1 and HIV-2 genomes have been determined,[14,15] making it possible to identify viral genes and some of the relationships between viral gene products and the clinical course of AIDS. The HIV genome is unique among retroviruses in its complexity. It has at least five regulatory genes (*tat*, *art/trs*, *sor*, *3'orf*, and *R*), in addition to the usual structural genes (*gag*, *pol*, and *env*; Fig. 26-2).

The *gag* (group antigen) gene codes for the core proteins. These proteins are cleaved from a large polypro-

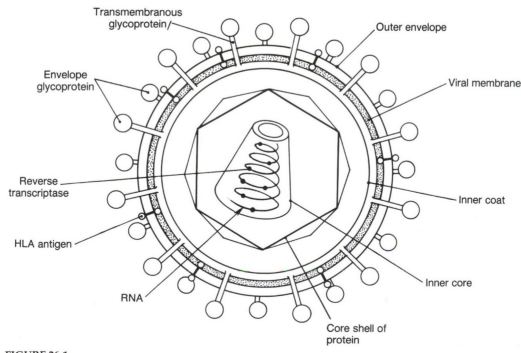

FIGURE 26-1
Structure of the HIV virion.

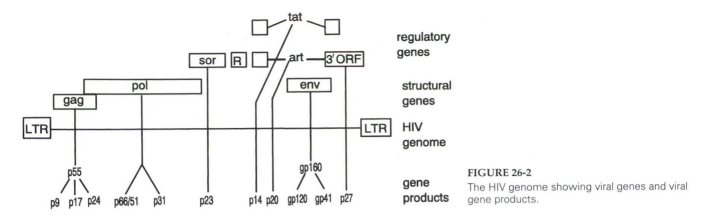

FIGURE 26-2
The HIV genome showing viral genes and viral gene products.

tein of 55 kDa, which is found in high levels in infected cells. The cleavage products form the three core structural proteins, p17, p24, and p9. The *pol* (*polymerase*) gene codes for four enzymes: reverse transcriptase, RNAse, protease, and integrase. Reverse transcriptase transcribes single-stranded RNA into double-stranded DNA. It is an immunogenic protein and is designated p66/51. RNAse is an enzyme that digests the RNA in RNA-DNA hybrids that form as intermediates in the creation of viral DNA. Protease (p31) cleaves itself from an initial polyprotein and cleaves other enzymes and structural proteins from their polyproteins. Integrase is responsible for inserting the viral DNA into the host DNA.

The *env* (*envelope*) gene codes for the glycoprotein gp160, which is found in infected cells. It is cleaved to form the two envelope glycoproteins gp120, found on the outside of the viral envelope, and gp41, which is embedded in the viral membrane. The *sor* (*short open reading frame*) gene is related to viral infectivity. It produces a protein, p23, which is present in the filtrate of virus-infected cultures and against which antibodies form in the serum of HIV-infected persons.[16] The *tat* (*trans-activation translation*) gene accelerates viral protein production and is required for viral replication. Without *tat* only minimal RNA is produced, and no virus particles are formed.[17] The protein produced by *tat* is p14.

Between *sor* and *tat* on the viral genome lies the *R* (*reading frame*) gene, which codes for an immunogenic product (p15) of unknown function.[18] The *art/trs* (*antirepression transactivator*) gene regulates the translation of the viral genome.[19] It produces an antirepression transactivator protein p20, which regulates the expression of viral gene components. The *B3'orf* (*3'open reading frame*) gene is responsible for the latency of the virus, slowing down viral reproduction 10-fold in CD4 cells. The p27 protein produced by *B3'orf* raises antibodies that have been found in infected persons.[20] At each end of the viral genome are identical sequences (LTR = *long terminal repeats*) containing a terminator, an enhancer, and a promoter for the process of transcription.

All the protein and glycoprotein gene products (p and gp in Fig. 26-2) appear to be specific for HIV and may induce an antibody response in an infected person. Studies indicate that the first antibody to be observed in HIV-infected persons is directed against the p24 core protein, followed by a mixture of antibodies, usually including antibodies to the gp41 envelope glycoprotein.[21] In enzyme linked immunosorbent assays (ELISA) and Western blot (WB) studies of 280 specimens from AIDS and AIDS-related complex (ARC) patients, 96% of patients had antibodies to p24 and 88% had antibodies to gp41.[22] These antibodies are typically seen in both symptomatic and asymptomatic HIV-seropositive individuals and act as markers of HIV infection. Declining p24 antibody titers occur in the late stages of AIDS, when patients clinically deteriorate (Fig. 26-3 on p. 260). Antibodies to the envelope gene products (gp160, gp120, and gp41) can be detected in nearly all HIV-positive patients, and antibodies to the polymerase gene products (p31, p51, and p66) are also commonly detected.[23] Other antibodies are detected less consistently.

The nucleotide sequences of the HIV-2 genome have also been determined. The HIV-2 genome structure is similar to that of HIV-1, but the structural genes code for different proteins (gene products) of different molecular weights than in HIV-1 (see Fig. 26-2). In HIV-2, the *gag* proteins are p15, p26, and p55; the *env* proteins are gp34, gp120, and gp140; and the *pol* gene products are p31 and p55/58/68.[4,8] The different gene products produced by the HIV-1 and HIV-2 strains make it possible to develop specific HIV-1 and HIV-2 antibody tests to differentiate infections caused by these two viruses.

HIV Life Cycle

The HIV genome carries within it the genetic information required to reproduce HIV viruses within infected host cells. HIV binds to host cells through a complexing of the gp120 molecule on the viral surface and a receptor molecule—the CD4 molecule on host cells. CD4 molecules are found on the surface of some immune cells (helper T lymphocytes, B cells, mono-

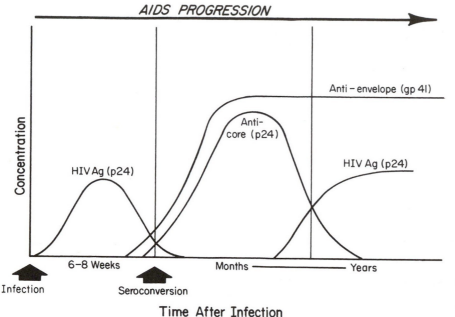

FIGURE 26-3

Antigen and antibody response in HIV infection.

cytes, and macrophages) and on some phagocytic cells found in the nervous system (monocytes and macrophages). Although CD4 receptors have also been identified on some glial cells and neuroleukin receptors have been identified on neurons that are capable of binding gp120, their clinical importance is still uncertain.

After HIV binds to the CD4-containing cell, it penetrates the host cell and loses its outer layers to expose the viral RNA. The viral RNA is transcribed into DNA and inserted into the host genome during cellular division or activation. Host cells can be activated by antigenic challenge or by allogenic stimulation after exposure to blood, semen, or allografts.

Once activated, transcription of viral proteins occurs. Viral RNA and proteins are then assembled at the host cell's cytoplasmic surface to produce a mature virion that escapes the host cell by budding from the host cell membrane (Fig. 26-4). When HIV replication occurs, the CD4 cell is killed, resulting in severe depletion of helper-inducer T lymphocytes. It is the depletion of these cells that correlates with the progressive severity of immune deficiency and with the increased susceptibility to opportunistic disease and malignancies seen in the clinical course of AIDS (Table 26-1).

EFFECT OF HIV
ON THE IMMUNE RESPONSE

Detailed information on the normal mechanisms of the immune response can be found in earlier chapters (see Chapter 3), and details of the effects of HIV on the im-

mune response can be found in the literature. HIV is so devastating primarily because of the destruction of CD4-containing cells and their central role in mediating the immune response. Helper T lymphocytes have a high concentration of CD4 molecules on their surface and are the major targets of HIV virions. The depletion of these cells as a result of HIV infection results in severe depression of the immune response (Table 26-2). The loss of CD4-positive cells correlates closely with the severity of the clinical course of AIDS.[24] Particularly important are the increased viral, protozoal, and fungal infections found in AIDS patients as a direct result of an impaired cell-mediated immune system (see Table 26-1). Cytotoxic-suppressor T cells expressing CD8 do not appear

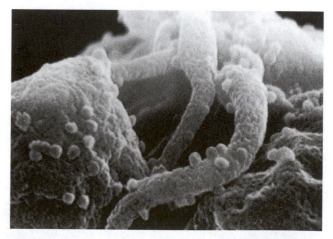

FIGURE 26-4

Scanning electron micrograph of HIV-infected CD4 lymphocytes showing virus budding from the plasma membrane of the lymphocytes. (Courtesy of CDC Archives.)

TABLE 26-1
Partial List of Conditions Included in the 1993 AIDS Surveillance Case Definition

OPPORTUNISTIC INFECTIONS

Bacteria

Mycobacterium avium-intracellulare

Mycobacterium kansasii

Mycobacterium tuberculosis

Salmonella species

Viruses

Cytomegalovirus

Herpes simplex virus

Protozoa

Pneumocystis carinii

Toxoplasma gondii

Cryptosporidium species

Isospora belli

Fungi

Candida albicans

Coccidioides immitis

Histoplasma capsulatum

Cryptococcus neoformans

NEOPLASMS

Kaposi sarcoma

Burkitt-like lymphoma

Undifferentiated non-Hodgkin's lymphoma

Invasive cervical cancer

Central nervous system lymphoma

Peripheral organ lymphoma

Immunoblastic sarcoma

Lymphocytic preleukemia

TABLE 26-2
Effect of HIV on the Immune Response

EFFECT ON T CELLS

Depletion of CD4 lymphocytes

Elevated, normal, or depressed suppressor CD8 lymphocytes

Increased susceptibility to opportunistic infections and neoplasms because of decreased T-cell function

Decreased delayed-type hypersensitivity

Decreased ability to promote help to B lymphocytes

Decreased production of interleukin-2

EFFECT ON B CELLS

Polyclonal hypergammaglobulinemia

Elevated circulating immune complexes

Inability to produce a serologic response to a new antigen or following immunization

Increased numbers of spontaneous Ig-secreting cells

Refractory to B-cell activation signals in vitro

EFFECT ON OTHER IMMUNE CELLS

Decreased natural killer cell activity

Defective chemotaxis in monocytes and macrophages

Enhanced release of interleukin-1 and cachectin by monocytes

OTHER SEROLOGIC ABNORMALITIES

Increased circulating α-interferon

Increased α_1-thymosin

Increased β_2-microglobulin

Increased serum and urinary neopterin

to be infected by HIV.[1] An early immunologic marker of HIV infection is an inverted helper-suppressor (CD4/CD8) cell ratio.

CLINICAL FEATURES

Epidemiology

As of 1993, there have been 400,000 reported cases of AIDS in the United States.[8] Adult AIDS victims can be broken down into the following groups: 49% homosexual or bisexual men, 27% intravenous (IV) drug users, 10% heterosexual men and women, 3% recipients of contaminated blood or blood-product transfusions (usually prior to 1985), 1% people with hemophilia or other coagulation disorders, and 3% unknown risk factors.[4,6] U.S. adult cases broken down by race are as follows: 59% white, 26% black, and 14% Hispanic.[6] Of the pediatric AIDS cases reported, 15% to 40% of the infections occurred perinatally, and most can be traced to IV drug use by the child's mother or father.[5,8]

HIV has been isolated from a variety of body fluids, cells, and tissues of infected persons: mononuclear cells, plasma, semen, cervical-vaginal secretions, saliva, tears, urine, breast milk, cerebrospinal fluid, lymph nodes, brain, and bone marrow.[25] Transmission of the virus has been documented by one of three routes: sexual transmission (heterosexual, bisexual, or homosexual), parenteral transmission (through blood or blood products or by sharing blood-contaminated drug paraphernalia), and perinatal transmission (transplacental transmission and possibly through breast milk).[25] There are no accounts of HIV infection transmitted by food, water, insects, or casual contact with HIV-infected individuals.[26]

HIV-2 was first identified in patients in West Africa in 1986.[8] It has since spread to Europe, India, and Brazil.[8] HIV-2 infection is rare in the United States, with approximately 50 cases reported by 1993 and linked to recent travel or contact with persons in endemic areas. HIV-2 infections are primarily transmitted through sexual contact, blood transfusions, or vertically from HIV-2–infected mothers to infants.[27] The clinical syndrome is similar to HIV-1 infection, but the clinical manifestations are less severe and the viral load is lower than in HIV-1 infection.[8] HIV-2 is estimated to be 3 times less efficiently transmitted sexually and 10 times less efficiently transmitted vertically than HIV-1.[8] Patients often appear asymptomatic but seropositive for HIV-2 antibodies. The rate of progression to full-blown AIDS symptomology is six to eight times higher in HIV-1 infection than in HIV-2.[4]

Clinical Manifestations

HIV infection results in a spectrum of disease presentations, from an apparently healthy state (asymptomatic infection), to symptomatic infection, to severe T-cell depletion with complicating opportunistic infections and cancers (AIDS). The intermediate state had been called AIDS-related complex (ARC). The symptoms of ARC are now considered as stages in HIV infection.

HIV infection generally manifests itself initially as a mononucleosis-like illness followed by either asymptomatic infection or chronic lymphadenopathy in HIV-antibody–positive, otherwise healthy individuals.[23] Estimates state that 25% to 50% of persons with subclinical HIV infections progress to full-blown AIDS over a 5 to 10 year period.[8,28] The disease then progresses to symptomatic infection with persistent lymphadenopathy and quantitative T-cell deficiencies (especially a decreased CD4-positive cell count and an inverted CD4/CD8 ratio), but without the typical opportunistic infections and cancers seen in AIDS. Patients typically present with prolonged constitutional symptoms of fatigue, night sweats, fever, diarrhea, and weight loss (HIV wasting syndrome).[28]

Beginning in 1993, the Revised Classification System for HIV Infection and Expanded AIDS Surveillance Case Definition for Adolescents and Adults was recommended by the Centers for Disease Control and Prevention.[29] The criteria of an HIV infection in a person ≥13 years of age includes: (1) repeatedly reactive screening tests for HIV antibody with specific antibody identified by a supplemental test, (2) direct identification of virus in host tissues by viral isolation, (3) HIV antigen detection, or (4) a positive result on any other highly specific licensed test for HIV. In an HIV-infected person, the CD4+ T-cell counts (or percentage) and clinical findings are used to classify the disease, as shown in Table 26-3.

The CD4+ T-cell category is used to gauge the degree of HIV-related immunosuppression and guides the clinical and therapeutic actions to manage the care of individuals infected with HIV. Clinical Category A consists of documented HIV infection that is asymptomatic or with persistent generalized lymphadenopathy or acute primary HIV infection. Clinical Category B consists of symptomatic conditions in an HIV-infected adolescent or adult not included in Category C and the conditions must be attributed to HIV infection, indicative of a defect in cell-mediated immunity, or must have a clinical course complicated by HIV infection. Clinical Category C consists of those conditions that are considered to be AIDS-indicator conditions and includes specific opportunistic infections and malignancies. A partial list is presented in Table 26-1.

The expanded AIDS surveillance case definition for adolescents and adults includes all persons in Clinical Category C and all persons with CD4+ T cells counts <200 cells/μL regardless of the clinical category. The reader is urged to consult the CDC guidelines for additional information.[4,29]

Therapy and Vaccine Development

Treatment of HIV infection has largely been limited to the treatment of opportunistic infections and cancers that are complications of AIDS.[30] With increased knowledge of the structure and replicative cycle of HIV, new drugs that inhibit HIV binding to CD4 receptors, inhibit viral replication, or reduce viral budding from cell membranes have been developed. The

---

TABLE 26-3
1993 Revised Classification System for HIV Infection and Expanded AIDS Surveillance Case Definition for Adolescents and Adults

CD4+ T-CELL CATEGORIES	CLINICAL CATEGORIES		
	Asymptomatic, acute (primary) HIV or PGL†	*Symptomatic, not (A) or (C) conditions**	*AIDS-indicator conditions**
(1) ≥500/μL	A1	B1	C1
(2) 200–499/μL	A2	B2	C2
(3) <200/μL AIDS-indicator T-cell count	A3	B3	C3

*The shaded cells illustrate the expanded AIDS surveillance case definition. Persons with AIDS-indicator conditions (Category C) as well as those with CD4+ T-lymphocyte counts <200/μL (Categories A3 or B3) will be reportable as AIDS cases in the United States and Territories, effective January 1, 1993.

†PGL = persistent generalized lymphadenopathy. Clinical Category A includes acute (primary) HIV infection.

(Centers for Disease Control and Prevention. 1993 revised classification system for HIV and expanded surveillance case definition for AIDS among adolescents and adults. MMWR 1992; 41[No. RR-17]:1–4.)

most widely administered drug is 3'azido-3'deoxythymidine, called zidovudine (formerly azidothymidine or AZT). This compound is an inhibitor of reverse transcriptase and is also a DNA chain terminator. Clinical trials have shown that zidovudine reduces mortality, morbidity, and the number of opportunistic infections in AIDS patients.[32] This drug is orally absorbed and crosses the blood-brain barrier. Side effects include megaloblastic anemia, neutropenia, nausea, insomnia, and myalgia.[30] Other drugs that inhibit reverse transcriptase and/or cause DNA chain termination include dideoxycytidine (ddC), dideoxyinosine (ddI), phosphonoformate, Zerit (d4T), epivir (3TC), and rifabutin.[4,33]

The inhibitors of reverse transciptase, ddI and ddC, are used in treating advanced cases of AIDS. ddI is used in treating adults infected with HIV who have received prolonged prior zidovudine therapy, and ddC is used in combination with zidovudine in advanced AIDS cases.[4] The drugs saquinavir (invirase), Ritonàvir, and Norvir are protease inhibitors that interfere with the reproductive cycle of HIV and slow the spread of the virus in the body. In one clinical trial, Ritonàvir decreased the mortality rate of advanced AIDS cases by 40% compared with a control group.[31] Ritonàvir side effects included diarrhea, nausea, vomiting, weakness, tingling, and an altered sense of taste.[31]

Another treatment strategy is to produce anti-idiotypic antibodies to the CD4 binding site or to create soluble CD4 (called rCD4) molecules that will block the CD4 binding site and prevent HIV binding to patient cells.[33] α-Interferon, which reduces viral budding from infected cell surfaces, has been shown to be of use in the treatment of Kaposi sarcoma.[34] All HIV drugs to date help to slow the progress of the disease but fail to evoke a cure.

Development of an effective HIV vaccine is problematic for two reasons: the antigenic diversity found among isolates of HIV and the lack of good animal models for vaccine trials. A good HIV vaccine should be able to protect against all viral strains and both viral types. However, the immunogenic envelope proteins of HIV-1 strains and HIV-2 show high degrees of antigenic variation.[35] A good vaccine strategy would be to develop a vaccine composed of single or multiple recombinant virus proteins derived from the more highly conserved shared core proteins of HIV-1 strains and HIV-2.[35] Animal models have been limited to the chimpanzee, which develops viremia followed by antibody production after infection but fails to develop immunodeficiency.[36] Chimpanzees are also rare and expensive, and this has limited animal trials.

Despite problems inherent in developing an HIV vaccine, many vaccines have been developed and several are in clinical trials. Three types of vaccines have been developed: genetically engineered HIV subunit vaccines (combined with adjuvant or in a virus vector), anti-idiotype vaccines (antibodies against CD4), and killed-virus vaccine.[36] These vaccines have been directed against HIV-1, HIV-2, or both viruses. Clinical trials are still being conducted to determine the effectiveness of these vaccines.

LABORATORY DIAGNOSIS

General Principles

Since the discovery of HIV, a variety of methods has been devised to isolate HIV, to detect HIV antibodies, and to detect HIV antigen in patients' blood and body fluids. Isolation of HIV and methods to detect HIV antigen are primarily used to detect early HIV infection before antibodies develop, to monitor the effectiveness of antiviral drugs, and to detect the progression of asymptomatic to symptomatic HIV infection by monitoring an increase in p24 antigen. In 1996, the U.S. Food and Drug Administration required that the blood supply be tested for p24. Detection of HIV antigen in patient samples indicates active HIV infection, whereas detection of antibodies to HIV denotes prior exposure to HIV.[24] HIV antibody tests are of two major classes: screening tests and supplementary tests.

ELISA tests to detect HIV antibodies were first developed to screen the nation's blood supply. AIDS is a clinical diagnosis based on the presence of signs and symptoms of the disease. One may have antibodies to HIV, signifying HIV exposure, and yet be healthy. These antibody-positive, asymptomatic persons harbor active virus and have the potential to transmit the virus to noninfected persons years before developing signs and symptoms of AIDS. The Centers for Disease Control and Prevention recommendations state that HIV-antibody–reactive persons should be regarded as capable of transmitting infection[37] and their blood and mucus secretions should be handled accordingly.

Since false positive and false negative tests occur with the ELISA screening test for a variety of reasons, all "repeatedly reactive" ELISA samples are confirmed by a supplementary test. A reactive supplementary test confirms the presence of HIV antibody and is therefore indicative of past exposure and, presumably, current HIV infection.[23] The most widely used supplemental tests are the Western blot assay and the indirect immunofluorescence assay.

Genetic probes for HIV viral RNA or proviral DNA for use in molecular hybridization techniques have been developed. The advantage of HIV probes is the ability to detect HIV genomes directly in cells infected with latent or actively replicating HIV viruses when other serologic markers may be absent.

Polymerase chain reaction (PCR) assays have been developed that detect nucleic acid gene sequences specific to HIV-1, HIV-2, or both viruses. These assays directly detect the proviral DNA sequences of the virus or the HIV RNA.[8] Their usefulness resides in resolving the infection status of individuals whose serum tests "indeterminate" in screening tests and for determining the infection status of infants born to HIV-infected women whose maternal antibody masks the infant's true serological response.

Detection of HIV-2 infections is currently possible by using crossreacting ELISA tests for HIV-1 and by modifying current methods to identify HIV-2 antibodies, proteins, and genes. HIV-1 and HIV-2 show genomic similarity in their *gag* and *pol* gene regions (56% and 66% nucleotide sequence homology, respectively).[38] Thus, HIV-2–positive sera may crossreact with HIV-1 core proteins, but probably not with HIV-1 envelope proteins. Because of crossreactive core proteins, five current HIV-1 ELISA tests have been shown to detect 42% to 92% of HIV-2 infections in blood samples.[39] Tests made more specific for detecting HIV-2 infections have been devised using HIV-2–derived recombinant proteins (especially envelope proteins in ELISA and Western blot tests), HIV-2–specific DNA probes, and PCR assays.

Although the number of HIV-2 infections in the United States remains low, the U.S. Food and Drug Administration recommended in 1992 that the U.S. blood supply (blood, blood components, plasma, or leukocytes) be routinely screened for HIV-2.[27] Blood donor screening in such situations can be performed by using a combination HIV-1/HIV-2 ELISA test or by a specific HIV-2 ELISA. Testing regimens follow those for diagnosing an HIV-1 infection in that repeatedly positive ELISA tests are subjected to supplemental HIV-1 specific tests. The most commonly used supplemental tests are HIV-2–specific Western blot assays or immunofluorescence assays. If a combination HIV-1/HIV-2 ELISA test is used as a screen, HIV-2 infection should be suspected when the ELISA screen is positive and the Western blot is indeterminate (or indeterminate but reactive for *gag* or *pol* only) or negative, or a supplemental immunofluorescence assay is negative. In situations other than blood bank testing, the CDC advises selective testing of patient sera for HIV-2 based on the clinical symptoms of the patient and patient risk factors.[27] Testing for HIV-2 is warranted in patients with opportunistic infections suggestive of AIDS yet with negative HIV tests; when HIV-1 Western blot assays are indeterminate; with patients of West African origin, sexual contact with West Africans, or blood transfusions in West Africa (or other affected regions of the world); or birth to an HIV-2–infected mother.[27]

All tests described in the next section refer to HIV-1 detection. However, the reader should keep in mind that, in combination HIV-1/HIV-2 ELISA tests, serologic crossreactions to HIV-2 can occur and that all test methods can be modified to produce specific HIV-2 tests.

Laboratory Methods

HIV ISOLATION

Isolation of HIV from patients' cells and body fluids is not routinely performed in medical laboratories. This procedure is costly (several hundred dollars), is time consuming (generally taking 15 to 30 days), requires adequate safety containment facilities, and may expose personnel to high virus concentrations.[23,40] Cocultivation is usually performed using patient and HIV-negative donor peripheral blood monocytes. Monocytes are collected from peripheral blood samples by Ficoll-Hypaque gradients. Donor monocytes are stimulated with phytohemagglutinin for 2 to 4 days before mixing with patient monocytes and interleukin-2. The cell mixture is cocultivated in tissue culture flasks with added cell culture medium for up to 1 month.[24] Culture fluid is removed on a weekly basis and tested for the presence of HIV by reverse transcriptase assays, antigen indirect immunofluorescence assay, antigen ELISA testing, or PCR assays. Isolation of HIV can also be performed in two cell lines found to support HIV growth, H9 cells and CEM cells. Isolation of HIV from patient specimens has two main purposes: to detect HIV antigen in early infection before antibodies form and to monitor antiviral drug therapy (successful therapy results in decreased viral isolation).

ENZYME-LINKED IMMUNOSORBENT ASSAY

The ELISA test is the most widely used screening test for HIV antibodies. It is simple to perform, relatively inexpensive, and adaptable to screening large numbers of specimens in a short time (4 hours). It is the test format of choice for screening the U.S. blood supply.

HIV antigens derived from either disrupted virus particles (first-generation assays), recombinant antigens, or chemically synthesized peptides (second- and third-generation assays) are immobilized onto microtiter wells or plastic or metal beads. Patient serum or plasma is then incubated with the fixed antigen and washed. Anti-IgG antibody, conjugated to either horseradish peroxidase, glucose oxidase, or alkaline phosphatase, is then added and allowed to incubate. After a washing step, the appropriate chromogenic enzymatic substrate is added and a color change occurs that is proportional to the amount of human IgG present. Results are read on a spectrophotometer by comparing values obtained from positive and negative controls with those from the test sample. This results in an absorbance cutoff value above which a reactive test is defined. IgM antibodies can also be detected if the ELISA test is modified to include a mixture of heavy- and light-chain antibodies to human immunoglobulin.

The ELISA test has also been modified into a competitive assay format for detecting HIV antibody. In this test, patient serum or plasma samples are incubated with enzyme-labeled HIV antibodies in microtiter wells coated with HIV antigens. Patient and enzyme-labeled HIV antibodies then compete for binding sites on the immobilized HIV antigens. The more unbound patient HIV antibody that binds to the antigen, the less labeled HIV antibody binds and the less color development occurs when the substrate is added. Therefore, color development is inversely proportional to the amount of HIV antibodies present in the patient's sample.

There are several potential sources of error in ELISA testing for HIV antibodies. In addition to technical error, false positive and negative reactions occur. False positive reactions occur in persons with autoimmune diseases (shared-membrane antigens between the HIV virion and the human host cell, i.e., T-cell antigens, HLA antigens, and nuclear and cellular antigens), alcoholism, lymphoproliferative diseases, adult T-cell leukemia-lymphoma, syphilis, and with no known risk.[23,41] False negative reactions occur during the incubation stages of HIV infection (between the time of infection and the development of detectable antibodies); in the late stages of AIDS, when antibody titers typically decrease; when envelope glycoproteins (i.e., gp41 and gp120) are lost during overstringent purification methods; or when there is insufficient p24 in antigen mixtures as a result of glycoprotein enrichment procedures.[42]

When an ELISA test is "reactive," it is repeated in duplicate to rule out technical error. If the specimen is reactive in two out of three tests, it is termed *repeatedly reactive* and a supplementary test is performed to confirm the positive ELISA result.

Although the sensitivity and specificity of ELISA antibody tests are better than 98% when compared with Western blot assays,[23] an important concept in ELISA testing is the predictive value positive (PVP) of a positive result. The PVP tells the probability of a positive (reactive) test being a true positive. It is dependent upon the prevalence of a disease in a given population. Populations having a low disease prevalence have a low PVP, and populations with a high disease prevalence have a high PVP. Therefore, a reactive ELISA test in a high-risk person or population is most likely indicative of true infection, whereas a reactive test result in a low-risk individual or population may indicate a false positive test.[42] For illustration, Reesink

et al. showed that the PVP of a positive ELISA test was 100% in a population of AIDS and ARC patients (a high-prevalence group) but was between 5% and 100% when blood donors (a low-prevalence group) were tested.[43]

ELISA tests have also been modified to detect HIV antigen in serum, plasma, culture fluids, and cerebrospinal fluid. In these tests an antibody sandwich technique is used in which monoclonal or polyclonal anti-HIV antibody is coated to the microwell or bead; a patient sample is added, incubated, and washed; and rabbit or goat anti-HIV antibody is added. If the patient's sample contains HIV antigen, an antibody-antigen-antibody complex is formed. Enzyme-conjugated antibody to rabbit or goat immunoglobulin is then added, followed by the appropriate substrate in a typical ELISA format. Because antibodies to p24 proteins have higher binding affinities to HIV antigen than other HIV antibodies, these ELISA kits primarily detect free p24 HIV antigens.[44]

If the ELISA antigen test is repeatedly reactive, an antibody neutralization assay is performed on the specimen.[23] In this assay the patient specimen is incubated with human antibody to HIV before performing the ELISA antigen test. If HIV antigen is present in the specimen, it will be neutralized by the human antibody and attachment to the ELISA antibody-coated microwell or bead will not occur. This results in a reduction in absorbance when compared with a concomitant nonabsorbed patient specimen. Specific p24 core antigen ELISA assays lack sensitivity because of the formation of immune complexes between p24 antigen and host antibodies. To increase the sensitivity of the p24 antigen assay, a procedure to dissociate the resultant immune complexes has been developed. This immune complex dissociation (ICD) procedure uses glycine buffer at pH 2.0 to preferentially denature host antibodies and to unmask the p24 antigen.[4] The p24 antigen is a marker of early (before host antibodies form) or late (immune system depletion and concomitant virus particle increase) HIV infections.[4] The ICD procedure is useful for following antigenemia in seropositive individuals or for diagnosis of infant infection when maternal antibodies are present.[4]

SLIDE AGGLUTINATION TESTS

Rapid slide agglutination (SA) tests for detecting the presence of HIV antibodies or antigens have been developed. These tests are being widely used in field work in Africa to detect HIV antibodies in blood products and patients. These screening tests offer distinct advantages over the currently used ELISA antibody tests because they are simple to perform, they require 5 minutes to 2 hours of technician time, heat inactivation of serum does not affect test results, all materials are portable, results can be read with the naked eye, and no costly equipment is needed.[45,46] In addition, SA tests simultaneously detect both IgG and IgM HIV antibodies.[45]

The principle of SA tests is that of an antigen-antibody reaction made visible on a slide by linking the detector antigens or antibodies to polystyrene or polyvinyl beads,[46] or to gelatin carriers.[45] When detector antigens (for HIV antibody tests) or antibodies (for HIV antigen tests) are mixed with the patient serum or plasma on a slide, a visible agglutination reaction is formed if the patient's sample contains HIV antibody or antigen, respectively.

WESTERN BLOT ASSAY

The Western blot (WB) assay is the most widely used supplementary test for confirming repeatedly reactive HIV ELISA antibody tests. In this assay HIV virus is disrupted and HIV proteins are separated by molecular weight into discrete bands by electrophoresis onto polyacrylamide gels.[47] The viral proteins are then transferred onto nitrocellulose sheets and cut into strips. Individual strips are incubated overnight with patient serum (HIV antibodies), washed, and incubated with anti–human immunoglobulin conjugated with enzymes or biotin. After addition of the appropriate substrate, color develops to show discrete bands where antigen-antibody reactions have occurred.

The WB assay is cumbersome to perform, is expensive, requires overnight incubation, and is difficult to interpret. Interpretation of positive tests varies between laboratories, depending on which recommendations are followed (i.e., CDC or commercial test kit manufacturers) and individual laboratory experiences. The CDC recommends that test results be called positive when two of three bands—p24, gp41, or gp 120/160—appear.[5] One commercial WB test kit (Biotech/DuPont HIV Western Blot Kit, Wilmington, DE) states that characteristic HIV bands at p24 and p31 plus either gp41 or gp160 must be present for a positive test.

WB tests are negative for HIV antibodies when no bands appear. Indeterminate results occur when there is either isolated reactivity to a single HIV protein (p24, p17, or p55 only) or a pattern of reactivity to multiple proteins from the same viral gene product (i.e., *gag* gene products: p24 and p55) appears.[4,48] When indeterminate results occur, a follow-up patient specimen should be collected in 6 months and the WB assay repeated. In this way, if the patient was in an early stage of HIV infection, additional antibody development should have occurred and a more accurate test interpretation can be made. Alternatively, a direct detection test may be used, such as a gene probe or PCR, to detect the presence of virus.

False positive WB reactions may occur in healthy persons, HTLV-1–infections, bilirubinemia, connective tissue disease, polyclonal gammopathies, and patients with HLA antibodies.[23]

INDIRECT IMMUNOFLUORESCENCE ASSAY

The indirect immunofluorescence assay (IFA) test is growing in popularity as a supplemental test for confirming reactive ELISA tests. The antigen is HIV-infected H9 or HUT 78 cells (malignant T-cell lines) dried and acetone fixed to wells of a glass slide.[49] Patient serum or plasma is then applied, followed by fluorescein-labeled anti–human globulin and washing with an Evans blue counterstain. Results are read on a fluorescence microscope by noting the degree of fluorescence intensity, the percentage of fluorescent cells, and localization of the fluorescence to cell surfaces. It is the envelope proteins gp160 and gp120 that are reacting in the IFA antibody test.[23] The advantages of using the IFA rather than WB as a supplemental test are the IFA's comparable sensitivity and specificity, the simplicity of the test, and rapid results (generally <2 hours).[23,40] Disadvantages include nonspecific staining, the use of expensive fluorescence microscopes, possibly difficult interpretation, the necessity for skilled technologists, and fluorescence that fades quickly so that slides cannot be stored.[23,40]

The IFA test can also be modified to detect HIV antigen in infected cells.[40] In this assay, HIV-infected cells are treated with polyclonal or monoclonal antibody raised against HIV proteins p17 or p24. The assay is then performed in a manner similar to the IFA antibody assay. The p24 IFA test can be combined with flow cytometric analysis to determine the level of viral antigens in patient cells and the frequency of cell expression of this viral antigen.[8] The level of p24 detected in patients' peripheral blood cells by flow cytometric analysis is inversely related to the patient CD4+ count.[8] Therefore, high p24 levels indicate low numbers of CD4+ cells and severe clinical disease.

RADIOIMMUNOASSAY

Radioimmunoassay (RIA) tests for detecting antibodies to HIV are rarely used in diagnostic laboratories because of the use of radioactive materials for labeling antibodies. The principle of the RIA antibody test is similar to that of the competitive binding ELISA test. Radioactively labeled (generally with ^{125}I) HIV antibodies compete with unlabeled patient serum (unlabeled antibody) for binding sites on solid-phase, fixed HIV antigen. Radioactivity of bound antibodies is measured in a gamma counter. The amount of HIV antibodies in the patient's sample is inversely proportional to the number of counts detected.[41]

RADIOIMMUNOPRECIPITATION ASSAY

The radioimmunoprecipitation assay (RIPA) test is mainly a research technique because it is expensive, time consuming, requires the use of radioisotopes, and requires the maintenance of infected cell lines.[23] The principle is that HIV-infected cells are exposed to a radioactive isotope, lysed, and centrifuged in an ultracentrifuge to obtain a cell lysate containing radiolabeled viral proteins. Patient serum is preabsorbed with protein A-Sepharose beads and then mixed with the cell lysate. Immunoprecipitates are formed by boiling in buffer, and the immunoprecipitate is separated by electrophoresis on sodium dodecyl sulfate-polyacrylamide gels. Banding patterns similar to those on WB are formed and interpreted.[23] RIPA tests for detecting viral antigens have also been developed. RIPA tests have been useful in distinguishing HIV-1 from HIV-2 infections.[8]

GENE PROBES

Gene probes that detect HIV genes rather than gene products or protein antigens have been developed. They have not yet gained popularity because of their low sensitivity in detecting HIV directly in cells and tissues. Both radioactively labeled DNA and RNA probes have been produced that can be used in molecular hybridization tests to detect if proviral HIV DNA or RNA is present in a sample. Further research is needed to perfect the use of HIV gene probes, but applications of more sensitive versions of these tests might be to detect latent virus or to monitor antiviral drug therapies.[40]

POLYMERASE CHAIN REACTION

The polymerase chain reaction (PCR) technique is a highly sensitive and specific assay for detecting HIV infection. PCR detects specific gene sequences of the virus, which are selected by forming short complementary nucleotide sequences (primers) that bind to the plus and minus strands of denatured proviral DNA or HIV RNA.[8] Viral genes are amplified in a series of denaturation, renaturation, and elongation of the primers in a reaction mediated by DNA polymerase and controlled temperatures.[8] The amplified gene sequences are then labeled to a radioactively labeled HIV probe, separated into bands based on molecular weight by polyacrylamide gel electrophoresis, and visualized by autoradiography.[8] Alternatively, biotinylated or chemiluminescent-labeled HIV probes may be used to detect the amplified PCR gene segments. PCR assays have been developed that directly detect viremia caused by HIV-1, HIV-2, or both viruses. Advantages of this technique are the ability to distinguish HIV-1 from HIV-2 infections, to diagnose the infection status of infants born to HIV-infected mothers, to detect nonreplicating (latent) virus, and to directly detect HIV in patient blood cells without the need for cocultivation assays.[8] Disadvantages include the complicated nature of the assay, the use of radioactive probes, incorrect selection of primers leading to false positive reactions, and cross-reaction with previously amplified contaminating nucleic acids resulting in false positive reactions.[8] In June, 1996, the first commercial reverse-transcriptase PCR kit, the Amplicor HIV Monitor Test Kit (Roche Molecular Systems, Alameda, CA), was licensed by the U.S. Food and Drug Administration as a surrogate marker to monitor HIV viral load.

PREVENTION OF HIV INFECTION IN HEALTH-CARE WORKERS

Since 1984 there have been reported cases of HIV infection in health-care workers with occupational exposure to HIV but without other known risk factors.[50] Cases involved accidental needle sticks, exposure of blood or body fluids to ungloved hands or skin lesions, exposure of lacerated fingers while working, or unknown exposure. Each day health-care workers are exposed to the blood and body fluids of patients during patient care or in the laboratory. Although the risk of transmission of HIV following a needle stick injury with HIV-contaminated blood is less than 1%,[8,51] health-care workers should take precautions to minimize this risk by appropriate use of protective clothing to minimize direct contact, frequent hand washing, proper use of equipment to prevent exposure to aerosols, and adoption of a policy of universal precautions for all patients (treating all patients and patient specimens as if HIV or hepatitis B infected). The Centers for Disease Control have published guidelines of recommended precautions for laboratory workers to help decrease the risk of HIV transmission in health care settings.[52] These recommendations are as follows:

1. Avoid contaminating the outside of containers upon specimen collection. The lid should be tight.
2. Wear gloves when processing patient specimens. Use masks and eyewear if splashing or aerosolization is anticipated. Change gloves and wash hands at the end of processing.
3. Use biological safety cabinets for blending, sonicating, and vigorous mixing.
4. No mouth pipetting.
5. Use precautions when handling needles. No bending, breaking, recapping, or removing of needles from disposable syringes. Place in puncture-resistant containers.
6. Decontaminate work surfaces with a chemical germicide after spills and when work is completed.

7. Dispose of contaminated materials in bags and in accordance with institutional policies for disposal of infective waste.
8. Decontaminate equipment before repair or shipping.
9. Wash hands and remove protective clothing before leaving the laboratory.

SUMMARY

HIV infection is the most serious infectious disease threatening humans today. To date, there are no effective vaccines, and antiviral therapies that slow the progress of the disease offer no cure. Extensive research has delineated the structure of the virus, its life cycle, its mode of transmission, and groups at risk of infection. HIV infection results in severe immunodeficiency of the host, with T-cell and humoral defenses being affected. Opportunistic infections and cancers are a confounding result of the severe immunosuppression of the host. A variety of methods to isolate HIV virus in vitro and to detect HIV antibodies and antigens have been developed and are in use today in research and medical laboratories.

Case Studies

Case Study 1

A 25-year-old male patient presents to his physician with complaints of prolonged fatigue, night sweats, fever, diarrhea, and weight loss. The physician orders an HIV test.

How should the lab proceed?

Case Study 2

A New York blood bank uses a combination HIV-1/HIV-2 ELISA test to screen blood donations. A recent blood donation tested repeatedly positive by this test.

What tests should the laboratory undertake next?

References

1. Ho DD, Pomerantz RJ, Kaplan JC: Pathogenesis of infection with human immune deficiency virus. N Engl J Med 317:278, 1987
2. McDougal JS, Mawle AC, Nicholson JKA: The immunology of AIDS. In Kaslow R, Francis D (eds): The Epidemiology of AIDS. Oxford, Oxford University Press
3. Shulman J, Blumberg HM, Kozarsky PE, et al: Acquired immunodeficiency syndrome (AIDS): An update for the clinician. Emory Univ J Med 1:157, 1987
4. Henrard, DR: Retrovirus Learning Guide: HIV, 2nd ed. Abbott Park IL, Abbott Diagnostics Educational Services, 1993
5. Centers for Disease Control: Pneumocystis pneumonia— Los Angeles. Surveill Summ 30:250, 1981
6. Heyward WL, Curran JW: The epidemiology of AIDS in the US. Sci Am Oct: 264:72, 1985
7. Stoops S. AIDS and human immunodeficiency virus infection. Horizons 1:1, 1995
8. Barker E, Barnett S: Human immunodeficiency viruses. In Murray PR, Baron EJ, Pfaller MA, et al (eds): Manual of Clinical Microbiology, 6th ed, p 1098. Washington, DC, American Society for Microbiology Press, 1995
9. Hardy AM: Characterization of long term survivors of AIDS. 27th Intersci Conf Antimicrobial Agents and Chemotherapy, American Society for Microbiology, Abstract 98, 1987
10. Clavel F, Mansinho K, Chamaret S, et al: Human immunodeficiency virus type 2 infection associated with AIDS in West Africa. N Engl J Med 316:1180, 1987
11. Barré-Sinoussi F, Chermann JC, Rey F, et al: Isolation of a T-lymphotrophic retrovirus from a patient at risk for acquired immunodeficiency syndrome (AIDS). Science 220:868, 1983
12. Popovic M, Sarngadharan MG, Read E, et al: Detection, isolation, and continuous production of cytopathic retroviruses (HTLV-III) from patients with AIDS and pre-AIDS. Science 224:497, 1984
13. Levy JA, Hoffman AD, Kramer SM, et al: Isolation of lymphocytotrophic retroviruses from San Francisco patients with AIDS. Science 225:840, 1984
14. Ratner L, Haseltine W, Patarca R, et al: Complete nucleotide sequence of the AIDS virus. Nature 313:277, 1985
15. Wain-Hobson S, Sonigo P, Danos O, et al: Nucleotide sequence of the AIDS virus, LAV. Cell 40:9, 1985
16. Aiya SK, Gallo RC: Three novel genes of human T-lymphotrophic virus type III: Immune reactivity of their products with sera from acquired immune deficiency syndrome patients. Proc Natl Acad Sci USA 83:1553, 1986
17. Fisher AG, Feinberg MB, Josephs SF, et al: The transactivation gene of HTLV-III is essential for virus replication. Nature 320:367, 1986
18. Wong-Staal F, Chanda P, Ghrayeb J: Human immunodeficiency virus: The eighth gene. AIDS Res Hum Retroviruses 3:33, 1987
19. Muesing MA, Smith DH, Capon DJ: Regulation of mRNA accumulation by a human immunodeficiency virus transactivation protein. Cell 48:691, 1987
20. Luciw PA, Cheng-Mayer C, Levy JA: Mutational analysis of the human immunodeficiency virus: The *orf*-B region down-regulates virus replication. Proc Natl Acad Sci USA 84:1434, 1987
21. Groopman JE, Chen FW, Hope JA, et al: Serological characterization of HTLV-III infection in AIDS and related disorders. J Infect Dis 153:736, 1986
22. Bowen DL, Lane HC, Fauci AS: Immunopathogenesis of the acquired immunodeficiency syndrome. Ann Intern Med 103:704, 1985
23. Jackson JB, Balfour HH Jr: Practical diagnostic testing for human immunodeficiency virus. Clin Microbiol Rev 1:124, 1988

24. Zagury D, Bernard J, Leonard R, et al: Long-term cultures of HTLV-III infected cells: A model of cytopathology of T-cell depletion in AIDS. Science 231:850, 1986

25. Redfield RR: The etiology and epidemiology of HTLV-III related disease. Abbott Park, IL, Abbott Diagnostics HTLV-III Education Series, 1987

26. Mann JM, Chin J, Piot P, Quinn T: The international epidemiology of AIDS. Sci Am 259:82, 1988

27. Coleman PF: Detecting and differentiating HIV-2. Am Clin Lab Oct:10, 1992

28. Hessol NA, Rutherford GW, O'Malley PM, et al: The natural history of human immunodeficiency virus infection in a cohort of homosexual and bisexual men: A seven year prospective study. Abstract M3.1, Third International Conference on AIDS, Washington, DC, 1987

29. Centers for Disease Control and Prevention: 1993 Revised Classification System for HIV Infection and Expanded Surveillance Case Definition for AIDS Among Adolescents and Adults. MMWR 41(RR-17):1–19, 1992

30. Weller IA: Treatment of infections and antiviral agents. Br Med J 295:200, 1987

31. Schwartz J: FDA approves drug ritonavir in 72 days. *Washington Post* p A8, March 2, 1996

32. Fischi MA, Richman DD, Grieco MH, et al: The efficacy of azidothymidine (AZT) in the treatment of patients with AIDS and AIDS-related complex. N Engl J Med 317:185, 1987

33. Yarchoan R, Mitsuya H, Broder S: AIDS therapies. Sci Am 259:110, 1988

34. Klatzman D, Montagnier L: Approaches to AIDS therapy. Nature 319:10, 1986

35. Seligmann M, Pinching AJ, Roger FS, et al: Immunology of human immunodeficiency virus infection and the acquired immunodeficiency syndrome. Ann Intern Med 107:234, 1987

36. Matthews TJ, Bolognes DP: AIDS vaccines. Sci Am 259:120, 1988

37. Additional recommendations to reduce sexual and drug abuse-related transmission of human T-lymphocyte virus type III (lymphadenopathy-associated virus). Surveill Summ 35:152, 1986

38. Guyader M, Emerman M, Sonigo P, et al: Genome organization and transactivation of the human immunodeficiency virus type 2. Nature 326:662, 1987

39. Denis F, Leonard G, Mounier M, et al: Efficacy of five enzyme immunoassays for antibody to HIV in detecting antibody to HTLV-IV. Lancet 1:324, 1987

40. Khan NC, Hunter E: Detection of human immunodeficiency virus type 1. American Clinical Product Review May:20, 1988

41. Janda WM: Serologic tests for HTLV-III antibodies: Methods and interpretations. Clin Microbiol Newslett 7:67, 1985

42. Papsidero LD, Montagna RA, Poiesz BJ: Acquired immune deficiency syndrome: Detection of viral exposure and infection. American Clinical Product Review :17, 1986

43. Reesink HW, Lelie PN, Huisman JG, et al: Evaluation of six enzyme immunoassays for antibody against human immunodeficiency virus. Lancet 2:483, 1986

44. Goudsmit J, Lange JMA, Paul DA, et al: Antigenemia and antibody titers to core and envelope antigens in AIDS, AIDS-related complex, and subclinical human immunodeficiency virus infection. J Infect Dis 155:558, 1987

45. Yoshida T, Matsui T, Kobayashi S, et al: Agglutination test for HIV antibody. J Clin Microbiol 25:1433, 1987

46. Riggin CH, Beltz GA, Hung CH, et al: Detection of antibodies to human immunodeficiency virus by latex agglutination with recombinant antigen. J Clin Microbiol 25:1772, 1987

47. Lombardo JM: HIV testing: An overview. American Clinical Product Review Nov:10, 1987

48. Kleinman S: The significance of indeterminate Western blots for HIV-1. Update, Ortho Diagnostic Systems, 2:1, 1988

49. Lennette ET, Karpatkin S, Levy JA: Indirect immunofluorescence assay for antibodies to human immunodeficiency virus. J Clin Microbiol 25:199, 1987

50. Carlson DA: AIDS risks and precautions for laboratory personnel. Med Lab Observ Jan 20:57, 1988

51. Centers for Disease Control: Recommendations for preventing transmission of infection with human T-lymphotrophic virus type III/lymphadenopathy-associated virus in the workplace. Surveill Summ 34:687, 1985

52. Centers for Disease Control: Recommendations for prevention of HIV transmission in health care settings. Surveill Summ 36:1, 1987

CHAPTER 27

Serology of Miscellaneous Infectious Diseases

Denise R. Zito

Objectives

Upon completion of the chapter, the reader will be able to:

1. List two reasons why serology evaluation may be preferred over culture for the diagnosis of infectious disease
2. List the four major rickettsia groups
3. Name the organisms that are the causative agents of the following: epidemic typhus, endemic typhus, scrub typhus, and Q fever
4. Describe the cold agglutinin test for mycoplasma
5. Describe the method of detection of fungal precipitin antibodies
6. List the two primary risk groups for toxoplasma infection
7. Describe the use of cytomegalovirus serology in blood banking
8. List the two clinical manifestations of HTLV-I infection

Serological assays are useful to diagnose diseases caused by organisms that are either difficult to culture or that grow at such a slow rate that diagnosis through culture would be delayed by weeks. Direct antigen detection for the organisms described in this chapter may be difficult because they are usually present in such low levels in the circulation. The polymerase chain reaction (PCR) is an extremely sensitive technique but is not yet available in most clinical laboratories. PCR may eventually be useful in detecting these organisms in the infected individual. Yet even PCR methods can take up to a week to complete, whereas serological techniques can be done in a few hours. Antibody detection provides a means of identifying individuals who have been exposed to a particular organism. Antibodies are relatively large molecules that are easily detected in serum. This makes serological techniques the method of choice to aid in the diagnosis of a variety of infectious diseases.

It is important to remember that in many cases, a single serological test result may not give the clinician enough information to make a diagnosis. Many serological tests indicate exposure to, rather than infection by, an organism. Often it is necessary to show a significant increase in antibody titer over several weeks to establish a current or recent infection. Immunosuppressed individuals may be unable to mount the usual antibody response. This situation will be seen with increasing frequency in laboratories that receive specimens from transplant patients.

Diseases caused by the organisms discussed in this chapter are usually detected using serological techniques. The nature of these tests requires that interpretation be done in the context of clinical history. For example, there are relatively few crossreactions or falsely positive or negative test results for hepatitis B serology, but cytomegalovirus infection may be difficult to diagnose solely through the use of serologic testing.

RICKETTSIA

These gram-negative cocci are dangerous when aerosolized and are difficult to culture because they will grow only in living cells. Therefore, serological testing is the preferred method to detect exposure and infection. Rickettsial diseases are transmitted primarily through tick bites or by mites and lice. Distribution of the rickettsial diseases is worldwide, and several of them are prevalent in the United States. Rickettsia can be divided into three groups: spotted fever, typhus, and scrub typhus.

Spotted Fever Group

Spotted fevers are caused by at least five different species of Rickettsia and are distributed worldwide. The most common disease in the United States is Rocky Mountain spotted fever (RMSF), caused by Rickettsia rickettsii. Like the other spotted fevers, the incubation period may be up to 14 days. Most patients experience an acute onset. High fever, chills, and myalgia are common, and a characteristic rash on the wrists, ankles, palms, soles, and forearms is seen. Later the rash extends to the axilla, buttocks, trunk, neck, and face. The disease is transmitted by ticks, but about 20% of patients fail to recall an instance of tick bite. The polymerase chain reaction (PCR) test, when widely available, will be an ideal test for RMSF because it allows the disease to be diagnosed before the patient is able to mount a detectable antibody response.[1]

Currently, the most common test performed is an indirect immunofluorescence antibody test. Rickettsial antigen isolates are applied to glass slides. Dilutions of patient serum are added to the slide and incubated. Following a wash step, a fluorescence-labeled anti–human immunoglobulin is added to each slide well and incubated. The slides are read using a fluorescence microscope. The sensitivity of these assays must be established in each laboratory using appropriate controls.

Patients with RMSF are treated with large doses of tetracycline until the patient improves and has been afebrile for 24 hours.

Typhus Group

Epidemic typhus, caused by R. prowazekii, is a serious illness carried by lice. It is prevalent in areas of South America and Africa. Symptoms include headache, chills, and fever, followed several days later by a skin rash. The disease can be fatal in up to 40% of those infected.[2] Sporadic typhus, caused by the same organism, has been reported in the United States in individuals who have had contact with flying squirrels.

Endemic typhus, a much milder form of typhus, is caused by R. typhi. The disease is flea borne and is also known as murine typhus. Its prevalence is worldwide. Scrub typhus is transmitted via chiggers carrying R. tsutsugamushi. Like the other rickettsial diseases, the symptoms include fever, headache, myalgia, and skin rash. This disease is most commonly seen in Asia, Australia, and the Pacific Islands.

In contrast to the rickettsial diseases already described, Q fever, caused by Coxiella burnetii, is transmitted by aerosol rather than through an arthropod vector. This is more of a systemic disease, causing cough, chest infiltrates, and hepatitis. Although Q fever is a rare malady, it is distributed worldwide.

There is significant crossreactivity between the typhus group antigens. The testing is usually performed at state laboratories, with antigen preparations obtained from the Centers for Disease Control and Prevention (CDC). Indirect immunofluorescence, as described earlier, is used to detect patient antibody.

MYCOPLASMA

Mycoplasma pneumoniae is the most common of the mycoplasmas, an unusual group of bacteria that lack a rigid cell wall. This property causes the organisms to escape detection using the Gram stain. M. pneumoniae most frequently causes a respiratory infection or a mild pneumonia. Because the organism is very fastidious in vitro, it is difficult to make the diagnosis using a culture.

Testing for antibodies against M. pneumoniae is difficult because of the problems with culturing that make the production of large amounts of antigen difficult.[3] The complement fixation method can be used but is not available in most clinical laboratories. Instead, laboratories have relied on the inexpensive cold agglutinin test, which measures the presence of cold-reacting antibodies against the I antigen on adult human red blood cells.

The blood specimen for the cold agglutinin testing should be held at room temperature until the serum can be separated from the clot. If the specimen is refrigerated prior to serum separation, the cold-reacting antibodies may bind to the red cells and be removed with the clot, resulting in a false negative test reaction. Serial dilutions of patient serum are incubated with 0.1 mL of a 1% solution of washed, human group O red blood cells. After a 1 hour incubation at 4°C, the tubes are read for agglutination. Agglutinated cells form a 'carpet' at the bottom of the test tube and are disrupted by gentle shaking. The endpoint of the reaction is the highest dilution showing agglutination after incubation in the cold. The agglutination must reverse when heated to 37°C in order to be considered a cold agglutinin–associated mycoplasmal infection. The minimum clinically significant titer is 64. Although the test is not specific for mycoplasma infection, it requires very simple reagents and can be performed in virtually any laboratory. A positive cold agglutinin test combined with a good clinical history can provide the diagnosis.

LEGIONELLA

Legionella pneumophila was first identified in 1976 during an outbreak of pneumonia that occurred in the participants at the American Legion Convention held in Philadelphia.[4] *Legionella* is a fastidious gram-negative, aerobic bacillus. The organisms are ubiquitous in the environment but can cause disease when aerosolized and inhaled by humans, for example, from an air-conditioning system. Legionnaire's disease is a fulminant pneumonia with fever and flulike symptoms. Diagnosis is made by culture because seroconversion occurs too long after the necessity for diagnosis. Serological tests are primarily used for epidemiological purposes. The method used is indirect immunofluorescence using bacteria fixed to a microscope slide. Dilutions of patient serum are incubated on the slides. Following washes, a fluorescent-labeled anti–human immunoglobulin is added. The secondary antibody binds to any patient antibody bound to the organisms, and detection is made using a fluorescence microscope. It is essential that paired sera taken early in the infection and several weeks later be used in testing. Legionnaire's disease is treated by administration of erythromycin. Immunocompromised individuals are also given rifampin.

FUNGI

Cellular immunity is the principal host response to fungal infections. Neutrophils, monocytes/macrophages, lymphocytes, and natural killer cells all respond to fungal antigens. Infection is most often observed in patients with impaired cellular immunity. With few exceptions, fungi are not killed by antibody and complement.

Fungal infections can be classified as superficial, cutaneous, subcutaneous, or systemic.[5] Superficial, cutaneous, and subcutaneous fungal infections produce visible nodules or other skin manifestations. Laboratory tests for these involve culture and examination of smears made from skin scrapings. Systemic infection usually results from inhalation, producing pulmonary symptoms and a flulike illness.

Although humoral immunity does not aid the host in fighting fungal infections, antibodies are produced and serological testing is useful in certain fungal infections, although they do not provide the definitive diagnosis. *Blastomyces dermatitidis*, *Histoplasma capsulatum*, and *Coccidioides immitis* infections are rare but may cause lung inflammation following inhalation of spores. All may cause cough, fever, and chest pain.

Precipitating antibodies are detected using the double diffusion technique described in Chapter 11. Purified antigens are placed in wells that surround the central well containing patient serum. Lines of precipitation indicate that the patient has formed antibodies against a given organism. However, the presence of antibody does not distinguish between active disease and remote infection; active disease requires the isolation of organisms from the infected site to confirm the diagnosis.[5] False positive results may occur because some individuals have antibodies without true infection. A false negative may result if the patient is tested too early in the infection, before seroconversion.

Candida albicans and *Aspergillus fumigatus* are considered opportunistic fungal infections because the organisms are ubiquitous in the environment but rarely cause infection until the host is immunocompromised. Serological tests for *Candida* are not useful; diagnosis can be made only through identification of multiple sites of infection. *Aspergillus* infections may result in the formation of IgG antibodies that are detectable through double diffusion.

Sporotrichosis schenckii infection is usually localized in skin following a scrape or cut that inoculates the organism deep in the skin. Gardeners are often affected because the organism is common on roses and in organic matter. Serologic testing is not helpful. Diagnosis is made through culture of the wound material.

Cryptococcus neoformans infection is usually caused by inhalation of fungus into the lungs. In immunocompromised individuals, especially those with AIDS, the infection may spread to the brain via the blood stream and cause meningitis. Diagnosis is made through culture and direct microscopy using an India ink–stained smear. Rapid testing is also available using a latex agglutination method that detects cryptococcal antigen in serum or cerebrospinal fluid. These tests frequently yield false positive results, so culture provides the definitive diagnosis.

Treatment varies according to the specific infectious agent. In general, systemic fungal infections require prolonged drug therapy to induce recovery. Amphotericin B is the most common antibiotic used in the treatment of these infections.

TOXOPLASMA

Toxoplasma gondii is a parasitic disease acquired through the ingestion of cysts or oocysts that are present in undercooked pork or lamb. Domestic cats may also be carriers. The organism exists in three forms: the trophozoite, tissue cyst, and oocyst. Infection in immunocompetent patients is usually asymptomatic and self-limiting. However, in immunocompromised patients, such as AIDS or transplant patients, the disease can have devastating consequences.[6] In these individuals the disease becomes disseminated, causing inflammation and necrosis. Infants are also considered to be immunocompromised, and infection can be transmitted in utero, with infection being most severe if contracted during the first trimester of the pregnancy. The disease in infants progresses similarly to infected adults and may also cause hydrocephalus. There are many reliable enzyme immunoassays available commercially. It is important in infants to test for IgM antibodies against *T. gondii*.

A combination of pyrimethamine plus sulfadiazine is used in the treatment of acute, reactivated, or congenital toxoplasmosis.[6] However, the cyst form is resistant to therapy, and recurrence is common after therapy ceases when tissues cysts break down, releasing more organisms. When this occurs, therapy is resumed.

VIRUSES

Cytomegalovirus

Cytomegalovirus (CMV) is a ubiquitous virus that is widespread in humans and generally causes asymptomatic infection. However, exposure to this virus is an important issue when dealing with immunocompromised patients, particularly those who have received organ transplants. Infants who need blood transfusions are susceptible to CMV infection and require CMV antibody–negative blood products. The presence of antibody in a patient's serum does not preclude reinfection, and this is of particular concern in transplant patients.

CMV testing in the clinical laboratory may be achieved through viral culture or serology. The most common serological technique is the enzyme-linked immunosorbent assay (ELISA) test, and many automated forms are commercially available. Beads or microtiter wells are coated with CMV and incubated with patient serum. CMV specific patient antibody will bind to the virus during the incubation period, following which the excess serum is washed away. An enzyme-labeled anti–human immunoglobulin reagent is added to the solid phase and binds to any patient antibody. Following a wash step, the enzyme substrate is added and a color reaction indicates the presence of virus–patient antibody–antibody "sandwich." The test can use a secondary antibody specific for IgM or IgG to distinguish recent infection from past infection.

Because of the possibility of active infection, even in the presence of IgG antibody, some laboratories have attempted to use PCR techniques to look for the presence of viral DNA. However, this assay must be carefully standardized in each laboratory because viral detection does not necessarily reflect active infection.

Ganciclovir is the treatment of choice in immunocompromised individuals with CMV retinitis.[7,8] Patients with CMV pneumonitis respond less well to this treatment. In these cases, ganciclovir is combined with CMV immune globulin treatment.

Human T-Cell Leukemia Virus I

Human T-cell leukemia virus I (HTLV-I) is a retrovirus that induces transformation and replication of T lymphocytes. It preferentially infects T helper cells. Infected individuals produce an antibody response that can be detected in the laboratory. When AIDS was first identified as a clinical syndrome, it was thought that it was caused by an HTLV-type virus. Further study revealed that although HTLV and HIV are both retroviruses, they have little sequence homology.

HTLV-I infection is usually asymptomatic but can cause two separate clinical entities: a form of T-cell leukemia and tropical spastic paraparesis.[9,10] The latter is a neurological disease manifested as spastic gait. Both of these diseases are common in the Caribbean and Japan but rare in the United States. The virus can be spread through blood contact, so all blood products are tested before they are transfused to patients.

Testing for HTLV-I is by routine ELISA, as described previously. Newer assays will also react with antibodies to HTLV-II. Although this virus causes no known disease, it can be transmitted by transfused blood products and so is of concern to the blood banking community. Confirmatory testing for presence of the virus is by Western blot analysis. In this assay, viral proteins are electrophoresed in a gel so that they align by increasing molecular weight. The proteins are then transferred to nitrocellulose to serve as the solid phase of the assay. A source of protein, usually milk powder, is incubated with each nitrocellulose strip to block any part of the strip that does not carry a viral protein. From here the assay resembles a straightforward ELISA. A nitrocellulose strip is then incubated with either a control or patient serum. Serum antibody, if present, will bind to the appropriate viral proteins on the strip. After washing, the strip is incubated with an enzyme-labeled anti–human immunoglobulin. Excess antibody is then removed by washing the strips. The substrate appropriate to the enzyme label is then incubated with each strip. Color will develop wherever serum antibody has reacted with viral proteins bound to the nitrocellulose strip. Interpretation of the test results is a visual evaluation of the band pattern compared with those produced with standard sera.

HTLV-I is not treated unless symptoms develop in the infected individual. There is no known chemotherapeutic regimen found to be effective in treating the resulting leukemia. Patient treatment consists of supportive measures only.

SUMMARY

Immunological methods have been extremely useful as an aid to diagnosis of diseases caused by organisms that are difficult to culture in the laboratory. Serological testing can differentiate recent infection through the detection of IgM specific antibody, from past exposure or infection through the detection of IgG specific antibody. Antibody techniques may also used for the direct detection of infecting organisms, as in acute *Cryptococcus* infections. Detecting patient antibody leads to rapid patient diagnosis because it eliminates the need to grow dangerous organisms in the laboratory. DNA probe technology will eventually replace the need for serology in the vast number of infectious diseases. Until the proper probes are identified, serology will remain an essential method of diagnosis.

Case Studies

Case 1

CH is a 52-year-old Japanese-American woman admitted to the hospital with a white blood cell count of 187,000/μL³. Her differential showed 69% blasts. Flow cytometric studies were performed and showed a predominance of CD3+, CD5+, and CD4+ cells. The case was signed out as a T-cell leukemia, with a helper T-cell phenotype.

What other serological tests should be done?

Case 2

JE is a 28-year-old Caucasian female with a history of sarcoidosis. She is visiting her doctor to follow up new symptoms that she is experiencing. She recalls going to other people's houses and becoming markedly ill hours afterward, including severe cough and fevers. Upon questioning she recalls seeing a black mold growing on her windowsills.

What further serological testing should be done?

References

1. Hechemy K: The immunoserology of rickettsiae. In Rose NR, DeMacario EC, Fahey JL, Friedman H, Penn GM (eds): Manual of Clinical Laboratory Immunology, 4th ed, p 776. Washington, DC, American Society for Microbiology, 1992
2. Duma RJ, Sonenshine DE, Bozeman FM, et al.: Epidemic typhus in the United States associated with flying squirrels. JAMA 25:2318–2323, 1981
3. Kenny GE: Immunologic methods for mycoplasmas and miscellaneous bacteria. In Rose NR, DeMacario ED, Fahey JL, Friedman H, Penn GM (eds): Manual of Clinical Laboratory Immunology, 4th ed, p 498. Washington, DC, American Society for Microbiology, 1992
4. Fraser DW, Tsai TR, Orenstein W, et al: Legionnaire's disease. Description of an epidemic of pneumonia. N Engl J Med 297:1189, 1977
5. Drutz DJ: Fungal diseases. In Stites DP, Stobo JD, Wells JV (eds): Basic and Clinical Immunology, 8th ed, p 649. Norwalk, CT, Appleton and Lange, 1994
6. Remington JS, Desmonts G: Toxoplasmosis. In Remington JS, Klein JO (eds): Infectious Diseases of the Fetus and Newborn Infant, p 143. Philadelphia, WB Saunders, 1983
7. Hirsch MS: Cytomegalovirus infection. In Wilson JD, Braunwald E, Isselbacher KJ, Petersdorf RG, Martin JB, Fauci AS, Root RK (eds): Principles of Internal Medicine, 12th ed., p 692. New York, McGraw-Hill, 1991
8. Onorato IM, Morens DM, Martone W, et al: Epidemiology of cytomegaloviral infections: Recommendations for prevention and control. Rev Infect Dis 7:479, 1985
9. Blattner WA, Takatsuki K, Gallo RC: Human T-cell leukemia-lymphoma virus and adult T-cell leukemia. JAMA 250:1074–1080, 1983
10. Gessain A, Barin F, Vernant JC, et al.: Antibodies to human T-lymphotropic virus type-I in patients with tropical spastic paraparesis. Lancet 2:407–410, 1985

Section B. Autoimmune Disease

CHAPTER 28

Immunologic Tolerance

Catherine Sheehan

Objectives

Upon completion of the chapter, the reader will be able to:

1. Define tolerance, anergy, and apoptosis
2. Discuss the relationship between immune activation and tolerance
3. Compare and contrast clonal deletion and anergy
4. Describe general mechanisms by which tolerance is broken
5. Explain the beneficial and deleterious effects of tolerance and broken tolerance

INTRODUCTION

Immunological tolerance is a physiologic state in which the immune system is nonresponsive to a specific antigen. Most importantly, tolerance is needed to prevent immune reaction against autoantigens.[1] It has long been recognized that the host avoids self-destructive reactions; this avoidance was originally described as "horror autotoxicus" by Ehrlich and Morgenroth.[2] Thus autoimmune disease is prevented. Autoimmune disease differs from autoreactivity and autoimmune mechanisms. The former are immune reactions that are harmful to the host, and the latter are simply processes that involve self-recognition without harmful consequences.

The immune system must balance its active role to defend the host from foreign intruders and its ability to tolerate autoantigens. Thus while immunocompetent, the host must selectively remain unresponsive to its own antigens. It is not surprising that this delicate balance depends on controlling T and B cells. Central tolerance affects immature lymphocytes encountering antigens, and peripheral tolerance affects mature lymphocytes encountering antigens, as shown in Figure 28-1. Many currently accepted ideas about tolerance are based primarily on experimental mouse studies and secondarily on human studies and observations are listed in Table 28-1. By more fully understanding the mechanisms of tolerance, the success of transplantation engraftment may improve and autoimmune diseases may be prevented or treated more effectively.

CENTRAL TOLERANCE

Medawar et al. first described the acquired nature of immunological tolerance when cellular antigens from one strain of mouse were administered to fetal mice of a different strain; subsequently the adult mice were exposed to skin grafts from the first strain and the graft

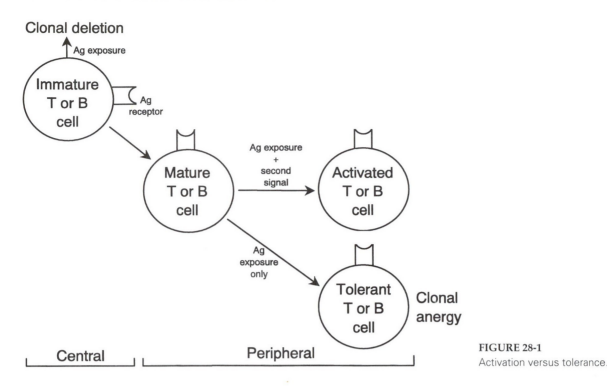

FIGURE 28-1
Activation versus tolerance.

was accepted.[3] Chimeras were also studied to evaluate the exposure of unrelated antigens between dizygotic (fraternal) twins during development. Each twin tolerated the genetically different tissue of the other twin.[4] Both studies suggested that early exposure to foreign antigens can prevent antibody formation. Clones of lymphocytes appeared to be eliminated during fetal development, and this resulted in tolerance.

T-Cell Clonal Deletion

Immature T cells are eliminated in the thymus by a process known as negative selection. The clone is most efficiently eliminated if the immature cell expresses

TABLE 28-1
Mechanisms of Immunologic Tolerance

CENTRAL TOLERANCE
 T-cell clonal deletion
 B-cell clonal deletion
PERIPHERAL TOLERANCE
 Anergy
  Antigen blockade (B lymphocyte)
  Lack of costimulation (T and B lymphocytes)
 Sequestered antigen
IMMUNOREGULATION
 Antibody mediated
 Idiotype network
 Suppressor T lymphocytes

both CD4 and CD8. Autoantigens must be transported to the thymus and then presented by dendritic or other cells during thymocyte development. If the T-cell receptor has a minimum affinity (commonly a low affinity) for the antigen and the cell is at an appropriate level of maturation, the clone will die by apoptosis. The usual morphologic changes associated with apoptosis are observed: cytoplasmic blebbing, chromatin condensation, and DNA fragmentation, all of which result in cell disintegration and phagocytosis by macrophages without inflammation. Evidence suggests that this requires the activation of a calcium-dependent endonuclease.[5]

Failure to induce complete tolerance may result when self-peptides do not reach the thymus, are hidden based on their spatial arrangement, or are not presented in the context of the MHC requirement.[6] Thus specific T-cell clones will not be eliminated and harmful autoimmune reactions are possible.

B-Cell Clonal Deletion

Although there is some debate about B-cell tolerance, most agree that it occurs in the bone marrow when nonhematologic cells present multivalent haptens to immature B cells. Crosslinking of surface immunoglobulin without T-lymphocyte help is required to induce tolerance by clonal deletion. High-affinity clones are preferentially eliminated. Immature B cells are more susceptible to tolerization and may require activation of specific genes to facilitate apoptosis in selected immature B cells.[7]

PERIPHERAL TOLERANCE

If immature autoreactive lymphocytes are not eliminated during maturation, then mature, competent lymphocytes are released from primary lymphoid tissues. At the local level, mechanisms to prevent harmful autoimmune reactions include anergy, receptor downregulation, and antigen sequestration.

Anergy

Nossal and Pike[8] coined the term anergy to refer to the functionally inactivated state induced in response to a substance (tolerogen). This is a reversible, antiproliferative state. One early explanation is that when the surface antigen receptors on B lymphocytes are overwhelmed by excessive antigen, antigen blockade prevents crosslinking of surface immunoglobulin, an event that is necessary for B-cell activation.[9] The number of B cells remains the same, making clonal deletion unlikely. The cells are anergic. Experimentally, in the state of B-cell anergy, the concentration of surface IgM (sIgM; the antigen receptor) is greatly reduced although surface IgD is normal. The decreased sIgM may prevent antigen binding, thus preventing a B-cell response and inducing tolerance of the antigen.[10] A similar mechanism has been investigated in T lymphocytes. When T cells are exposed to high doses of antigen by antigen-presenting cells, downregulation of the T-cell receptor occurs and the T-cell loses responsiveness.

Antigen that binds to a specific lymphocyte receptor is only one of at least two signals required to activate lymphocytes. The lack of a second stimulatory molecule prevents activation of the lymphocyte, even in the presence of specific antigen. For T-cell activation, the antigen must be presented in association with MHC Class II peptides and interaction with additional surface molecules is necessary. The antigen-presenting cell must express B7, which binds to CD28 on the T-cell surface. This then initiates metabolic events in the T cell to increase the expression of high-affinity IL-2 receptors, to increase cell size, and to synthesize and release IL-2. Without costimulation, IL-2 is not produced and T cells do not proliferate; the T cell is anergic.[11]

A similar two-signal model has been proposed for B lymphocytes.[12] Antigen presentation in the absence of T-cell–derived IL-4, IL-5, IL-6, and IL-10 will render the B cell anergic. Some evidence suggests that interaction between surface molecules (CD40 on B cells and the CD40 ligand on T cells) is necessary to induce metabolic changes for antibody synthesis.

Sequestered Antigens

Some anatomic sites, such as the brain, testis, and anterior chamber of the eye, are less likely to be involved in immunologic reactions and more easily accept grafts.[13] Early thinking suggested that antigen in these sites was sequestered and that lymphocytes did not ordinarily gain access to these privileged sites, so these antigens were tolerated. Now it is more likely that low levels of MHC expression prevent immune activation.

IMMUNOREGULATION

Mechanisms that regulate immune activation may also be important in immune tolerance. Antibody-mediated tolerance, idiotype network regulation, and suppressor T-cell activity are three mechanisms that contribute to tolerance.

Antibody-mediated tolerance can be demonstrated when antibody is passively transferred prior to antigen exposure.[14] After antigen is administered, immune complexes form and are eliminated by the mononuclear phagocyte system, thus preventing activation or priming of the immune system. Clinically, following accidental exposure to the hepatitis B virus, hepatitis B immune globulin is administered to prevent infection and sensitization. Effectively, the antibody binds the virus and the complex is eliminated without infection. A second example relates to maternal stimulation during pregnancy in which the D antigen was expressed on fetal red blood cells and not by the mother. Rh immune globulin containing D antibody is administered to the mother within 72 hours after a miscarriage or birth to prevent the mother from responding to the D antigen. The mother then fails to produce antibody that may interfere in subsequent pregnancies.

The idiotype network is believed to exert its control via anti-idiotype antibodies reacting with the variable regions of antibody or T-cell receptors (TCR).[15] By reacting with antibody or TCR, antigen cannot bind or sIg is not crosslinked, rendering the cell tolerant. Some evidence suggests that idiotype antibody reacting with the TCR may activate CD8+ cells to lyse the targeted T cell. Finally, some evidence suggests suppressor T cells are involved in tolerance, but the mechanisms are poorly understood.

FACTORS AFFECTING TOLERANCE

Dosage and route of administration of the antigen affect the ability of cells to respond. Generally a low dose of antigen induces T-cell tolerance and a high dose induces B-cell tolerance. For tolerance to be sustained when new cells emerge from primary lymphoid tissue, the antigen exposure must be persistent. Subcutaneous injection favors immunity, while intravenous and oral exposure favors tolerance. When different cells are exposed to antigen via different routes of administration, different cytokines are produced and different mechanisms are activated.

Fetal-maternal tolerance is unique. By genetic rules, one half of the chromosomes in fetal cells are inherited from the father; therefore, significant antigenic differences exist between the fetus and mother. The potential maternal reaction to these differences should be high, but the fetus is usually well tolerated by the mother. Several mechanisms exist to prevent a harmful reaction: Syncytioblasts (cells of the placenta) do not express MHC Class I or II peptides, thus preventing immune activation; increased steroid hormone production induces transient thymus involution; and the fetus produces immunosuppressive chemicals (alpha fetoprotein, progesterone, and transforming growth factor β).

DISRUPTION OF TOLERANCE

As listed in Table 28-2, autoimmune disease results when tolerance is broken by one of four general mechanisms: genetic mutation, loss of tolerance to an organ-specific antigen, antigen-specific B-cell response, or persistent organ-specific autoimmune disease. A genetic mutation may contribute to systemic, non–organ-specific autoimmune disease. This mutation may affect the survival or function of lymphocytes.

An alteration in a tissue that leads to selective activation of immune mechanisms is likely to be responsible for organ-specific autoimmune disease. Some initiating event (such as a drug interaction or viral infection) may alter the antigens expressed on the cell surface such that the cell becomes sufficiently different and escapes tolerance. Sometimes upregulation of MHC peptides can turn the state of tolerance into an immune response.

B-cell autoimmunity may occur when antibody is produced in response to one antigen and that antibody crossreacts with an autoantigen. When the offending organism is eliminated, the autoimmune damage is reversed. The classic example is rheumatic fever, in which the M protein of some streptococci stimulate antibody formation, which also reacts with cardiac myosin.

Finally, when T-cell tolerance is broken, persistent organ-specific autoimmune disease may follow. The in-

flammation and resultant damage may be caused by chronic cytokine action localized in an organ.

CONCLUSIONS

Immune tolerance is needed to distinguish self from non-self, thereby preventing harmful reactions to autoantigens. Some autoreactive lymphocytes are deleted during development, and others are rendered tolerant when mature. Peripheral tolerance may be induced by incomplete cell signaling and antigen sequestration, and will vary based on the route of administration and dosage of antigen. Disruption of tolerance can result in autoimmune disease.

Review Questions

1. Failure of the immune system to tolerate autoantigens may result in

   a. transplantation rejection
   b. autoimmune disease
   c. tumor production
   d. chronic infections

2. The immunologic state in which a mature lymphocyte is unresponsive to an antigen is known as

   a. mimicry
   b. anergy
   c. antigen blockade
   d. clonal deletion

3. Ninety to ninety-five percent of thymocytes die intrathymically. This results in

   a. B-cell tolerance
   b. T-cell clonal deletion
   c. receptor downregulation
   d. sequestered antigens

4. Administration of Rh immune globulin prevents maternal sensitization by fetal blood by

   a. inducing thymic involution
   b. steroid suppression of the immune response
   c. stimulating suppressor T-cell activation
   d. forming immune complexes that are rapidly cleared

5. Antibodies to spermatozoa are not commonly produced by the host because

   a. spermatozoa are not immunogenic
   b. B cells do not produce the necessary signal
   c. lymphocytes cannot enter the testis
   d. inadequate MHC peptides are expressed

TABLE 28-2
Possible Mechanisms of Autoimmune Disease

Genetic mutation: systemic, non–organ-specific

Peripheral loss of tolerance: organ-specific

Mimicry: acute, organ-specific

Persistent broken T-cell tolerance: chronic, organ-specific

References

1. Schwartz RH: Immunological tolerance. In Paul WE (ed): Fundamental Immunology, 3rd ed, p 677. New York, Raven Press, 1993

2. Ehrlich P, Morgenroth J: On haemolysins: Third and fifth communications. In The Collected Papers of Paul Ehrlich, Vol 2, pp 205–212, 246–255. London, Pergamon, 1957

3. Billingham RE, Brent L, Medawar PB: Actively acquired tolerance of foreign cells. Nature 172:603–606, 1953

4. Owen RD: Immunogenetic consequences of vascular anastomoses between bovine twins. Science 102:400–401, 1945

5. Wyllie AH, Morries RG, Smith AL, Dunlop D: Chromatin cleavage in apoptosis: Association with condensed chromatin morphology and dependence on macromolecular synthesis. J Pathol 142:67–77, 1984

6. Schild H, Rotzschke O, Kalbacher H, Rammensee HG: Limit of T cell tolerance to self protein by peptide presentation. Science 247:1587–1589, 1990

7. Metcalf ES, Linman NR: In vitro tolerance induction of neonatal murine B cells. J Exp Med 143:1327–1340, 1976

8. Nossal GJV, Pike BL: Clonal anergy: Persistence in tolerant mice of antigen-binding B lymphocytes incapable of responding to antigen or mitogen. Proc Natl Acad Sci USA 77:1602–1606, 1980

9. Howard JG, Mitchison NA: Immunological tolerance. Prog Allergy 18:68–72, 1975

10. Goodnow CC, Crosbie J, Adelstein S, et al: Altered immunoglobulin expression and functional silencing of self-reactive B lymphocytes in transgenic mice. Nature 334:676–682, 1988

11. LaSalle JM, Tolentino PJ, Freeman GJ, Nadler LM, Hafler DA: Early signaling defects in human T cells anergized by T cell presentation of autoantigen. J Exp Med 176:177–186, 1992

12. Bretscher P, Cohn M: A theory of self-nonself discrimination: Paralysis and induction involve the recognition of one and two determinants on an antigen, respectively. Science 169:1042–1049, 1970

13. Barker CF, Billingham RE: Immunologically privileged sites. Adv Immunol 25:1–54, 1977

14. Uhr JW, Moller G: Regulatory effect of antibody on the immune response. Adv Immunol 8:81–127, 1968

15. Jerne N: Toward a network theory of the immune system. Ann Immunol (Paris) 125C:373–389, 1974

CHAPTER 29

Non–Organ-Specific Autoimmune Disease

Dorothy J. Fike

Objectives

Upon completion of the chapter, the reader will be able to:

1. Define autoimmunity
2. Discuss the general mechanism of autoimmunity
3. Explain the theories that cause autoantibody production
4. Describe the patterns seen when antinuclear antibody is detected by indirect immunofluorescence
5. List the marker antibodies and explain the significance of each
6. State the immunofluorescent pattern associated with the major nuclear antigens discussed in this chapter
7. Define rheumatoid factor
8. For each of the following diseases, state the general abnormality and major serologic changes:
    Systemic lupus erythematosus
    Rheumatoid arthritis
    Sjögren's syndrome
    Progressive systemic sclerosis
    Polymyositis-dermatomyositis
    Autoimmune hemolytic anemia

AUTOIMMUNITY

Autoimmunity is a general term to describe an immune response generated by the body against its own cells or tissues. Protective immunity requires specific and nonspecific immune mechanisms that recognize and eliminate foreign configurations. Under normal circumstances, the host tolerates autoantigens, thus avoiding immune-mediated injury to itself. Detrimental or abnormal autoimmunity represents a failure to tolerate autoantigens.

The general mechanisms of harmful autoimmunity include:

1. Interaction of antibodies with cell-surface components (e.g., in myasthenia gravis, antibodies bind to acetylcholine receptors).
2. Formation of autoantigen-autoantibody complexes in fluids with or without deposition in tissue (e.g.,

immune complex–mediated glomerulonephritis in systemic lupus erythematosus).
3. Sensitization of T cells (e.g., the lymphocyte infiltrate associated with Hashimoto's thyroiditis).

These autoimmune mechanisms may be primary (an immunologic abnormality alone) or secondary (the immune abnormality resulting from another underlying condition).

Evidence suggests that some autoimmunity is beneficial and is essential to the host. Three beneficial mechanisms use the ability of immune cells and antibodies to recognize autoantigens. First, to initiate an immune response, major histocompatibility complex (MHC) Class II molecules and antigens must be coexpressed on an antigen-presenting cell to activate helper T (T_H) cells. MHC Class I molecules associated with antigen are needed to activate cytotoxic T (T_C) cells. Second, regulation of an immune response occurs by an idiotype–anti-idiotype interaction. In 1974 Jerne proposed an idiotype network based on the ability of B lymphocytes to recognize the idiotype (antigenic determinants within the antigen binding site in the variable region) of an antibody molecule and to produce an anti-idiotype antibody. This anti-idiotype antibody can then modulate the activity of T cells and B cells.[1] A third type of beneficial autoimmunity removes aged red blood cells from the circulatory system. As red cells age, a new membrane antigen is formed from another membrane protein found on younger red cells. This new antigen is produced by removing a portion of the original membrane protein; the new membrane antigen is not tolerated as self and old red blood cells are removed from circulation.[2]

THEORIES TO EXPLAIN HARMFUL AUTOIMMUNE REACTIONS

At the beginning of the century, Paul Ehrlich described the central immunologic concept of tolerance in his dictum *horror autotoxicus*. Experimentally he introduced soluble autologous constituents into the host and no immune reaction was detected. Apparently, the host was incapable of mounting an immune response to itself. Because autoimmune diseases occur spontaneously in nature, an explanation was needed.

Theories proposed to explain the mechanism of autoimmune disease include (1) the forbidden-clone theory, (2) the sequestered-antigen theory, and (3) the immunologic deficiency theory (Table 29-1).[4] The forbidden-clone theory was originally postulated by Burnet. In Burnet's model, antibodies on the surface of

TABLE 29-1
Theories to Explain Harmful Autoimmune Reactions

Forbidden-clone theory
Clonal anergy
Sequestered-antigen theory
Immunologic deficiency theory

immune cells served as receptors for specific antigens. When the specific antigen is present, the corresponding cell is stimulated to eliminate the specific antigen. Stimulated cells proliferated, establishing a clone of identical cells. Some cells of the clone became antibody-secreting cells; others became memory cells. Thus, clonal selection and expansion was a normal response to foreign antigens. When an error in self-recognition occurs during fetal life and lymphocytes directed against an autoantigen are not eliminated, this allows the expression of immune products against self—autoimmunity. Refinement of the forbidden-clone model led to the concept of clonal anergy. During fetal development, clones encountering fetal antigens would not be eliminated but would be unresponsive to low doses of the antigen. Thus, the ability to respond to higher doses of antigens later in life would be preserved.

According to the sequestered-antigen theory, some antigens are hidden from cells of the immune system; thus, the immune system never encounters these antigens and tolerance results. If the tissue is damaged, sequestered antigens are exposed and an autoimmune reaction can occur. This theory explains some autoimmune reactions, such as the development of antibodies against spermatozoa following vasectomy and against the lens after eye injury. In these cases, the autoimmune response is usually short lived and disappears before clinical symptoms develop.[5]

The immunologic deficiency theory relates the increased frequency of autoantibodies and increased immune system deficiency to increasing age. Normally, suppressor T lymphocytes prevent expression of antibody and cellular reactions by suppressing the activity of B lymphocytes and T lymphocytes. When there is a decline in the activity of the suppressor T-lymphocyte population, the response to an antigen can continue uncontrolled and can result in an autoimmune response.

The immunologic deficiency theory has evolved to reflect the current understanding of immunoregulation.[6] Control of the immune response requires both T and B lymphocytes. After an antigen is recognized, a coordinated response results via intercellular signals. As shown in Figure 29-1, the balanced interaction

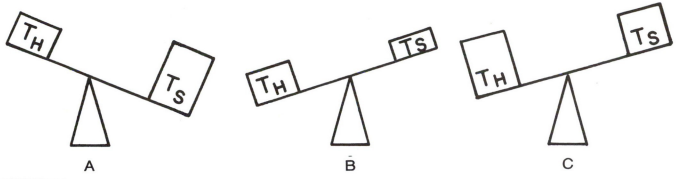

FIGURE 29-1

Autoimmunity: immunologic deficiency. (**A**) No overt autoimmune reaction occurs when suppressor T cells (T_s) dominate over helper T cells (T_H), preventing the expression of a harmful autoimmune response. (**B**) An overt autoimmune reaction may occur when hypoactive T_s fail to turn off a T_H reaction to an autologous antigen. (**C**) An overt autoimmune reaction may occur when hyperactive T_H cells dominate and encourage an inappropriate response.

between helper T cells and suppressor T cells determines whether an immune response will occur and to what extent. The helper T cells induce other T cells and B cells to react to the antigen, whereas suppressor T cells prevent other T cells and B cells from reacting. Hyperactive helper T cells can encourage an inappropriate autoimmune response, and hypoactive suppressor T cells may fail to turn off a response. Either mechanism of impaired function results in the impaired regulation of an immune response and can produce an autoimmune reaction, expressed by a variety of antibodies to common autoantigens.

Lack of appropriate immune regulation is caused by another mechanism and contributes to some autoimmune diseases.[7,8] As shown in Figure 29-2, the idiotype is immunogenic and stimulates the production of an antibody, an anti-idiotype antibody. When the anti-idiotype antibodies and the idiotype are produced by the same host, the anti-idiotype antibody is called an auto–anti-idiotype. Auto–anti-idiotypes are believed to be important in regulating a normal immune response by interacting with the idiotypic area of the antibody. However, if an anti-idiotype behaves as an autoantibody, autoimmunity can result. The best

example is Graves' disease, an autoimmune disease of the thyroid gland.[6]

SEROLOGIC FINDINGS COMMON TO NON–ORGAN-SPECIFIC AUTOIMMUNE DISEASE

Anti-Nuclear Antibodies

Antibodies to nuclear antigens (ANA) are antibodies directed against components of the cell nucleus, such as nucleoproteins and nucleic acids. ANA are associated with many systemic diseases, including systemic lupus erythematosus (SLE), mixed connective tissue disease (MCTD), and rheumatoid arthritis (RA). ANA can be used as a diagnostic indicator, a prognostic indicator, or as a means to monitor the effectiveness of therapy.

The antinuclear factor was first recognized by Hargraves when he described the lupus erythematosus (LE) cell in patients with SLE.[9] The LE cell, seen primarily in vitro, requires cells to be damaged and to release nuclear material. The nuclear chromatin is altered by the LE factor and complement. When the altered chromatin is phagocytozed by an intact neutrophil, the altered chromatin appears homogeneous. The LE factor is now known to be an anti-nuclear antibody directed against deoxyribonucleoprotein. It is found predominantly in individuals with systemic lupus erythematosus but is also detected in other systemic rheumatic diseases.

There are several techniques used to screen for ANA: agglutination, indirect immunofluorescence, light microscopy, fluorescence immunoassay, and enzyme immunoassay. The development of the immunofluorescence technique and its application to detect antinuclear antibodies provided greater sensitivity and specificity, allowed semiquantitation, and was easier to

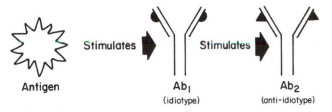

FIGURE 29-2

Idiotype network. The antigen stimulates the production of a specific antibody (Ab_1) or the idiotype. The variable region of Ab_1 is immunogenic and stimulates the production of a second antibody (Ab_2) or the anti-idiotype. When Ab_1 and Ab_2 are produced in the same individual, Ab_2 is an auto–anti-idiotype. Some anti-idiotype antibodies mimic the antigen and stimulate the production of more idiotype antibody.

perform than the LE cell preparation. Indirect immunofluorescence is still the method of choice to screen for ANA, although enzyme immunoassay appeals to laboratories preferring automation.

A representative protocol for the indirect fluorescence technique follows: Fixed substrate containing nuclei (tissue culture cells or mouse kidney) is incubated with patient or control serum. After washing, the tissue is incubated with anti–human immunoglobulin conjugated with fluorescein; following a second wash, the slide is viewed with a fluorescence microscope. The pattern and titer of the reaction are recorded.

Several patterns of nuclear fluorescence are described and are shown in Figure 29-3 (see also Color Plates 6–12). If a human epithelial tissue culture cell line, such as HEp-2 or KB cells, is used as the substrate, the patterns observed are diffuse, peripheral, speckled, nucleolar, centromere, and spindle fiber. The diffuse, or homogeneous, pattern evenly stains the nuclei and is associated with deoxyribonucleoprotein; the peripheral, or rim, pattern appears as bright fluorescence near the edge of the nuclei and is associated with native DNA; the speckled pattern appears as numerous evenly distributed speckles of fluorescence within the nuclei and is associated with many saline-extractable nuclear antigens; and the nucleolar pattern appears as two or three large, nearly round fluorescent areas within the nucleus and is associated with nucleolar RNA. The centromere and spindle-fiber patterns are present in cells that are actively replicating. The centromere pattern has a characteristic discrete speckled pattern as the centromere fluoresces, while the spindle-fiber pattern has fluorescence of only the spindle fiber. When mouse kidney is used, only the diffuse, peripheral, speckled, and nucleolar patterns of fluorescence are observed. A summary of the immunofluorescence patterns and nuclear antigens is presented in Table 29-2.[10] Sometimes there is fluorescent staining in the cytoplasm or the connective tissue between cells (Fig. 29-4, Color Plates 13–16). These staining patterns may be indicative of other autoimmune diseases. An anti-mitochondrial pattern appears as numerous speckles in the cytoplasm and is associated with primary biliary cirrhosis, while anti–smooth-muscle antibody staining of the cytoplasm is more diffuse and is associated with chronic active hepatitis.

Thus, from the indirect immunofluorescence procedure, not only can the titer of an ANA be measured, but the pattern of fluorescence can also be described. Multiple ANAs can be present in the patient sample and may be demonstrated by more than one pattern. Each pattern and its titer should be reported. The pattern, although generally not a diagnostic marker for any specific disease, may suggest the specificity of the antibody or antibodies present. Further testing can confirm the antibody specificity.

The ANA enzyme immunoassay procedure uses nuclear antigens immobilized onto a solid phase, such as the microplate well or membrane. Patient or control serum is added. After incubation, the solid phase is washed and incubated with conjugated enzyme anti–human immunoglobulin; after washing, the enzyme substrate is added. The colored product can be read visually or spectrophotometrically. The enzyme immunoassay allows for quantitation of the antibody present, but there are no patterns of reactivity. Any positive ANA result requires further testing to identify its specificity.

Each specific ANA and its antigen is listed in Table 29–3. Some apecific ANA associated with the diagnosis of systemic rheumatic diseases are marker antibodies.[10,11] The antibody directed against the nonhistone antigen, Sm antigen, is a marker antibody found in 30% to 40% of patients with SLE. Some SLE patients also have an antibody that reacts only with double-stranded DNA; this antibody is present when SLE is active and is rarely seen in other diseases. A second marker antibody is directed against the nonhistone antigen Scl-70 and is present in 15% to 20% of patients with progressive systemic sclerosis (scleroderma). The centromere antibody is a marker antibody found in a subset of progressive systemic sclerosis, CREST, with a frequency of 70% to 90%.

The frequency and association of other specific antibodies are presented in Table 29-4. Note the considerable overlap of the presence of an antibody with several diseases; for diagnostic purposes, a panel of antibodies is useful. The principal methodologies to characterize the ANA specificity include double diffusion, passive hemagglutination, enzyme immunoassay, radioimmunoassay (RIA), indirect immunofluorescence (IIF), and immunoblotting. Native DNA (n-DNA) antibodies can be detected by RIA or IIF techniques.[10] The RIA method, or Farr technique, uses radiolabeled DNA to capture the n-DNA antibody; the complex is then precipitated with saturated ammonium sulfate. Following centrifugation, the radioactivity in the precipitate is measured and is directly related to the amount of n-DNA antibody present. The IIF method uses *Crithidia luciliae* as the substrate because a strand of unbroken n-DNA is present in its kinetoplast. After incubating with fluorescent-labeled anti–human globulin and final washing, the slide is viewed with a fluorescence microscope. As seen in Figure 29-5 (see also Color Plates 17 and 18), specific fluorescence of the kinetoplast indicates the presence of n-DNA antibodies.

Either double diffusion or enzyme immunoassay may be used to detect antibodies against the saline-extractable nuclear antigens, such as Sm, SSA, SSB, Jo-1, Scl-70, and ribonucleoprotein (RNP). In the double

(*Text continues on p. 289*)

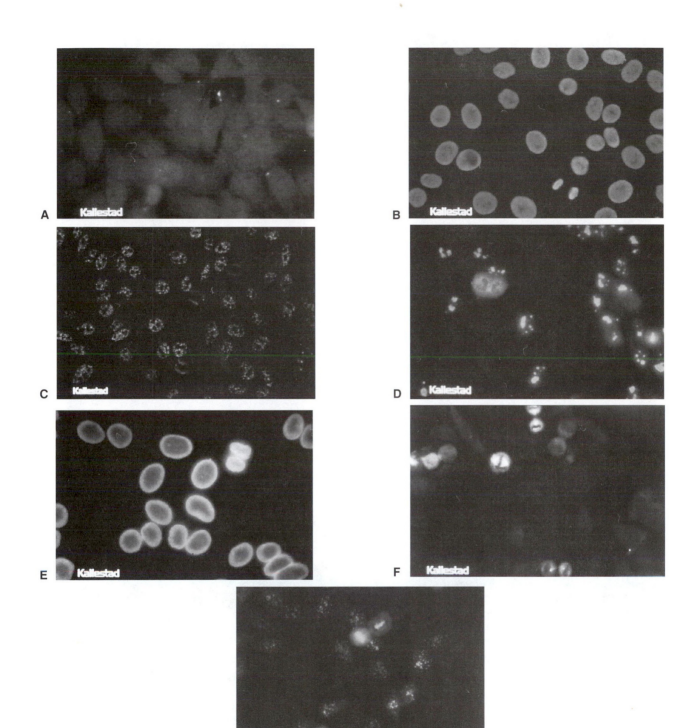

FIGURE 29-3 (COLOR PLATES 6–12)

Nuclear patterns observed in ANA testing. The indirect immunofluorescence technique uses HEp2 tissure culture cells as the substrate. The magnification is 400×. (**A**) Negative test result with no fluorescence. (**B**) Homogeneous pattern with chromosome positive. (**C**) Speckled pattern with Sm antibodies and chromosome negative. (**D**) Nucleolar pattern with chromosome-negative staining. (**E**) Peripheral pattern with chromosome-positive staining. (**F**) Spindle pattern with chromosome-negative staining. (**G**) Centromere (discrete speckled) with chromosome-positive staining. (Reproduced with permission from Sanofi Diagnostics Pasteur, Chaska, MN.)

TABLE 29-2
Nuclear Antigens and Associated Immunofluorescence Patterns

NUCLEAR ANTIGEN	PATTERN
ds-DNA	Peripheral and/or homogeneous
ssDNA	Negative
Histone	Homogeneous
RNP (U1)	Coarse speckled
Sm	Fine speckled
SS-A	Fine speckled
SS-B	Fine speckled
Scl-70	Fine speckled
Centromere	Discrete speckled
Jo-1	?Cytoplasmic
Nucleolar	Nucleolar
Spindle fiber	Spindle fiber

TABLE 29-3
Antinuclear Antibody Specificities

ANTIBODY	NATURE OF ANTIGEN
ds-DNA	Native DNA
Histone	Histones
Sm	Core proteins of nuclear ribonucleoprotein (Smith antigen)
Anti–nuclear RNP	Ribonucleoprotein (U1RNP)
SS-A	Ribonucleoprotein
SS-B	Ribonucleoprotein
Scl-70	DNA topoisomerase I
Centromere	Centromere proteins
Jo-1	Histidyl-t-RNA synthetase
Nucleolar	RNA polymerase I, fibrillarin, nucleolar organizing protein

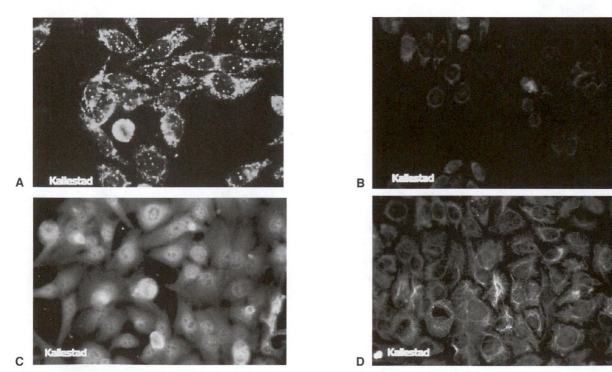

FIGURE 29-4 (COLOR PLATES 13–16)
Non-nuclear patterns in ANA testing. The HEp2 tissue culture cells may also exhibit non-nuclear staining in the indirect immunofluorescence technique. (**A**) Anti-mitochondral antibody (AMA) pattern with chromosome-negative staining. (**B**) Antiribosomal P protein pattern staining. (**C**) Anti–smooth-muscle (anti-actin) pattern staining. (**D**) Anti–smooth-muscle (anti-cytokeratin) pattern staining. (Reproduced with permission from Sanofi Diagnostics Pasteur, Chaska, MN.)

TABLE 29-4
Antibody Specificity and Disease Association

ANTIBODY	SLE	DRUG-INDUCED SLE	SS	SCLERODERMA	CREST	MYO	RA
		DISEASE (PERCENT POSITIVE)					
ds-DNA	40–60	<5	<5	<5	<5	<5	+
Histone	50–70	>95	<5	<5	<5	<5	ND
Sm	20–30	<5	<5	<5	<5	<5	ND
Nuclear RNP	30–40	<5	<5	15	10	<5	+
SS-A	30–50	<5	70–95	<5	<5	10	ND
SS-B	10–15	<5	60–90	<5	<5	<5	ND
Scl-70	<5	<5	<5	30–70	10–20	<5	ND
Centromere	<5	<5	<5	20–35	90	<5	ND
Jo-1	<5	<5	<5	<5	<5	25	ND
Nucleolar	+			+			

SLE, systemic lupus erythematosus; SS, Sjögren's syndrome; CREST, a variant of scleroderma; MYO, polymyositis; RA, rheumatoid arthritis; ND, not done. RA, rheumatoid arthritis.

diffusion method, the antigen, an extract of calf or rabbit thymus, and placed in the center well. The prototype (known positive) serum, known negative serum, and unknown patient serum are placed in the surrounding wells. During incubation, the antigen and antibody diffuse toward each other and form a precip-

itin line when the reactants meet. A line of identity between the positive serum control reaction with the patient serum reaction defines the antibody. In Figure 29-6, a line of identity confirms the presence of anti-Sm antibody in patient A and anti-RNP antibody in patient B.

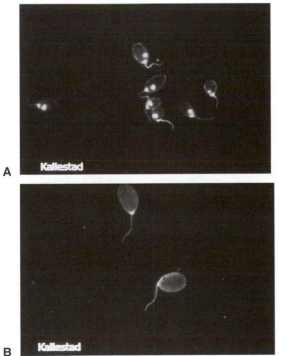

A Kallestad

B Kallestad

FIGURE 29-5 (COLOR PLATES 17 and 18)
Patterns observed in DNA testing. Indirect immunofluorescence technique using *Crithidia luciliae* and 1000× magnification. (**A**) Positive staining demonstrating anti–native-DNA antibody. The kinetoplast contains unaltered double-stranded DNA. (**B**) Negative reaction with no staining of the kinetoplast. (Reproduced with permission from Sanofi Diagnostics Pasteur, Chaska, MN.)

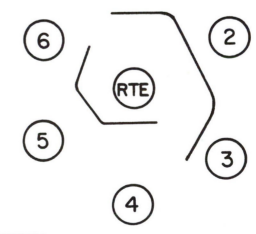

FIGURE 29-6
Immunodiffusion to identify Sm and RNP antibodies.
Well 1: anti-Sm prototype serum.
Wells 2 and 3: patient A serum.
Well 4: anti-U1-RNP prototype serum.
Wells 5 and 6: patient B serum.
The center well contains the antigens from rabbit thymus extract. Note the precipitin reaction of identity with wells 1 and 2 (patient A serum contains the Sm antibody); note the precipitin reaction of identity with wells 4 and 5 (patient B serum contains the U1-RNP antibody).

The enzyme immunoassay procedure is the same as the ANA screening procedure, except that the microwell is coated with a specific antigen. The antigen may be an extract of calf or rabbit thymus, as in the double diffusion method, or it may be a recombinant antigen. The latter antigen is slowly gaining acceptance for its use in the clinical laboratory.

Rheumatoid Factor

Rheumatoid factor (RF) is an immunoglobulin that reacts with the Fc portion of an IgG molecule; therefore, RF is an anti-antibody. In vivo, RF can be of the IgA, IgG, or IgM class; however, only RF of the IgM class is serologically detectable. RF is not species specific.[12]

Two agglutination methods are commercially available to measure RF: latex agglutination (or latex fixation) and hemagglutination. The latex agglutination method originally described by Singer and Plotz utilizes a latex particle coated with Cohn fraction II of human IgG.[13] When patient serum is heat inactivated and mixed with the human IgG-coated latex particles, macroscopic agglutination occurs when RF is present. Using a slide or tube method, semiquantitation of positive sera results in the titer; weakly positive sera have titers from 20 to 40, whereas a titer greater than 80 is considered suggestive of rheumatoid arthritis. Although this test is easy to perform, there are some disadvantages associated with it. Low titers of RF are seen in the absence of disease and with greater frequency with increasing age. False positive reactions can occur when excess lipids, microbial contamination, or C1q are present in the serum.

The other commercially available method, the Rose-Waaler test, uses sheep red blood cells coated with hemolysin, an anti-sheep erythrocyte IgG antibody produced in rabbits.[14,15] Sera containing RF will react with the rabbit IgG-coated sheep red blood cells and cause macroscopic agglutination. The hemagglutination method exhibits fewer false positive reactions with serum from normal individuals than the latex agglutination method and exhibits more specificity for those RF associated with rheumatoid arthritis. Because this assay uses sheep cells, heterophile antibodies may interfere, causing a false positive reaction.

Nephelometry can also be used to detect RF. This procedure uses the free Fc antibody fragments to detect the presence of RF. If the patient has the RF, the RF will combine with the antibody fragment and scatter light.[12] Nephelometry is easily automated and quantitated.

RF reference preparations are commercially available and are used to convert a tube titer into International Units/mL. The preparation has an assigned value that was determined by comparing its performance with that of the Bureau of Laboratories Provisional Reference Preparation for Rheumatoid Arthritis. To quantitate the amount of RF in an unknown sample, the commercial reference preparation is assayed along with the unknown sample. The concentration of RF in the unknown sample is calculated by multiplying the stated concentration of the reference preparation times the titer of the unknown, which is then divided by the titer of the reference preparation.[16]

Cryoglobulins

Cryoglobulins are proteins that reversibly precipitate or gel at 0° to 4°C. They are classified as follows: Type I cryoglobulins are monoclonal immunoglobulins, Type II represent mixed cryoglobulins in which a monoclonal immunoglobulin is directed against a polyclonal immunoglobulin, and Type III cryoglobulins are polyclonal and consist of one or more immunoglobulins, none of which are homogeneous. Types I and II cryoglobulins are associated with monoclonal gammopathies, a group of diseases in which a monoclonal protein is produced by neoplastic plasma cells or lymphocytes. Types II and III cryoglobulins are circulating immune complexes produced in response to a variety of antigens, including viral, bacterial, and autologous antigens.[17,18]

The tendency of cryoglobulins to precipitate at low temperatures may occlude blood vessels; symptoms include Raynaud's phenomenon, vascular purpura, bleeding tendencies, cold-induced urticaria, pain, and cyanosis. The cryoglobulin concentration, the temperature at which the protein precipitates, and the ability of the cryoglobulin to bind complement determine the extent of symptomatology. Essential mixed cryoglobulinemia is an idiopathic disease with arthralgia, purpura, and weakness, and frequently lymphadenopathy, hepatosplenomegaly, and renal failure. This disease can progress and may result in death.

Cryoglobulins can be detected and characterized in the clinical laboratory. Blood should be collected, allowed to clot, and centrifuged at 37°C; the serum should be separated at 37°C to ensure that the cryoglobulins will remain in the serum. If the serum is then refrigerated, cryoglobulin will appear as a white precipitate or gel. The serum should be refrigerated for a minimum of 72 hours, although 7 days is better to detect the presence of cryoglobulin. Warming the serum to 37°C will reverse the precipitation. The cryoglobulin can be quantitated by filling a hematocrit tube with serum, incubating at 1°C, centrifuging at 1°C at 750 g for 30 minutes, and reading the cryocrit. To characterize the cryoprotein, remove the supernatant and wash the precipitate three times using cold normal saline. Redissolve the cryoprecipitate by adding saline and then warming the suspension to 37°C for 30 minutes. Immunoelectrophoresis of the protein solution will identify the immunoglobulin class or classes present.[18]

Cryoglobulins can interfere in a number of laboratory tests. Complement activation can occur when C1q binds to immune complexes, causing in vitro consumption. When using optical methods to detect fibrinogen, the concentration can be falsely increased due to the presence of cryoglobulins, especially if the sample is spun at room temperature.[17]

Immune Complexes

After antigen combines with antibody, they circulate in the blood and are known as circulating immune complexes (CIC). It is a nonspecific indicator of immune activation and is commonly found in autoimmune diseases. Immune complexes lodged in tissue often result in damage. Methods to quantitate CIC are based on the physical properties of CIC, and some are shown in Figure 29-7. One method relies on the ability of CIC to bind C1q, while another relies on the interaction of the immunoglobulin portion of the immune complex to bind to rheumatoid factors. A third method relies on the property of CIC to bind Raji cells (a cultured human lymphoblastoid cell line from Burkitt's lymphoma with receptors for C3d, iC3b, and C1q).[19,20]

The clinical utility of quantitating circulating immune complexes has been questioned because of the lack of reliable assays and clinical significance. Newer commercially available ELISA tests for CIC may resolve some of these problems. These tests detect both C3d and IgG. Although various methods detect different characteristics of immune complexes, lack of a stable, reproducible calibrator has hampered the standardization of quantitative assays. Interfering substances also prevent standardization. For instance, antilymphocyte antibodies can react with Raji cells.[20] Circulating immune complexes represent a diverse group of substances containing antigen and antibody; some methods may preferentially measure one type of complex over another. The dynamics of the presence of CIC, degree of disease activity, and immune complex deposition in tissue require further investigation to assess clinical usefulness.

NON–ORGAN-SPECIFIC AUTOIMMUNE DISEASES

Systemic Lupus Erythematosus

Systemic lupus erythematosus (SLE) is a chronic, noninfectious, inflammatory disease that may involve many organs. Episodes of exacerbation alternate with remission. The onset of the disease can be insidious or acute, and the course of the disease is variable. Women are nine times more likely than men to develop SLE, particularly during the childbearing years, although the diagnosis has been made in patients aged 2 to 97 years. There is a higher incidence in African Americans than in Caucasians.[21]

SLE is an immune complex disease. Tissue injury is mediated by immune complexes that when deposited in tissue can initiate an inflammatory response. Evidence suggests that depressed suppressor T-cell function allows the overproduction or inappropriate production of autoantibodies; these autoantibodies combine with common autoantigens and form immune complexes.[22] Most important is the production of DNA–anti-DNA complexes.

The cause of SLE is unknown, but the expression of the autoimmune reaction is influenced genetically. In identical twins, if one twin has SLE, 50% to 60% of the other twins will also have the disease,[21] and in first-degree relatives of patients with SLE, the incidence of SLE is more than 200 times greater than that in the general population.[23] There is an association between SLE and the presence of HLA-DR3.[5] Recent evidence suggests that asymptomatic first-degree relatives with SLE have impaired suppressor T-cell function.[24] The increased frequency of SLE in women of childbearing age suggests that hormones influence the disease; the production of DNA antibodies appears to be enhanced by estrogens.[20]

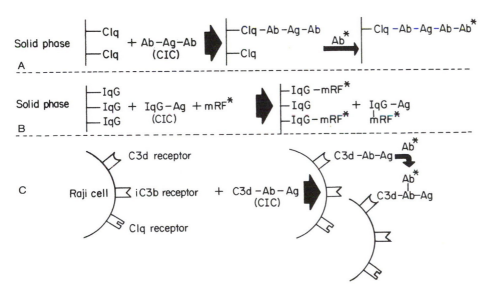

FIGURE 29-7

Methods to detect circulating immune complexes. (**A**) Solid-phase sandwich assay. Circulating immune complexes (CICs) bind to solid-phase C1q. The labeled immunoglobulin (Ab*) is quantitated and is directly related to the bound CICs. (**B**) Competitive inhibition radioimmunoassay. Unlabeled rheumatoid factor competes for binding sites on immobilized IgG and on the CICs. The labeled rheumatoid factor (mRF*) is quantitated and is inversely related to the bound CICs. (**C**) Raji cell assay. CICs bind to the cell surface receptors of the lymphoblastoid cell line, Raji cell. The labeled immunoglobulin (Ab*) is quantitated and is directly related to the bound CICs.

As in many immune diseases, the severity of the disease varies from one individual to another; there is no single, common clinical pattern. Preliminary criteria for the classification of SLE were prepared by the American Rheumatism Association in 1971 and revised in 1982. These criteria were developed to identify patients to be included in clinical studies. The presence of 4 of 11 criteria is sufficient for inclusion. The patient history and symptoms are often insufficient; when serologic and immunopathologic tests are included in the criteria, there is greater chance to establish a diagnosis.[23]

Clinical manifestations may include signs and symptoms related to any organ system. General manifestations include fever, weight loss, malaise, and weakness. Arthritis is the most common manifestation of SLE and may precede multisystem involvement. Joint involvement is SLE is symmetrical, rarely deforming, and can involve almost any joint.

Skin lesions and photosensitivity are the next most common findings in SLE. Usually the rash is erythematous and primarily involves areas exposed to ultraviolet radiation. The classic butterfly rash (malar rash) found in a minority of patients is diagnostically useful. Direct immunofluorescence performed on a skin biopsy to demonstrate immunoglobulin (usually IgG or IgM) and complement at the epidermal-dermal junction is the lupus band test. Immune complexes can be demonstrated in lesional skin in discoid lupus erythematosus, a skin disease that may exist independent of or in conjunction with SLE.

The systemic nature of SLE is apparent from the presence of immune complexes in skin biopsies from areas without an active rash and in non–sun-exposed skin. The presence and nature of the lupus band test has been used to predict the presence of renal disease, a serious manifestation of SLE. A negative lupus band test or one with IgM only is associated with a low incidence of lupus nephritis, whereas the presence of IgG, with or without other immunoglobulins, is associated with a greater incidence of renal disease. Active immune complex disease process in SLE is associated with hypocomplementemia and the presence of anti-DNA antibodies.[23,25]

Renal involvement occurs in the majority of patients with SLE. According to the World Health Organizations's Classification of Lupus Nephropathy, five classes of glomerulonephritis are associated with SLE.[21] In Class I (normal), there are no changes seen in a kidney biopsy when it is evaluated by light microscopy, electron microscopy, and immunofluorescence microscopy. The renal function is normal and the urine sediment may be normal, or a minimal amount of protein may be excreted. In Class II (mesangial changes), immune complexes in mesangium are seen by electron microscopy and direct immunofluorescence. There may be hypercellularity of the mesangial region when evaluated by light microscopy. There is slightly abnormal renal function, with the presence of hematuria, pyuria, and slight proteinuria being present. In Class III (focal and segmental proliferative, necrotizing, or sclerosing glomerulonephritis), there is hypercellularity of the mesangial region, and focal and segmental proliferation of intercapillary and extracapillary cells are seen in less than 50% of the glomeruli or less than 50% of the glomerular surface when evaluated by light microscopy. Subendothelial and mesangial deposits are seen by electron microscopy and immunofluorescence microscopy. With these changes, there is increased abnormal renal function. Nearly all patients show proteinuria, and some have nephrotic syndrome. In Class IV (diffuse proliferative glomerulonephritis), the light microscopy findings are the same as in Class III, except that greater than 50% of the glomeruli or greater than 50% of the glomerular surface is involved. Abundant subendothelial deposits are present in fluorescence microscopy. These changes are the most severe, with azotemia, hematuria, pyuria, and proteinuria being present in nearly all patients, and two thirds have nephrotic syndrome. Renal failure may occur. In Class V (membranous glomerulonephritis), a diffused uniform thickening of the glomerular capillary walls is present owing to intramembranous immune deposits. These deposits may be seen with fluorescence microscopy. All of the patients with Class V changes have proteinuria, most have nephrotic syndrome, and some have azotemia, hematuria, and pyuria.

Almost any organ system can be involved in SLE. Clinical features may include pleurisy, pericarditis, seizures, psychosis, ocular changes, pancreatitis, and small-vessel vasculitis. Hematologic findings are normochromic, normocytic anemia, leukopenia, thrombocytopenia, and deficiency in the function of suppressor T cells.[23] Although the LE factor can be demonstrated in most patients with SLE and is shown by a high titer of an IgG antibody directed against deoxyribonucleoprotein, the insensitivity and labor-intensive nature of the test has made it impractical; the ANA test is preferred.

Screening tests for ANA may be performed by fluorescence microscopy, light microscopy, and enzyme immunoassay. Virtually all patients with SLE have a high titer of ANA (≥160) with the fluorescence or light microscopy immunoassay methods. Although the IIF pattern may be diffuse, peripheral, or speckled, sera may contain multiple ANA, evidenced by detecting more than one pattern. One pattern may be masked by another (the speckled pattern can be masked by the diffuse pattern). Multiple antibodies may be present in different concentrations; thus, the pattern may change as the titer changes. Specific characterization of the ANA can be useful in making a diagnosis of SLE. Antibodies to double-stranded DNA (ds-DNA) and to the Sm antigen are nearly specific for SLE. In patients with active disease, approximately 60% to 75% have anti–ds-DNA antibodies, and 25% have Sm antibodies.[11,22] ds-DNA antibodies are strongly associated with SLE, especially at high levels. Some evidence also suggests that this antibody is associated with renal disease. Sm antibodies represent a marker for SLE: They are present in SLE and not in other rheumatic diseases. Sm antibodies can be detected by immunodiffusion, counterimmunoelectrophoresis, hemagglutination, and enzyme immunoassay.[10]

The immunologic nature of SLE is supported by the presence of numerous serum antibodies directed against other self antigens. Red blood cell antibodies are detected by the direct antiglobulin test and may cause hemolytic anemia. Lymphocyte antibodies are associated with lymphocytopenia. Platelet antibodies occur in 75% to 80% of patients with SLE and are believed to be responsible for thrombocytopenia. The lupus anticoagulant is a phospholipid antibody that interferes with coagulation and prolongs the partial thromboplastin and prothrombin times. The lupus anticoagulant is also responsible for the biological false positive non-treponemal tests for syphilis (RPR or VDRL). The antiphospholipid antibody occurs in about 15% of patients with SLE. Rheumatoid factor is another autoantibody present in low titers in nearly 30% of patients with SLE.[23]

During the active phase of the disease, complement is decreased. The immune complexes activate the complement cascade, thereby decreasing the serum complement components C3 and C4 and the functional activity when serum CH50 is measured. Cryoglobulins and circulating immune complexes may be detected in serum. The erythrocyte sedimentation rate also increases, indicating an inflammatory response. Acute-phase reactants, such as C-reactive protein, are also elevated.[26]

Rheumatoid Arthritis

Rheumatoid arthritis (RA) is a chronic noninfectious systemic inflammatory disease of unknown etiology that primarily affects the joints. Women are affected two to three times more often than men. The frequency of the disease increases with age, and the peak incidence occurs in women between 30 and 50 years of age.[23]

Pathogenetically, RA is believed to begin with the production of IgG by lymphocytes in the synovium, although the stimulus is unknown. The IgG is recognized as foreign, stimulating the production of rheumatoid factors (RF). Most RF are of the IgG and IgM (both monomeric and pentameric forms) classes, both of which can recognize the Fc portion of the IgG molecule. Immune complexes are formed, either IgG aggregates or IgM-IgG complexes, and the classical pathway of complement is activated and amplified by the alternative pathway of complement. The inflammatory response proceeds via the bioactive complement fragments, and the inflammatory cells enter the synovial space and release intracellular products (e.g., the lysosomal content, prostaglandins, and leukotrienes) that damage the synovium. T cells contribute to the inflammatory process. A consequence of the inflammatory response in the joint is the production of a pannus, an abnormal growth of synovial cells following enzymatic destruction of the cartilage. The pannus continues to grow with erosion of the cartilage and cyst formation. The final stage of rheumatoid arthritis is ankylosing (immobilization and fixing) of the joint.[24,27] The clinical course of the disease varies but usually the disease progression is slow, affecting small joints before large joints.[27]

Clinical manifestations of RA include nonspecific findings of fatigue, weight loss, weakness, mild fever, and anorexia. Morning stiffness and joint pain that improve during the day are present in all patients with RA. The inflammatory joint changes, most often in the small joints, may result in loss of function and permanent deformity. Extra-articular manifestations, most common in patients with high titers of RF, include vasculitis, rheumatoid nodules, and Sjögren's syndrome. Rheumatoid nodules, found in approximately 20% to 25% of patients with RA, especially the more severe forms, are round or oval firm masses located in the subcutaneous tissue near the joints. These are areas of collagen necrosis surrounded by a granulomatous inflammation with histiocytes, lymphocytes, and plasma cells. Sjögren's syndrome is present in approximately 30% of patients with RA. The association of splenomegaly, neutropenia, and rheumatoid arthritis is referred to as Felty's syndrome.[23]

Laboratory findings in RA include a normochromic, normocytic anemia and thrombocytosis. The erythrocyte sedimentation rate is commonly elevated, as is the concentration of C-reactive protein. RF is detected serologically in about 70% of patients with RA. The RF may be detected by latex agglutination, hemagglutination, nephelometry, and enzyme immunoassay. The hemagglutination method is more specific for RA than the latex agglutination test because it is more likely to be negative in conditions other than RA, such as hypergammaglobulinemia, syphilis, and old age. In seronegative RA, RF cannot be detected by conventional serologic methods; this may be due to the presence of RF that are IgG, monomeric IgM, IgA, or RF complexed to the IgG.[28] Cryoglobulins may also be present, but serum complement levels are usually normal.

Low titers of ANA are also present in 20% to 70% of patients with RA.[23]

During active disease, the synovial fluid has the characteristics of an inflammatory exudate; it is cloudy, with a cell count usually between 5000 and 20,000/uL, most of which are neutrophils. The protein concentration is elevated; depolymerization of hyaluronate reduces the viscosity of the fluid and causes a poor mucin clot. Complement is often decreased, and RF may be detected.[28]

Sjögren's Syndrome

Sjögren's syndrome is an inflammation of salivary and lacrimal glands causing decreased secretion from these glands that results in dryness of the mouth and eyes. Sjögren's syndrome can occur alone (primary Sjögren's syndrome) or in conjunction with other diseases (such as rheumatoid arthritis). Serologic findings that may be observed are polyclonal hypergammaglobulinemia (50% of patients); rheumatoid factor (90%); ANA (70%), usually a speckled or diffuse pattern; and autoantibodies directed against the salivary duct. Specific ANA include SS-B (in primary Sjögren's syndrome), SS-A (associated with SLE), and rheumatoid arthritis nuclear antigen (associated with rheumatoid arthritis).[10,21,23,29]

Progressive Systemic Sclerosis (Scleroderma)

Progressive systemic sclerosis (PSS) is a systemic disease in which fibrosis and degenerative changes occur in the skin, synovium, and some internal organs. PSS may be associated with Sjögren's syndrome and thyroiditis. The disease may be severe, with generalized skin and internal organ involvement, or more benign, restricted to the skin. CREST syndrome is the milder form of scleroderma manifested by *c*alcinosis, *R*aynaud's phenomenon, *e*sophageal dysmotility, *s*clerodactyly, and *t*elangiectases. Raynaud's phenomenon, pain in the extremities when exposed to cold temperatures, is the most common symptom of the disease (>90% of patients). Laboratory findings include polyclonal hypergammaglobulinemia and ANA (70% of patients) with a speckled or nucleolar pattern. Scl-70 antibody is a marker ANA detected in 15% to 20% of patients with PSS, whereas centromere antibody is a marker antibody for the CREST variant, with a frequency of 70% to 90%.[10,21,29]

Polymyositis-Dermatomyositis

This group of diseases shows acute or chronic inflammatory changes in muscle and skin. Laboratory findings include polyclonal hypergammaglobuline-mia, rheumatoid factor, antinuclear antibody, myoglobinemia, increased erythrocyte sedimentation rate, elevated creatine kinase from striated muscle, and elevated urine creatine.[28] Specific ANA are PM-1, associated with polymyositis-progressive systemic sclerosis overlap syndrome, and Jo-1, which is the serum antibody most often detected in patients with polymyositis.[10,21,29]

Autoimmune Hemolytic Anemia

Autoimmune hemolytic anemia is a systemic disorder in which there is an increased rate of destruction of red blood cells. The resulting anemia is normocytic and normochromic. Autoantibody can be directed against a number of red cell antigens, including Rh antigens.[30] The disease may be primary or secondary, as seen in chronic myelogenous leukemia. The direct antiglobulin test will detect IgG antibodies and/or C3 components that have attached to the red cells. The destruction of the red cell is generally extravascular so that complement levels are normal.

Case Studies

Case 1

SM is a 23-year-old female who felt tired for several months, had pain in the joints of her fingers, and recently developed dermatitis following exposure to the sun. The following test results were obtained on a blood sample drawn during the initial evaluation:

Total protein: 8.4 g/dL (6.0–8.0 g/dL)
ANA: 320 speckled pattern
CRP: positive
C3: 40 mg/dL (80–180 mg/dL)
C4: 5 mg/dL (15–45 mg/dL)

Case 1 Study Questions

1. Based on clinical and laboratory findings, what disease is suspected?

2. For each clinical finding and each abnormal laboratory finding, explain how it is related to the disease.

3. What additional tests should be done to further evaluate this patient?

Case 2

RP is a 36-year-old male with morning stiffness for greater than 6 months. The pain in small joints improves during the day. RP has lost 10 lbs during the last year and has noticed a decrease in his general level of energy. The following screening tests were performed:

ANA: 40 diffuse
CRP: positive
RF: negative
C3: 105 mg/dL (80–180 mg/dL)
C4: 30 mg/dL (15–45 mg/dL)

Case 2 Study Questions

1. Based on clinical and laboratory findings, what disease is suspected?

2. For each clinical finding and each abnormal laboratory finding, explain how it is related to the disease.

3. What additional tests should be done to further evaluate this patient?

References

1. Jerne NK: Towards a network theory of the immune system. Ann Immuno (Paris) 125C:3373, 1974
2. Tizard IR: Immunology, An Introduction, 3rd ed, p 476. Philadelphia, Saunders, 1992
3. Roitt I, Brostoff J, Male D: Immunology, 4th ed, p 12.1. London, CV Mosby, 1996
4. Abbas AK, Lichtman AH, Pober JS: Cellular and Molecular Immunology, 2nd ed, p 377. Philadelphia, Saunders, 1994
5. Theofilopoulos AN: Autoimmunity. In Stites DP, Stobo JD, Wells JV (eds): Basic and Clinical Immunology, 6th ed, p 128. Norwalk, CT, Appleton and Lange, 1987
6. Shoenfeld Y, Schwartz RS: Immunologic and genetic factors in autoimmune diseases. N Engl J Med 311:16, 1984
7. Burdette S, Schwartz RS: Idiotypes and idiotypic networks. N Engl J Med 317:219, 1987
8. Kennedy RC: Anti-idiotype antibodies: Prospects in clinical and laboratory medicine. Lab Management 8:33, 1987
9. Zweiman B, Lisak RP: Autoantibodies: Autoimmunity and immune complexes. In Henry JB (ed): Clinical Diagnosis and Management by Laboratory Methods, 17th ed, p 924. Philadelphia, Saunders, 1984
10. Nakamura RM, Peebles CL, Moldern DP, et al: Autoantibodies to Nuclear Antigens, 2nd ed. Chicago, American Society of Clinical Pathologists Press, 1985
11. Isenberg DA, Maddison PJ: Detection of antibodies to double stranded DNA and extractable nuclear antigen (Broadsheet 117). J Clin Pathol 40:1374, 1987
12. Cook L, Agnello V: Tests for detection of rheumatoid factor. In Rose NR, DeMacario EC, Fahey JL, Friedman H, Penn GM (eds): Manual of Clinical Laboratory Immunology, 4th ed, p 762. Washington, DC, American Society for Microbiology, 1992
13. Singer JM, Plotz CM: The latex fixation test. I. Applications to the serologic diagnosis of rheumatoid arthritis. Am J Med 21:888, 1956
14. Waaler E: On the occurrence of a factor in human serum activating the specific agglutination of sheep blood corpuscles. Acta Pathol Microbiol Scand 17:172, 1940
15. Rose HM, Ragan C, Pearce E, et al: Differential agglutination of normal and sensitized sheep erythrocytes by sera of patients with rheumatoid arthritis. Proc Soc Exp Biol Med 68:1, 1948
16. Anderson SG, Bentzon MW, Houba V, Krag P: International Reference Preparation of Rheumatoid Arthritis Serum. Bull WHO 42:311–318, 1970
17. Zweiman B, Lisak RP: Autoantibodies: Autoimmunity and immune complexes. In Henry JB (ed): Clinical Diagnosis and Management by Laboratory Methods, 17th ed, p 885. Philadelphia, WB Saunders, 1991
18. Stites DP, Rodgers RPC: Clinical laboratory methods for detection of antigens and antibodies. In Stites DP, Stobo JD, Wells JV (eds): Basic and Clinical Immunology, 6th ed, p 241. Norwalk, CT, Appleton and Lange, 1987
19. Cook L, Agnello V: Detection of immune complexes. In Rose NR, DeMacario EC, Fahey JL, Friedman H, Penn GM (eds): Manual of Clinical Laboratory Immunology, 4th ed, p 110. Washington DC, American Society for Microbiology, 1992
20. Theofilopoulos AN, Aguado MT, McDougal JS: Assay for detection of complement-fixing immune complexes: Raji cells, conglutinin and anti-C3 assays. In Rose NR, DeMacario EC, Fahey JL, Friedman H, Penn GM (eds): Manual of Clinical Laboratory Immunology, 4th ed, p 104. Washington, DC, American Society for Microbiology, 1992
21. Coltran RS, Kumar V, Robbins SL (eds): Robbins Pathologic Basis of Disease, 5th ed, p 199. Philadelphia, WB Saunders, 1994
22. Miller KB, Schwartz RS: Autoimmunity and suppressor T lymphocytes. Adv Intern Med 227:281, 1982
23. Schumacher HR: Primer on the Rheumatic Diseases, 9th ed. Atlanta, Arthritis Foundation, 1988
24. Miller KB, Schwartz RS: Familial abnormalities of suppressor-cell function in systemic lupus erythematosus. N Engl J Med 301:803, 1979
25. Diaz LA, Provost TT: Dermatologic diseases. In Stites DP, Stobo JD, Wells JV (eds): Basic and Clinical Immunology, 6th ed, p 516. Norwalk, CT, Appleton and Lange, 1987
26. Tucker ES, Nakumura RM: Laboratory studies for the evaluation of systemic lupus erythematosus and related disorders. Lab Med 11:717, 1980
27. Rosenberg AE: Skeletal system and soft tissue tumors. In Coltran RS, Kumar V, Robbins SL (eds): Robbins Patho-

logic Basis of Disease, 5th ed, p 1249. Philadelphia, WB Saunders, 1994

28. Fye KH, Sack KE: Rheumatic diseases. In Stites DP, Stobo JD, Wells JV (eds): Basic and Clinical Immunology, 6th ed, p 516. Norwalk, CT, Appleton and Lange, 1987

29. Nakamura RM, Tan EM: Update on autoantibodies to intracellular antigens in systemic rheumatic diseases. Clin Lab Med 12:1, 1992

30. Walker RH (ed): Technical Manual, 11th ed, p 355. Bethesda, MD, American Association of Blood Banks, 1993

CHAPTER 30

Organ-Specific Autoimmune Disease

Dorothy J. Fike

Objectives

Upon completion of the chapter, the reader will be able to:

1. Discuss the differences between non–organ-specific and organ-specific autoimmune diseases
2. List the laboratory test procedures used to diagnose thyroid autoimmune diseases
3. Describe the differences between Graves' disease and Hashimoto's thyroiditis
4. List the laboratory test procedures used to diagnose liver autoimmune diseases
5. Describe the differences between autoimmune chronic active hepatitis and primary biliary cirrhosis
6. Discuss spinal fluid immunoglobulin quantitation in multiple sclerosis
7. Identify autoimmune antibodies and immunologic changes associated with myasthenia gravis, diabetes mellitus, idiopathic adrenal failure, autoimmune bullous skin diseases, Good-pasture's syndrome, and spermatozoa antibody-mediated infertility.

ORGAN VERSUS NON-ORGAN SPECIFICITY

The spectrum of autoimmune diseases ranges from organ-specific to non–organ-specific to non–species-specific. In organ-specific autoimmune diseases, autoantibody and cellular reactions take place in only one organ or type of tissue, for example, in the thyroid gland in Hashimoto's thyroiditis. At the other end of the spectrum are those autoimmune diseases in which multiple antibodies affect multiple organs; systemic lupus erythematosus is the classic example and was discussed in Chapter 29. Table 30-1 lists autoimmune diseases based on the extent of organ specificity. Some autoimmune diseases are in between the extremes and occur primarily in one organ but exhibit multiple antibodies. The pathogenesis of organ-specific autoimmune diseases is the same as that of systemic autoimmune diseases.

TABLE 30-1
Spectrum of Autoimmune Disease

ORGAN-SPECIFIC	INTERMEDIATE	NON–ORGAN-SPECIFIC
Hashimoto's thyroiditis	1° biliary cirrhosis	SLE
Graves' disease	Sjögren's syndrome	Rheumatoid arthritis
Pernicious anemia	Myasthenia gravis	PSS
Insulin-dependent diabetes mellitus	Goodpasture's syndrome	MCTD
	Chronic active hepatitis	

SLE, systemic lupus erythematosus; PSS, progressive systemic sclerosis; MCTD, mixed connective tissue disease.

ORGAN-SPECIFIC AUTOIMMUNE DISEASES

Autoimmune Thyroiditis

Two common autoimmune diseases of the thyroid gland are chronic lymphocytic thyroiditis and Graves' disease. Chronic lymphocytic thyroiditis or Hashimoto's thyroiditis most often appears in women between 30 and 60 years of age, with a 5:1 female-to-male ratio.[1] Both humoral and cellular immunity are activated in Hashimoto's thyroiditis, as demonstrated by serum antibodies to multiple thyroid antigens and a prominent lymphocytic infiltrate. The lymphocytic infiltrate is predominantly B cells and CD4+ T cells; germinal centers are seen because the architecture of the thyroid resembles that of a lymph node. Destruction of normal thyroid tissue leads to hypothyroidism, loss of thyroid function and low levels of circulating thyroid hormones. The inflammatory response in the thyroid gland is probably initiated by antibody-dependent cell-mediated lymphocytotoxicity.[1]

The thyroid autoantibodies detectable in the serum are directed against three thyroid antigens: thyroglobulin in the follicle, thyroid peroxidase (previously known as the microsomal antigen) in the cytoplasm of the epithelial cells, and the second colloid antigen (CA-2) in the follicle.[2] Approximately 75% of patients with Hashimoto's thyroiditis demonstrate thyroglobulin antibodies, 70% thyroid peroxidase antibodies, and 40% CA-2. Nearly all (97%) patients with Hashimoto's thyroiditis have at least one of these three antibodies, often in very high titers. The classic screening test for thyroid autoantibodies is the indirect immunofluorescence method using primate thyroid sections as the substrate. Using sections fixed in methanol, the presence of thyroglobulin antibodies will cause the follicle to appear flocculent and CA-2 antibodies to appear diffuse; unfixed sections are used to detect thyroid peroxidase antibodies in which the cytoplasmic staining of the epithelial cells is granular (Fig. 30-1, Color Plates 19 and 20). Although the indirect fluorescence test was the first method used, passive hemagglutination to detect thyroglobulin and thyroid peroxidase antibodies is

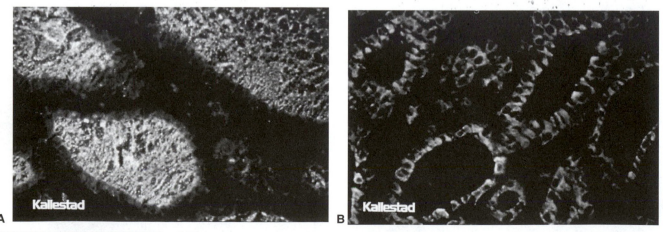

FIGURE 30-1 (COLOR PLATES 19 and 20)
Using fixed primate thyroid as the substrate, thyroglobulin antibody is shown in **A** as diffuse staining of the colloid in the follicle. The thyroid peroxidase antibody is shown in **B** as granular cytoplasmic staining of the unfixed epithelial cells surrounding the follicle. (Reproduced with permission from Sanofi Diagnostics Pasteur, Chaska, MN.)

more commonly used. The need for pure antigen in this test and heterophile antibody interference are disadvantages, but its ease of performance and greater sensitivity are advantages compared with the indirect immunofluorescence method. Further refinements have enhanced specificity and shortened the turnaround time.[1,3] Use of recombinant antigens aids in specific antibody detection, whereas the dot-blot immunoassay format allows multiple antibodies to be detected simultaneously. The prozone effect can be monitored by testing patient serum with more than one concentration of thyroid antigen.[2]

In Graves' disease the thyroid gland is overstimulated, causing diffuse hyperplasia and the development of a diffuse goiter. The continuous stimulation results in hyperthyroidism (thyrotoxicosis) with elevated serum concentrations of thyroid hormones (free and total T3 and T4) and decreased thyroid stimulating hormone. Exophthalmos and infiltrative dermopathy are common findings in Graves' disease.

In normal function, the thyroid gland is stimulated by thyroid stimulating hormone (TSH) to release thyroid hormones. When a sufficient serum level of thyroid hormone is achieved, TSH is no longer secreted by the anterior pituitary. Consequently, the thyroid is no longer stimulated and stops releasing the thyroid hormones. In Graves' disease an autoantibody mimics the thyroid stimulating hormone and reacts with the TSH receptor on thyroid cells. Some of these autoantibodies stimulate the thyroid and have been called long-acting thyroid stimulator (LATS) and thyroid-stimulating antibodies (TSab); other antibodies inhibit the action of TSH receptor and have been called thyrotropin binding-inhibiting immunoglobulin (TBII). To clarify the terminology for antibodies that react with the TSH receptor, the American Thyroid Association recommended the term TSH receptor antibody (TRAb) be used to describe all antibodies reacting with the TSH receptor.[4] Experimental evidence suggests that the autoantibody in Graves' disease is an anti-idiotype antibody. When TSH antibodies are used to produce anti-TSH antibodies that are anti-idiotype antibodies, the anti-idiotype antibody stimulates thyroid cells in tissue culture, mimicking the metabolic events in spontaneous Graves' disease.[5]

Two different methods have evolved to measure TRAb. One measures the ability of the antibody to stimulate the thyroid, and the other measures the ability of the antibody to compete with TSH for receptor binding. The ability of some TRAb to stimulate the thyroid gland while others do not suggests that different epitopes on the TSH receptor are recognized. TRAb directed against the glycoprotein portion of the TSH receptor fails to stimulate the gland, whereas antibodies against the ganglioside portion of the receptor are stimulatory for the thyroid.[6,7] Other thyroid autoantibodies may also be present in a significant number of patients with Graves' disease: thyroglobulin antibodies in 40%, thyroid peroxidase antibodies in 50%, and CA-2 antibodies in 5%.[2]

Autoimmune Disease of the Liver

A loss of tolerance against autologous liver tissue appears to be the principal pathogenetic mechanism in autoimmune diseases of the liver. Even though there are diagnostic antibodies used to detect autoimmune chronic active hepatitis (AI-CAH) and primary biliary cirrhosis (PBC), the exact mechanisms responsible for the tissue destruction are not completely known.[8]

AUTOIMMUNE CHRONIC ACTIVE HEPATITIS

Of the many forms of chronic active hepatitis, evidence for autoimmune factors is prominent in one type, autoimmune chronic active hepatitis (AI-CAH). Histologic changes include intraportal and periportal infiltration of lymphocytes and plasma cells. The diminished number and function of suppressor T cells explain the polyclonal increase in serum immunoglobulin (especially IgG) and the presence of autoantibodies to different organs. Because anti-nuclear antibodies (ANA) are commonly present, this disease is also known as lupoid chronic active hepatitis. The ANA test is an appropriate test to support the diagnosis, although no specific ANA has been characterized for AI-CAH. Smooth-muscle antibodies are present, usually in high titer. To test for smooth-muscle antibodies, the indirect immunofluorescence test uses smooth muscle from one of several organs and species as the substrate. The major antigen in the smooth muscle is actin, and the antibodies produced are IgG. Actin antibodies can be seen as non-nuclear staining of the HEp-2 cells used in the indirect immunofluorescence method to detect ANA.[9]

PRIMARY BILIARY CIRRHOSIS

Primary biliary cirrhosis (PBC) affects small intrahepatic bile ducts and eventually leads to liver failure. Nearly all patients (99%) with PBC have high-titer mitochondrial antibody, although this antibody may be found less frequently and in lower titers in other liver diseases. There are nine mitochondrial antigens, designated M1 to M9. M2 appears to have specificity for PBC.[2] The mitochondrial antigen is a lipoprotein located on the inner mitochondrial membrane. Detection of the mitochondrial antibody is most often accomplished by indirect immunofluorescence on rat kidney substrate, in which the tubular epithelial cells serve as the source rich in mitochondria. As with AI-CAH, non-nuclear staining occurs in the indirect immunofluorescence method to detect ANA using HEp-2 cells. Extrahepatic manifestations of the disease—arthritis, arteritis, and glomerulonephritis—are probably related to circulating immune complexes. Reduction in the number and function of suppressor T cells leads to the overproduction of monomeric IgM and the failure to switch to IgG production. Patients with primary biliary cirrhosis are severely anergic.[9,10]

Myasthenia Gravis

Myasthenia gravis is a neuromuscular disease in which the innervation of muscles is impaired. Muscle weakness results, especially after sustained exercise, when acetylcholine is prevented from stimulating muscle to contract. Antibodies to acetylcholine receptors, present in approximately 90% of patients with myasthenia gravis, are believed to bind to the acetylcholine receptors, causing endocytosis of the receptors; thus, acetylcholine cannot bind to the receptor and does not stimulate the muscle. Other findings contribute to the immunologic basis of the disease: thymic hyperplasia with an increased number of germinal centers and increased B cells (70%), thymoma (a tumor of epithelial cells in the thymus gland; 10%), smooth-muscle antibodies, and a greater than expected association with other autoimmune disorders.[11] Experimentally, an acetylcholine receptor antibody that is an anti-idiotype antibody produces a myasthenia-like syndrome in rabbits and mice;[12,13] this has led to the speculation that in human myasthenia gravis, the increased number of B cells in germinal centers in the thymus produce an auto-acetylcholine receptor antibody that is responsible for the impaired neuromuscular transmission.[14] Following thymectomy, two thirds of patients with myasthenia gravis improve, further supporting the role of the thymus in the production of acetylcholine receptor antibodies and the pathogenesis of myasthenia gravis.[11]

Multiple Sclerosis

Multiple sclerosis, a chronic progressive inflammatory disease, is associated with demyelination of the white matter of the central nervous system. Affecting primarily young adults, there is a familial association and a geographic distribution of the disease. The etiology of this disease is unknown; however, an immunologic mechanism is suggested by the presence of lymphocytes in early lesions and plasma cells, lymphocytes, and macrophages in older lesions. Increased globulin concentrations in cerebrospinal fluid (CSF) are detected in 60% to 80% of multiple sclerosis patients. Faulty T-cell immunoregulation is present in multiple sclerosis; decreased suppressor T-cell function during active disease episodes can explain the increased CSF concentration of IgG.[11] The active lesions of multiple sclerosis, also called *plaques*, contain suppressor T cells, helper T

cells, and macrophages that actively break down myelin basic protein, releasing it into CSF: A concentration greater than 4 ng/mL is associated with multiple sclerosis and other demyelinating diseases.[15]

Increased immunoglobulin concentrations in CSF are present in the majority of patients with multiple sclerosis. Two methods to evaluate central nervous system production of immunoglobulins are the IgG index and CSF protein electrophoresis. The IgG index can determine if the increase in CSF IgG is caused by local IgG production or by a change in the permeability of the blood-brain barrier.

$$IgG\ index\ =\ \frac{CSF\ IgG/serum\ IgG}{CSF\ albumin/serum\ albumin}.$$

The normal range for the IgG index is 0.4 to 0.53. An index greater than 0.7 is considered elevated and indicates that IgG production originates in the central nervous system.

The second method to evaluate the source of immunoglobulin production is high-resolution agarose gel electrophoresis of CSF. Oligoclonal banding in the gamma globulin region suggests local IgG synthesis. Oligoclonal banding is seen as several discrete protein bands in the gamma globulin region and represents immunoglobulins produced by several clones of lymphocytes (Fig. 30-2, Color Plate 21). Ninety percent of multiple sclerosis patients have oligoclonal banding; however, it is not specific for multiple sclerosis because it can also be demonstrated in viral meningitis, neurosyphilis, SLE with central nervous system involve-

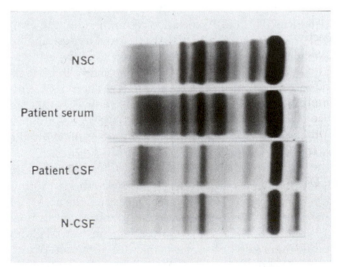

FIGURE 30-2 (COLOR PLATE 21)
Using high-resolution protein electrophoresis, note the oligoclonal banding seen in the CSF from a patient with multiple sclerosis (Patient CSF) compared with the normal CSF (N-CSF). The gamma region is on the left. The patient serum and normal serum control (NSC) do not show oligoclonal banding which is consistent with multiple sclerosis. (Used with permission of Helena Laboratories.)

ment, and other immunologic disease of the central nervous system.[16]

Diabetes Mellitus

Insulin-dependent or type I diabetes mellitus (IDDM) is associated with islet cell antibodies early in the disease. The National Diabetes Data Group of the National Institutes of Health classified IDDM as having an early onset (<20 years of age), the presence of islet cell antibodies, commonly ketoacidosis, and a genetic component.[17] The pathogenesis of IDDM is autoimmunity with early insulitis. Marked atrophy and fibrosis of the islet cells causes severe insulin deficiency and beta-cell depletion. Three mechanisms contribute to IDDM: environmental insult, genetic susceptibility, and autoimmunity. The environmental insult that triggers the autoimmune response is unknown, but viruses are suspected to be initiators; there is a seasonal trend in the diagnosis. After outbreaks of mumps, measles, rubella, coxsackie B virus, and infectious mononucleosis in a community, there is an increase in new cases of IDDM. Early ingestion of cow's milk may be another environmental insult; antibodies to bovine serum albumin (BSA) are present in patients with IDDM. Because BSA and islet cells have a 17 amino-acid peptide in common, BSA antibody may crossreact with islet cell antigens and initiate an immunologic reaction.[18]

MHC Class II antigens contribute to the genetic susceptibility of IDDM. The most common antigen in Caucasians is HLA-DQ3.2, which is present in 70% of the patients. Individuals with this gene have an eight-fold risk of developing IDDM. HLA-DR3 also has an increased frequency in IDDM. When both HLA-DQ3.2 and HLA-DR3 are present, an individual has a 20-fold risk of developing IDDM. HLA genes can also be protective; individuals with HLA-DQ1.2 have a decreased risk of developing IDDM.[18]

By indirect immunofluorescence, approximately 60% to 85% of patients with insulin-dependent diabetes mellitus have cytoplasmic staining of the beta cells of the pancreas, even before impaired glucose tolerance. Other evidence of an autoimmune pathogenesis which is frequently observed in recent-onset cases of IDDM is the presence of lymphocytic infiltrates, containing CD4+ and CD8+ T cells in the pancreas. In animal models, CD4+ T cells of diseased animals can transfer IDDM to normal animals, thus establishing that T cells mediate autoimmunity in IDDM. Approximately 10% of individuals with IDDM also have other organ-specific autoimmune disorders, such as Graves' disease and pernicious anemia. In these individuals there is a major derangement of immunoregulation.[18]

Diabetics are more susceptible to infections such as pyelonephritis, tuberculosis, pneumonia, and dermatitis. These infections result in approximately 5% of the deaths in diabetic patients. Impaired leukocyte functions and poor blood supply secondary to vascular disease predispose diabetics to these infections.[18]

Idiopathic Adrenal Failure

The idiopathic form of Addison's disease (adrenocortical failure) is associated with the production of antibodies directed against the microsomal component of adrenal cortical cells in approximately 50% of the patients.[3] These antibodies are detected by the indirect immunofluorescence method. Adrenal insufficiency is often accompanied by other autoimmune disorders, such as Hashimoto's thyroiditis, Graves' disease, pernicious anemia, diabetes mellitus, or hypoparathyroidism.[2]

Chronic Atrophic Gastritis with Pernicious Anemia

Atrophy of the stomach mucosa results in decreased pepsinogen secretion by the chief cells and decreased secretion of hydrochloric acid and intrinsic factor by the parietal cells. Pepsinogens are hydrolytic enzymes necessary to digest protein; hydrochloric acid reduces the pH in the stomach, and intrinsic factor is necessary for vitamin B_{12} absorption. Vitamin B_{12} deficiency results in pernicious anemia.[9] Pernicious anemia is a megaloblastic anemia caused by defective DNA synthesis; vitamin B_{12} is required for folic acid to produce DNA. Three types of humoral antibodies are frequently associated with pernicious anemia: parietal cell antibodies and two antibodies reactive with intrinsic factor. Parietal cell antibodies, detected by indirect immunofluorescence, appear as granular, cytoplasmic staining of parietal cells. This granular appearance mimics the staining pattern of mitochondrial antibodies but can be distinguished from it by comparing the reactivity on two tissue substrates, gastric mucosal and renal epithelial cells. Parietal cell antibody will react with the lipoprotein antigen of the parietal cell but not with the mitochondria of epithelial cells of the renal tubules, whereas the mitochondrial antibody will react with mitochondria in both parietal cells and renal tubular epithelial cells.[9]

There are two intrinsic factor antibodies: a blocking antibody (type I) that prevents vitamin B_{12} from binding to intrinsic factor and a binding antibody (type II) that reacts with intrinsic factor or intrinsic factor–vitamin B_{12} complexes. The blocking antibody occurs twice as frequently as the binding antibody. In patients with pernicious anemia, approximately 90% have parietal cell antibodies, and 60% to 70% have intrinsic factor antibodies.[9] Parietal cell antibodies are detected in other diseases, such as atrophic gastritis without hematologic changes (60%), chronic thyroiditis (30%), thyrotoxicosis

(25%), and diabetes mellitus (21%).[2,9] Intrinsic factor antibodies, however, are found nearly exclusively in pernicious anemia. Low levels of thyroid antibodies may also be present in patients with pernicious anemia.

Goodpasture's Syndrome

In Goodpasture's syndrome, circulating antibodies directed against Type IV collagen combine with alveolar basement membrane and the glomerular basement membrane to initiate an autoimmune reaction. Following complement activation, tissue damage results in pulmonary hemorrhage and progressive glomerulonephritis. Complement components and anti–basement membrane antibodies can be demonstrated by direct immunofluorescence in a kidney biopsy (Fig. 30-3). The fluorescence pattern is linear and appears smooth, in contrast to the granular pattern associated with immune complex glomerulonephritis. Circulating anti–glomerular basement membrane antibodies of the IgG class can be demonstrated in approximately 89% of patients with Goodpasture's syndrome by indirect immunofluorescence,[19] but enzyme immunoassay is preferred because of its greater sensitivity.

Autoimmune Bullous Skin Diseases

Pemphigus vulgaris, bullous pemphigoid, and dermatitis herpetiformis are blistering autoimmune skin diseases.[20] Pemphigus vulgaris is characterized by an intraepidermal blister caused by damage to the intercellular bridges (desmosomes) of the prickle cells in the epidermis. Using direct immunofluorescence on a biopsy of perilesional skin, the intercellular space consistently demonstrates the presence of IgG. Circulating serum autoantibodies directed against the intercellular substance can be demonstrated by indirect immunofluorescence using monkey esophagus as the substrate.

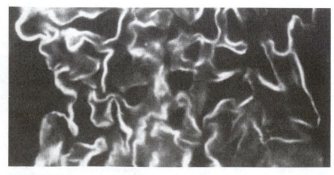

FIGURE 30-3
Goodpasture's syndrome shows linear fluorescent staining of the glomerular basement membrane. (Charlesworth JA, Pussell BA, [1986]. Clinical Immunology Illustrated, JV Wells and DS Nelson [eds.]. Williams and Wilkins, 191, used with permission.)

These autoantibodies are of the IgG class and are present in approximately 90% of patients with pemphigus vulgaris. There is a close association between pemphigus and HLA-DR4.

Bullous pemphigoid is a subepidermal blistering disease in which IgG and C3 can be demonstrated by direct immunofluorescence in biopsies of perilesional skin. The staining pattern is linear, indicated by smooth, continuous fluorescence. By immunoelectronmicroscopy the immune complexes are located in the lamina lucida of the basement membrane. Serum autoantibodies directed against the basement membrane are found in approximately 80% of patients with bullous pemphigoid. These autoantibodies are detected by indirect immunofluorescence and are of the IgG class.[20]

Dermatitis herpetiformis is a chronic bullous disease in which a granular pattern of IgA deposition in perilesional skin can be demonstrated by direct immunofluorescence. Circulating IgA autoantibodies are absent. Dermatitis herpetiformis is nearly always associated with gluten-sensitive enteropathy. A current pathogenetic hypothesis suggests that gluten, or another dietary substance, damages the small intestine and stimulates antibody production. The antibody combines with its antigen and forms circulating immune complexes that lodge in the skin. The alternative pathway of complement is activated, and the resulting production of inflammatory mediators is responsible for the blister formation. Restriction of dietary gluten improves the skin disease. There is a strong association between dermatitis herpetiformis and HLA-DR3.[20]

Spermatozoa Antibody-Mediated Infertility

Two immune mechanisms may lead to infertility: antisperm antibodies found in females and autoimmune disease of the gonads found in males.[21] Sperm antibodies incapacitate spermatozoa by complement-dependent cytotoxicity, interfering with their transport in the female genital tract, or by cellular interaction in the fertilization process. In most patients there appears to be a spontaneous formation of autoantibodies to sperm, but formation of these autoantibodies may also form after vasoligation in men. When the spermatozoa antibodies are produced systemically, antibody will be found in the serum; when they are produced in the mucosal tissue, antibodies are found only in the gonads.

The class of immunoglobulin has a predictive value on fertility. IgM sperm antibodies are commonly found in serum samples but not in seminal plasma. IgM antibody that binds to the spermatozoa tail is commonly found in fertile couples. The presence and concentration of IgG and IgA sperm antibodies are more predictive of fertility reduction.[21]

There are many methods that may be used to detect these antibodies, such as direct and indirect immunobead, mixed antiglobulin reaction, and microscopic spermatozoa agglutination. Even though there are methods to detect sperm antibodies, the clinical significance of these antibodies is incomplete; methods for detecting sperm antibodies are not quantitative, and no prospective double-blind studies on the significance of antibodies have been performed.[21]

CONCLUSION

Autoimmunity is an immune process involving recognition of autoantigens. A summary of these antigens and associated diseases is listed in Table 30-2. Both humoral immunity and cell-mediated immunity may contribute to host damage. Evidence of an autoimmune process may be documented by identifying circulating or tissue-lodged immune complexes, circulating auto-

antibodies, complement consumption or activation, or histologic changes.

Case Studies

Case 1

GN, a 45-year-old male, went to his physician because he was feeling tired all the time. The physical examination revealed a goiter and slight lid lag and stare. From these symptoms, the physician suspected a thyroid disorder.

Case 1 Study Questions

1. What two autoimmune disorders might the physician suspect?

2. What are the tests that the physician would order to detect an autoimmune thyroid disorder?

3. What would the test results be for each of these disorders?

Case 2

AL, a 34-year-old male, went to his physician because he was not feeling well and noticed that his eyes looked a little yellow.

Case 2 Study Questions

1. What are two autoimmune liver disorders?

2. What tests would be used to detect autoimmune liver disorders?

3. What would be the test results for each of these disorders?

TABLE 30-2
Representative Organ-Specific Autoantibodies

ORGAN	ANTIBODY
Thyroid	
Graves' disease	Thyroid peroxidase, TRAb, LATS
Hashimoto's thyroiditis (chronic lymphocytic)	Thyroid peroxidase, thyroglobulin, CA-2
Liver	
Autoimmune chronic active hepatitis	ANA, smooth muscle (actin)
Primary biliary cirrhosis	Mitochondrial
Nervous system	
Myasthenia gravis	Acetylcholine receptor
Multiple sclerosis	Cellular response, antibody unknown
Pancreas	
Diabetes mellitus	Islet cell
Stomach	
Pernicious anemia	Parietal cell, intrinsic factor (2)
Kidney	
Goodpasture's syndrome	Type IV collagen
Skin	
Pemphigus vulgaris	Intercellular cement substance
Bullous pemphigoid	Component of skin basement membrane
Dermatitis herpetiformis	Gliadin, reticulin
Gonads	
Spermatozoa	Spermatozoa

References

1. Rose NR, Lorenzi M, Lewis M: Endocrine diseases. In Stites DP, Stobo JD, Wells JV (eds): Basic and Clinical Immunology, 6th ed, p 582. Norwalk, CT, Appleton and Lange, 1987

2. Zweiman B, Lisak RP: Autoantibodies, autoimmunity and immune complexes. In Henry JB (ed): Clinical Diagnosis and Management by Laboratory Methods, 18th ed, p 885. Philadelphia, Saunders, 1991

3. Bigazzi PE, Burek CL, Rose NR: Antibodies to tissue-specific endocrine, gastrointestinal, and surface-receptor antigens. In Rose NR, DeMacario EC, Fahey JL, Friedman H, Penn GM (eds): Manual of Clinical Laboratory Immunology, 4th ed, p 765. Washington, DC, American Society for Microbiology, 1992

4. Larsen PR, Alexander NM, Chopra IJ, et al: Revised nomenclature for tests of thyroid hormones and thyroid-related proteins in serum. J Clin Endocrinol Metab 46:1089, 1987

5. Shoenfield T, Schwarryz RS: Immunologic and genetic factors in autoimmune diseases. N Engl J Med 311:16, 1984

6. Valente WA, Vitti P, Rotella CM, et al: Antibodies that promote thyroid growth: A distinct population of thyroid-stimulating autoantibodies. N Engl J Med 309:1028, 1983

7. Yavin E, Yavin Z, Schneider MD, et al: Monoclonal antibodies to the thyrotropin receptor: Implications for receptor structure and the action of autoantibodies in Graves' disease. Proc Natl Acad Sci USA 78:3180, 1981

8. Crawford JM: The liver and the biliary tract. In Cotran RS, Kumar V, Robbins SL (eds): Robbins Pathologic Basis of Disease, 5th ed, p 853. Philadelphia, Saunders, 1994

9. Taylor KB, Thomas HC: Gastrointestinal and liver diseases. In Stites DP, Stobo JD, Wells JV (eds): Basic and Clinical Immunology, 6th ed, p 457. Norwalk, CT, Appleton and Lange, 1987

10. McMillan SA, Alderdice JM, McKee CM, et al: Diversity of autoantibodies in patients with antimitochondrial antibody and their diagnostic value. J Clin Pathol 40:232, 1987

11. Hoffman PM, Panitch HS: Neurologic diseases. In Stites DP, Stobo JD, Wells JV (eds): Basic and Clinical Immunology, 6th ed, p 598. Norwalk, CT, Appleton and Lange, 1987

12. Wasserman NH, Penn AS, Freimuth PI, et al: Anti-idiotypic route to anti-acetylcholine receptor antibodies and experimental myasthenia gravis. Proc Natl Acad Sci USA 79:4810, 1982

13. Cleveland WL, Wasserman NH, Sarangarajan R, et al: Monoclonal antibodies to the acetylcholine receptor by a normally functioning auto-anti-idiotypic mechanism. Nature 305:56, 1983

14. Vincent A, Scadding GK, Thomas HC, et al: In vitro synthesis of anti-acetylcholine-receptor antibody by thymic lymphocytes in myasthenia gravis. Lancet 1:305, 1978

15. Gerson BS, Cohen R, Gerson IM, et al: Myelin basic protein, oligoclonal bands, and IgG in cerebrospinal fluid as indicators of multiple sclerosis. Clin Chem 27:1974, 1981

16. Caron J, Penn GM: Electrophoretic and immunochemical characteristics of immunoglobulins. In Rose NR, De Macario EC, Fahey JL, Friedman H, Penn GM (eds): Manual of Clinical Laboratory Immunology, 4th ed, p 84. Washington, DC, American Society for Microbiology, 1992

17. Bennett PH: The diagnosis of diabetes: New internal classification and diagnostic criteria. Annu Rev Med 34:295, 1983

18. Crawford JM, Coltran RS: The pancreas. In Coltran RS, Kumar V, Robbins SL (eds): Robbins Pathologic Basis of Disease, 5th ed, p 909. Philadelphia, Saunders, 1994

19. Wilson CB, Yamamoto T, Ward DM: Renal diseases. In Stites DP, Stobo JD, Wells JV (eds): Basic and Clinical Immunology, 6th ed, p 495. Norwalk, CT, Appleton and Lange, 1987

20. Murphy GF, Mihm MC: The skin. In Cotran RS, Kumar V, Robbins SL (eds): Robbins Pathologic Basis of Disease, 5th ed, p 1201. Philadelphia, Saunders, 1994

21. Bronson RA, Tung KSK: Human spermatozoa antibodies: Detection and clinical significance. In Rose NR, DeMacario EC, Fahey JL, Friedman H, Penn GM (eds): Manual of Clinical Laboratory Immunology, 4th ed, p 775. Washington, DC, American Society for Microbiology, 1992

Section C. Immune Deficiencies

CHAPTER 31

Immune Deficiency

Therese B. Datiles
Richard L. Humphrey

Objectives

Upon completion of the chapter, the reader will be able to:

1. Differentiate between primary and secondary immune deficiencies (ID)
2. Understand the location of defects in the immune system causing the ID and in the pathways of normal lymphocyte differentiation
3. Classify selected immune deficiencies as humoral, cellular, or combined
4. Discuss the information generated from each of the laboratory tests described in the chapter and how they are used to evaluate immunocompetence
5. Suggest the most likely type of immune deficiency when provided with laboratory and clinical data

Immune system deficiencies had been considered rare until the emergence of acquired immune deficiency syndrome (AIDS). Apart from AIDS, the most common deficiencies of cellular and/or humoral immunity are secondary to some underlying abnormality or dis-ease process. For example, immune deficiency (ID) states are observed in acquired lymphoreticular proliferative diseases (e.g., myeloma, lymphoma) or occur after prolonged treatment with cytotoxic and immunosuppressive drugs. The hereditary or primary immunodeficiency states are quite rare.

Despite their rarity, careful study of these conditions provides important insights into the organization and function of the normal immune system. A schematic diagram of the organization of the immune system is provided in Figure 31-1, which depicts the development and differentiation of the immune system into two main compartments, the cellular immune system and the humoral immune system. In the cellular arm, the main effector agent is the T cell; in the humoral arm, it is the antibody molecule (immunoglobulin [Ig]).

The ID state is caused by an impairment of various host defense mechanisms, resulting in decreased resistance to infectious agents (e.g., bacteria, viruses, fungi, parasites). This impairment could be due to abnormalities of stem cells, thymus, gut-associated lymphoid tissue (GALT), T and B lymphocytes, and phagocytes; or impairment of the complement system and other amplifying systems (e.g., production of interferons, interleukins, or cytokines); or impairment of general health status (e.g., starvation, diabetes, uremia).

Primary ID are grouped according to whether the defect is chiefly humoral or cellular, or whether there is a combination of defects. Figure 31-2 shows the approximate distribution, that is, 50% antibody deficient, 10% cellular deficient, 20% combined cellular and antibody deficient, 18% phagocyte deficient, and 2% complement deficient.[1]

Humoral ID or agammaglobulinemia is characterized by recurrent bacterial infection. Patients are chronically ill. Children usually have retarded growth. Tonsils and lymph nodes are small and serum immunoglobulin levels are low or absent.

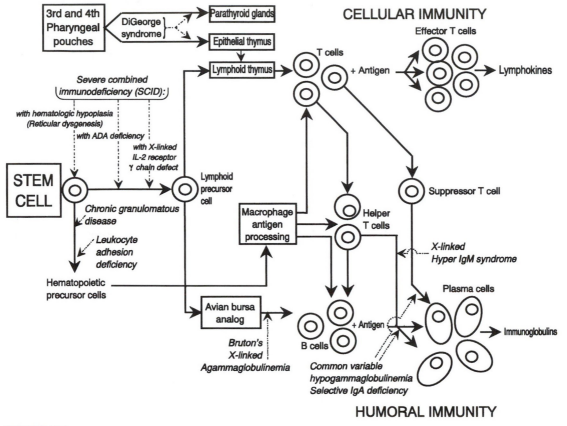

FIGURE 31-1
Diagrammatic representation of the ontogeny and organization of the mammalian immune system, emphasizing its two main functional divisions, cellular immunity and humoral immunity. The dashed lines indicate the possible locus of the defects responsible for some of the prototype immune deficiency states discussed in the text.

Cellular ID is characterized by severe viral or fungal infections. Patients are chronically ill and growth may be retarded. Tonsils and lymph nodes are small and the thymus is absent. Disseminated vaccinia occurs when there is vaccination against smallpox. Similar dissemination may occur if other live vaccines, such as bacillus Calmette-Guérin (BCG) or polio, are used. The graft-versus-host reaction may develop if live immunocompetent cells are transferred by blood or platelet transfusion.

The severe combined ID (SCID) is characterized by severe deficiency of both T and B lymphocytes, which may be caused by underlying defects in stem cells. Survival is limited to a few days after birth to a few months and is characterized by recurrent, severe, and overwhelming infections.

With all forms of the primary immunodeficiency disorders, early infant deaths or similarly affected siblings may be observed in the family history. Some laboratory tests used to evaluate humoral and cell immu-

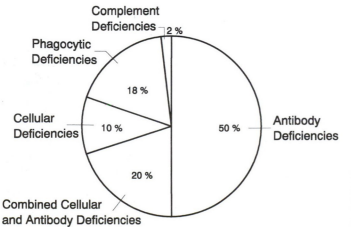

FIGURE 31-2
Pie chart showing the approximate distribution of the primary immunodeficiency disorders. (Modified from Stiehm ER: Immunologic Disorders, 4th ed. Philadelphia, WB Saunders, p 203, 1996, with permission.)

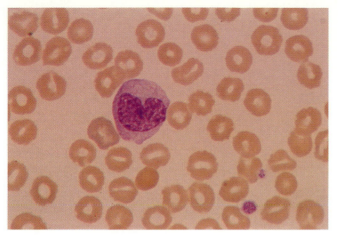

COLOR PLATE 1 (FIGURE 2-1)
Monocytes are found in the peripheral blood. When they migrate to the tissue, changes occur in their size and cytoplasm, and the cell is known as a macrophage. (From Lotspeich-Steininger CA, Steine-Martin EA, Koepke JA. Clinical hematology. Philadelphia, JB Lippincott Company, 1992.)

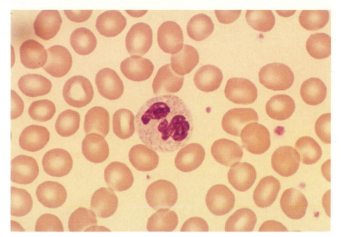

COLOR PLATE 2 (FIGURE 2-2)
The granules of the neutrophil are small. The nucleus of a mature neutrophil is segmented into three or more lobes. (From Lotspeich-Steininger CA, Steine-Martin EA, Koepke JA. Clinical hematology. Philadelphia, JB Lippincott Company, 1992.)

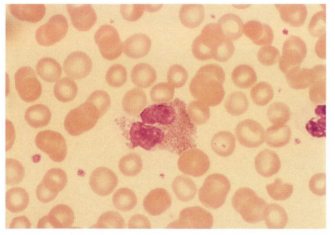

COLOR PLATE 3 (FIGURE 2-3)
The eosinophil is a granulocyte. Note that the granules of this cell are stained red and the nucleus is segmented into two lobes. (From Lotspeich-Steininger CA, Steine-Martin EA, Koepke JA. Clinical hematology. Philadelphia, JB Lippincott Company, 1992.)

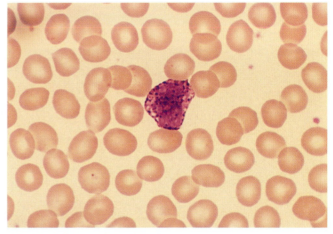

COLOR PLATE 4 (FIGURE 2-4)
The basophil is a granulocytic cell. The granules of this cell stain with basic dyes and are larger than the granules of neutrophils and eosinophils. The granules obscure the nucleus of the cells. (From Lotspeich-Steininger CA, Steine-Martin EA, Koepke JA. Clinical hematology. Philadelphia, JB Lippincott Company, 1992.)

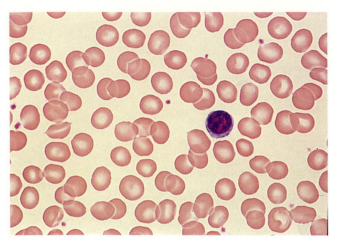

COLOR PLATE 5 (FIGURE 2-5)
Lymphocytes vary in size. A small lymphocyte that contains very little cytoplasm is shown. (From Lotspeich-Steininger CA, Steine-Martin EA, Koepke JA. Clinical hematology. Philadelphia, JB Lippincott Company, 1992.)

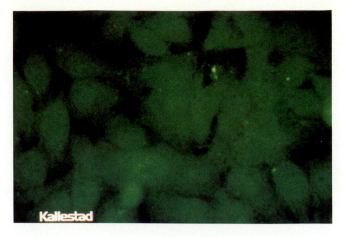

COLOR PLATE 6 (FIGURE 29-3A)
HEp2–negative ANA pattern and chromosome negative. (Reproduced with permission from Sanofi Diagnostics Pasteur, Chaska, MN.)

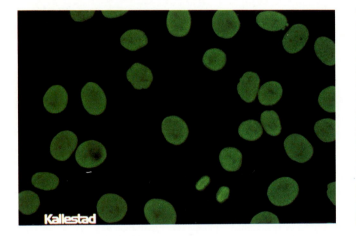

COLOR PLATE 7 (FIGURE 29-3B)
HEp2–homogenous ANA pattern and chromosome positive. (Reproduced with permission from Sanofi Diagnostics Pasteur, Chaska, MN.)

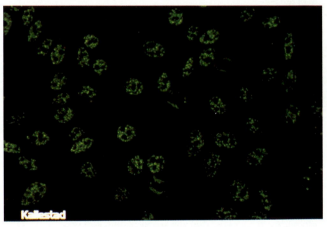

COLOR PLATE 8 (FIGURE 29-3C)
HEp2–speckled ANA pattern with Sm antibodies and chromosome negative. (Reproduced with permission from Sanofi Diagnostics Pasteur, Chaska, MN.)

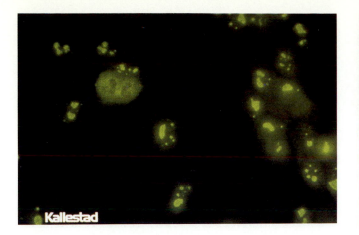

COLOR PLATE 9 (FIGURE 29-3D)
Hep2–nucleolar ANA pattern with chromosome negative staining. (Reproduced with permission from Sanofi Diagnostics Pasteur, Chaska, MN.)

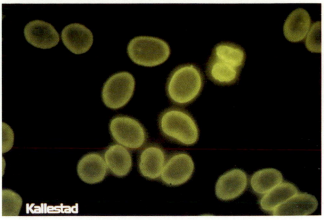

COLOR PLATE 10 (FIGURE 29-3E)
HEp2–peripheral ANA pattern with chromosome positive staining. (Reproduced with permission from Sanofi Diagnostics Pasteur, Chaska, MN.)

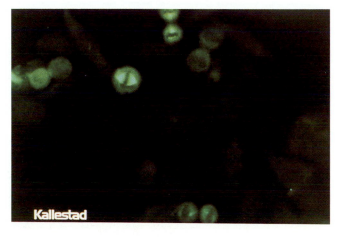

COLOR PLATE 11 (FIGURE 29-3F)
HEp2–spindle pattern with chromosome negative staining. (Reproduced with permission from Sanofi Diagnostics Pasteur, Chaska, MN.)

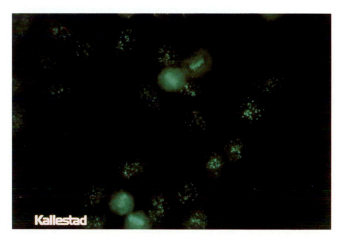

COLOR PLATE 12 (FIGURE 29-3G)
HEp2–centromere (discrete speckled) ANA pattern with chromosome positive staining. (Reproduced with permission from Sanofi Diagnostics Pasteur, Chaska, MN.)

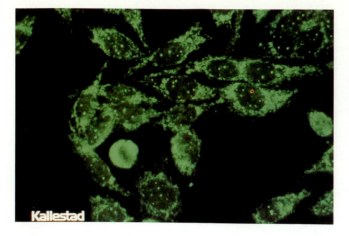

COLOR PLATE 13 (FIGURE 29-4A)
HEp2–anti-mitochondrial antibody pattern with chromosome negative staining. (Reproduced with permission from Sanofi Diagnostics Pasteur, Chaska, MN.)

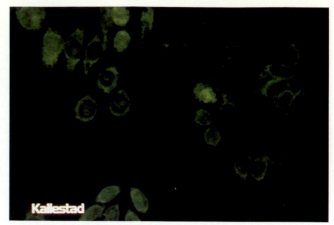

COLOR PLATE 14 (FIGURE 29-4B)
HEp2–anti-ribosomal P protein pattern staining. (Reproduced with permission from Sanofi Diagnostics Pasteur, Chaska, MN.)

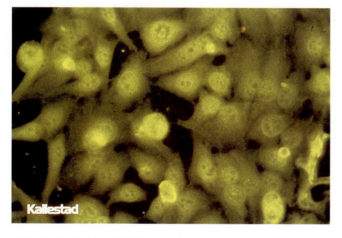

COLOR PLATE 15 (FIGURE 29-4C)
HEp2–anti-smooth muscle (anti-actin) pattern staining. (Reproduced with permission from Sanofi Diagnostics Pasteur, Chaska, MN.)

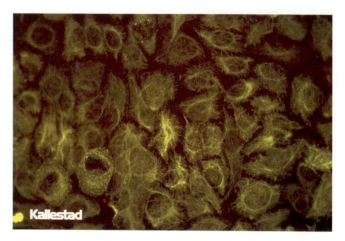

COLOR PLATE 16 (FIGURE 29-4D)
HEp2–anti-smooth muscle (anti-cytokeratin) pattern staining. (Reproduced with permission from Sanofi Diagnostics Pasteur, Chaska, MN.)

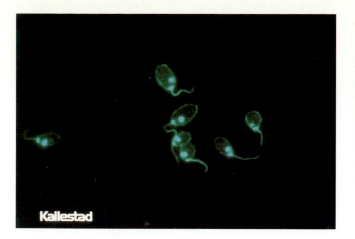

COLOR PLATE 17 (FIGURE 29-5A)
Crithidea luciliae positive staining demonstrating anti–native-DNA antibody. (Reproduced with permission from Sanofi Diagnostics Pasteur, Chaska, MN.)

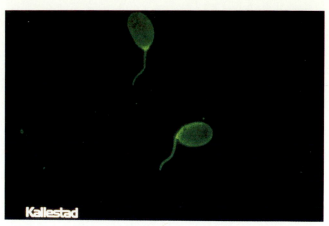

COLOR PLATE 18 (FIGURE 29-5B)
Crithidea luciliae negative reaction with no staining of the kineto-plast. (Reproduced with permission from Sanofi Diagnostics Pasteur, Chaska, M.N.)

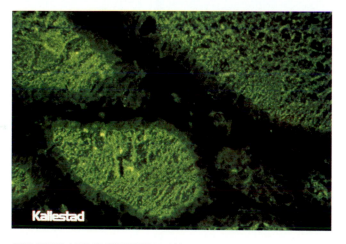

COLOR PLATE 19 (FIGURE 30-1A)
Using fixed primate thyroid as the substrate, thyroglobulin antibody is shown as diffuse staining of the colloid in the follicle. (Reprinted with permission from Sanofi Diagnostics Pasteur, Chaska, MN.)

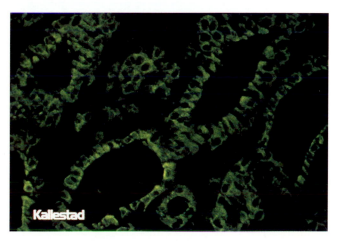

COLOR PLATE 20 (FIGURE 30-1B)
The thyroid peroxidase antibody is shown as granular cytoplasmic staining of the unfixed epithelial cells surrounding the follicle in primate thyroid. (Reprinted with permission from Sanofi Diagnostics Pasteur, Chaska, MN.)

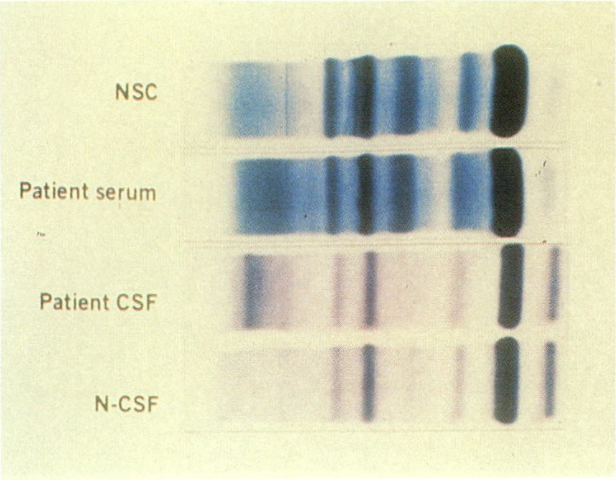

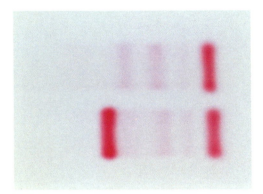

COLOR PLATE 21 (FIGURE 30-2)
Using high-resolution protein electrophoresis, note the oligoclonal banding seen in the CSF from a patient with multiple sclerosis (Patient CSF) compared with the normal CSF (N-CSF). The gamma region is on the left. The patient serum and normal serum control (NSC) do not show oligoclonal banding which is consistent with multiple sclerosis. (Used with permission of Helena Laboratories.)

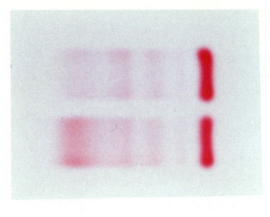

COLOR PLATE 22 (FIGURE 32-3A)
Cellulose acetate membrane comparing a normal serum (top lane) with a polyclonal hypergammaglobulinemia serum (bottom lane). Note the disappearance of the normal immunoglobulins in the hypergammaglobulinemia serum, with the gamma region approaching the baseline levels in the scan. (See Fig. 32-11 for SPE pattern.)

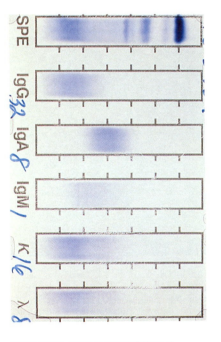

COLOR PLATE 23 (FIGURE 32-4A)
Cellulose acetate membrane comparing a hypogammaglobulinemia serum (top lane) with a monoclonal hypergammaglobulinemia serum (bottom lane).

COLOR PLATE 24 (FIGURE 32-5)
Serum immunofixation electrophoresis (SIFE) revealing a polyclonal hypergammaglobulinemia involving all three major classes of Ig (G, A, and M) and both light-chain types (κ and λ). The point of application seen in most of the lanes in the γ region should not be confused with a monoclonal band.

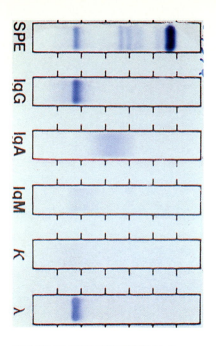

COLOR PLATE 25 (FIGURE 32-6)
SIFE of a patient's serum with a IgG lambda monoclonal gammopathy. Note the restricted electrophoretic mobility of the band seen in the IgG and lambda lanes, and the marked reductions of the other Igs.

COLOR PLATE 26 (FIGURE 32-9A)
Electrophoresis of a concentrated urine specimen on a cellulose acetate membrane demonstrating a restricted band in the β region.

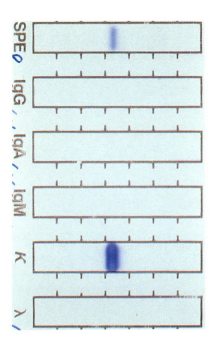

COLOR PLATE 27 (FIGURE 32-10)
UIFE revealing the presence of a markedly increased band of restricted electrophoretic mobility in the κ lane (kappa Bence Jones proteinuria).

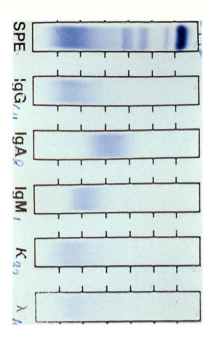

COLOR PLATE 28 (FIGURE 32-15)

Serum immunofixation electrophoresis for case 1. To avoid antigen excess and to optimize the visualization of each of the IFE lanes, the patient's serum has been appropriately diluted according to the concentration of Ig (quantitative measurement) in order to proportionately correspond to the strength of the antisera used. The numbers written next to the labels of the lane indicate the dilution used in each lane. For example, the IgG lane has been loaded with serum diluted to 1:64, the kappa lane diluted at 1:32, and so forth. The SPE lane is loaded at a 1:2 dilution. These careful choices of the respective dilutions used permit the demonstration of the polyclonal nature of the Ig and prevent misinterpretation due to antigen excess in any lane.

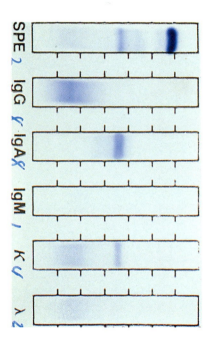

COLOR PLATE 29 (FIGURE 32-17)

Serum immunofixation electrophoresis for case 2. Note the pale appearance of the monoclonal band as revealed in the κ lane in spite of the serum load being twice the concentration (1:4) compared with the serum loaded on the IgA lane (1:8). This emphasizes the need to balance the strength of the antiserum with the antigen concentration in each lane.

TABLE 31-1
Laboratory Evaluation of Immunocompetence

TEST	COMMENT
Humoral Immunity	
1. Immunoglobulin survey (serum protein electrophoresis, Ig quantitation, immunofixation electrophoresis, IgG subclass levels)	1. General assessment of B-cell function
2. Isohemagglutinatin titer (anti-A, anti-B)	2. General indicator of IgM production
3. Titers before and after immunization with a specific vaccine (tetanus toxoid, Pneumovax™, typhoid-paratyphoid)	3. Demonstrates the in vivo ability to respond to a known antigen (tests both the afferent and efferent loops of B-cell function)
4. B-cell enumeration by flow cytometry (CD19)	4. Measures the number of circulating B cells (normally 10% to 20% of the total peripheral blood lymphocytes)
5. Biopsy of bone marrow, lymph node, or gut	5. Assessment of the presence and/or location of lymphocytes (germinal centers, plasma cells)
Cell-Mediated Immunity	
1. Peripheral lymphocyte count and morphology	1. General assessment of T-cell presence (normally 80% to 90% of total blood lymphocytes)
2. T-cell enumeration by flow cytometry (CD3)	2. Measures the total number of T cells in the peripheral blood (normally, >1200 cells/μL)
3. Enumeration of T-cell subsets (CD4, CD8) by flow cytometry	3. The CD4/CD8 ratio is usually 2:1
4. Delayed hypersensitivity skin testing to recall antigens (PPD, histoplasmin, trichophytin, *Candida*, mumps, streptokinase-streptodornase)	4. Assessment of the in vivo ability of T cells to respond to a previously encountered antigen (tests the efferent loop of T-cell function)
5. Dinitrochlorobenzene skin (DNCB) sensitization	5. Assessment of the in vivo function of T cells to respond to a newly encountered antigen (tests both the afferent and efferent loops of T-cell function)
6. Measurement of lymphokine production	6. Assessment of the T-cell ability to secrete lymphokines
7. Biopsy of lymph node	7. Assessment of the presence of T cells in thymus-dependent areas

nity are presented in Table 31-1. The changes in the number and type of lymphocytes in selected immune deficiencies are summarized in Table 31-2 (on p. 308). In the following sections some of the more common and well-understood examples of these disorders are described as prototypes to illustrate the major features of this group of diseases. More than 70 ID syndromes have been described, some involving only a few patients. This emphasizes the complex web of cells and their interactions in the normal immune system and illustrates that there are a great many ways in which the system can become impaired. These complex relationships are suggested in Figure 31-1, which is necessarily a schematic over simplification. A number of comprehensive reviews are available for further study.[1-5]

PRIMARY IMMUNE DEFICIENCIES

Humoral Immune Deficiencies

BRUTON'S X-LINKED AGAMMAGLOBULINEMIA

X-linked agammaglobulinemia, a congenital inherited disorder, was first reported in a male infant by Bruton in 1952. When maternal immunoglobulins (Igs) are ca-

tabolized and fall below protective levels at about 6 months of age and are not replaced by the infant's own humoral immune system, a deficiency in all classes of Ig becomes apparent. As a result of this lack of antibodies, recurrent life-threatening pyogenic infections are observed. Pyogenic organisms most often involved are *Streptococcus pneumoniae* and *Haemophilus influenzae*, and the recurrent infections are pneumonia, sinusitis, bronchitis, otitis, furunculosis, meningitis, and septicemia. Fungal infections are usually not a significant problem. *Pneumocystis carinii* pneumonia rarely occurs unless neutropenia also is present.

Infections with viruses usually do not cause severe complications, with the exceptions of viral hepatitis and enterovirus infections, which can be fulminant and even fatal. Fatal central nervous system infections have occurred with echoviruses. Live virus vaccines are usually handled normally. Paralysis has occurred in several patients after polio vaccination, possibly caused by mutation of this vaccine from an enterovirus to a more neurotropic form. Serum concentrations of IgG, IgA, and IgM are markedly reduced, and functional levels of antibody are absent. Antigenic stimulation by bacterial infections or by injected soluble or particulate antigens produces no demonstrable antibody response.

T-cell subset percentages are usually normal, although the total number of T cells is usually increased.

TABLE 31-2
Lymphocytes in Selected Immunodeficiency Diseases

	T-CELL MARKER				B-CELL MARKER
	CD3	CD4	CD8	CD4/8	CD19
I. Primary immunodeficiency					
A. Humoral					
1. Bruton's X-linked agammaglobulinemia (XLA)	N-↑	↓-N	N	N	0-↓↓
2. Selective IgA deficiency	N	↓-N	N-↑	20%↑ 10%↓	N
3. Common variable ID	↓-N	↓-N-↑	↓-N-↑	25%↓ 15%↑	↓↓-N
4. Hyper IgM (HIM)	N	N	N	N	N
B. Cellular					
1. DiGeorge anomaly	0-↓↓	↓↓	↓↓	N	↑
2. Nezelof's syndrome	↓↓	↓	↓	N	N
C. Combined humoral and cellular					
1. Severe					
a. SCID (autosomal recessive)	0-↓↓	↓↓	↓↓	N	N-↑
b. SCID (with hematopoietic hypoplasia)	0-↓↓	↓↓	↓↓	N	↓↓
2. Combined Immune Deficiency (CID)	N	↓	N-↑	↓	N
3. Partial					
a. Wiskott-Aldrich	↓	↓	↓	N	N
b. Ataxia-telangiectasia	↓	↓	N-↑	↓	N
D. Phagocytic deficiencies	N	N	N	N	N
E. Complement deficiencies	N	N	N	N	N
II. Secondary immunodeficiency					
A. AIDS	N-↓	↓↓	N-↑	↓↓	N-↓

N, normal; ↑, increased; ↓, decreased

The thymus is histologically normal; however, B cells are markedly decreased or absent. The XLA gene defect is intrinsic to the B-cell lineage, and the gene involved is called the Btk gene (Bruton's tyrosine kinase).[6] A number of mutations in the Btk gene have been described that seem to have the common effect of preventing normal signal transduction in the B-cell lineage. This prevents the maturation of pre-B cells to B cells, and results in markedly reduced numbers of circulating B cells. The lymph nodes, adenoids, and tonsils are small, hypoplastic, and lack germinal centers. Plasma cells are completely absent from the lymph nodes, Peyer's patches, the appendix, and the bone marrow.

Treatment consists of prompt use of appropriate antimicrobials (when a patient has an infection) and chronic administration of intravenous gammaglobulin. The prophylactic use of antibiotics is not advisable because it is not likely to prevent most infections and may result in colonization with antibiotic-resistant bacteria. Long-term results are fairly good, but these patients often develop chronic lung disease because of destruction of lung parenchyma by repeated infections. They are also prone to develop leukemia and lymphoma.

SELECTIVE IgA DEFICIENCY

The incidence of isolated IgA deficiency in the general population is about one case per 600 to 800.[7] A study done with Tennessee blood donors demonstrated a ratio of IgA deficiency to normals of 1:333. Almost or complete absence of serum and secretory IgA (<10 mg/dL) is the hallmark of this disorder. The mode of inheritance varies among families. In some families it seems to be a recessive trait; others have a dominant form of transmission. Equal occurrence in the male and female suggests autosomal inheritance. Selective IgA deficiency can be caused by some drugs (e.g., phenytoin sodium and penicillamine); however, the disorder is corrected when these drugs are stopped.

Most of these individuals are asymptomatic, but some individuals suffer from recurrent infections. These infections commonly occur in the respiratory, gastrointestinal, and urogenital tracts. This deficiency is associated with other syndromes, such as allergies, autoimmune disorders, various malignancies, malabsorption, and mental retardation.

A serious difficulty for some patients is the presence of anti-IgA antibodies (the incidence of which is as high as 44% in some series), which can lead to gastrointestinal symptoms after milk ingestion. These anti-IgA antibodies may interfere with the laboratory measurement of IgA. Patients with such antibodies may face serious allergic complications (e.g., anaphylaxis) when blood or plasma that contains IgA is administered. Similarly, if IgA is administered in a blood product, antibodies may develop so that life-threatening anaphylaxis may result later when another blood product is administered. Patients with IgA deficiency should be warned to avoid exposure to IgA and hence to avoid being immunized against this immunoglobulin.

Meticulous sinopulmonary hygiene and prompt and specific antibiotic therapy for infections as they occur are currently the only available treatment. No commercial source of IgA is available for administration. In addition, there would be serious reservations about its use because anaphylaxis may result, and without the secretory component the IgA would not be transported to the mucous membrane surface, where its presence and function are needed. The defect in this disorder is thought to be related to that in common variable immunodeficiency[8] and may be caused by an abnormality in the regulation of immunoglobulin class switching.

COMMON VARIABLE IMMUNODEFICIENCY (CVID)

Immunodeficiency may occur in adults with a history of previous good health. The presumption is that their immune system was previously normal and that it is therefore a late-onset disorder. This is a heterogeneous group of disorders[9] with both autosomal dominant and recessive, as well as X-linked, inheritance. However, most cases occur without an inherited background. Clinically, this ID is similar to the X-linked agammaglobulinemia, as shown by the marked decrease in serum Ig concentration and similar infections caused by *S. pneumoniae* and *H. influenzae*. The main differences are the adult onset (15 to 35 years), less severe infections, equal sex distribution, normal-sized or enlarged tonsils and lymph nodes, and splenomegaly.

Other conditions that may develop are autoimmune disorders (rheumatoid arthritis, dermatomyosi-

tis), malabsorption (*Giardia lamblia*; more common in this disorder than in X-linked agammaglobulinemia), hemolytic anemia, pernicious anemia, bronchiectasis, gastric carcinoma, lymphoreticular malignancy, and cholelithiasis. Recurrent infections of the paranasal sinuses and middle ear and bacterial conjunctivitis are also common. Although bacterial infection responds well to antibiotic treatment, the frequent recurrence of infections constitutes a problem.

Most patients have decreased numbers of B cells. In most patients, the lymphocytes can be stimulated to transform into plasma cells to produce Ig. However, the B cells are immature, suggesting failure of in vivo activation. Family members have been shown to have an increased incidence of selective IgA deficiency.

Normal levels of the T-cell subsets are usually found, but their ability to function may be reduced in some patients. Some studies indicate that for some patients the defect is overactive suppressor T cells, and this observation may lead to new ways to treat or control the disorder. Other studies indicate that the defect in T cells resides in their failure to mediate normal B-cell differentiation. Difficulties in the interpretation of T-cell activation studies may be caused by recurrent infections or intravenous immunoglobulin (IV-Ig) therapy. Chronic administration of gammaglobulin, specific antibiotics and supportive care during acute infections are the current standards of therapy. Approximately 8% of these patients develop malignancy, including leukemia, lymphomas, and epithelial cell tumors.

HYPER-IgM SYNDROME (HIM)

This syndrome resembles XLA; however, the predominant defect is characterized by markedly elevated serum IgM, markedly decreased IgG, and absent IgA. This syndrome was initially thought to be X-linked until female patients were identified, which established at least two modes of inheritance. Seventy percent of these patients have the X-linked form of HIM, designated as XHIM. Clinically, these patients are susceptible to pyogenic infections but, in addition, have an increased incidence of opportunistic infections (e.g., *Pneumocystis carinii*), and they are prone to autoimmune diseases (e.g., autoimmune hemolytic anemia, thrombocytopenia purpura, and neutropenia).

Treatment is usually administration of IV-Ig and granulocyte-macrophage colony stimulating factor (GM-CSF). A recent case was successfully treated by bone marrow transplantation (BMT).[10] The defect in the X-linked form of HIM is a failure of the patient's T cells to synthesize CD40 ligand, which is a part of the signal required by the B cells to undergo Ig class switching from IgM to IgG or IgA. A number of different mutations have been shown to occur in the

CD40 ligand gene, which maps on the long arm of the X chromosome.[11]

Cellular Immune Deficiencies

THYMIC HYPOPLASIA (DiGEORGE ANOMALY)

The presenting feature of DiGeorge anomaly is often the appearance of hypocalcemic tetany shortly after birth as a result of the failure of the parathyroids and thymus to develop normally from the third and fourth pharyngeal pouches during embryonic development. This disorder occurs in both males and females, and does not seem to be inherited. Familial cases and chromosome abnormalities are rare. There are often a number of associated physical abnormalities, including hyperteliorism (wide-set eyes), an antimongoloid slant of the eyes, low-set and notched ears, micrognathia (small jaw), a short philtrum of the upper lip, mandibular hypoplasia, and cardiac and aortic arch anomalies (tetralogy of Fallot).

The thymus is absent, and T lymphocytes are absent from the blood and from the thymus-dependent areas of the lymph nodes and spleen. However, humoral-mediated immunity develops normally. Characteristically, these patients are very susceptible to infections with opportunistic pathogens (e.g., fungi, virus, *Pneumocystis carinii*) and are prone to develop graft-versus-host disease (GVHD) from lymphocytes transferred by the transfusion of nonirradiated blood products.

Serum Ig levels are usually normal, although IgA may be decreased and IgE may be increased. The total B-cell percentage is increased, and the total T-cell percentage is decreased; however, the ratio of helper T cells to suppressor T cells is normal. T-cell function may be normal. Delayed hypersensitivity skin test reactions will be absent or reduced, and exposure to sensitizing antigens, such as dinitrochlorobenzene, fails to stimulate a delayed hypersensitivity reaction. Correction has been achieved by means of early (14 weeks gestational age) fetal thymus transplants, with the beneficial effect mediated by thymosin produced by the epithelial cells in the transplanted thymus. Bone marrow transplantation has also been helpful in correcting this disorder.

NEZELOF'S SYNDROME (CELLULAR IMMUNODEFICIENCY WITH NORMAL OR INCREASED IMMUNOGLOBULINS)

Characteristic of Nezelof's syndrome is profound T-cell dysfunction with abnormal immunoglobulin synthesis. Children with this disease usually have chronic pulmonary infection, failure to thrive, oral or cutaneous candidiasis, chronic diarrhea, recurrent skin infection, gram-negative sepsis, urinary tract infection, and severe progressive varicella. Patients usually have lymphopenia, diminished lymphoid tissue, abnormal thymus architecture, normal numbers of B cells, and the presence of normal or elevated serum concentrations of most of the five classes of Igs. Frequently, IgA is deficient and IgD and IgE levels are elevated. Unresponsiveness to delayed hypersensitivity skin tests and a decreased to absent lymphocyte response to mitogens and allogeneic cells have been noted in the cellular immune function studies.

Because of the presence of normal Ig levels, the following features may be useful to differentiate Nezelof's syndrome from acquired immunodeficiency syndrome (AIDS): (1) There is a marked decrease of total T cells and the T-cell subset has a normal ratio of helper (CD_4) to suppressor (CD_8) T cells, whereas in AIDS there is an inverse CD_4/CD_8 ratio, caused by a marked decrease of CD_4 cells.[2] There is paracortical lymphocyte reduction and hypoplastic peripheral lymphoid tissue compared with lymphadenopathy in AIDS. The thymus is small and has little corticomedullary differentiation and no Hassall's corpuscles, yet thymic epithelium is present. This is in contrast to patients with AIDS, who show marked atrophy of thymic epithelium. Except for appropriate supportive measures, including antibiotics, no treatment has been curative, except for patients treated with HLA-matched bone marrow transplantation.

Combined Humoral and Cellular Immune Deficiencies

SEVERE COMBINED IMMUNE DEFICIENCY (SCID)

Severe combined immune deficiency was first described in 1958; however, later characterization showed this to be a collection of immune deficiency syndromes showing a diversity of genetic, enzymatic, dermatologic, and immunologic features. Basically, these disorders are characterized by a failure to develop lymphoid stem cells, which results in the absence of both the cellular and humoral components of the immune response. This syndrome is the most severe of the recognized immunodeficiencies, and survival for more than a few months is unlikely because of recurrent severe infections.

Successful treatment with correction of all these abnormalities has been achieved using histocompatible bone marrow transplantation from sibling donors. Stable engraftment has also been achieved after administration of T-cell–depleted bone marrow transplantation from unrelated closely matched donors. Depending on the specific nature of the SCID syndrome, enzyme replacement and gene therapy also seem promising for long-term therapy.

Autosomal Recessive SCID (Swiss-Type Lymphopenic Agammaglobulinemia) with or Without Adenosine Deaminase Deficiency

In 1958 Swiss workers reported the first SCID syndrome. These infants initially appear to grow normally, but extreme wasting develops after diarrhea and infections begin (e.g., otitis, pneumonia, sepsis, dermatitis). Death is caused by infections with opportunistic organisms (e.g., *Candida albicans, P. carinii,* varicella, measles, and cytomegalovirus [CMV]) and by dissemination of live organisms used for vaccination (e.g., BCG, poliovirus, and vaccinia).

These infants have a markedly decreased percentage of T cells (but rarely have the inverted helper-suppressor ratio seen in AIDS patients, and this observation can help in the differential diagnosis), but many have increased B-cell percentages. However, both T and B cells are largely nonfunctional. Immunologic findings include profound lymphopenia, delayed hypersensitivity anergy, and failure to reject transplants, thereby increasing their risk for graft-versus-host disease from maternal lymphocytes acquired in utero or inadvertently transferred by blood transfusions. Serum immunoglobulin concentrations are extremely low, and antibody is not formed after immunization.

Natural killer (NK) cell function is absent in most SCID patients; however, a recent study reported a new phenotype in two SCID infants who had large granular lymphocytes with an NK cell phenotype and function, further confirming the heterogeneity of these disorders at a cellular level. (NK cells are similar to T cells morphologically and mature in the thymus gland; however, they appear to be capable of mediating a cytotoxic reaction without the need for prior antigen sensitization). In SCID patients the thymus is atrophic with absent Hassall's corpuscles but with normal-appearing thymic epithelium. This latter observation may help to differentiate SCID from AIDS, because thymic epithelium is markedly atrophic in AIDS patients. The best treatment is to reconstitute the lymphoid cell populations by a histocompatible bone marrow transplant. The ideal donor is an HLA-matched sibling.

Approximately 40% of the autosomal recessive form of SCID has been observed to have adenosine deaminase (ADA) deficiency. ADA deficiency causes abnormal purine metabolism, leading to combined T- and B-cell immunodeficiency. The presence of rib cage abnormalities similar to a rachitic rosary and multiple skeletal abnormalities (chondro-osseous dysplasia) are characteristic. Enzyme replacement therapy has been accomplished by the administration of polyethylene glycol–modified bovine ADA. Bone marrow transplantation has also been used. Early studies of gene insertion therapy appear to be successful.[12] Inserting the missing gene into mature T cells provides the missing ADA enzyme. This therapy is very attractive because it eliminates the complications of immune reactions to foreign ADA and the risk of graft-versus-host disease. Strategies for the insertion of ADA enzyme by transfer of cDNA by means of bone marrow and umbilical cord stem cells are in clinical trials.

X-Linked Recessive SCID

X-linked recessive SCID is clinically, immunologically, and histopathologically indistinguishable from the autosomal recessive form described earlier and seems to be the most common form of SCID in the United States. The fact that different genetic loci can be involved and yet lead to very similar syndromes reveals that the immune system is dependent on and under the control and regulation of many different genes, any one of which, if defective, can have profound consequences. This heterogeneity also suggests that the different mechanisms involved may require elucidation before individualized treatment strategies can be devised. The defect in this disorder has been shown to be a mutation in the gamma chain of the IL-2 receptor. This gamma chain is also a component of the receptors for IL-4, IL-7, IL-11, and IL-15, which helps to account for the global nature and severity of this immunodeficiency.[6,13]

SCID with Hematopoietic Hypoplasia

Characteristic of SCID with hematopoietic hypoplasia (reticular dysgenesis) is the severe deficiency of both T and B lymphocytes and failure to develop granulocytes. Most of the few reported cases have died of overwhelming infection within the first 3 months of life. Rare patients have been treated with bone marrow transplantation and have achieved immunologic reconstitution. The thymus gland is small, weighing <1 g; Hassall's corpuscles are absent; and thymocytes are rarely observed. Its inheritance is thought to be autosomal recessive. A total failure of stem cells is not entirely satisfactory as an explanation for the defect because heterogeneity among these patients has been observed, with a few cases having very low numbers of normal-appearing granulocytes and rare patients having a normal percentage of nonfunctional T cells in cord blood. Bone marrow transplantation would be the treatment of choice but would almost require prenatal diagnosis of the affected child to accomplish the procedure promptly after birth.

COMBINED IMMUNODEFICIENCY (CID)—MHC CLASS DEFICIENCY

In this disorder, formerly known as bare-lymphocyte syndrome, the defects are in the expression of the major histocompatibility complex (MHC).[14] The deficiency is characterized by severe and protracted diarrhea, frequently associated with candidiasis and cryptosporidiosis, sclerosing cholangitis, frequent severe upper respiratory tract infection and pneumonia, and failure to thrive.

The MHC Class II deficiency is an inherited autosomal recessive trait. A study of North African children with this disorder showed that these children have insufficient numbers of CD4+ T cells and are unable to mount delayed hypersensitivity reactions. Although the B cells are normal, the children are hypogammaglobulinemic. The genetic defect is in the regulation of the transcription of the major MHC Class II molecules HLA-DP, -DQ, and -DR. This deficiency is less clinically severe than SCID, but it can be fatal in the first or second decade of life. Bone marrow transplantation has resulted in long-term survival.

MHC Class I deficiency is characterized by recurrent and severe bacterial pulmonary infection starting in late childhood. This rare genetic defect was recently studied in a Moroccan family, and the gene was found to have a mutation in the transporter protein, TAP 2. The affected children were deficient in CD8+ T cells.

PARTIAL COMBINED IMMUNE DEFICIENCY

Wiskott-Aldrich Syndrome

Patients with Wiskott-Aldrich syndrome,[15] an X-linked recessive disorder, are characterized by the presence of eczema, thrombocytopenic purpura, and increased susceptibility to infection. Clinically, the eczema is similar to infantile atopic dermatitis. Petechiae, prolonged oozing from the umbilicus or circumcision, or bloody diarrhea may call attention to the thrombocytopenia. Normal megakaryocytes are found in the bone marrow, suggesting the presence of an intrinsic defect in the platelets. In the early phases of the disorder, recurrent infections, such as pneumonia, meningitis, otitis, and sepsis, occur with pyogenic encapsulated bacteria at fault. Later on, as cellular immune function declines, infection with *P. carinii* and the herpesviruses become more of a problem. Death results from infection and bleeding. There is also a 12% incidence of malignancy. Survival beyond the teens is rare.

There are multiple immune defects. Humoral response to polysaccharide antigens is impaired. Anamnestic responses are poor or absent. Dysgammaglobulinemia with decreased IgM, elevated IgA and IgE, and normal or low levels of IgG is often seen. Ig synthesis is actually increased, with hypercatabolism of IgG, IgA, IgM, and albumin. This explains the high degree of variation in Ig concentration seen in different patients as well as within a single patient when measured over time. There is a low percentage of total T, helper T, and suppressor T cells, but the helper/suppressor ratio is usually normal.

Some patients with uncontrollable bleeding have been helped by splenectomy. Long-term survival has been possible with carefully maintained antibiotic therapy. Antibody replacement therapy by intravenous administration of gammaglobulin has been useful. Both platelet and immunologic abnormalities have been successfully treated by HLA-identical sibling bone marrow transplants.

Ataxia-Telangiectasia

The characteristics of ataxia-telangiectasia, an autosomal recessive disorder, include ataxia, telangiectasia, recurrent sinopulmonary infections, a high incidence of malignancy, and variable defects of humoral and cellular immunity. Ataxia is often not noticed until the child begins to walk. From then on, it is progressive, with the child often confined to a wheelchair by 10 to 12 years of age. Telangiectasia is observed by 3 to 6 years of age and progresses slowly. Chronic sinopulmonary infection is observed in about 80% of patients. Malignancy is most often of the lymphoreticular type, but a high incidence of adenocarcinomas has been reported in patients' normal relatives. Patients show a selective absence of serum and secretory IgA, which in 50% to 80% of cases may be caused by hypercatabolism of IgA. The serum concentration of IgA2 and IgG4 may be decreased in some patients. In others IgE is absent, and serum IgM may be of the low molecular-weight (monomeric) type. Cellular immunity is impaired. The total number of T cells and the helper cell percentage are low, but normal or high percentages of suppressor cells are observed.

Ig synthesis studies show defects in B cells and helper T cells. The thymus is hypoplastic, with poor organization and a deficiency of Hassall's corpuscles. To date, treatment attempts have been unsatisfactory.

The gene responsible for this syndrome has recently been identified and has been named the ATM gene.[16] It is thought that this gene plays an important role in signal transduction networks that activate multiple cellular functions in response to DNA damage. The failure of these normal repair mechanisms and the triggering of programmed cell death (apoptosis) in a variety of tissues and organs leads to this complex syndrome.

PHAGOCYTIC DEFICIENCIES

Phagocytic defects can be in the quantity or in the function of the polymorphonuclear (PMN) leukocyte system and/or the mononuclear phagocyte system. Functional defects can include locomotion, extravasation, chemotaxis, attachment, phagocytosis, intracellular killing, and digestion of the microorganism. Any disorder or malfunction in this system affects the defense mechanism, and thereby results in recurrent infection or ineffective antibiotic therapy.

Leukocyte-Adhesion Defect (LAD)

This impairment of leukocytes results from their inability to adhere to endothelial surfaces and to other cell membranes, thus being unable to migrate into the site of infection. Patients with LAD are unable to form pus and, as a result, there is an impairment of wound healing (see Chapter 4).

Chronic Granulomatous Disease (CGD)

The production of microbicidal oxidants by phagocytes is important in the intracellular killing of ingested microorganisms. In CGD patients, there is an impairment in the ability of the phagocytes to produce oxygen radicals and hydrogen peroxide, which are important for killing ingested bacteria (especially catalase-positive organisms) and fungi. As a result, these microorganisms remain alive in phagocytes and granulomas are formed. CGD patients develop pneumonia, lymphadenitis, abscesses in the skin, liver, and other viscera. Approximately 65% are X-link inherited and 35% are autosomal recessive. Diverse mutations, deletions, insertions, point mutations, and multiple gene defects have been identified (see Chapter 4).

COMPLEMENT DEFICIENCIES

Defects resulting in the decreased synthesis or increased consumption of serum complement components cause a predisposition to infection and to autoimmune diseases. The inherited form has been called the autosomal codominant pattern. Any disorder (e.g. biochemical enzymatic reactions and control mechanisms) in the balanced interplay of the 11 complement components of the classical pathway or the three factors in the alternate pathway can result in an increased susceptibility to infection or other disease process (see Chapter 4).

Autoimmune Diseases

Decreased protein synthesis of the early complement components of the classical pathway, caused by an inherited homozygous deficiency, results in an increased incidence of immune complex diseases, for example, systemic lupus erythematosus, glomerulonephritis, and vasculitis. The patients with C1q, C1r, C1s, C4, and C2 deficiencies are unable to generate C3b, which is crucial for clearing immune complexes.

Recurrent Bacterial Infection

The early complement components of the classical and alternate pathways mediate localized inflammatory response, opsonization, and phagocytosis of bacteria. Patients deficient in these components are predisposed to recurrent pyogenic or *Neisseria* infections. Primary selective deficiencies in C1q, C1r, C1s, C4, C2, Factor D, and C3 have been associated with pyogenic infections.

The membrane attack component (MAC) of the classical pathway has an important role in the intracellular destruction and lysis of bacteria, especially gram-negative bacteria. Patients with homozygous deficiencies in the terminal components C5, C6, C7, and C8 are susceptible to recurrent meningococcal and gonococcal infections by the *Neisseria* species. There are little or no clinical findings for individuals with C9 deficiency. In the alternate pathway, Factor D or properdin deficiency has also been associated with increased susceptibility to *Neisseria* infections as well as other pyogenic organisms.

Hereditary Angioedema (HAE)

The deficiency or the dysfunction of the C1 inhibitor (C1INH), a complement regulatory protein, results in the clinically most important deficiency of the complement system. C1INH prevents the excessive activation of C4 and C2. The clinical manifestation of the disease is swelling or edema involving various parts of the body, for example, the face and upper respiratory airway (which could be a medical emergency because the patient could choke to death). Edema can also occur in the abdomen and intestines (which can cause severe abdominal pain). HAE is an autosomal dominant inherited disorder. One type has the defect in the gene resulting in the absence of the C1INH. The second type has a point mutation in the C1INH gene resulting in a dysfunctional C1INH protein.

SECONDARY IMMUNE DEFICIENCIES

The secondary immunodeficiency states occur in previously healthy individuals, who are therefore considered to have had a normal immune system. They result from an underlying illness and may be more or less reversible, depending on how completely the underlying illness can be controlled. Almost any severe illness can lead to an impairment in immune function. Examples include diabetes, uremia, starvation, cystic fibrosis, burns, rheumatic heart disease, indwelling catheters and other foreign bodies, splenectomy, viral infections, prematurity, and so on. A few selected examples are described to illustrate some of the disorders involved.

Transient Hypogammaglobulinemia of Infancy

Transient hypogammaglobulinemia is an uncommon disorder occurring in about 0.1% of newborns. The disorder is characterized by an abnormal prolongation and accentuation of the decline in serum Ig concentrations, which is normally seen during the first 3 to 7 months of life. Despite this delay, by 6 to 11 months of age all cases are able to synthesize normal amounts of antibodies to human type A and B erythrocytes, and also to diphtheria and tetanus toxoids. This occurs well before the Ig concentrations themselves become normal and helps to distinguish these patients from those with other primary immunodeficiency diseases, such as Bruton's X-linked agammaglobulinemia. The normal percentages of the different lymphoid cell subpopulations are observed along with normal responses to mitogens.

These patients can be divided into two groups. One group has no significant health problems during infancy; the other group has recurrent infections. Most patients in the first group later develop normal serum Ig levels. However, the second group's serum Ig levels remain below the normal range, although significantly higher than during infancy. Follow-up studies show that these patients did not have any subsequent serious infections, even though none received Ig replacement therapy. Gammaglobulin replacement therapy is not indicated in this condition because the passively administered immunoglobulin could suppress the patient's own antibody formation. Other than careful management of recurrent infections, no other specific therapy is required. Careful differentiation from the other, more serious immune deficiency states is required so that the parents can be reassured that the infant will outgrow the problem with no lasting consequences.

Malignancy

A number of cancers (if not most of them) clearly show a suppressive effect on normal immune function. Defects in T-cell function are well known in Hodgkin's disease, and functional impairment of antibody formation is seen with many lymphomas, chronic lymphocytic leukemia, and multiple myeloma. More subtle defects can be elicited (e.g., a failure to respond to delayed hypersensitivity skin testing) in many patients with a variety of metastatic cancers (e.g., melanoma, breast, colon). The converse is also true: Suppression of the immune system can lead both to an abnormal incidence of cancer and to unusual types of cancer (e.g., Kaposi sarcoma in AIDS patients, central nervous system lymphomas in renal transplant patients).

These considerations clearly reveal the interdependency and the interaction of the immune system with the development of malignancies. This interaction has led to the postulation that there is constant surveillance by the immune system, which eliminates newly developed malignant cells. For example, when a primary or secondary immune defect or other special circumstance is present, a cancer cell can evade this immune elimination. The newly developed cancer will become established and the immune system is no longer effective in eliminating the cancer. Efforts to overcome this and to enhance the specific immune elimination of cancer cells (e.g., the use of interferon, IL-2, LAK cells, etc.) are currently areas of intense interest and active research, with the hope that new forms of cancer therapy will emerge.

Viral Disease

It is widely appreciated that a variety of viral illnesses can impair the proper functioning of the immune system. AIDS can be thought of as representing a more recently recognized and severe form of this immune suppression, and a great deal has already been learned about the molecular biology of this interaction. Older observations of bacterial infections (e.g., pneumonia) following on the heels of influenza epidemics are still valid, although the availability of modern antibiotics has served to ameliorate much of the resulting mortality, if not the morbidity, of this association. The exact molecular nature of the viral-induced impairment of the immune system is not well understood but may share some features with the more dramatic effects of the HIV virus in AIDS patients. Viruses, such as those that cause the common cold, the herpes family of viruses, cytomegalovirus (CMV), and Epstein-Barr virus, also affect host defense mechanisms and are, of course, more prevalent and dangerous when host resistance is impaired (e.g., by chemotherapy, immunosuppressive therapy, stress). It is likely that the knowledge gained in the current intensive investigations of AIDS will have a dramatic impact on our understanding of these viral, host, and immune system interactions.

Bone Marrow Transplantation and Graft-Versus-Host Disease

Although in some ways the use of bone marrow transplantation is an attempt to re-create the immune system, there are a number of ways in which the transplanted immune system does not follow normal ontogeny. The normal development of the immune system in the fetus has some very special features. Immune system development occurs under the influence of the thymus and the mammalian equivalent of the bursa, and during this development it is protected from encounters with antigens. Ratios of the various cellular elements are maintained as the immune system matures, and regulation occurs to eliminate autoimmune reactions. Altogether, the protected environment in which the fetus develops provides a very elegant system for keeping the development of the immune system on target and in balance.

Bone marrow transplantation recreates few, if any, of these features of normal immune system development. The donor cell population is only a minor sample of the whole immune system as represented by its presence in the bone marrow. The cells are not naive, that is, antigen abounds in the donor and a whole new universe of antigen is encountered in the recipient. There is no active thymus present in the recipient, and the bursal equivalent is also probably much different from that of the fetus. It is remarkable that the immune system reconstitution proceeds as well as it does under these very altered circumstances. Recovery of the immunoglobulins, especially IgG and IgM, occurs but may take several months, and regulation is not precise. Frequent monoclonal immunoglobulins are observed, including Bence Jones proteinuria, but their presence has not yet been shown to proceed to a plasma cell malignancy. They are usually transient, being replaced by more normal polyclonal immunoglobulins. IgA recovery tends to be very delayed, and very low levels of IgA can be observed for several years. T-cell function is also impaired and may persist for prolonged periods.

These abnormalities account for the pattern and frequency of post-transplant infections, with CMV and the herpesviruses predominating. In addition, the minor differences between the graft and host may very well set up a chronic rejection reaction of the host by the transplanted immunocompetent cells (graft-versus-host disease). When severe, the gut (diarrhea), the skin (exfoliation), and the liver (hepatitis) can be fatally affected. Minor degrees of rejection also occur, which can also be associated with significant morbidity. Better means of suppression of these reactions have been developed (e.g., cyclosporin), but this in turn also leads to host defense impairment as well as other host side effects.

Despite these drawbacks, a great deal has been learned about immune system functioning and its manipulation that makes bone marrow transplantation the treatment of choice for a number of otherwise fatal diseases (e.g., aplastic anemia, relapsing acute leukemia), and the technology is sure to be improved in the future, extending it to other disease processes.

Case Studies

Case 1

The patient is a 14-month-old boy with a normal family history. He was admitted with a very high fever of 105°C and had a positive blood culture for *Streptococcus pneumoniae*. He was given penicillin for 10 days. He recovered and was discharged. In the next several months, this infection recurred twice, responding each time to penicillin treatment.

Physical examination was normal except for inflamed tonsils. Routine laboratory tests were entirely normal. On each occasion, positive blood cultures revealed different types of pneumococcus. However, no antibodies against the pneumococcus were detected in his blood.

Additional laboratory findings revealed a marked reduction of the gamma region in the serum protein electrophoresis, and there were no immunoglobulins detected by quantitative nephelometry. The patient was treated monthly with IV gammaglobulin infusion and no further infections were observed.

Case 1 Study Questions

1. What type of immune deficiency (primary or secondary) is this consistent with?

2. With what immunodeficiency disease state is this case consistent?

3. What is the mode of inheritance?

4. If his parents have other children, what are the chances of his sisters being affected? His brothers?

5. Will he be able to live a normal life?

Case 2

The patient is a 60-year-old male with an initial presentation of generalized lymphadenopathy, anemia, thrombocytopenia, and a recent history of recurrent pulmonary infections. The spleen was significantly enlarged. Laboratory findings showed a marked reduction of the gamma region in the serum protein electrophoresis and a markedly decreased immunoglobulin quantitation of IgG, IgA, and IgM by nephelometry. The white blood count (WBC) was 68,000/μL with 98% small, well-differentiated lymphocytes.

Case 2 Study Questions

1. What type of immune deficiency (primary or secondary) is this case consistent with?

2. What additional laboratory tests would be helpful?

3. How can additional infections be prevented?

4. Why are pyogenic infections such as *Streptococcus pneumoniae* so serious a problem in this patient?

5. Would immunization with Pneumovax be helpful?

References

1. Conley ME, Stiehm ER: Immunodeficiency disorders: General considerations. In Stiehm ER (ed): Immunologic Disorders in Infants and Children, 4th ed, p 201. Philadelphia, WB Saunders, 1996

2. Rosen FS, Seligmann M (eds): Immunodeficiencies, Philadelphia, Harwood Academic, 1993

3. Rosen FS, Cooper MD, Wedgwood RJP: The primary immunodeficiencies. N Engl J Med 333:431, 1995

4. Buckley RH: Breakthrough in the understanding and therapy of primary immunodeficiency. Pediatr Clin North Am 41:665, 1994

5. Eibl MM, Wolf HM: Primary immunodeficiency disorders—pathogenesis and treatment. Clin Immunotherapeutics 5:137, 1996

6. Leonard WJ: The molecular basis of X-linked severe combined immunodeficiency—defective cytokine receptor signaling. Ann Rev Med 47:229, 1996

7. Truedsson L, Baskin B, Pan Q, et al: Genetics of IgA deficiency. APMIS 103:833, 1995

8. Vorechovsky I, Zetterquist H, Paganelli R, et al: Family and linkage study of selective IgA deficiency and common variable immunodeficiency. Clin Immunol Immunopathol 77:185, 1995

9. Cunningham-Rundles C: Clinical and immunologic studies of common variable immunodeficiency. Curr Opin Pediatr 6:676, 1994

10. Thomas C, de Saint Basile G, Le Deist F, et al: Brief report: Correction of X-linked hyper-IgM syndrome by allogeneic bone marrow transplantation. N Engl J Med 333:426, 1995

11. Ochs HD, Hollenbaugh D, Aruffo A: The role of CD40L (gp39)/CD40 in T/B cell interaction and primary immunodeficiency. Semin Immunol 6:337, 1994

12. Thrasher A, Kinnon C: Gene therapy for primary immunodeficiency. Gene Ther 2:601, 1995

13. Noguchi M, Yi H, Rosenblatt HM, et al: Interleukin-2 receptor γ chain mutation results in X-linked severe combined immunodeficiency in humans. Cell 73:147, 1993

14. Mach B, Steimle V, Martinezsoria E, Reith W: Regulation of MHC class II genes—lessons from a disease. Annu Rev Immunol 14:301, 1996

15. Kolluri R, Shehabeldin A, Peacocke M, et al: Identification of WASP mutations in patients with Wiskott-Aldrich syndrome and isolated thrombocytopenia reveals allelic heterogeneity at the WAS locus. Hum Mol Genet 4:1119, 1995

16. Meyn MS: Ataxia-telangiectasia and cellular responses to DNA damage. Cancer Res 55:5991, 1995

17. Wahn U: Evaluation of the child with suspected primary immunodeficiency. Pediatr Allergy Immunol 6:71, 1995

Section D. Proliferative Disease

CHAPTER 32

Hypergammaglobulinemia

Therese B. Datiles
Richard L. Humphrey

Objectives

Upon completion of the chapter, the reader will be able to:

1. Characterize the laboratory findings of hypergammaglobulinemia as monoclonal or polyclonal based on serum protein electrophoresis, immunoelectrophoresis, immunofixation electrophoresis, and quantitation of immunoglobulin classes
2. Identify abnormal laboratory results
3. Compare and contrast polyclonal and monoclonal gammopathies with respect to cellular processes, the concentration of immunoglobulin, and the appearance on immunofixation electrophoresis (or immunoelectrophoresis)
4. Classify each of the following diseases or conditions as a monoclonal gammopathy or a polyclonal gammopathy and describe the expected changes on serum protein electrophoresis, immunoelectrophoresis, immunofixation electrophoresis, and quantitation of immunoglobulin:
    Chronic infection
    Multiple myeloma
    Connective tissue disease
    Primary amyloidosis
    Waldenström's macroglobulinemia
    Heavy-chain disease
    Liver disease
    HIV infection

INTRODUCTION

Hypergammaglobulinemia is the term used to describe the laboratory finding of elevated gammaglobulins on serum protein electrophoresis. The process known as *gammopathy* results from the increased production of immunoglobulins by plasma cells. It can involve many clones of plasma cells and hence be a polyclonal process, or it may result from a single clone and thus be a monoclonal process. Hypergammaglobulinemia usually is either polyclonal or monoclonal in character, but infrequently both may coexist. This chapter discusses the cellular basis of hypergammaglobulinemia, the associated laboratory and clinical findings, and the clinical and laboratory correlation.

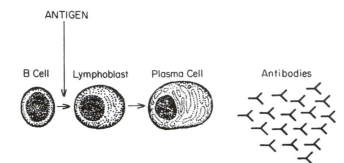

FIGURE 32-1
An antigen interacts with a B cell and triggers its transformation into a lymphoblast, which then multiplies by cell division and differentiates into a plasma cell. The plasma cell synthesizes and secretes antibodies, which bind to the triggering antigen, inactivates it, and helps the body to clear it.

CELLULAR BASIS

B lymphocytes that are appropriately stimulated by an antigen are transformed into plasma cells that synthesize and secrete immunoglobulin (Ig), as shown in Figure 32-1. These antibodies bind to the stimulating antigen and aid in its elimination or the neutralization of harmful properties. Five classes of Igs are recognized by their structural and antigenic differences, functional properties, etc. (see Chapter 8 for additional information). The secreted Ig is found in the blood and other body fluids, and can be characterized by immunologic methods. Throughout life, an individual is continuously exposed to diverse antigens, thereby stimulating the production of a mixture of antibodies composed of different isotypes and idiotypes (as defined in Chapter 8). Normally, in an adult, IgG constitutes about 65% of total serum Ig, IgA about 20%, and IgM about 15% (Fig. 32-2). IgD and IgE are present in very small (ng/mL) quantities. Overproduction of Ig is termed hypergammaglobulinemia and can be classified as polyclonal or monoclonal, depending on the pathophysiology of the process.

Polyclonal Hypergammaglobulinemia

Exposure to a complex antigen (Ag) transforms many clones of B cells, causing them to produce many different antibodies; hence, there is a polyclonal response. Each clone will synthesize an antibody with a different specificity, corresponding to different epitopes on the complex antigen. A polyclonal antibody response is usually composed of one or more classes and subclasses of immunoglobulin, and also involves both light-chain types. Polyclonal hypergammaglobulinemia (gammopathy) results when this normal interplay between the Ag and the Ig response is either unregulated or exaggerated. Polyclonal gammopathy can be observed in a variety of clinical situations (e.g., acute and chronic infections, AIDS, sarcoidosis, autoimmune disorders, and liver diseases, and is shown in Fig. 32-3 and Color Plate 22).

Monoclonal Hypergammaglobulinemia

In contrast to the regulated antigenic transformation of many B cells in a polyclonal response, an autonomous, antigen-independent, "malignant" transformation of one specific clone of B cells results in the production of one immunoglobulin restricted to one choice of heavy chain and one choice of light chain. These monoclonal Ig molecules usually have a normal immunoglobulin structure, that is, for IgG the molecule will have two identical heavy chains and two identical light chains, with all the expected constant domains (isotype) and variable domains (idiotype). The hypervariable regions of the heavy chain and light chain co-operate to create an antigen combining site, although the complementary antigen is

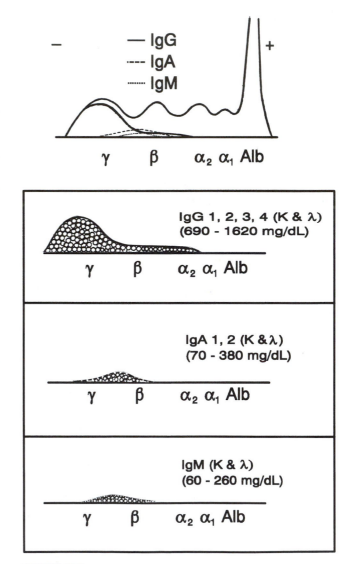

FIGURE 32-2
Serum protein electrophoretogram (SPE) with normal Ig (IgG, IgA, IgM) migrating from the α_2-region through the γ-region. The major portion of the γ-region is contributed by IgG (solid line). The relative electrophoretic mobility and concentration are indicated by the areas under the respective curves. The small circles filling the area under the curve are a diagrammatic representation of the number of plasma cells producing these classes. The normal range in mg/dL for each of these three principal classes is also shown.

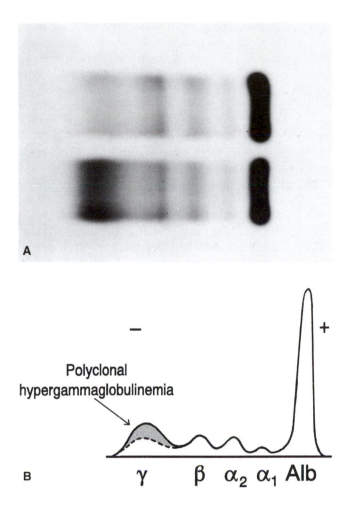

FIGURE 32-3 (COLOR PLATE 22)
(**A**) Cellulose acetate membrane comparing a normal serum (top lane) with a polyclonal hypergammaglobulinemia serum (bottom lane). (**B**) The normal SPE scan is depicted by the open area (dashed line), in contrast to the polyclonal gammopathy, which is illustrated by the dark area. The polyclonal pattern is characterized by a broad-based, diffuse increase in the γ-region.

	NORMAL (g/dL) (open Area)	REFERENCE RANGE (g/dL)
Total protein	7.4	(6.0–8.0)
Albumin	4.4	(3.1–5.4)
Alpha 1 globulin	0.2	(0.1–0.4)
Alpha 2 globulin	0.7	(0.4–1.1)
Beta globulin	1.1	(0.5–1.2)
Gamma globulin	1.1	(0.7–1.7)

	POLYCLONAL HYPERGAMMA-GLOBULINEMIA (g/dL) (DARK AREA)	REFERENCE RANGE (g/dL)
Total protein	9.6↑	(6.0–8.0)
Albumin	4.2	(3.1–5.4)
Alpha 1 globulin	0.3	(0.1–0.4)
Alpha 2 globulin	0.8	(0.4–1.1)
Beta globulin	1.2	(0.5–1.2)
Gamma globulin	3.1↑	(0.7–1.7)

usually unknown.[1] Every immunoglobulin (Ig) molecule produced as a result of the expansion of this single clone is identical and is therefore homogeneous, and is called a monoclonal immunoglobulin or an *M component* (MC), as shown in Figure 32-4 (on p. 320; see also Color Plate 23). "M" used this way represents "monoclonal" and should not be confused with the IgM class of immunoglobulins. The plasma cell disorders that result in the production of a monoclonal immunoglobulin are termed the plasma cell dyscrasias.[2] Another commonly used synonym is monoclonal gammopathies.[3]

Monoclonal Ig or M components may be found in malignant, benign, or transient disorders. The malignant processes include multiple myeloma,[4,5] Waldenström's macroglobulinemia,[6] the heavy-chain diseases,[7] and primary amyloidosis.[8] Sometimes a monoclonal protein is detected in other lymphoreticular neoplasms (e.g., chronic lymphocytic leukemia and B-cell lymphomas). Occasionally, a monoclonal Ig is detected in elderly patients in the absence of a progressive disease; this process is called *monoclonal gammopathy of undetermined significance (MGUS)*, previously known as benign monoclonal gammopathy.[9]

LABORATORY EVALUATION

Three test methodologies can be used to assess, study, and interpret the polyclonal or monoclonal nature of serum Ig response and to relate the results to a disease state. The three tests are

1. Protein electrophoresis: performed on serum (SPE), urine (UPE), or cerebrospinal fluid (CSF-PE)
2. Immunoglobulin quantitative measurement (Ig Q): performed on serum or CSF
3. Immunofixation electrophoresis: performed on serum (SIFE), urine (UIFE), or cerebrospinal fluid (CSF-IFE). An earlier method, immunoelectrophoresis (IEP), is still in use in some laboratories.

Protein Electrophoresis

Electrophoresis is the separation of charged molecules, such as serum proteins, in an electrical field.[10] Serum protein is applied to a solid support medium, such as cellulose acetate or agarose gel. All serum proteins will have a net negative charge at pH 8.6, which is the standard buffer system. Albumin, α_1 globulins, α_2 globulins, and β globulins will migrate toward the positive pole (anode), whereas most gamma globulins will migrate toward the negative pole (cathode). After electrophoresis, the separated proteins are fixed and stained, and the membrane is cleared so that the protein bands can be visualized, scanned, and quantitated by densitometry (see Figs. 32-2 and 32-3). Protein electrophoresis can be performed using diluted or undiluted serum (depending on the procedure used), con-

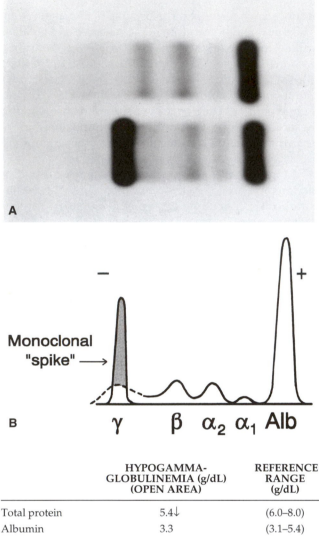

FIGURE 32-4 (COLOR PLATE 23)
(**A**) Cellulose acetate membrane comparing a hypogammaglobu-linemia serum (top lane) with a monoclonal hypergammaglobuline-mia serum (bottom lane). Note the disappearance of the normal immunoglobulins in the hypogammaglobulinemia serum, with the gamma region approaching the baseline levels in the scan. (See Figure 32-11 for SPE pattern.) (**B**) In contrast with the normal pat-tern (dashed line), the monoclonal gammopathy results in a single, sharply defined, narrow-based peak or "spike," illustrated here by the dark area in the γ-region.

	HYPOGAMMA-GLOBULINEMIA (g/dL) (OPEN AREA)	REFERENCE RANGE (g/dL)
Total protein	5.4↓	(6.0–8.0)
Albumin	3.3	(3.1–5.4)
Alpha 1 globulin	0.2	(0.1–0.4)
Alpha 2 globulin	0.8	(0.4–1.1)
Beta globulin	0.7	(0.5–1.2)
Gamma globulin	0.3↓	(0.7–1.7)

	MONOCLONAL HYPERGAMMA-GLOBULINEMIA(g/dL) (DARK AREA)	REFERENCE RANGE (g/dL)
Total protein	9.9↑	(6.0–8.0)
Albumin	3.5	(3.1–5.4)
Alpha 1 globulin	0.4	(0.1–0.4)
Alpha 2 globulin	1.0	(0.4–1.1)
Beta globulin	0.5	(0.5–1.2)
Gamma globulin	4.5↑	(0.7–1.7)

centrated urine, or concentrated cerebrospinal fluid. Urine and CSF have a lower protein concentration and therefore require concentration, usually 100-fold prior to electrophoresis. A commonly used method to con-centrate a protein solution is to pass the fluid through a membrane with a proper pore size that will retain pro-teins and other large molecules but allow smaller mol-ecules (e.g., water and salt) to easily pass through.

Serum protein electrophoresis performed on a cellu-lose acetate membrane is illustrated in Figure 32-3A and 32-4A, while densitometric scans are shown in Figures 32-2, 32-3B, and 32-4B. Protein fractions reading from the right (anode, +) to the left (cathode, −) are albumin, alpha-1, alpha-2, beta, and gamma. The qualitative vi-sual interpretation of the symmetry of each protein frac-tion is carefully assessed. Any asymmetry should be noted. The quantitative measurement of each fraction is calculated from the total protein concentration obtained from the biuret or other quantitative method. Multiply-ing the total protein concentration times the percent of each of the fractions yields the concentration of the frac-tion. The normal serum adult reference ranges are listed in Figure 32-3B and 32-4B. It is extremely important that the interpretation include *both* the qualitative pattern *and* the quantitative concentration measurements of each fraction because both are necessary to detect an early monoclonal process or other disease process, for exam-ple, immunodeficiency. It is possible to have a normal quantitative protein fraction and yet an abnormal quali-tative pattern, which might indicate an early-onset or low-concentration monoclonal gammopathy.

Immunoglobulin Quantitative Measurement

Immunoglobulin measurement can be performed in a liquid phase (e.g., rate nephelometry) or semisolid phase (radial immunodiffusion [RID]). Nephelometry measures light scattering resulting from immune com-plex formation. For example, patient IgG reacts with the reagent anti-IgG, producing an IgG–anti-IgG complex. This complex is relatively large in size and scatters light, which can be detected and quantitated electronically. The amount of light scatter is directly proportional to the amount of Ig present in the patient's sample. (Neph-elometry is more fully discussed in Chapter 16.)

Radial immunodiffusion is a precipitation reaction in which soluble patient Ig reacts with anti-Ig in the semisolid agarose, and a precipitin ring forms at the zone of equivalence. The diameter of the precipitin ring is directly proportional to the concentration of patient Ig. (RID is discussed in detail in Chapter 11.)

Immunoelectrophoresis (IEP)

Immunoelectrophoresis (IEP) is one of the original methods developed to identify and characterize Ig through antigenic determinants found on heavy and light chains. IEP consists of two phases: electrophoresis and immunodiffusion/precipitation. In the electrophoretic phase, proteins are applied to the agarose gel and separated in an electrical field, as described earlier in the section on protein electrophoresis. Next the trough parallel to the direction of the electrophoretic separation is filled with a specific antiserum (anti-IgG, -IgA, -IgM, -κ, or -λ) and is allowed to incubate overnight. The electrophoretically separated serum proteins and antisera diffuse toward each other through the agarose, and when the antiserum binds to its antigen, an Ig–anti-Ig complex precipitates and forms an arc. Unprecipitated proteins are removed by washing. The arcs can be visualized by indirect lighting, or interpretation can follow when the gel is dried and stained, which produces a permanent record. The shape and position of the precipitin arcs are interpreted by comparing them with the arcs formed by the normal serum control. IEP is discussed in detail in Chapter 11.

Immunofixation Electrophoresis

Immunofixation electrophoresis (IFE), a more sensitive method that is easier to interpret than IEP, has replaced IEP in many clinical laboratories.[3,11–13] IFE is composed of two phases: electrophoresis, to separate the proteins, and fixation, to precipitate the proteins. Serum or other fluid is applied to the agarose gel, and the proteins are separated during electrophoresis. Specific proteins are then fixed in place by covering the area of separated proteins with antiserum specific for the protein to be visualized. The antiserum fixes the selected specific protein by precipitation. Unprecipitated proteins are removed by washing. After drying, the precipitated protein-antisera complex can be stained and visualized. In order to optimize the bands, the serum (or urine, or CSF) concentration is often adjusted. This serves to balance the protein concentration with the antisera being used and brings the immunologic reaction into the zone

of equivalence. Attention is paid to the diffuse or restricted nature of the band, which permits characterization of the band as polyclonal or monoclonal. A diffuse band recognized by the specific antiserum suggests a heterogeneous group of proteins (i.e., a polyclonal hypergammaglobulinemia; Fig. 32-5; Color Plate 24). In contrast, a homogeneous protein will migrate in a very narrow region, demonstrating electrophoretic restriction. This is the expected pattern of a monoclonal protein (Fig. 32-6; Color Plate 25).

The combined use of high-resolution electrophoresis, immunoglobulin quantitation, and immunofixation has resulted in the detection of low-concentration monoclonal abnormalities that would have been overlooked with prior, less sensitive techniques.[14]

CLINICAL CORRELATION

This section describes the different clinical manifestations of disease states causing polyclonal or monoclonal hypergammaglobulinemia. Polyclonal gammopathy (see Figs. 32-3 and 32-5) results from an exaggerated or unregulated immune response, for example, acute or chronic infections, AIDS, connective tissue disorders, and liver disease. Monoclonal gammopathy (see Figs. 32-4 and 32-6) results from an unregulated proliferation and accumulation of a single plasma cell clone. This process can be malignant (e.g., multiple myeloma, Waldenström's macroglobulinemia, heavy-chain disease, primary amyloidosis, and other lymphoreticular neoplasms), benign (e.g. about 70% of MGUS), or transient (e.g. bone marrow transplant).

Polyclonal Hypergammaglobulinemia

INFECTIOUS DISEASES

Chronic antigenic stimulation, which occurs in a variety of clinical conditions, such as chronic infection, sarcoidosis, and autoimmune disorders, usually causes

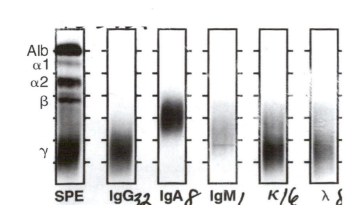

FIGURE 32-5 (COLOR PLATE 24)
Serum immunofixation electrophoresis (SIFE) revealing a polyclonal hypergammaglobulinemia involving all three major classes of Ig (G, A, and M) and both light-chain types (κ and λ). The point of application seen in most of the lanes in the γ region should not be confused with a monoclonal band.

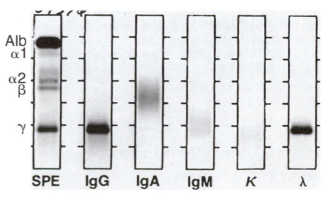

FIGURE 32-6 (COLOR PLATE 25)
SIFE of a patient's serum with an IgG lambda monoclonal gammopathy. Note the restricted electrophoretic mobility of the band seen in the IgG and lambda lanes, and the marked reductions of the other Igs.

polyclonal hypergammaglobulinemia (Fig. 32-3). A typical serum protein electrophoresis pattern shows a broad-based, diffuse (heterogeneous) increase of the proteins in the γ region (see Fig. 32-3). The quantitative SPE gamma fraction is moderately to markedly increased compared with normal serum. On occasion, the γ region becomes very accentuated and may either obscure or mimic a monoclonal Ig (M component). Quantitative Ig measurement will show an increased concentration of one or more Ig classes. The polyclonal nature of the abnormality can be confirmed by performing an IFE. The IFE pattern in polyclonal hypergammaglobulinemia is characterized by a diffuse and heterogeneous band in each of the IFE lanes (see Fig. 32-5)

INFLAMMATORY PROCESSES

During tissue destruction and acute inflammation, the concentration of acute-phase reactants increases, which leads to an increase in the α_2 region of serum protein electrophoresis and, to a lesser extent, an increase in α_1 and a decrease in albumin. With persistent inflammation, the laboratory findings, that is, the electrophoretic pattern, the Ig Q, and the IFE results, can overlap and share features with the pattern seen with chronic antigenic stimulation (see Fig. 32-3).

LIVER DISEASE

The electrophoretic pattern seen in chronic liver disease also is characterized by a polyclonal increase in the γ region. In addition, there often is a polyclonal increase in IgA, which results in a bridging or obliteration of the space usually present between the β and γ regions. Additional features often include a stair-step–like decrease from the γ to β to α_2 to α_1 regions and a reduction in the albumin concentration (Fig. 32-7). This pattern overlaps with and is a variation of that seen with chronic antigenic stimulation (compare with Fig. 32-3). However, the following four characteristics often help to establish chronic liver disease: (1) decreased albumin; (2) stair-step decrease ranging from the γ region to the α_1 region; (3) bridging between the β and γ regions; and (4) a polyclonal increase in the γ region. The Ig Q and IFE lab findings are similar to the chronic antigenic stimulation pattern but often with disproportionate accentuation of the polyclonal IgA increase.

Monoclonal Hypergammaglobulinemia

MULTIPLE MYELOMA

Multiple myeloma is a lymphoproliferative disease that results from the uncontrolled proliferation of a single clone of plasma cells that produces a homoge-

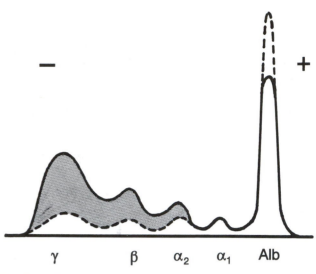

FIGURE 32-7
Liver disease pattern. SPE shows decreased albumin (Alb); stair-step decrease from γ to α_1; bridging between β and γ regions; and polyclonal increase in the γ region. Compare with Figure 32-3B.

neous immunoglobulin or immunoglobulin fragment.[2,3,5] Traditionally, multiple myeloma is subclassified according to the heavy-chain class and light-chain type of the monoclonal protein (Table 32-1). IgG myeloma is the most common form, accounting for 50% of all myeloma. IgA myeloma accounts for 25%. IgD myeloma rarely occurs (<1%), and IgE myeloma is extremely rare. In some instances malignant plasma cells lose the ability to synthesize the heavy chain and can produce only the light chain (see Table 32-1, line F.L.C.).[15] This accounts for about 24% of myeloma cases and is called light-chain disease or light-chain myeloma. Approximately 1% of the cases are nonsecretory myeloma, in which neither the heavy nor the light chain is produced. In approximately half of IgG and IgA myeloma patients light chains are overproduced relative to heavy chains (unbalanced synthesis). This free or unattached light chain circulates in the blood and is easily filtered by the glomeruli because of its low molecular weight (20 kDa). Thus, free light chains can be found in the urine and are called Bence Jones protein, in honor of the man who first described the unusual properties of this protein (see Table 32-1, line F.L.C.). Taken together, the 24% of the myeloma cases that produce only light chain plus the 26% of cases in which light chain production is unbalanced (in association with either a serum IgG or IgA monoclonal protein) result in about 50% of myeloma patients with detectable free light chain in their urine (Bence Jones proteinuria). When free light chain is produced, it is sometimes nephrotoxic for the kidney, which causes renal damage and may result in renal failure.[16]

TABLE 32-1
Patterns of Monoclonal Gammopathies in Multiple Myeloma

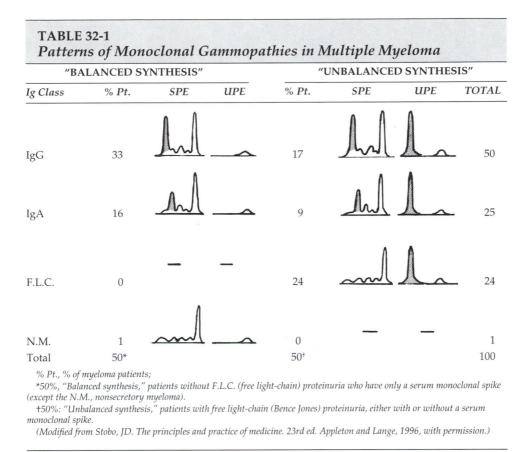

| Ig Class | "BALANCED SYNTHESIS" | | | "UNBALANCED SYNTHESIS" | | | |
	% Pt.	SPE	UPE	% Pt.	SPE	UPE	TOTAL
IgG	33			17			50
IgA	16			9			25
F.L.C.	0	—		24			24
N.M.	1			0	—	—	1
Total	50*			50†			100

% Pt., % of myeloma patients;

*50%, "Balanced synthesis," patients without F.L.C. (free light-chain) proteinuria who have only a serum monoclonal spike (except the N.M., nonsecretory myeloma).

†50%: "Unbalanced synthesis," patients with free light-chain (Bence Jones) proteinuria, either with or without a serum monoclonal spike.

(Modified from Stobo, JD. The principles and practice of medicine. 23rd ed. Appleton and Lange, 1996, with permission.)

The incidence of multiple myeloma is about 5 per 100,000 in the general population, with a median age of approximately 60 years. Although the pathogenesis in humans is unknown, epidemiologic studies show an increased incidence of myeloma following radiation and some chemical exposures. The prevalence is about the same for men and women. For unknown reasons, the incidence is greater in blacks and the onset is at a somewhat earlier age.

The clinical findings include weakness, anorexia, and weight loss, suggesting a chronic, progressive, systemic illness. As the disease advances, bone involvement with skeletal destruction (Fig. 32-8) and pain, anemia, renal insufficiency, various neurologic deficits, and recurrent bacterial infections often occur.

Laboratory findings in multiple myeloma include demonstration and characterization of the monoclonal Ig. As seen in Table 32-1, three quarters of the patients with multiple myeloma (lines: IgG and IgA) with both balanced and unbalanced synthesis show a peak or spike of variable size in the γ or β region on SPE (see Fig. 32-4B). The Ig class of the monoclonal protein is usually quantitatively increased, whereas the normal, uninvolved Ig classes are commonly decreased. Serum IEP shows an abnormal position, density, and/or shape of a precipitin arc, restricted to one heavy-chain

class and one light-chain type. The shape of the abnormal precipitin arc of the heavy chain is identical to that of the light chain because each antiserum detects different antigenic determinants (epitopes) on the same Ig molecule. Similarly, the serum IFE will identify a band of restricted electrophoretic mobility with the

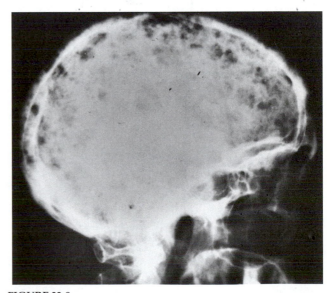

FIGURE 32-8
Skull x-ray of a patient with multiple myeloma showing osteolytic "punched-out" lesions.

anti–heavy-chain antisera that is identical to that revealed by the light-chain antisera (see Fig. 32-6). When there is unbalanced synthesis (see Table 32-1, lines: IgG, IgA, and F.L.C.), free light chain can be demonstrated in the urine by protein electrophoresis (Fig. 32-9; Color Plate 26). The free light chain also can be identified and typed by IEP or IFE (Fig. 32-10; Color Plate 27).

Light-chain myeloma is the production of a monoclonal light chain without a corresponding heavy chain (see Table 32-1, line: F.L.C.—unbalanced synthesis). The quantitative measurement of serum Igs is often in the low normal range or can be markedly decreased. As a result of this suppression of normal Ig production, the SPE may show a hypogammaglobulinemia pattern; for example, a markedly reduced γ region is shown in Figure 32-11. Occasionally, the monoclonal light chain can be detected by serum IFE because this procedure is much more sensitive than SPE. Taken together, free light chains can be found in the urine by protein electrophoresis or can be detected by urine IEP or IFE in approximately 50% of myeloma patients (see Table 32-1, lines: IgG, IgA, F.L.C.—unbalanced synthesis; footnote).

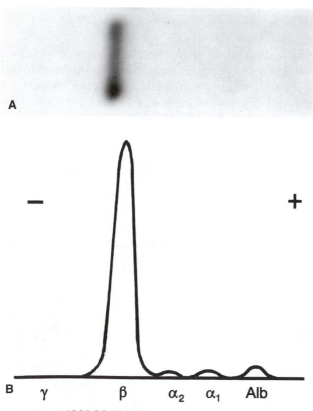

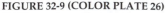

A

B   γ   β   α₂   α₁   Alb

FIGURE 32-9 (COLOR PLATE 26)
(**A**) Electrophoresis of a concentrated urine specimen on a cellulose acetate membrane demonstrating a restricted band in the β region. (**B**) UPE shows a markedly increased narrow band or "spike" in the β-region. This pattern represents a free light chain (Bence Jones) proteinuria.

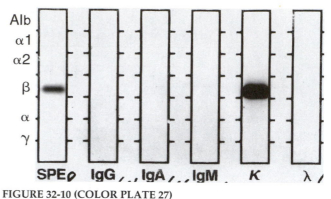

FIGURE 32-10 (COLOR PLATE 27)
UIFE revealing the presence of a markedly increased band of restricted electrophoretic mobility in the κ lane. (kappa Bence Jones proteinuria.)

Multiple myeloma is a malignant tumor of plasma cells. The plasma cells typically are diffusely present in the bone marrow and less commonly in other tissues; rarely, localized tumor masses develop (plasmacytoma; Fig. 32-12). A typical plasma cell infiltrate of the bone marrow is shown in Figure 32-13. Osteolytic lesions are associated with bone pain and fractures, and appear as "punched-out" areas when evaluated by x-ray. The skull is commonly affected, as shown in Figure 32-8. Treatment of multiple myeloma includes local radiation therapy of myelomatous tumors and systemic chemotherapy to reduce the plasmacytosis of the bone marrow. Alkylating agents (such as melphalan and cyclophosphamide) are commonly used and work by interfering with cell replication. Responding patients have a median survival expectancy of about 3 to 4 years, whereas unresponsive patients have a median survival of 12 to 18 months. Recent attempts to intensify treatments followed by bone marrow transplantation may provide long-term control (cure?) of the disease for some patients.

WALDENSTRÖM'S MACROGLOBULINEMIA

Waldenström's macroglobulinemia is a relatively rare disorder characterized by uncontrolled proliferation of a single clone of lymphoid cells that synthesize a homogeneous IgM. It represents one form of several related lymphoproliferative disorders characterized by their production of a monoclonal IgM.[6] It is usually observed in individuals over age 50, with the incidence peaking in the sixth decade. The frequency in men is about one and one half times that in women.

Clinical findings include weakness, fatigability, headache, and weight loss. As the disorder progresses, the features associated with the hyperviscosity syndrome develop. These features can cause abnormalities of the cardiovascular (congestive heart failure), neurologic (headache, dizziness), ocular (partial or total loss

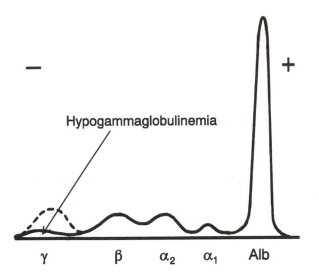

Hypogammaglobulinemia

γ   β   α₂   α₁   Alb

FIGURE 32-11
Hypogammaglobulinemia. SPE shows marked reduction of the γ-region compared to the normal pattern (dashed line). Refer to the cellulose acetate membrane in Fig. 32-4A, top lane.

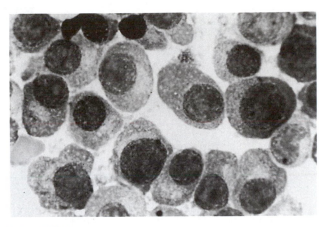

FIGURE 32-13
Oil-immersion micrograph of a bone marrow smear stained with Wright's stain taken from a patient with multiple myeloma. The malignant plasma cells are characterized by abundant cytoplasm and eccentrically placed nuclei. They have a finely vacuolated cytoplasm that represents the dilated endoplasmic reticulum caused by the active synthesis of the monoclonal Ig. A zone of reduced staining is often seen next to the nucleus, the perinuclear clear zone.

of visual acuity), and hematopoietic (bleeding, anemia) systems.

Laboratory findings include a spike in the β or γ region on serum protein electrophoretogram (SPE). The serum IgM is quantitatively increased, whereas IgG and IgA are often decreased. Serum IEP and IFE

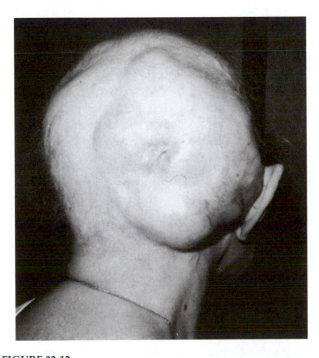

FIGURE 32-12
Localized plasmacytoma of the skull in a patient with far-advanced multiple myeloma.

demonstrate a monoclonal IgMκ or IgMλ protein. In the presence of hyperviscosity, the relative plasma viscosity is elevated. Relative plasma viscosity is a comparison of the time it takes for a standard volume of saline to pass through a capillary tube with the time required for the patient's plasma to do the same. The relative plasma viscosity is an indication of the resistance of the plasma to flow and, when markedly increased, results in the symptoms of the hyperviscosity syndrome. The threshold for symptoms often occurs when the relative viscosity is greater than 3.0 (normal, 1.5 to 1.9) but will differ among patients. The hyperviscosity syndrome in Waldenström's macroglobulinemia is caused by excess monoclonal IgM production because IgM is a very large molecule (close to one million daltons) and is quite asymmetric in shape.[17]

The diagnosis of Waldenström's macroglobulinemia centers on the presence of the monoclonal IgM and the abnormal accumulation of plasmacytoid lymphocytes in bone marrow and other tissues. Kyle and Garton[6] arbitrarily set the level of the monoclonal IgM as ≥3000 mg/dL in order to discriminate between Waldenström's macroglobulinemia and the other related lymphoproliferative disorders characterized by the presence of a monoclonal IgM. When defined in this way, the median survival expectancy is about 6 years. When it occurs, death is related to infection, bone marrow failure, or uncontrolled hyperviscosity. Initial treatment centers on rapid control of the hyperviscosity by the removal of the monoclonal IgM from the serum by plasmapheresis. Longer term control of the production of the IgM is often achieved by chemotherapy with alkylating agents, such as chlorambucil or cyclophosphamide, and, more recently, by nucleoside analogs. When treatment is successful, the plasmapheresis requirement can often be reduced or eliminated.

HEAVY-CHAIN DISEASES

The heavy-chain diseases are rare lymphoproliferative disorders characterized by the presence of fragments of the heavy (H) chains without light chain.[7] The H chains of the α, γ, and μ classes have been involved and serve as a convenient way to classify these disorders. Although the clinical syndromes differ, the proteins are characterized by major deletions in the variable (VH) and first constant domain (CH₁) of the Ig molecule. These deletions preclude the attachment of the light chains.

α-Heavy-chain disease is the most common, occurring predominantly among young Arabs and non-Ashkenazi Jews in the Middle East. The disease is characterized by abdominal pain, severe diarrhea, and malabsorption caused by lymphoid and plasma cell infiltration of the small intestines and mesenteric lymph nodes. Early-stage patients have responded to treatment with antibiotics. Late-stage patients may also require chemotherapy.

γ-Heavy-chain disease is characterized by fever, malaise, weight loss, peculiar edema and erythema of the palate and uvula, generalized lymphadenopathy, and hepatosplenomegaly. The survival is variable, from a few weeks to more than 5 years after the onset of symptoms. Chemotherapy has been successful in some instances.

μ-Heavy-chain disease is characterized by hepatosplenomegaly and lymphadenopathy. The lymphocytoid-plasma cells are often characterized by vacuolated cytoplasm and sometimes circulate in high numbers, causing this disease to mimic chronic lymphocytic leukemia.

Although these syndromes vary in their clinical expression, in the laboratory they are characterized by the following features:

1. SPE: A monoclonal "spike" may be present in the beta or gamma region
2. Ig Q: There may be increased IgG (γ-heavy chain disease, HCD); increased IgM (μ-HCD), or increased IgA (α-HCD) quantitative measurements
3. IFE: Often a band of restricted electrophoretic mobility that is identical in both serum and urine is found in the IgG, IgA, or IgM lanes. This band is identified by antisera directed against the involved heavy chain but does not react with light-chain antisera. The band may be detectable in both the serum and urine because the large deletion (VH and CH₁) reduces the molecular size of the remaining fragment (about 40,000 Da) to the point where it can be filtered by normal glomeruli into

the urine. Confirmation of the diagnosis rests on the measurement of the molecular weight of the heavy-chain fragment and biochemical proof of the absence of the light chain.

PRIMARY AMYLOIDOSIS

Primary amyloidosis is a rare disorder occurring in less than 1% of autopsies in general hospitals. It is characterized by the accumulation of a complex extracellular proteinaceous substance that is dominated by a fibrillar component visualized by electron microscopy. Amyloidosis is diagnosed by the histologic examination of a biopsy of an involved tissue, such as the tongue, gingiva, nerve, muscle, skin, liver, bone marrow, rectum, kidney, or heart. Congo red staining of affected tissues when examined under polarized light reveals the characteristic apple-green to yellow birefringence. The course of the disease varies with the organs most involved.

In the primary and myeloma-related form of the disease, the fibril has been shown to be an immunoglobulin fragment, usually the variable end of the light chain. It is produced by a clone of plasma cells that is usually present in the bone marrow but not in sufficient numbers or with the skeletal destruction seen in multiple myeloma. However, amyloid deposition can complicate myeloma as well as other plasma cell disorders. Other forms of amyloidosis exist with the biochemical structure of the fibril unrelated to immunoglobulin. For example, the secondary form occurs after prolonged infection (e.g., tuberculosis, osteomyelitis) or in association with chronic inflammatory processes such as rheumatoid arthritis. The fibril is called amyloid A and is related to an acute-phase reaction protein. There are also a number of inherited forms of amyloidosis, which also are caused by the deposition of fibrils that are unrelated to Ig.

In the laboratory, primary amyloidosis can often be suspected because of the frequently associated abnormalities of the serum immunoglobulins. Many cases are characterized by hypogammaglobulinemia (see Fig. 32-11) which can be markedly reduced, often involving more than one of the major Ig classes. Frequently, a low-concentration monoclonal gammopathy is detected in the serum, with associated free light chains found in the urine. On occasion, the abnormalities are subtle and not easy to detect by UPE. This can be especially true when there is kidney damage caused by the amyloidosis, leading to substantial proteinuria, which may obscure the detection of low-concentration monoclonal free light chain in the urine. Under these circumstances, the UIFE often proves to be of enormous help in detecting, identifying, and characterizing the monoclonal Ig.

MONOCLONAL GAMMOPATHY OF UNDETERMINED SIGNIFICANCE (MGUS)

Sometimes a monoclonal protein in serum or urine is present without other manifestations of a plasma cell disorder. The frequency of this finding increases with age and has been estimated at about 10% in persons greater than 60 years of age. Some patients may demonstrate progression over time, that is, 17% in 10 years and 33% in 20 years, but some do not.[9] It is important to distinguish between early detection of a malignant, progressive process and MGUS, which can behave in a benign fashion for years. Unfortunately, there is no easy, reliable way to predict whether or when a given patient will progress. The quantity, class, or type of the monoclonal gammopathy or the presence of free light-chain (Bence Jones) protein fails to predict which patient's disease process will progress. All patients with benign monoclonal gammopathy should be monitored indefinitely for the possible emergence of malignant behavior.

Case Studies

Case 1

The patient was a 44-year-old male known to be an I.V. drug user and also known to be hepatitis C positive and HIV positive. He was transferred from another hospital with respiratory and metabolic acidosis as well as mental confusion, thought to be secondary to pneumonia in the upper right lobe of unclear etiology. Despite the use of broad-spectrum antibiotics, he remained confused, and multiple blood cultures were negative. He underwent bronchoscopy with bronchoalveolar lavage to try to identify the causative organisms, but the results were negative.

The chemistry screening tests revealed increased total serum protein and globulins but low normal albumin. Because of these findings, serum protein electrophoresis was performed, which revealed a broad-based increase in the gamma region with beta-gamma bridging. Immunoglobulin quantitation by nephelometry showed an IgG level of 3650 mg/dL (reference range, 690–1620 mg/dL), IgA level of 777 mg/dL (70–380 mg/dL), and IgM level of 248 mg/dL (60–260 mg/dL). Despite the use of broad-spectrum antibiotics and oxygen, the patient expired from respiratory failure.

Case 1 Study Questions

1. Interpret the SPE pattern in Figure 32-14, describing each of the protein fractions.

2. What type of gammopathy does this SPE pattern suggest?

3. Interpret the IFE pattern in Figure 32-15, describing each of the Ig lanes observed on the IFE membrane.

4. What type of gammopathy does this IFE pattern suggest?

5. What clinical conditions or disease states would correlate with these SPE and IFE patterns?

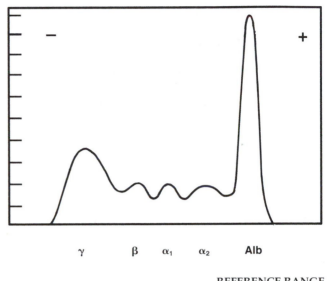

	CASE 1	REFERENCE RANGE (g/dL)
Total protein	8.2↑	(6.0–8.0)
Albumin	3.2	(3.1–5.4)
Alpha 1	0.1	(0.1–0.4)
Alpha 2	0.9	(0.4–1.1)
Beta	0.9	(0.5–1.2)
Gamma	3.1↑	(0.7–1.7)

FIGURE 32-14

Serum protein electrophoresis scan for case 1

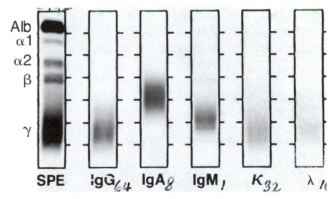

FIGURE 32-15 (COLOR PLATE 28)

Serum immunofixation electrophoresis for case 1. To avoid antigen excess and to optimize the visualization of each of the IFE lanes, the patient's serum has been appropriately diluted according to the concentration of Ig (quantitative measurement) in order to proportionately correspond to the strength of the antisera used. The numbers written next to the labels of the lane indicate the dilution used in each lane. For example, the IgG lane has been loaded with serum diluted to 1:64, the kappa lane diluted at 1:32, and so forth. The SPE lane is loaded at a 1:2 dilution. These careful choices of the respective dilutions used permit the demonstration of the polyclonal nature of the Ig and prevent misinterpretation due to antigen excess in any lane.

Case 2

The patient is a 76-year-old man with an initial presentation of back pain, 20-pound weight loss over a 3-month period, and increasing generalized weakness. His hematocrit was markedly low, his serum calcium level was high, and his total serum protein and albumin were normal. Plain radiographs of his skeleton showed osteolytic lesions, and the bone marrow aspirate showed increased plasma cells.

Case 2 Study Questions

1. Interpret the SPE pattern in Figure 32-16, describing each of the protein fractions.

2. What type of gammopathy does this SPE pattern suggest?

3. Interpret the IFE pattern in Figure 32-17, describing each of the Ig lanes in the IFE membrane.

4. What type of gammopathy does this IFE pattern suggest?

5. What clinical conditions or disease states would correlate with these SPE and IFE patterns?

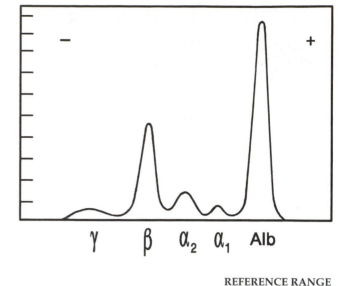

	CASE 2 (g/dL)	REFERENCE RANGE (g/dL)
Total protein	7.6	(6.0–8.0)
Albumin	3.9	(3.1–5.4)
Alpha 1	0.3	(0.1–0.4)
Alpha 2	0.9	(0.4–1.1)
Beta	1.9↑	(0.5–1.2)
Gamma	0.6↓	(0.7–1.7)

Immunoglobulin Quantitation
(nephelometric assay)

	CASE 2	REFERENCE RANGE (mg/dl)
IgG	720	690–1620
IgA	970↑	70–380
IgM	54↓	60–260

FIGURE 32-16
Serum protein electrophoresis for case 2.

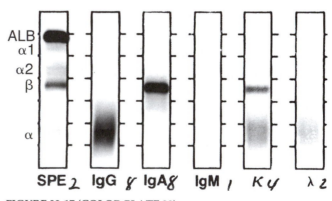

FIGURE 32-17 (COLOR PLATE 29)
Serum immunofixation electrophoresis for case 2. Note the pale appearance of the monoclonal band as revealed in the κ lane in spite of the serum load being twice the concentration (1:4) compared with the serum loaded on the IgA lane (1:8). This emphasizes the need to balance the strength of the antisera with the antigen concentration in each lane. Review the discussion of the need to balance the antibody and the antigen provided in Fig. 32-15.

References

1. Duggan DB, Schattner A: Unusual manifestations of monoclonal gammopathies, autoimmune and idiopathic syndromes. Am J Med 81:864, 1986
2. Humphrey RL: Plasma cell dyscrasias. In Stobo JD, Hellmann DB, Ladenson PW, Petty BG, Traill TA (eds): The Principles and Practice of Medicine, 23rd ed, p 802. Stamford, CT, Appleton and Lange, 1996
3. Kyle RA: The monoclonal gammopathies. Clin Chem 40:2154, 1994
4. Kyle RA: Multiple myeloma: How did it begin? Mayo Clin Proc 69:680, 1994
5. Seiden MV, Anderson KC: Multiple myeloma. Curr Opin Oncol 6:41, 1994
6. Kyle RA, Garton JP: The spectrum of IgM monoclonal gammopathy in 430 cases. Mayo Clin Proc 62:719, 1987
7. Wahner-Roedler DL, Kyle RA: Heavy chain diseases. In Wiernik PH, Canellos GP, Dutcher JP, Kyle RA (eds): Neoplastic Diseases of the Blood, 3rd ed, p 613. New York, Churchill Livingston, 1996
8. Gertz MA, Kyle RA: Primary systemic amyloidosis—a diagnostic primer. Mayo Clin Proc 64:1505, 1989
9. Kyle RA: Monoclonal gammopathy of undetermined significance. Blood Rev 8:135, 1994
10. Briere RO, Mull JD: Electrophoresis of serum protein with cellulose acetate: A method for quantitation. Am J Clin Pathol 42:547, 1964
11. Ritchie RF, Smith R: Immunofixation. I. General principles and application to agarose gel electrophoresis. Clin Chem 22:497, 1976
12. Ritchie RF, Smith R: Immunofixation. III. Application to the study of monoclonal proteins. Clin Chem 22:1982, 1976
13. Whicher JT, Calvin J, Riches P, Warren C: The laboratory investigation of paraproteinemia. Ann Clin Biochem 24:119, 1987
14. Keren DF, Warren JS, Lowe JB: Strategy to diagnose monoclonal gammopathies in serum, high-resolution electrophoresis, immunofixation and κ/λ quantification. Clin Chem 34:2196, 1988
15. Solomon A: Clinical implications of monoclonal light chains. Semin Oncol 13:341, 1986
16. Sanders PW: Pathogenesis and treatment of myeloma kidney. J Lab Clin Med 124:484, 1994
17. Bloch KJ, Maki DG: Hyperviscosity syndromes associated with immunoglobulin abnormalities. Semin Hematol 10:113, 1973

CHAPTER 33

Lymphocytic Leukemia and Lymphoma

J. Patrick Reed

Objectives

Upon completion of the chapter, the reader will be able to:

1. Describe the principal differences between lymphoma and leukemia
2. Identify commonly used lymphocyte markers that are used in the classification of leukemias and lymphomas
3. Distinguish between Hodgkin's disease and non-Hodgkin's lymphoma
4. Describe the criteria used in the diagnosis of Hodgkin's disease, including the Reed-Sternberg cell
5. List the four subtypes of Hodgkin's disease used in the Rye classification system
6. Name three classification systems for the identification of non-Hodgkin's lymphoma
7. Describe the subtypes of lymphoma identified by the working formulation of the NCI
8. Identify a form of cutaneous T-cell lymphoma
9. Identify the major characteristics of the three forms of leukemia classified as chronic lymphoproliferative leukemic disorders
10. Characterize the major findings in acute lymphocytic leukemia using the FAB system and immunological system of identification

INTRODUCTION

The cells of the immune system are subject to the same neoplastic potential as other cells of the body. Neoplastic diseases of the immune system, known as lymphoproliferative diseases, are a set of disorders in which a clone of cells has undergone malignant transformation and expansion. Typically, the cells in the clone are arrested at a particular maturational or activation stage, and the accumulation of malignant cells, most frequently lymphocytes, expresses common lymphocyte markers. This phenomenon is known as maturational arrest. The neoplastic lymphocytes maintain most, if not all, of the biological properties of normal lymphocytes in addition to malignant properties, such as tumor formation, invasiveness, and metastatic capability. The biological properties of malignant lymphocytes are exceedingly useful for the diagnosis and classification of lymphoproliferative diseases. For example, B-cell neoplasms usually express B-cell markers, such as HLA-DR and surface immunoglobulin, and home to B-cell domains in lymphoid organs.

Lymphoproliferative diseases are subdivided into two categories of malignancies: leukemia and lymphoma. Lymphomas arise from lymph node cells and are further categorized into Hodgkin's and non-Hodgkin's lymphoma based on cell characteristics, prognosis, and treatment response. In the leukemias, cells from the bone marrow circulate in the peripheral blood. There is, however, overlap between lymphoma and leukemia. Occasionally, lymphomas may develop a leukemic phase, and lymphocytic leukemias frequently have lymph node manifestations.

LYMPHOCYTE MARKERS AND CELL IDENTIFICATION

Lymphocyte marker analysis is used in conjunction with morphologic observations to diagnose lymphoid malignancy; in some cases, marker analysis is the primary tool used to identify specific malignancies. The multiparametric analysis uses cytochemical and immunological methods to phenotype the malignant lymphoid cells. Specific disease diagnosis and subsequent therapy depend on such analysis.[1] Because malignant cells express markers that correspond to those of normal cells, some insight into the maturation state of the malignant cell is obtained by the marker study (Fig. 33-1; refer to Chapter 2 for a discussion of lymphocyte markers.) Identification of the cell type and characterization of the maturation stage are essential components of the diagnosis of lymphoproliferative diseases because the prognosis and therapeutic response significantly depend on the subpopulation of malignant lymphoid cells involved.

Cluster of differentiation (CD) analysis can be determined by a variety of methods, but flow cytometry methods are rapidly becoming the norm because they are rapid, specific, and sensitive.[2] In these procedures, cells are mixed with reagents containing monoclonal antibodies (MAb) to specific cell surface markers that are labeled with a fluorescent chromophore. Cells are then passed single file through a laser optical detection system, in which the size, granularity, and specific marker fluorescence intensity are evaluated by the instrument and the data and statistics of the cell populations are available for further calculation. Subpopulations within the sample can be analyzed individually using electronic "gating" to select the desired cells.[3] See

Tables 33-1 and 33-2 for CD profiles of lymphocytic cells.

CD10, also called the common acute lymphoblastic leukemia associated antigen (CALLA), was originally defined by an antibody produced by rabbits that were immunized with non-T, non-B lymphoblastic leukemic cells. CALLA is a 100 kDa glycoprotein[4,5] that is associated with approximately 75% of non-T, non-B acute lymphoblastic leukemias (ALL), 40% of lymphoblastic lymphomas, and some follicular lymphoma cells.[6-8] A small percentage of bone marrow cells also express CALLA and are presumed to be lymphopoietic precursor cells.[9]

Immunoglobulin (Ig) is one of the most specific markers for B-cell malignancy. The Ig expressed in or on malignant B cells corresponds to the maturational stage.[10] Thus, a B-cell neoplasm with small resting B-cell morphology expresses surface immunoglobulin with little or no cytoplasmic immunoglobulin, whereas malignant plasma cells contain cytoplasmic immunoglobulin without expressing surface immunoglobulin. Between these two extremes are neoplasms that are arrested at different stages of maturation, and the cells express varying amounts of surface and/or cytoplasmic immunoglobulin. Furthermore, because the clonal expansion of a single transformed B cell is inherent in the malignant process, light-chain expression is restricted and is a strong indicator of malignancy. Neoplastic B-cell proliferation can be readily distinguished from a normal polyclonal B-cell proliferation with confidence. The B cells in the latter condition express the normal ratio of light chains, whereas in malignant conditions the B cells have restricted light-chain expression (i.e., either kappa or lambda light chain) and a subsequent altered light chain ratio.

Terminal deoxynucleotidyl transferase (TdT) is a nuclear enzyme that catalyzes the addition of deoxynucleotide triphosphate to the 3'-hydroxyl end of oligonucleotides and polydeoxynucleotides without template instruction.[11] TdT is present in thymocytes and bone marrow cells (<5%) but is absent from mature lymphocytes.[12] TdT is identified in all cases of ALL except for B-ALL and Burkitt's lymphoma. Frequently, TdT-positive leukemic cells appear during the blast crisis of chronic myelogenic leukemia. TdT-positive cells

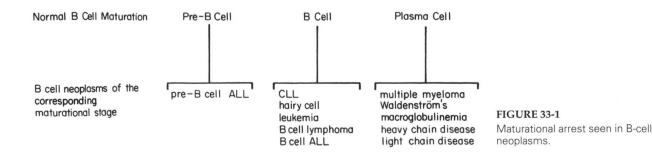

FIGURE 33-1
Maturational arrest seen in B-cell neoplasms.

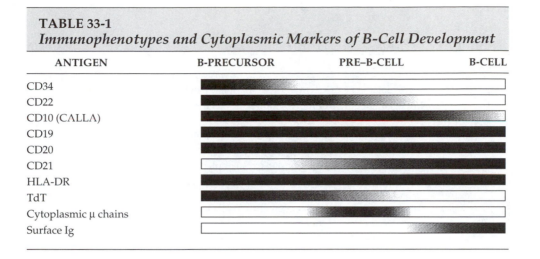

TABLE 33-1
Immunophenotypes and Cytoplasmic Markers of B-Cell Development

ANTIGEN	B-PRECURSOR	PRE–B-CELL	B-CELL
CD34			
CD22			
CD10 (CALLA)			
CD19			
CD20			
CD21			
HLA-DR			
TdT			
Cytoplasmic μ chains			
Surface Ig			

during blast crisis are more likely to respond to combination chemotherapy consisting of vincristine and prednisone than TdT-negative cells.[13] TdT is also observed in T-lymphoblastic lymphoma.[6]

Expression of functional receptors by T or B cells (i.e., T-cell antigen receptor heterodimer and B-cell surface immunoglobulin) requires sequential gene arrangement during cell maturation. Study of clonal rearrangement of these genes using polymerase chain reaction (PCR) methods is a sensitive tool that can be used to identify and characterize lymphoid malignancies.[14,15]

LYMPHOMA

Lymphoma is used to describe a malignant disease that arises from cells of the lymphatic system and is manifest primarily in the lymph nodes. Lymphadenopathy is a common finding. Spread of the disease is predominantly from one lymph node to another; lymphoma cells are generally not seen in the peripheral blood and bone marrow until late in the disease.

Lymphomas are divided into two major types: Hodgkin's disease or Hodgkin's lymphoma (HD) and non-Hodgkin's lymphoma (NHL). The type of lymphoma is based on lymph-node biopsy examination. The two forms of the disease are distinguished by the presence of the Reed-Sternberg cell in the lymph nodes of Hodgkin's disease patients. This cell is identified by its morphology (a large cell with bilobed nucleus containing prominent nucleoli) and positive reaction for CD30. In HD the cell-infiltration patterns within the lymph nodes are variable, whereas in NHL they are more uniform. NHL often appears in several noncontiguous nodes at the time of diagnosis and spreads to nonlymphatic tissue more readily than does HD. There is a different response to therapeutic treatment: HD responds well to radiation and standard chemotherapy and has a low relapse rate, and NHL is generally resis-

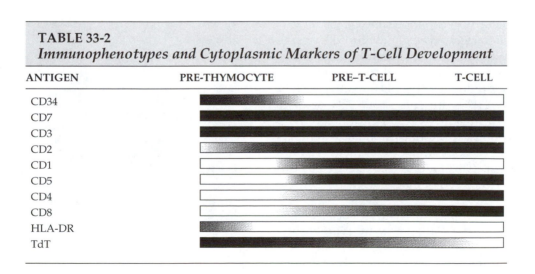

TABLE 33-2
Immunophenotypes and Cytoplasmic Markers of T-Cell Development

ANTIGEN	PRE-THYMOCYTE	PRE–T-CELL	T-CELL
CD34			
CD7			
CD3			
CD2			
CD1			
CD5			
CD4			
CD8			
HLA-DR			
TdT			

TABLE 33-3
Ann Arbor Staging System for HD and NHL[16]

STAGE	CRITERIA
I	Involvement of single lymph node *or* a single extralymphatic site (I_e)
II	Involvement of two or more lymph nodes on the same side of the diaphragm *or* involvement of a contiguous extralymphatic site (II_e)
III	Involvement of nodes on both sides of the diaphragm
	III_s indicates splenic involvement
	III_{sc} indicates both splenic and extralymphatic site involvement
IV	Diffuse disease involving nodes and extralymphatic organs on both sides of the diaphragm

Any stage can be given the additional suffix A or B. A indicates the presence of no other symptoms. B indicates the presence of fever, night sweats, or weight loss.

tant or refractory to most forms of therapy and has a higher relapse rate. In addition to nodal cell infiltration, lymphomas are staged using the Ann Arbor Staging System, which characterizes the severity of the spread of the disease.[16] See Table 33-3 for details of the staging criteria.

Hodgkin's Disease

The hallmark of HD is the Reed-Sternberg cell, a large cell with a bilobate nucleus with prominent nucleoli, often resembling owl eyes (Fig. 33-2). Although these cells are always found in the lymph nodes of HD patients, the origin of these neoplastic cells remains uncertain. Currently, Hodgkin's lymphoma is classified by the Rye classification scheme, which uses histological observations of the lymph node to subdivide the disease into four major subtypes.[17,18] The four subtypes are lymphocyte predominant, nodular sclerosing, mixed cellularity, and lymphocyte depletion.[19] Lymphocyte-predominant HD is characterized by a diffuse infiltrate of small, mature lymphocytes. Although uncommon (about 5% of cases), it has a good prognosis and is seen predominantly in young males. Nodular sclerosing HD is the most common subtype (about 65% of cases) and is characterized by nodal fibrosis that subdivides the lymph node into nodules containing normal lymphocytes, macrophages, and granulocytes. The lymphocytes are predominantly CD4-positive T cells. Mixed-cellularity HD represents about 25% of cases and is associated with a mixed-cell infiltration of lymphocytes, neutrophils, eosinophils, and large numbers of Reed-Sternberg cells. Lymphocyte-depleted HD has a relatively poor prognosis and is characterized by diffuse fibrosis and decreased numbers of lymphocytes in the lymph node.

A strong host immune response is associated with a favorable prognosis. Patients with lymphocyte-predominant subtype are generally younger and have limited disease at the time of diagnosis. They have a more favorable prognosis when compared with patients with the lymphocyte-depleted subtype, who tend to be associated with widespread disease and a poor prognosis. The cell-mediated immune response is frequently compromised in patients with Hodgkin's disease. Skin anergy is a common finding.[20]

Non-Hodgkin's Lymphoma

Non-Hodgkin's lymphoma is a heterogeneous group of neoplasms whose exact classification has frustrated investigators and clinicians alike. In the 1960s the histopathologic classification proposed by Rappaport was widely accepted to diagnose this malignancy.[21] As the modern concept of the immune system emerged, new classifications were proposed that combine lymphocyte morphology, lymph node architecture, and immune system physiology. The Lukes-Collins classification system incorporated both the histology of the node and the immunological phenotype of the predominant infiltrating cell.[22] In 1982, a Working Formu-

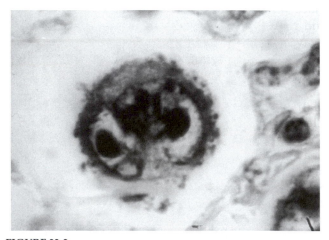

FIGURE 33-2
Reed-Sternberg cell in Hodgkin's disease (×1000). (Courtesy of BH Tindle, MD.)

lation was proposed as a result of the study led by the National Cancer Institute.[6] In this formulation the prognosis as determined by survival is correlated with the morphology and immunology of the tumors. Recently, an additional system based on histologic, immunologic, and genetic evaluation of the tumor cells has been proposed by a group of American and European hematopathologists.[23] Three major categories recognized in this revised European-American classification are B-cell neoplasms, T-cell neoplasms, and Hodgkin's disease. Although clinicians use aspects of different classification systems, the Working Formulation proposed by the NCI is the classification system used most frequently and is discussed in detail in this chapter.[6] Three major groups are identified: low grade, intermediate grade, and high grade. Each is associated with a favorable, intermediate, and unfavorable prognosis, respectively.

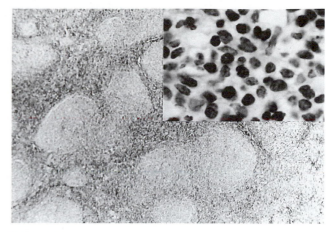

FIGURE 33-3
Follicular lymphoma with predominantly small, cleaved cells (low grade, ×250). *Insert*: Small, cleaved lymphocytes (×1000). (Courtesy of BH Tindle, MD.)

LOW-GRADE LYMPHOMA

Malignant Lymphoma: Small Lymphocytic Cell

In general, small lymphocytic (SL) malignant lymphoma has a diffuse lymph node architecture. The cells are round and the size varies from small to medium. Mitotic activity is scant or absent. The presence of plasmacytoid lymphocytes may be associated with a monoclonal gammopathy. Chronic lymphocytic leukemia may present with a similar morphology and must be ruled out. This is mainly a B-cell neoplasm, with the malignant cells expressing surface immunoglobulin, Fc receptors, complement receptors, and MHC Class II molecules.

Malignant Lymphoma: Follicular, Predominantly Small Cleaved Cells

In follicular, predominantly small cleaved cell (FSC) lymphoma, the involved lymph node is usually replaced by follicles that are relatively uniform in size and shape. The cells are predominantly small with a cleaved nucleus (indentation of the nuclear membrane) (Fig. 33-3). The neoplastic B cells express surface immunoglobulin, CALLA, and MHC Class II molecules.

Malignant Lymphoma: Follicular, Mixed Small Cleaved, and Large Cells

The lymph node architecture in follicular, mixed small cleaved and large cell (FM) lymphoma is similar to that in FSC, except that the cells in the follicles are a mixture of small cleaved and large cells. The small cleaved cells are surface immunoglobulin positive, whereas the large cells tend to be surface immunoglobulin negative but may be cytoplasmic immunoglobulin positive. Both small cleaved cells and large cells are positive for MHC Class II molecules and CALLA.

INTERMEDIATE-GRADE LYMPHOMA

Malignant Lymphoma: Follicular, Predominantly Large Cells

The lymph node architecture in follicular, predominantly large cell (FL) lymphoma is similar to that in FM; however, the predominant cells are large and noncleaved. There are numerous mitotic figures. Most often the neoplastic cells express surface immunoglobulin, MHC Class II molecules, and CALLA.

Malignant Lymphoma: Diffuse, Small Cleaved Cells, and Diffuse, Mixed Small and Large Cells

Diffuse, small cleaved cells (DSC) and diffuse, mixed small and large cells (DM) lymphoma represent diffuse counterparts of FSC and FM, respectively. The neoplastic cells express surface immunoglobulin and MHC Class II molecules. However, unlike their follicular counterparts, the cells do not usually express CALLA.

Malignant Lymphoma: Diffuse, Large Cells

In diffuse, large cell lymphoma (DL) the normal lymph node architecture is entirely replaced by a diffuse proliferation of malignant cells (Fig. 33-4). The cell population may be composed of large cleaved and noncleaved cells. The large cleaved cells may have minimal cytoplasm and inconspicuous nucleoli, whereas large noncleaved cells possess a rim of cytoplasm and one or more prominent nucleoli. The malignant cells of the majority of cases express surface immunoglobulin and MHC Class II molecules.

HIGH-GRADE LYMPHOMA

Malignant Lymphoma: Large-Cell, Immunoblastic

Large-cell immunoblastic lymphoma (IBL) is divided into three categories: plasmacytoid, clear cell, and poly-

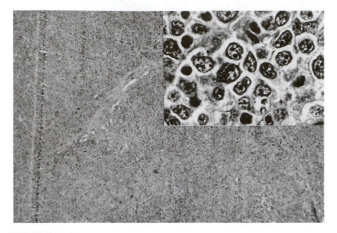

FIGURE 33-4
Diffuse lymphoma with large noncleaved cells (intermediate grade, ×250). *Insert*: Large cleaved lymphocytes (×1000). (Courtesy of BH Tindle, MD.)

morphous immunoblastic lymphoma. The cells of the plasmacytoid variant possess eccentric nuclei with abundant cytoplasmic immunoglobulin. The clear-cell type and polymorphous variant appear to be of T-cell lineage.

Malignant Lymphoma: Lymphoblastic

In lymphoblastic lymphoma (LBL), the lymph node is typically associated with a diffuse architecture pattern. A "starry-sky" pattern caused by evenly distributed macrophages may be prominent. The neoplastic cells may have convoluted nuclei with scant cytoplasm. There are invariably numerous mitotic figures. The neoplastic cells are of T-cell lineage based on their ability to rosette sheep red blood cells and to be labeled with CD2 monoclonal antibodies. Approximately one third of childhood and 5% of adult non-Hodgkin's lymphomas are identified as LBL. The disease is more prevalent in males and often is associated with a mediastinal mass. In some cases, the disease may evolve into a leukemic phase that is frequently indistinguishable from T-cell acute lymphoblastic leukemia.

Malignant Lymphoma: Small Noncleaved Cell

Small noncleaved cell (SNC) malignant lymphoma includes Burkitt's lymphoma and other high-grade undifferentiated non-Burkitt's lymphomas. Most cases of Burkitt's lymphoma seen in patients in Africa are associated with Epstein-Barr virus (EBV) infection; however, most Burkitt's lymphoma cases seen in the United States are not associated with EBV and may reflect a different etiology. Cells of Burkitt's lymphoma associated with EBV express Fc receptors, receptor for complement (C3b), and receptors for Epstein-Barr virus. Conversely, none of the preceding markers is expressed by the malignant cells of Burkitt's lymphoma seen in patients in the United States. The Burkitt's lymphoma

cells usually do not express CALLA, although some express surface IgM, suggesting some degree of differentiation.

Cutaneous T-Cell Lymphoma

Cutaneous T-cell lymphoma is a rare form of lymphoma, also called mycosis fungoides. The leukemic phase is referred to as Sézary cell leukemia. The prominent clinical feature of this disease is the skin lesion that varies from limited plaques to generalized plaques, tumors, and generalized erythroderma. In the skin the malignant cells are referred to as mycosis fungoides cells; in the peripheral blood they are called Sézary cells. Both cell types form rosettes with sheep red blood cells and are CD2 positive. In most reported cases the malignant T cells are CD4 positive and are able to help B-cells synthesize antibodies in vitro.[24-26]

LEUKEMIA

In general the diagnosis of leukemia is made from bone marrow analysis of the expanded neoplastic cell. Leukemia is usually classified as chronic or acute in nature. Chronic leukemias present as an indolent disease, with differentiated cells, and often resist therapy. Acute leukemias present with a rapid onset, minimal differentiation of immature forms, and a higher response rate to therapy. Specific lymphocytic leukemias are classified as part of chronic lymphoproliferative leukemic disorders (CLLD) or acute lymphocytic leukemias.

Chronic Lymphoproliferative Leukemic Disorders

CLLD are a diverse group of diseases that involve B cells nearly 99% of the time. Specific diseases include chronic lymphocytic leukemia (CLL), prolymphocytic leukemia (PPL), and hairy cell leukemia (HCL).

CHRONIC LYMPHOCYTIC LEUKEMIA

Classical chronic lymphocytic leukemia (CLL) is a disease of clonal expansion of B cells that involves the proliferation and accumulation of these cells in the peripheral blood, bone marrow, spleen, lymph nodes, and other organs. It is rarely seen in patients less than 45 years old and has a male predominance of 2:1. Patients usually present with an elevated peripheral white blood cell count, an absolute lymphocyte count of over $10 \times 10^9/L$, and bone marrow alterations that include increased lymphocyte populations and hypercellularity. The malignant B cells appear as small mature lymphocytes (Fig. 33-5). They express weak surface immunoglobulin that is invariably restricted to one light

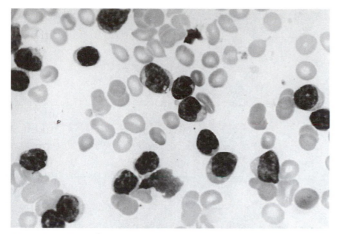

FIGURE 33-5
Chronic lymphocytic leukemia (CLL) (peripheral blood, ×1000). (Courtesy of BH Tindle, MD.)

chain, either kappa or lambda. Complement receptors, Fc receptors, and MHC Class II molecules are also expressed by the malignant cells. Less than 5% of CLL are reported to be of the T-cell type, commonly involving the skin and central nervous system.[27,28]

PROLYMPHOCYTIC LEUKEMIA

Prolymphocytic leukemia (PLL) is a variant of CLL in which many cells are relatively large lymphoid cells with a round to oval nucleus containing coarse nuclear chromatin and one to two nucleoli. Absolute lymphocyte counts in the blood are usually very high, with many patients presenting with values over 100×10^9/L. Immunologic deficiencies, such as low levels of immunoglobulins, are frequently found. PLL is often refractory to therapy and represents a poor prognosis.[29,30]

HAIRY CELL LEUKEMIA

Hairy cell leukemia (HCL), previously referred to as leukemic reticuloendotheliosis, is a rare, insidious disease characterized by infiltration of bone marrow and spleen by leukemic cells without peripheral lymphadenopathy. The disease occurs in patients from 20 to over 80 years of age, with a male predominance of 4:1. The majority of patients initially present with pancytopenia (granulocytopenia, thrombocytopenia, and anemia), but with mild lymphocytosis. The malignant cells usually have irregular or "hairy" cytoplasmic projections (hairy cells).[31] Monoclonal surface immunoglobulin with restricted light chain is frequently detected on the surface of hairy cells. Therefore, hairy cell leukemia is most consistent with a B-cell malignancy.[32] These cells also contain cytoplasmic tartrate-resistant acid phosphatase (TRAP), which is useful in the laboratory identification of hairy cells.[33] Splenectomy and

the use of alpha-interferon have been proven effective therapy for this disease.

Acute Lymphocytic Leukemia

Acute lymphocytic leukemia (ALL), also called acute lymphoblastic leukemia, is characterized by the presence of increased blast cells in the bone marrow that frequently disseminate to the peripheral blood. Although their rate of proliferation is often slower than that of normal blast cells in the bone marrow, the leukemic blast cells maintain their ability to divide for a long period of time. There is little maturational development seen in these cells (Fig. 33-6). Large numbers of these cells accumulate and infiltrate the spleen, liver, meninges, testes, kidney, and skin, disrupting the function of these organs.[34]

Cases of ALL are most often seen in children from ages 2 to 14 and represent the form of leukemia affecting the majority of patients in this age group. Advances in therapy over the last 20 years have produced a success rate of cure approaching 60% to 70%, making childhood ALL the most treatable leukemia of all. Relatively few cases of ALL are seen in adults, and when it does affect this older population, the response to therapy is reduced and the prognosis is poor.[35]

ALL consists of a heterogeneous group of diseases that is divided into three major types by the French-American-British (FAB) classification system—L1, L2, and L3—which are defined by cytologic criteria that consider cell size, heterogeneity, and morphological features of the cells.[36,37] L1 presents with predominantly small blasts that are generally uniform in size, with finely distributed chromatin in a regularly shaped nucleus. L2 is similar to L1, but there is striking heterogeneity in cell size, with considerable nuclear variations, which include clefting and prominent nucleoli.

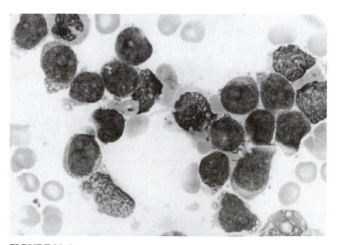

FIGURE 33-6
T-cell acute lymphocytic leukemia (ALL) (bone marrow, ×1000). (Courtesy of BH Tindle, MD.)

L3 is a B-cell leukemic phase of Burkitt's lymphoma in which the blasts express a basophilic cytoplasm and multiple vacuoles (Fig. 33-7).

More recently, the classification of ALL using immunological markers has gained preeminence with three major divisions recognized: T-cell ALL, B-cell ALL, and non-T, non-B ALL.[38] The non-T, non-B ALL is further classified into common ALL (CALL), which is CALLA positive, and "null-cell" ALL, which is CALLA negative. The preceding grouping predicts the prognosis in terms of survival; thus, CALL has the most favorable prognosis, followed by null-cell ALL, T-cell ALL, and B-cell ALL. The markers frequently used in a clinical laboratory to type ALLs are listed in Table 33-4.

T-CELL ALL

T-cell ALL represents approximately 15% to 25% of all cases. The characteristic clinical features include a high blast cell count, predominance in males over the age of 20, and the presence of a mediastinal mass. The leukemic cells form rosettes with sheep red blood cells, are CD2 positive, lack MHC Class II molecules, and contain TdT. Approximately 10% to 25% of T-cell ALL cases express CALLA.

B-CELL ALL

B-cell ALL represents less than 3% of ALL cases. B-cell ALL in children is probably a leukemic phase of Burkitt's lymphoma. The leukemic cells express surface immunoglobulin, Fc receptor, and complement receptors (C3d and C3b), indicating that the malignant cells derive from the follicular center. Pre–B-cell ALL is a unique malignancy in which the neoplastic B cells are arrested at the maturational stage in which only the heavy-chain gene rearrangement has occurred. Therefore, the cells are able to synthesize only IgM heavy chain (μ chain) but not a light chain. These malignant

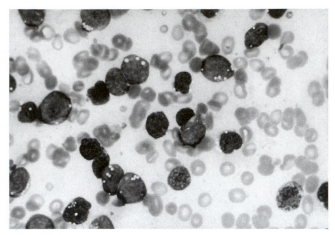

FIGURE 33-7
Acute lymphocytic leukemia, type L3 by FAB (Burkitt's type) (bone marrow, ×650). (Courtesy of BH Tindle, MD.)

cells are identified by the presence of cytoplasmic μ chains. They also express CALLA, TdT, and MHC Class II molecules.

NON-T, NON-B ALL

Non-T, non-B ALL does not express any conventional T- or B-cell markers. Based on the expression of CALLA, these are divided into two groups: Common ALL (CALL) is CALLA positive, whereas null-cell ALL is CALLA negative. However, both groups express MHC Class II molecules, Fc receptor, and nuclear TdT. Approximately 70% of ALL cases are CALL. The clinical features of CALL include a younger patient population and markedly elevated leukocyte count. The disease is not usually associated with mediastinal mass, lymphadenopathy, or hepatosplenomegaly. Null-cell ALL is CALLA negative, with a prognosis next to that of CALL.

TABLE 33-4
Cell Markers Frequently Used for ALL Typing

	HLA-DR	CALLA	IgGR	Cμ	SIg	TdT	CD2
Common ALL	+	+	+	−	−	+	−
Null ALL	+	−	+	−	−	+	−
Pre–B-cell ALL	+	+	+	+	−	+	−
B-cell ALL	+	+	+	−	+	−	−
T-cell ALL	−	+/−	−	−	−	+	+/−

CALLA, Common acute lymphoblastic leukemia associated antigen; IgGR, Receptor for IgG; Cμ, Cytoplasmic IgM heavy chain; SIg, Surface immunoglobulin; TdT, Terminal deoxynucleotidyl transferase; CD2, Sheep red blood cell receptor.

Case Studies

(All case studies are courtesy of B. MacPherson, MD.)

Case 1

A 42-year-old female was seen by her physician for complaints of a non-painful swelling under her left armpit. She denied having had weight loss, night sweats, or other swellings. Upon examining the patient, the physician palpated and identified a firm nodular mass in the left axilla and requested a biopsy. A single lymph node measuring 2.5 × 1.0 × 1.0 cm was removed and sent to the laboratory for further analysis.

Case 1 Study Questions

1. Microscopic analysis of the lymph node showed nodules containing primarily small, cleaved follicular center cells. Flow-cytometric analysis of these cells showed the following reactions: CD19+, CD20+, CD22+, HLA-DR+. Are these T cells or B cells?

2. The kappa/lambda ratio was 1:2.5 with fluorescence intensity brighter for the lambda-positive cells. Is this a normal ratio?

3. CD10 was expressed on a majority of the cells as well. What is the other name for this cell marker?

4. With what diagnosis are the above observations consistent?

Case 2

A 3-year-old boy was brought to his pediatrician by his mother because he had been complaining of pain in his knees and elbows, and a few bruises developed on his arms and legs. His mother stated that he was not his usual energetic self and appeared rather listless, something she had noticed for several weeks. Upon examining the boy, the physician noticed a pallor of the skin and slight splenomegaly. He ordered a complete blood count (CBC), which showed the following: Hb 6.6 g/dL, Hct 21.1 L/L (low values), WBC count 5.1 × 10⁹/L (normal value), and platelet count 28 × 10⁹/L (low value). The differential count of the peripheral blood WBCs showed that 25% of the WBC cells were undifferentiated cells called *blasts*. A bone marrow aspirate was ordered that showed a hypercellular marrow with an M/E ratio of 1:3, and a predom-

inant cell population of blasts (67% of all marrow cells) displaying a variation in size and irregular nuclear contours with fine nuclear chromatin and prominent nucleoli. The cells were Sudan black and non-specific esterase negative, and TdT positive. Immunologic analysis using a flow cytometer showed these cells to be CD10 (CALLA)+, CD34+, CD19+, CD 38+, and HLA-DR+. Neither lambda nor kappa light chains were expressed in these cells.

Case 2 Study Questions

1. Which CBC results show altered values? What do they indicate?

2. What is a normal M/E ratio in bone marrow? What percent of bone marrow cells do blasts comprise?

3. Sudan black and non-specific esterase stains are positive for which blood cell type?

4. What cells have the pattern of markers shown in the flow cytometer analysis on this patient?

5. What is the diagnosis?

Case 3

A 64-year-old male with several "swellings" in his neck was evaluated by his physician. He had been in good health for many years, living with his wife in a condominium unit in a resort town where they enjoyed social and outdoor activities. On physical exam he had slight splenomegaly and four non-painful enlarged lymph nodes in his neck. He did not appear anemic, and this was confirmed by laboratory tests. His Hb was 16.6 g/dL, Hct 47.2 L/L, WBC count 87.7 × 10⁹/L, and platelet count 264 × 10⁹/L. Differential WBC identification showed 78% mature lymphocytes. Analysis of his bone marrow showed slight hypercellularity, an M/E ratio of 2:1, and a few focal lymphoid aggregates, composed mainly of small lymphocytes with round or mildly irregular nuclei. Thirty-nine percent of the marrow cells were of this type. Only 1% of the bone marrow cells were blasts. The lymphocytes taken for analysis were CD19+, CD20+, and HLA-DR+, expressing lambda light chains. CD10 (CALLA) was negative.

Case 3 Study Questions

1. What diagnosis is consistent with the above history and data?

2. Are the marrow cells of T- or B-cell type?

Case 4

A 22-year-old female college student was seen in the student health clinic, complaining of an unexplained weight loss of 20 pounds and the occurrence of night sweats that disturbed her sleep. The physician noted several enlarged axillary and cervical lymph nodes. A hilar mass was observed on a CT scan. Biopsy of the mass showed a cell population comprised predominantly of small lymphocytes mixed with a significant number of larger cells with clear cytoplasm, a polyploid nuclear configuration, and small nucleoli, strongly suggestive of Reed-Sternberg cells. These cells showed no immunoreactivity with either B- or T-cell antibodies. Immunological studies showed the small lymphocytes to be CD2+, CD3+ CD5+ with an excess of CD4+ cells (CD4+ = 89%, CD8+ = 7%).

Case 4 Study Questions

1. On the basis of the information provided, what is the probable diagnosis?

2. What lymphocyte type do the immunological studies show?

References

1. Coon JS, Landay AL, Weinstein RS: Biology of disease—advances in flow cytometry for diagnostic pathology. Lab Invest 57:453, 1987
2. Keren DF: History and evolution of surface marker assays. In Keren DF, Hanson CA, Hurtubise PE (ed). Flow Cytometry and Clinical Diagnosis, p 1. Chicago, IL, ASCP Press, 1994
3. Kipps TJ, Meisenholder G, Robbins BA: New developments in flow cytometric analysis of lymphocyte markers. Clin Lab Med 12:237, 1992
4. Greaves MF, Brown G, Rapson NT, et al: Antisera to acute lymphoblastic leukemia cells. Clin Immunol Immunopathol 4:67, 1975
5. Foon KA, Todd RF: Review: Immunologic classification of leukemia and lymphoma. Blood 68:1, 1986
6. The non-Hodgkin's Lymphoma Pathologic Classification Project: National Cancer Institute sponsored study of classification of non-Hodgkin's lymphomas: Summary and description of a working formulation for clinical usage. Cancer 49:2112, 1982
7. Hoffman-Fizer G, Knapp W, Thierfelder S: Anatomical distribution of CALL antigen-expressing cells in normal tissue and in lymphoma. Leuk Res 6:761, 1982
8. Stein H, Gerdes J, Lemke H, et al: The normal and malignant germinal center. Clin Haematol 11:531, 1982
9. Greaves M, Delia D, Janossy G, et al: Acute lymphoblastic leukemia associated antigen. IV Expression on nonleukemic lymphoid cells. Leuk Res 4:15, 1980
10. Korsmeyer S, Hieter P, Ravetch J, et al: Developmental hierarchy of immunoglobulin gene rearrangements in leukemic pre-B cells. Proc Natl Acad Sci USA 78:7096, 1981
11. Bollum FJ: Terminal deoxynucleotidyl transferase. In Boyer PD (ed): The Enzyme, Vol 10, p 145. Orlando, FL, Academic Press, 1974
12. Greenwood MF, Coleman MS, Hutton JJ, et al: Terminal deoxynucleotidyl transferase distribution in neoplastic and hematopoietic cells. J Clin Invest 59:889, 1977
13. Marks SM, Baltimore D, McCaffrey R: Terminal transferase as a prediction of initial responsiveness to vincristine and prednisone in blastic chronic myelogenous leukemia. N Engl J Med 298:812, 1978
14. Korsmeyer S, Arnold A, Bakhshi A, et al: Immunoglobulin gene rearrangement and cell surface antigen expression in acute lymphocytic leukemias of T-cell and B-cell precursor origins. J Clin Invest 71:301, 1983
15. Tawa A, Hozumi N, Minden M, et al: Rearrangements of the T-cell receptor beta chain gene in non-T-cell, non-B-cell acute lymphoblastic leukemia of childhood. N Engl J Med 313:1033, 1985
16. Carbone P, Kaplan HS, Mushoff K, et al: Report of the Committee on Hodgkin's Disease Staging Classification. Cancer Res 31:1707, 1971
17. Lukes RL, Butler JJ, Hicks EB: Natural history of Hodgkin's disease as related to its pathologic picture. Cancer 19:317, 1966
18. Lukes RL, Craver LF, Hall TC, et al: Report of the nomenclature committee. Cancer Res 26:1311, 1966
19. Thomas MG: Hodgkin's disease. In Jaffe ES (ed): Surgical Pathology of the Lymph Nodes and Related Organs, p 86. Philadelphia, WB Saunders, 1985
20. Kaplan HS: Review: Hodgkin's disease: Biology, treatment, and prognosis. Blood 57:813, 1981
21. Rappaport H: Tumors of the hematopoietic system. In Atlas of Tumor Pathology, Section 3, Fascicle 8. Washington, DC, US Armed Forces Institute of Pathology, 1966
22. Lukes RL, Collins R: Immunologic characterization of human malignant lymphomas. Cancer 49:1488, 1974
23. Harris NL, Jaffe ES, Stein PM, et al: A revised European-American classification of lymphoid neoplasms: A proposal from the International Lymphoma Study Group. Blood 84:1361, 1994

24. Edelson RL: Cutaneous T-cell lymphoma: Mycosis fungoides, Sézary syndrome, and other variants. J Am Acad Dermatol 2:89, 1980

25. Harris TJ, Bhan AK, Murphy E, et al: Lymphomatoid papulosis and lymphomatoid granulomatosis: T-cell subset populations. Refined microscopic morphology and direct immunofluorescence observations. Clin Res 29:579, 1981

26. McMillan EM, Wasik R, Beeman K, et al: In situ immunologic phenotyping of mycosis fungoides. J Am Acad Dermatol 6:888, 1982

27. Van der Reigden HJ, Van der Gaag R, Pinkster J, et al: Chronic lymphocytic leukemia: Immunologic markers and functional properties of the leukemic cells. Cancer 50:2826, 1982

28. Huhn D, Theil E, Rodt H, et al: Subtype of T-cell chronic lymphocytic leukemia. Cancer 51:1434, 1983

29. Galton D, Goldman J, Wiltshaw E, et al: Prolymphocytic leukemia. Br J Haematol 27:7, 1974

30. Melo J, Catovsky D, Galton D: The relationship bewteen chronic lymphocytic leukemia and prolymphocytic leukemia. Br J Haematol 63:377, 1985

31. Golomb HM: Hairy cell leukemia: Lesson learned in twenty-five years. J Clin Oncol 1:652, 1983

32. Golomb HM, Davis S, Wilson C, et al: Surface immunoglobulin in hairy cells of 55 patients with hairy cell leukemia. Am J Hematol 12:397, 1982

33. Variakojis D, Vardiman JW, Golomb HM: Cytochemistry of hairy cells. Cancer 45:72, 1980

34. Shumacker HR, Garven DF, Triplett DA: Acute leukemia. In Introduction to Laboratory Hematology and Hematopathology, p 109. New York, Alan R Liss, 1984

35. Hoelzer D, Theil E, Loffler H, et al: Prognostic factors in a multicenter study for treatment of acute lymphoblastic leukemia in adults. Blood 711:123, 1988

36. Bennett JM, Catovsky D, Daniel MT, et al: Proposal for the classification of adult leukemia. Br J Haematol 33:451, 1976

37. Bennet JM, Catovosky D, Daniel MT, et al: The morphological classification of acute lymphoblastic leukemia: Concordance among observers and clinical correlations. Br J Haematol 47:553, 1981

38. Foon Ka, Gale RP, Todd RF: Recent advances in the immunologic classification of leukemia. Semin Hematol 23:257, 1986

Section E. Transplantation

CHAPTER 34

Transplantation Immunology

Catherine Sheehan

TYPES OF GRAFTS
GRAFT ACCEPTANCE AND REJECTION
CLINICAL MANIFESTATIONS
TISSUE TYPING
IMMUNOSUPPRESSION
TRANSPLANTATION
COMPLICATIONS OF TRANSPLANTATION

Objectives

Upon completion of the chapter, the reader will be able to:

1. Classify a graft as autologous, syngeneic, allogeneic, or xenogeneic
2. Compare and contrast hyperacute rejection, first-set rejection, and second-set rejection
3. Explain why ABO and HLA compatibility are important in clinical transplantation
4. Describe the cellular and humoral events that lead to graft rejection
5. Describe the tests used to phenotype the ABO blood group and HLA-A, HLA-B, HLA-D, and HLA-DR
6. State the general immunosuppressive effect of azathioprine, cyclophosphamide, corticosteroids, cyclosporin A, FK506, anti-lymphocyte serum, irradiation, and monoclonal antibodies
7. Explain the difference between allogeneic bone marrow, autologous bone marrrow, and peripheral blood stem cells

8. State in what general conditions bone marrow or peripheral blood stem cells are transplanted
9. List and explain the complications of transplantation
10. Compare and contrast acute and chronic graft-versus-host disease

TYPES OF GRAFTS

Transplantation is the transfer of cells, tissues, or organs from one site to another. The success of the transplantation is related to the degree of genetic similarity between the donor and the recipient. When a graft is identical or similar to the recipient, the likelihood of engraftment is best. When the graft is dissimilar, the recipient (host) immune system recognizes that it is not recipient tissue and responds to eliminate the donor (foreign) transplant. The type of graft, as defined by the relationship of the graft to the recipient, greatly influences the extent of the immune response.

An autograft is the transfer from one site to another within an individual. For instance, healthy skin from one location may be moved to a burned area. An isograft is a graft between genetically identical (syngeneic) individuals, such as would occur between monozygotic twins. In both autografts and isografts, the donor and recipient are genetically identical so that there is little, if any, rejection. The most common type of graft is the allograft, which is the transfer between two members of the same species. The degree of genetic difference between the two members determines the rate of rejection. Finally, xenografts are those between different species. Because the genetic differences are greatest in xenografts, the immune response is strongest, and this explains why xenografts have been unsuccessful to date.

GRAFT ACCEPTANCE AND REJECTION

When a graft is accepted, as can be demonstrated in an autologous skin graft, the processes of revascularization and healing lead to resolution of the repair in approximately 2 weeks. When a graft initiates an immune response, as seen in allogeneic skin graft transplantation, first-set rejection or second-set rejection can occur. The first time a graft is encountered and rejected, it is known as the primary graft rejection and is called first-set rejection. After initial revascularization of a skin graft, lymphocytes, monocytes, and other inflammatory cells enter the area and lead to decreased vascularization; thrombosis and necrosis follow. This rejection usually occurs within 10 to 14 days after transplantion. If a secondary immune response occurs (which could occur when the recipient receives a second graft from the same or a closely related donor), rejection is accelerated and occurs within 6 days. This is the second-set rejection. Specificity and memory are active in second-set graft rejection, as shown by the accelerated rate of rejection. Mechanisms of specific cellular immunity mediated by T lymphocytes are more important than specific humoral immunity or nonspecific immune responses to reject a graft.[1] The same types of rejection occur with other transplanted tissues, although the time lines may vary.

The immune system responds to antigens present in the donor graft that are not expressed by the recipient; when the antigenic differences are sufficient, the tissue is histoincompatible and will be rejected by the recipient. Those antigens that are expressed by the donor graft and lead to rejection are called transplantation antigens. Although numerous transplanation antigen systems are present, the most influential is the major histocompatibility complex (MHC); in humans, this is the HLA complex. (Refer to Chapter 5 for additional information about HLA.) The MHC molecules are required to stimulate the helper T (T_H) cells and the cytotoxic T (T_C) cells to initiate a strong response. If the MHC of the donor and recipient are identical and transplant rejection still occurs, it is caused by mismatched minor histocompatibility antigens that are detected by the recipient's immune system. The donor minor histocompatibility antigens are recognized in association with the recipient's MHC molecules.[1]

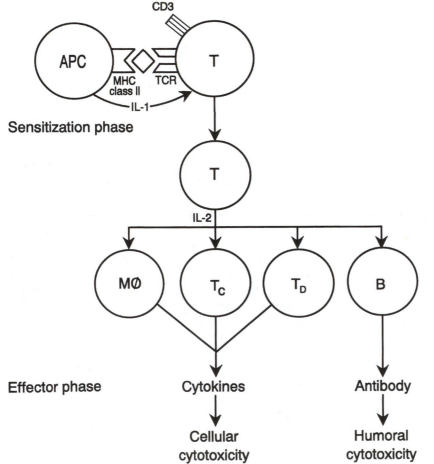

FIGURE 34-1

In the sensitization phase, the antigen-presenting cell (APC) presents the transplantation antigen (◇) to the T cell. The T cell becomes activated and, in turn, activates effector mechanisms. (1) Direct cellular cytotoxic mechanisms of cytotoxic T (T_C) cells, delayed hypersensitivity T (T_D) cells, and macrophages (M) and (2) humoral cytotoxic mechanisms of antibody-dependent cellular cytotoxicity (ADCC) and complement-dependent cytolysis.

Selected immune mechanisms that are activated to sensitize the recipient and then to reject the graft are shown in Figure 34-1. During the sensitization phase, the T-cell–mediated immune response expands the number of cells responding to the graft. After cellular proliferation, the cells perform their specific effector mechanisms, rejecting the graft and generating memory cells.

To begin the sensitization phase, an antigen-presenting cell (APC) will present transplantation antigens in association with MHC molecules to the T_H. Various APC (dendritic cells, passenger leukocytes, and Langerhans' cells) can present the donor alloantigens to the recipient's immune cells. Often this presentation takes place in a lymph node or the spleen. After antigen and other necessary signals stimulate the T_H cell, the T_H cell secretes cytokines (especially important are IL-2, IL-4, IL-5, and IL-6, interferon gamma, and tumor necrosis factor β [TNF β]) to activate T_C, B cells, and T cells involved in delayed hypersensitivity. The cellular infiltrate (predominantly T cells, macrophages, and natural killer [NK] cells) seen in graft rejection appears to be that seen in Type IV delayed hypersensitivity. T cells damage the graft by the action of TNF β and interferon gamma, while the activated macrophages release other toxic cytokines and may damage the graft via proteolytic enzymes. The T_C cells may directly cause membrane damage and may lyse the cells in the graft. B-cell proliferation and differentiation directed by T_H cells leads to antibody production, which can result in complement-dependent cytolysis and antibody-dependent cellular cytotoxicity. The immune response to graft cells is primarily cellular rather than humoral in nature.[1]

CLINICAL MANIFESTATIONS

Types of graft rejection are based on the time taken to reject the organ. A hyperacute reaction occurs within 24 hours of the transplantation. Acute rejection occurs within weeks of the transplantation, and chronic rejection occurs months to years after transplantation. The time varies based on the type of tissue transplanted and the level of immune stimulation and response.

Hyperacute rejection is humoral rejection caused by a pre-existing antibody to an antigen expressed by the graft. As shown in Figure 34-2, recipient antibody enters the graft, binds to graft antigen, and activates complement. Neutrophils infiltrate the area, and inflammation leads to clot formation that occludes capillaries, preventing vascularization. ABO antibodies and MHC Class I antibodies have been shown to cause hyperacute rejection. Alloimmunization can lead to alloantibody production in individuals who have received multiple transfusions, who have been pregnant, or who have been previously transplanted. This led to the recommendation that a crossmatch should be performed for solid organ transplantation to identify these preformed antibodies. In the crossmatch, the serum of the recipient is mixed with mononuclear cells of the donor, and evidence of cytotoxicity is monitored.[2]

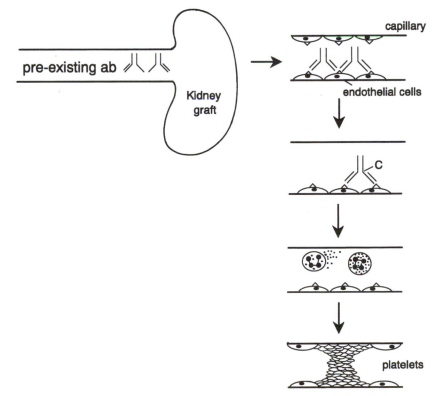

FIGURE 34-2
Pre-existing antibody enters the graft and binds to transplantation antigens. Complement (C) is activated by the local immune complexes. Biologically active complement fragments recruit neutrophils to the area. Proteolytic enzymes from the neutrophils damage the endothelium. Platelets adhere to the damaged endothelium and form a plug, which occludes the capillary.

While the crossmatch can reduce humoral rejection, it does not address the issue of cellular rejection. Thus acute and chronic rejection are not prevented. Acute rejection usually occurs within 10 days of the transplantation and results from T_H activation. Chronic rejection is a mixture of both cellular and humoral immune mechanisms, and may be difficult to control. To prevent rejection, the best strategy is to find the donor organ that is immunogenically closest to the recipient.

TISSUE TYPING

Allograft transplantation requires typing and matching the donor and recipient for ABO and HLA antigens. The ABO blood group system is composed of antigens present on red blood cells, epithelial cells, and endothelial cells. It is possible for an individual to express the A antigen (and thus to be classified as blood group A), B antigen (blood group B), both A and B antigens (blood group AB), or neither antigen (blood group O), as determined by the inherited alleles. An allele can code for an enzyme that attaches a sugar to an altered precursor substance that is part of the cell membrane; the sugar determines the specificity of the A or B antigen. In addition, an individual will produce antibody to the A or B antigen, provided it is not expressed on cells. For example, a person with a blood group A will express the A antigen on cells and will have serum antibody to the B antigen. The antibody is produced in response to normal flora of the gut that express epitopes similar to those of the ABO system. These antibodies are sometimes called isohemagglutinins and are of the IgM class. It is essential to match the donor and recipient for the ABO blood group system to prevent recipient isohemagglutinins from reacting with ABO antigens on the graft. Forward ABO blood grouping is accomplished by mixing red blood cells with reagent antiserum; clumping indicates the presence of the antigen on the cell surface.

Matching HLA phenotypes is useful to reduce the immune response to the graft and to reduce the rate of organ rejection. Early work studying kidney transplants from living related donors showed that HLA-identical donors had the lowest rate of rejection, followed by one haplotype match donors, followed by unmatched donors. Kidneys, usually cadaver kidneys, are donated by an unrelated person, and even with identical matching are less well accepted than kidneys from living related donors. The rate of rejection decreases as the match between the cadaver kidney and the recipient increases. Currently a six-antigen match (2 HLA-A, 2 HLA-B, and 2 HLA-DR) is required before a kidney is shipped to a recipient by the United Network for Organ Sharing. Matching for HLA-DR is most important, followed by HLA-B, then HLA-A. The extent of HLA typing is necessarily limited by the time interval between organ removal from the donor and placement in the recipient.[2] To type for HLA-A, HLA-B, and HLA-DR, the microcytotoxicity test is used. Known antiserum reagent is placed in microtitration wells. Purified lymphocytes are added. The antibody identifies the HLA antigen specificity and binds to the cell. Reagent complement is added, is activated by the antigen-antibody complex, and results in cell lysis. The dead cell then takes up a dye.

Theoretically, for a living related donor the one-way mixed-lymphocyte reaction can be used to evaluate the level of MHC Class II matching. Donor cells irradiated or treated with mitomycin C are used as the stimulator cells. The donor cells are mixed with recipient lymphocytes (responder cells). The responder cells proliferate and incorporate tritiated thymidine into their DNA. The greater the response by the recipient lymphocytes, the poorer the match for the graft. This test is unavailable when the organ is from a cadaver because the test requires 6 days to perform.

IMMUNOSUPPRESSION

All allogeneic transplantation require some degree of immunosuppression if the organ is to survive. The goal is to prevent the recipient from responding to the graft, yet to maintain sufficient recipient immune responsiveness to prevent infection. Chemicals, biologic agents, and radiation have been used to limit a generalized immune response; new therapies are more focused to specifically interfere with allograft rejection. Table 34-1 is a summary of selected immunosuppressive agents.

One group of chemical agents, the mitotic inhibitors, interfere with nucleic acid metabolism. Azathioprine, cyclophosphamide; and methotrexate be-

---

TABLE 34-1
Immunosuppression in Transplantation

CHEMICAL AGENTS
    Mitotic inhibitors
        Azathioprine
        Cyclophosphamide
        Methotrexate
    Corticosteroids
    Protein synthesis inhibitors
        Cyclosporin A
        FK506
        Rapamycin
BIOLOGIC AGENTS
    Anti-lymphocyte serum
    Monoclonal antibody
RADIATION

long to this group. Azathioprine decreases T- and B-cell proliferation by arresting cell division by preventing the synthesis of inosine, a precursor required to generate adenine and guanine. Cyclophosphamide is an alkylating agent that disrupts the DNA chain by interfering with DNA crosslinking. Methotrexate is a folic acid antagonist that prevents purine synthesis.[1]

Corticosteroids are anti-inflammatory drugs with a multifaceted impact on the immune system. The number of circulating lymphocytes decreases by presumably altering the circulation patterns of the lymphocytes. Phagocytic and cytotoxic capabilities of macrophages and neutrophils are also decreased. Chemotaxis is limited so that the number of cells infiltrating an area decreases. The lysosomal membranes are stabilized, thus decreasing the release of proteolytic enzymes at the site of inflammation. The expression of MHC Class II molecules and the production of IL-1 by macrophages is decreased, thus limiting the T-cell–driven immune response.[1]

A dramatic improvement in graft survival was noted when cyclosporin A (CsA) was evaluated for kidney transplantation. CsA prevents T_H activation by inhibiting transcription of genes necessary to synthesize IL-2 and IL-2 receptors. FK506 and rapamycin are newer drugs that also inhibit the transcription step necessary to synthesize IL-2 and IL-2 receptors. The nephrotoxicity of CsA, narrow therapeutic range, and variable effectiveness between patients can limit its use. Because FK506 is 100 times more potent than CsA, it may be used in lower dosages and may avoid some toxicity.[3]

Anti-lymphocyte serum contains antibodies that target lymphocytes for elimination. The serum is prepared by injecting human lymphocytes into a rabbit or a horse; the animal responds by making lymphocyte-specific antibody that is subsequently processed and administered along with chemical immunosuppressive agents at the time of transplantation. The number of circulating lymphocytes decreases, as does cell-mediated responsiveness. Because foreign proteins are injected, it is possible for the recipient to respond to the animal protein, thus causing serum sickness or anaphylaxis.

Irradiation is another strategy. Lymphocytes are sensitive to x-irradiation and thus can be depleted prior to transplantation by multiple exposures to irradiation. The bone marrow is not irradiated; thus new autologous lymphocytes are generated. These new lymphocytes appear to be more tolerant of the graft.

Newer strategies attempt to better target the immune system. Monoclonal antibodies directed against the CD3, IL-2 receptor, CD4, and adhesion molecules have been used to suppress T-cell responses. CD3 antibody binds to the T cell and causes it to be eliminated, probably by phagocytosis. Antibody to high-affinity IL-2R will block activation of selected T cells that were responding, presumably to alloantigens of the graft.

More specifically, the T_H cells can be targeted for immunosuppression by using antibody directed against CD4. In addition, antibody to adhesion molecules can prevent adhesion and signal transduction, thus preventing lymphocytes and other cells from infiltrating a graft and from becoming metabolically activated. In the future, monoclonal antibodies to specific cytokines will provide a new strategy to prolong graft survival.[1]

TRANSPLANTATION

The discussion to this point applies to solid organ transplantation. Kidney and cornea are commonly performed with high rates of success. Heart, lung, and liver transplantations are performed at lower success rates. Bone marrow and pancreas transplantations are performed when traditional therapy fails. One-year survival rates of selected transplanted organs are presented in Table 34-2.[4]

The nature and increasing frequency of bone marrow transplantation (BMT) require some additional comments. Bone marrow is a liquid tissue that is rich in hematopoietic precursors for red blood cells, granulocytes, platelets, lymphocytes, and monocytes/ macrophages. Bone marrow can be used to replace diseased or to reconstitute deficient bone marrow. Initially allogeneic BMT was performed to replace diseased bone marrow, such as in leukemia. The first successful allogeneic transplant in humans occurred in 1968.[5] The HLA match between bone marrow donor and recipient proved to be critical, even more important than in solid organ transplantation at the time. Thus the rejection rate was higher, even if the match was better and the degree of immunosuppression was greater. Successful autologous BMT in humans followed in 1978 and now is performed more frequently than allogeneic BMT.[6,7] The bone marrow cells can be frozen and stored until needed. More recently, it has become known that hematopoietic stem cells (CD 34–positive cells) circulate in the peripheral blood. These circulat-

TABLE 34-2
One-Year Survival Rates for Allografts in Humans

ORGAN	PERCENT
Kidney (sibling)	90
Kidney (cadaver)	80
Heart	80
Heart-lung	74
Liver	70
Pancreas	40

ing cells can now be used as the source of hematopoietic precursors instead of bone marrow.[8] After the donor cells are administered and the bone marrow is reconstituted, lymphocytes recover, leave the bone marrow, and may attack the host; this is known as a graft-versus-host reaction or disease.

BMT or peripheral blood stem cell transplantation is used to treat malignant and nonmalignant hematologic diseases, to rescue patients from lethal doses of chemotherapy administered to treat solid tumors, and to treat some immunodeficiencies. Allogeneic or autologous bone marrow is collected from multiple needle aspirations of the donor anterior or posterior iliac crests while under local or general anesthesia. The bone marrow is filtered to remove bone chips and fat. Subsequently, it may be treated to remove undesired cells, such as red blood cells, T cells, or tumor cells. Removing red cells may prevent a hemolytic reaction if the donor and recipient are ABO incompatible. Removing allogeneic T cells may minimize graft-versus-host disease (GVHD). Removing autologous tumor cells may prevent relapse of the cancer. It is interesting to note that partial removal of allogeneic graft T cells is preferred because the graft T cells appear to prevent sensitization of the host against the graft (thus improving the success of engraftment) and graft T cells seek and destroy host tumor cells.[7]

Peripheral blood stem cells (PBSCs) are collected by continuous flow pheresis in which whole blood is removed from the donor, the nucleated white cells are collected, and the plasma and non-nucleated cells are returned to the donor. Because PBSCs are rare in the peripheral circulation, stategies to mobilize the number of PBSCs collected during pheresis have been used; ultimately, this increases the rate of successful engraftment.[9] Chemotherapy or hematopoietic growth factors (such as granulocyte colony-stimulating factor or granulocyte-macrophage colony-stimulating factor, or a combination of both) have been used to mobilize the CD34 positive stem cells from the bone marrow into the peripheral blood. It is possible to obtain sufficient cells for engraftment in as few as one to three pheresis sessions. In autologous transplantation, the rate of engraftment and neutrophil recovery (indicated by the absolute neutrophil count in the peripheral blood) occurs best with mobilized PBSCs, followed by BMT administered with hematopoietic growth factors, followed by BMT alone.[10] The ease of collection and the success rate make PBSC transplantation attractive.[11]

The bone marrow or stem cells are intravenously transfused to the recipient, and the cells home to the bone marrow space. Early hematopoietic cells are believed to be captured by selectins (a class of cell adhesion molecules) expressed on endothelial cells in the bone marrow.

COMPLICATIONS OF TRANSPLANTATION

Whether chemotherapy, radiation therapy, or a combination of both are used to lessen the tumor mass or to suppress the host immune response, concern remains about the risk of infection and the lack of immune response to resolve an infection. Bacterial, fungal, viral, and parasitic infections are all possible. Treatment with prophylactic drugs, immune globulin, and granulocyte transfusions may prevent infection. In addition, the reduced immune response may allow the development or recurrence of tumors.

Chemotherapy or radiotherapy may be directly toxic to the liver, lungs, bladder, skin, heart, and other organs. Narcotics may be administered to alleviate the pain associated with chemotherapy or radiotherapy. When cyclosporin is administered after total body irradiation to ablate the bone marrow, clonal deletion of T cells in the thymus is interrupted and an autoimmune reaction occurs, notably in the skin.[12]

Of special concern related to BMT or PBSC transplantation is the reaction that occurs when donor lymphocytes are released from the newly reconstituted bone marrow. The lymphocytes, predominantly T cells, mount a cellular immune reaction against the host antigens. This reaction is known as graft-versus-host disease (GVHD).[13] GVHD is classified as acute if it occurs within 3 months after transplantation and as chronic if it persists or occurs more than 3 months after transplantation.

The findings in acute GVHD are related to immunologic reactions in the skin (pruritic, erythematous maculopapular rash, often on the palms and soles), intestine (anorexia and diarrhea), and liver (increased bilirubin, alkaline phosphatase, and transferases). The time of onset and the frequency of acute GVHD is related to the age of the patient, the degree of immunosuppression, the number of T lymphocytes in the graft, and the degree of histoincompatibility between the graft and donor. Acute GVHD is treated with methotrexate and cyclosporin.

The findings in chronic GVHD resemble collagen vascular disease and may be limited or extensive. There are various changes in the skin, chronic cholestatic liver disease, sicca syndrome, and thrombocytopenia. Prednisone and/or cyclosporin are most often used to treat chronic GVHD.

As can be seen from the discussion in this chapter, successful transplantation requires adequate similarity between the donor and recipient, sufficient immunosuppression, and careful monitoring to identify any complications of transplantation. When successful, the benefits are enormous. Transplantation continues to rapidly evolve to improve graft survival time, to increase the rate of graft acceptance, to increase the number of donors, and to decrease the risk of immunosuppression.

Case Study

Mrs. Smith, a 38-year-old woman, was diagnosed with progressive glomerulonephritis based on a needle kidney biopsy. She had a history of proteinuria, hematuria, increased blood pressure, and moderately high serum urea and creatinine. Other physical findings were unremarkable. Treatment with antihypertensive drugs and hemodialysis were insufficient and her kidney disease worsened. It was decided that a kidney transplant was needed.

Mrs. Smith's HLA and ABO phenotypes were tested. Her husband, three children, and sister were unacceptable donors. Finally an acceptable, unrelated cadaveric kidney donor was found. The transplantation surgery was successful and the immunosuppressive therapy of prednisolone, cyclosporin, and azathioprine was initiated. Renal function, urine output, and blood pressure returned to a satisfactory level. Six days post-transplant, Mrs. Smith began to feel tired and lacked energy. Fever, proteinuria, oliguria, increased urine lymphocytes, increased blood pressure, and increased serum urea nitrogen and creatinine developed. The graft was tender and a biopsy revealed a mononuclear infiltrate. Despite increased dosages of corticosteroids, the graft was rejected.

Case Study Questions

1. Classify the graft rejection as primary set, secondary set, or hyperacute. Defend your answer.

2. An HLA antibody was detected in Mrs. Smith's serum on day 6 post-transplant. What is the most likely event that led to sensitization?

3. Explain why her sister could be the most likely acceptable donor compared with her husband and children.

4. A second transplant is to be performed. What can be done to increase the chance of a successful graft?

References

1. Ruby J: Immunology, 2nd ed. pp 559–578. New York, WH Freeman, 1995
2. Perkins HA: Transplantation immunology. In Anderson KC, Ness (eds): Scientific Basis of Transfusion Medicine: Implications for clinical practice, pp 455–466. Philadelphia, WB Saunders, 1994
3. Warty VS, Venkataramanan R: New approaches in transplantation therapy. Clin Lab News 20:39, 1994
4. Batchelor JR, Chai YL: Prog Immunol 6:1002, 1986
5. Gatti RA, Meuwissen HJ, Allen HD, et al: Immunological reconstitution of sex-linked lymphocytopenic immunological deficiency. Lancet 2:1366–1369, 1968
6. Appelbaum FR, Herzig GP, Zielger JL, et al: Successful engraftment of cryopreserved autologous bone marrow in patients with malignant lymphoma. Blood 52:85–95, 1978
7. Appelbaum FR: The use of bone marrow and peripheral blood stem cell transplantation in the treatment of cancer. CA Cancer Clin 46:142–163, 1996
8. Inwards D, Kessinger A: Peripheral blood stem cell transplantation: Historical perspective, current status, and prospects for the future. Transfus Med Rev 6:183–190, 1992
9. Gillespie TW, Hillyer CD: Periperal blood progenitor cells for marrow reconstitution: Mobilization and collection strategies. Transfusion 36:611–624. 1996
10. Bensinger WI, Longin K, Appelbaum FR, et al: Peripheral blood stem cells (PBSCs) collected after recombinant granulocyte colony stimulating factor (rhG-CSF): An analysis of factors correlating with the tempo of engraftment after transplantion. Br J Haematol 87:825–831, 1994
11. Lane TA: Allogeneic marrow reconstitution using peripheral blood stem cells: The dawn of a new era. Transfusion 36:585–589, 1996
12. Horn TD: Acute cutaneous eruptions after marrow ablation: Roses by other names? J Cutan Pathol 21:385–392, 1994
13. Ferrara JLM, Deeg HJ: Graft-versus-host disease. N Engl J Med 324:667–674, 1991

Answers to Review Questions and Case Study Discussions

CHAPTER 1

Review Question Answers
1. a
2. b
3. c
4. a
5. b
6. a
7. d

CHAPTER 2

Review Question Answers
1. c
2. 2 a
   4 b
   1 c
   3 d
   5 e
3. b
4. 2 a
   4 b
   1 c
   5 d
   3 e
5. a

CHAPTER 3

Review Question Answers
1. d   6. b
2. b   7. c
3. a   8. b
4. a   9. b
5. b   10. b

CHAPTER 4

Review Question Answers
1. b   5. b
2. a   6. c
3. d   7. d
4. a   8. c

CHAPTER 5

Review Question Answers
1. a
2. b
3. b
4. a
5. The haplotypes of the mother are A2, B38 and A10, B27
6. b
7. d

CHAPTER 6

Review Question Answers
1. d
2. a
3. d
4. a
5. c
6. b

CHAPTER 7

Review Question Answers
1. b
2. a
3. a
4. d
5. b
6. a

CHAPTER 8

Review Question Answers
1. c
2. e
3. c
4. e
5. a. 3
   b. 5
   c. 1
   d. 2
6. false

CHAPTER 9

Review Question Answers
1. d
2. d
3. c
4. a
5. a
6. d
7. d

CHAPTER 10

Review Question Answers
1. d
2. d
3. c
4. d
5. c

CHAPTER 11

Review Question Answers
1. c
2. d
3. a
4. b
5. a

CHAPTER 12

Review Question Answers
1. c
2. c
3. a
4. b
5. b

CHAPTER 13

Review Question Answers
1. a
2. a
3. a
4. c
5. a

CHAPTER 14

Review Question Answers
1. Enzyme-linked immunosorbent assay
2. Rubella antibody of the IgM class
3. Heterogeneous
4. Noncompetitive
5. Alkaline phosphatase
6. Labeled rabbit anti–human IgM
7. PNPP is the substrate.
8. More absorbance
9. The absorbance values will be erroneously elevated.

CHAPTER 15

Review Question Answers
1. a
2. b
3. c
4. c
5. c

CHAPTER 16

Review Question Answers
1. b
2. e
3. a, b
4. a
5. c, d
6. d

CHAPTER 17

Review Question Answers
1. a
2. b
3. d
4. c
5. c
6. d
7. b

CHAPTER 18

Review Question Answers
1. b
2. c
3. b
4. a
5. 5 a
   1 b
   3 c
   2 d
   4 e
6. c

CHAPTER 19

Review Question Answers
1. c
2. c
3. d
4. b
5. d
6. b
7. c
8. b

CHAPTER 20

Discussion of Case Study
Rheumatic fever can occur at any age, although it is less common among the 20-year-old population than some other age groups. The oropharyngitis was actually a strep throat infection. Although there was no culture, the physician prescribed an appropriate therapeutic an-

tibiotic, that is, penicillin. Because the antimicrobial regime was not completed, the streptococcal infection continued beyond the disease, thus allowing for the development of the antibodies that are involved in the production of rheumatic fever. The elevated ASO titers (700 Todd Units on July 28 and 500 Todd Units on August 7) indicated a recent streptococcal infection in which significant antibodies were produced. Therapeutic treatment in this case consisted of aspirin to suppress the inflammation (swollen knee) and penicillin for treatment of any residual streptococci.

Effective prevention of RF depends on recognition of streptococcal oropharyngeal infections and effective antimicrobial treatment of them. Recurrences of RF can generally be avoided by prophylactic use of an appropriate antibiotic to prevent colonization of the throat with group A streptococci.[24]

CHAPTER 21

Discussion of Case Studies
Case Study 1

One would titer the serum using the rapid plasma reagin test. This titer would be used to monitor the effectiveness of subsequent patient therapy (effective therapy should show decreasing titers over time). Simultaneously, one would confirm the diagnosis using a treponemal antibody test such as the fluororescent treponemal antibody absorption test. This patient is presenting with secondary syphilis.

Case Study 2

Apparently, the mother was inadequately treated for syphilis during her pregnancy. A direct microscopic examination of cutaneous lesion material or nasal discharge is performed. If the result shows the presence of *T. pallidum*, the diagnosis of congenital syphilis is definitive. If not, a presumptive diagnosis can be made (a) if the mother is confirmed to have been inadequately treated, (b) if the infant has clinical signs or symptoms of congenital syphilis and reactive treponemal serology, and (c) if there is a reactive VDRL-CSF test or (d) a reactive IgM antibody test.

CHAPTER 22

Discussion of Case Study

Prior to her visit to the clinic, the patient exhibited a 104°C fever, which was later followed by headache, arthralgia, and a maculopapular rash. These symptoms are consistent with the early stage of Lyme disease, during which approximately 60% of patients exhibit erythema chronicum migrans. The negative throat culture rules out a streptococcal infection; negative results for rheumatoid factor and anti-nuclear antibody rule out autoimmune diseases, all of which could cause arthralgia. The laboratory diagnosis of Lyme disease is based on detecting antibody to the organism in patient serum.

CHAPTER 23

Discussion of Case Study

A rubella IgG titer of 512 indicates past or recent infection with the rubella virus or previous vaccination. A rubella titer performed on a second serum sample obtained 5 to 7 days after the first would be used to determine a recent infection. A fourfold rise in antibody titer between the acute and convalescent sera is diagnostic of a recent rubella infection. The infant's IgM titer is diagnostic of congenital infection because these antibodies do not cross the placenta. The IgG titer after 11 months indicates that antibody is being produced by the baby and is retrospective evidence of congenital infection. Low birthweight, cataracts, and neurosensory hearing loss are characteristic symptoms of congenital rubella.

CHAPTER 24

Discussion of Case Study

The Epstein-Barr virus specific serology indicates an acute primary infection. The presence of lgG anti-EA and lgM anti-VCA are most helpful to diagnose an acute primary infection. Some people never produce heteophile antibody; this occurs more frequently when the primary infection occurs at a young age. Antibodies to EBNA occur later in the disease, after the acute primary infection.

CHAPTER 25

Discussion of Case Studies
Case Study 1

The diagnosis is an acute hepatitis B infection. The vague symptoms are consistent with viral hepatitis. The IV drug use suggests HBV, HCV, or HDV because of a parental route of transmission. HBV is confirmed by the serologic evidence of HBV antigen (HB_sAg) and an early immune response (HB_c antibody of the IgM class). HAV and HCV infections are ruled out because there is no serologic evidence to support recent exposure to either. HDV infection is unlikely because of the severity of symptoms, though it cannot be ruled out.

Case Study 2

The patient is a chronic hepatitis B carrier. The physician may wish to test for hepatitis D virus using an anti-HDV antibody test. The presence of HDV infection suggests this patient's clinical course may lead to progressive liver damage and death.

CHAPTER 26

Discussion of Case Studies
Case Study 1
The patient's serum should be tested with a combination HIV-1/HIV-2 ELISA test or an HIV-1 ELISA test. If the test is reactive, it should be repeated to rule out a false positive ELISA reaction, using the same ELISA test or, preferably, an ELISA test developed against specific HIV-1 antigens. If this test is also reactive, a supplemental Western blot assay for HIV-1 is performed. The Western blot assay is positive and confirmatory for HIV-1 if HIV-1 antibody bands appear in the correct pattern (see the text). If the Western blot assay is negative for HIV antibodies, the patient does not have an HIV infection and the ELISA test was a false positive reaction. If the Western blot is indeterminate, patient serum should be retested by the Western blot assay after a period of 6 months.

Case Study 2
Because the combination HIV-1/HIV-2 ELISA screen was repeatedly reactive, the blood could contain either HIV-1 or HIV-2. The laboratorian should choose to perform a supplemental Western blot assay to confirm the ELISA test reaction and to determine the infection status of the blood. An HIV-1 Western blot assay should be chosen because the overwhelming majority of U.S. HIV cases are caused by HIV-1 virus infections. If the test is positive, the blood is contaminated by HIV-1 virus and must be destroyed. If the test is negative or indeterminate, an HIV-2–specific Western blot should be performed to rule out the presence of HIV-2.

CHAPTER 27

Discussion of Case Studies
Case Study 1
Leukemias and lymphomas of T-helper cell (CD4+) lineage are associated with infection from human T-cell leukemia virus I (HTLV-I). Antibodies to this virus are found in high frequency in persons with this disease as well as in patients with tropical spastic paraparesis and HTLV-I-associated myelopathy (TSP/HAM). HTLV-I is endemic in Japan and in the Caribbean. This patient had spent her childhood in Japan. She was tested and found to be positive for HTLV-I antibody. It is important to note that only 1% to 3% of patients with positive HTLV-I antibodies will develop T-cell leukemia/lymphoma. In the United States, only a small percentage of T-cell leukemia/lymphoma patients are positive for HTLV-I antibody. However, in the endemic areas most T-cell leukemia patients are HTLV-I antibody positive. Although HTLV-I is a retrovirus, there is no association with human immunodeficiency virus 1 or 2 (HIV-1/HIV-2).

Case Study 2
Sarcoidosis is a chronic disease of unknown etiology that may affect multiple organs but most often causes lung problems. Patients with lung involvement suffer from respiratory problems. The disease is characterized by an accumulation of T lymphocytes and mononuclear phagocytes in the affected organs and generalized decrease in cellular immunity. Sarcoidosis is often confused with tuberculosis and fungal infections of the lung. In this patient, fungal antibody tests showed positive precipitating antibody against *Aspergillus fumigatus* 1 and 6, and the patient's serum grew *Aspergillus*. The patient was seen by an allergist and had a positive skin test to *Aspergillus*. Also, flow cytometric studies of the lymphocytes from a bronchoalveolar lavage showed a decreased helper to suppressor T-lymphocyte ratio, a finding consistent with hypersensitivity pneumonitis. The patient indeed suffered from sarcoidosis but developed fungal precipitins as a result of repeated exposure and as a result of decreased cellular immunity. She was treated with corticosteroids and recovered.

CHAPTER 28

Study Question Answers
1. b
2. b
3. b
4. d
5. d

CHAPTER 29

Discussion of Case Studies
Case Study 1
1. Systemic lupus erythematosus (SLE) is suspected. The disease occurs most frequently in women of childbearing age, as is the case with SM.
2. Lethargy, arthritis, and photosensitivity are classic findings in SLE. Lethargy is related to the anemia (decreased RBC count). The arthritis and photosensitivity are immune complex mediated. Decreased C3 and C4 indicate an active immune process. The ANA is a high titer as expected in SLE. The CRP indicates an inflammatory response, as expected in SLE. The increased total protein is consistent with the polyclonal hypergammaglobulinemia associated with SLE.
3. Additional tests include further evaluation to characterize the specific ANA and to monitor the ANA are appropriate.

Case Study 2
1. Rheumatoid arthritis (RA) is suspected.
2. The finding of small joint pain that improves during the day is a classic finding in early RA. Weight loss and lethargy are also commonly seen

in RA. The positive CRP indicates an inflammatory response. The normal C3 and C4 indicate that the complement pathways are not activated or that the acute-phase response counteracts the complement consumption. A low titer ANA is present, as is frequently seen in patients with RA. The lack of serologically detectable RF occurs in 30% of patients with RA and does not exclude the diagnosis of RA.

3. The extent of inflammation of the joint can be determined radiographically. Other diseases associated with RA, such as Sjögren's syndrome and Felty's syndrome, should be evaluated.

CHAPTER 30

Discussion of Case Studies

Case Study 1

1. Hashimoto's thyroiditis and Graves' disease might be suspected as causes of autoimmune thyroid disease.
2. Tests for thyroid autoantibodies include anti–thyroid peroxidase and anti-thyroglobulin antibody tests for routine thyroid antibody screening procedures. Additional specific antibody tests include detection of CA-2, TSab, TBII, or TRAb antibodies.
3. The anti–thyroid peroxidase and anti-thyroglobulin antibody tests may be positive in both disorders. The CA-2 antibody is present only in Hashimoto's thyroiditis, while the TSab, TBII, and TRAb are present only in Graves' disease.

Case Study 2

1. Primary biliary cirrhosis and autoimmune chronic active hepatitis are two autoimmune liver diseases.
2. Mitochondrial and smooth muscle antibody tests detect autoimmune liver disease.
3. Mitochondrial antibodies would be found in primary biliary cirrhosis, while smooth muscle antibodies are detected in autoimmune chronic active hepatitis.

CHAPTER 31

Discussion of Case Studies

Case Study 1

1. This is a primary immune deficiency because the child is otherwise normal and the onset is early childhood.
2. Because the patient is in the right age range and is a male, the possibility of Bruton's X-linked agammaglobulinemia needs to be considered.
3. The mode of inheritance is X-linked recessive.
4. His sisters will have normal immune function because they will each receive a normal X

chromosome from their father. However, each brother will have a 50-50 chance of also being agammaglobulinemic, because the mother has one normal X chromosome and one abnormal X chromosome, and will pass one or the other to each of her sons.

5. With good medical care of any subsequent infections and regular (compulsive) administration of monthly IV Ig, he should be able to have a fully normal life. However, all of his daughters will be carriers for the syndrome. None of his sons will be affected.

Brief Discussion

This case illustrates the crucial features that should lead the pediatrician to suspect an immunodeficiency syndrome. These include repeated severe and otherwise unexplained infections. Any child can have one episode of pneumonia or otitis media or other infection. It is the repeated episodes of infection that indicate this child is not normal and needs to be worked up for a possible primary immunodeficiency state.[17]

Case Study 2

1. This is a secondary immune deficiency.
2. Bone-marrow aspiration and/or lymph-node biopsy might be considered, but the diagnosis of chronic lymphocytic leukemia (CLL) is quite certain based on the data given above. Flow cytometry might be considered and would confirm the diagnosis by showing that the cells are clonal (i.e., they have either kappa or lambda on their cell surfaces). In addition, either CD19 or CD20 is expressed on the cell surface with coexpression of CD5.
3. Intravenous Ig infusions on a monthly basis may be helpful in preventing recurrent pneumonia. Careful pulmonary hygiene and prompt antibiotic treatment at this first sign of infection will also be helpful.
4. With hypogammaglobulinemic states, attachment of the antibodies to the capsular polysaccharide and subsequent phagocytosis of the bacteria are markedly impaired or absent.
5. No, immunization with Pneumovax will not be useful because the patient's immune system will not be able to respond normally to the immunization and specific antibodies will be lacking, even after repeated exposure to the antigens in the Pneumovax.

Brief Discussion

This case exemplifies a secondary immune deficiency because of the onset of recurrent infections in later life. The previous good health of the patient indicates prior normal development and functioning of the immune system. Chemotherapy directed at reducing and controlling the CLL may be very helpful in controlling the patient's symptoms and restoring health. Long-term solution (cure) of the disease with current knowledge would require very aggressive treatment followed by bone marrow transplantation.

CHAPTER 32

Discussion of Case Studies
Case Study 1
1. Quantitatively, the total protein is slightly increased. The γ fraction is markedly increased. Qualitatively, the pattern shows a broad-based increase in the γ region and a stair-step appearance descending from the γ region to the α-1 region. In addition, there is a bridging between the β and γ regions. All of the fractions are symmetric.
2. The serum protein electrophoresis patterns suggest a polyclonal gammopathy.
3. Broad-based, diffuse bands are seen in each of the lanes: IgG, IgM, IgA, κ, and in the immuno-fixation electrophoresis
4. The immunofixation electrophoresis pattern also suggests a polyclonal gammopathy.
5. The clinical conditions suggested are AIDS, chronic infection, autoimmune diseases, and liver diseases.

Additional history obtained from the patient's family revealed IV drug abuse. On further testing, antibodies to hepatitis C virus and HIV were detected. His immunodeficiency state led to increased susceptibility to infection and death.

Case Study 2
1. Quantitatively, all of the fractions are within the reference range, except for a moderate increase in the β fraction, and a borderline low γ fraction. Qualitatively, all fractions have a symmetric contour except for the β fraction, which rises to a very prominent peak or "spike."
2. The serum protein electrophoresis suggests a monoclonal gammopathy.
3. Interpretation of IFE: Ig quantitation by nephelometry reveals a markedly increased IgA, a decreased IgM, and a normal level of IgG. IFE reveals a striking band of restricted electrophoretic mobility in the IgA lane with a corresponding band in the kappa lane.
4. The immunofixation electrophoresis pattern suggests an IgA kappa monoclonal gammopathy.
5. These results suggest multiple myeloma.

Brief Discussion
The patient's urine also revealed free kappa light chain (Bence Jones) proteinuria. (See Figs. 32-9A, B and 32-10.) He was treated with melphalan and prednisone,

and after one cycle of therapy his serum calcium level returned to normal and his back pain improved. After several cycles of therapy, his appetite returned, he gained weight, and his hematocrit climbed to the low end of the normal range.

CHAPTER 33

Discussion of Case Studies
Case Study 1
1. These are B cells because the positive markers are B-cell markers.
2. A kappa/lambda ratio of 1:25 is not normal. It is reversed from the normal ratio, which is usually 23:1.
3. The other name for CD10 is CALLA (common acute lymphocytic leukemia antigen).
4. The results are consistent with malignant lymphoma of B-cell-lambda lineage, probably of follicular center cell origin.

Case Study 2
1. The CBC values indicate anemia (the low Hb and Hct values) and severe thrombocytopenia.
2. A normal M/E ratio in a patient this age is 3:1, and blasts should comprise less than 5% of bone marrow cells.
3. These cytochemical stains are positive in neutrophils and monocytes. They are negative in lymphocytes and lymphocyte blasts.
4. These markers show the cells to be precursor B-cell type.
5. The results indicate a diagnosis of acute lymphocytic leukemia (ALL), of pre–B-cell type.

Case Study 3
1. The history and laboratory result are consistent with a diagnosis of chronic lymphocytic leukemia (CLL).
2. These cells are developed B cells.

Case Study 4
1. A diagnosis of Hodgkin's lymphoma is consistent with this history, probably nodular sclerosing type.
2. The immunological studies show these cells to be T cells.

CHAPTER 34

Discussion of Case Study
1. The timing (6 days post-transplant) suggests a second-set rejection. Hyperacute rejection occurs within 24 hours and first-set rejection usually occurs between 10 and 14 days. The loss of renal function (increased blood urea and creatinine, proteinuria, and oliguria) with an immune reaction (fever and increased urine lymphocytes

with mononuclear infiltrate) suggests rejection. Of course, it is always necessary to rule out an infectious process.

2. She was most likely exposed to different HLA antigens during pregnancy. Remember that the fetus is genetically 50% different than the mother because 50% of the genetic information is inherited from the father.

3. Genetically related people (father-offspring, mother-offspring, and sibling-sibling) are more likely to share more genetic information than genetically unrelated people. Husband and wife are genetically unrelated. An offspring can at best share one haplotype. Between siblings there is a 25% chance of sharing two haplotypes.

4. Select a donor that matches the phenotype of the recipient as well as that of her husband. This may prevent another second-set rejection caused by previous alloimmunization during pregnancy.

Glossary

Absorb: To take in.

Acquired immunodeficiency syndrome (AIDS): A secondary immune deficiency caused by the human immunodeficiency virus (HIV).

Active immunity: The immune response produced by an immunocompetent individual following exposure to a challenge.

Acute glomerulonephritis: Inflammation of the glomerulus that results in impaired renal filtration.

Acute lymphocytic leukemia (ALL): A malignant disease characterized by an increased concentration of lymphoblasts in the bone marrow which are frequently seen in the peripheral blood.

Acute phase: In infectious disease, the most severe signs and symptoms specifically related to the disease.

Acute-phase proteins: Plasma proteins whose concentration increases or decreases during inflammation.

Adaptive immunity: Immunity that is acquired or learned by an individual only after a challenge is encountered.

Adjuvants: Agents that potentiate or enhance an immune response.

Adoptive immunity: The transfer of immunocompetent cells from one individual to a second individual to establish immunocompetence in the second individual.

Adsorption: The attraction of material on the surface.

Affinity: The strength of one epitope to bind to an antigen combining site.

Affinity maturation: A phenomenon in which antibodies produced later in the secondary immune response have a higher affinity for the antigen than those produced earlier.

Agarose: A neutral derivative of seaweed used in immunologic procedures.

Agglutinin: Antibody that participates in agglutination reactions.

Agglutination: A serologic reaction in which a particulate antigen (or antibody) reacts with soluble antibody (or antigen) to yield detectable clumping.

Agglutination inhibition: A serologic technique in which soluble antigen in the patient's sample reacts with known antibody reagent to form an invisible complex; the antibody reagent is then unavailable to react with the particulate antigen reagent; no agglutination means antigen is present in the patient sample.

Agglutinogens: Antigens that participate in agglutination reactions.

AIDS: See acquired immunodeficiency syndrome.

Allergens: Exogenous antigens that stimulate an overproduction of IgE.

Allergy: A harmful reaction experienced by some people to commonly encountered environmental antigen; caused by the overproduction of IgE.

Allogeneic: Belonging to the same species, yet genetically different.

Allograft: Tissue transplanted between members of the same species.

Allotype: Antigenic variation within a species of the constant region of the heavy or light chain of an immunoglobulin molecule.

α heavy chain disease: The most common heavy chain disease characterized by an infiltration of lymphoid and plasma cells into the small intestines; the disease in common in the Middle East.

α_1-antitrypsin: An acute-phase protein that is a serine protease inhibitor.

α_2-macroglobulin: An acute-phase protein that is a protease inhibitor.

Alpha-fetoprotein (AFP): An oncofetal protein normally produced by fetal liver; in adults, elevated serum levels may indicate a hepatoma, testicular teratoblastomas, or inflammatory diseases.

Amboceptor: Sheep red blood cell antibody that causes hemolysis of sheep red cells in the presence of complement.

Amplification: The generation of C3b in the complement pathway, by either the classical or alternative pathway, to provide a feedback loop to increase the activation of C3 through C9.

Amyloid: An abnormal fibrillar protein that accumulates in tissue; one form resembles an immunoglobulin fragment and is monoclonal.

Anamnestic response: The secondary immune response in which the immune system remembers previous antigenic exposure.

Anaphylatoxin: Biologically active peptides that mediate inflammation by inducing the release of histamine, contracting smooth muscles, and increasing vascular permeability.

Anaphylaxis: Systemic immediate hypersensitivity that occurs when mast cell and basophil mediators affect more than one organ and may cause life threatening respiratory distress.

Anergy: Generalized immunologic unresponsiveness to many antigens.

Antibody: A protein produced by B lymphocytes and plasma cells that can bind to an epitope; often used as a synonym for immunoglobulin.

Anti-deoxyribonuclease B test: A neutralization test in which antibodies in patient serum will prevent the enzyme DNAse B from depolymerizing DNA.

Anti-human globulin: An antibody preparation that contains antibody to a range of globulins (polyspecific) or to a single globulin (monospecific, such as anti-C3b) used to detect sensitized red blood cells.

Anti-hyaluronidase test: A neutralization assay in which antibodies inactivate hyaluronidase and prevent subsequent enzymatic breakdown of the substrate by hyaluronidase.

Anti-lymphocyte serum (globulin): A form of immune suppression in which serum containing antibodies directed against lymphocytes leads to decreased lymphocyte responsiveness.

Anti-nuclear antibody: An autoantibody directed against a component of nucleus, commonly found in systemic lupus erythematosus.

Antibody-dependent cell-mediated cytolysis (ADCC): An effector mechanism in which cells coated with antibody react with the Fc receptors to cause target cell damage.

Antigen: A substance that is capable of reacting with products of the specific immune response.

Antigen-antibody complex: The union of an antibody with an antigen.

Antigen-presenting cells (APCs): Accessory cells that present antigen to lymphocytes in conjunction with MHC Class II molecules; APCs are required in the initial step of a T-dependent immune response.

Antigen valency: The number of antigenic determinants present on an antigen.

Antigenic determinant (epitope): The portion of the immunogen molecule that can bind with antibody.

Antigenicity: The ability of a substance to react with immune products.

APC: See antigen presenting cells.

Apoptosis: Programmed cell death.

Arthus reaction: A type III hypersensitivity reaction, induced experimentally by the intradermal injection of the sensitizing antigen, that allows pre-existing antibody to combine with the antigen and causes localized destructive inflammation at the site of immune complex formation.

ASO neutralization test: An enzyme inhibition reaction in which streptolysin O antibodies neutralize the streptolysin O reagent, thus preventing hemolysis of human group O red blood cells by the streptolysin O reagent.

Ataxia-telangiectasia: An autosomal recessive immunodeficiency characterized by variable humoral and cellular immune defects, as well as sinopulmonary infection and ataxia.

Atopy: A genetically determined hypersensitivity usually referring to allergic patients who produce an abnormally large amount of specific IgE when exposed to small concentrations of antigen.

Atypical (reactive) lymphocytes: In infectious mononucleosis, suppressor and cytotoxic T lymphocytes capable of recognizing and killing B lymphocytes infected with the Epstein-Barr virus.

Autofluorescence: The natural fluorescence of a tissue or substrate.

Autograft: Tissue transplanted from one site to another within the same individual.

Avidity: The cumulative binding strength of all antibody-epitope pairs which results from multivalent antigen and antibody.

Azathioprine: An immunosuppressive drug that inhibits purine metabolism and DNA proliferation so that cell divison is prevented.

Azidothymidine (AZT): Used to treat HIV infection, this purine analog inhibits reverse transcriptase, thus preventing viral RNA from being converted to DNA.

Becquerel (Bq): A standardized unit of radioactivity that equals one disintegration per second.

Bence Jones protein: Free light chains.

β_2 microglobulin: The small peptide that is noncovalently associated with all classical MHC Class I heavy chains.

β particles: Particles emitted from radioisotopes that are negatively charged electrons (negatrons).

Bruton's X-linked agammaglobulinemia: A congenital X-linked defect in which B cells fail to mature and secrete immunoglobulin.

Burkitt's lymphoma: A malignant neoplasm of B lymphocytes associated with Epstein-Barr virus infection and found primarily among children in a restricted area of Africa and in New Guinea.

C-reactive protein: An acute-phase protein produced by the liver in early inflammatory response, capable of precipitating the C-polysaccharide extract of pneumococcus.

Cachectin: Identical to tumor necrosis factor alpha, this monokine mediates inflammation and cell death.

CALLA: See common acute lymphoblastic leukemia antigen.

Carcinoembryonic antigen (CEA): A glycoprotein normally synthesized, secreted, and excreted by the fetal gastrointestinal tract; however, it can be detected in serum in disorders of the gastrointestinal tract. For tumors that secrete CEA, CEA measurements are used to monitor the efficacy of therapy and the recurrence of disease.

Carrier: A molecule that when coupled to a hapten renders the hapten immunogenic.

cDNA: Complementary DNA; the DNA synthesized from RNA.

Cell-mediated immunity: A form of adaptive immunity in which T lymphocytes recognize and react with a challenge through direct cell-to-cell interaction of lymphokines.

Ceruloplasmin: An acute-phase protein that is the principal copper-transporting protein in human plasma.

CH$_{50}$ assay: A hemolytic assay used to assess the function of the classical pathway of complement. Sheep red blood cells coated with rabbit anti-sheep red blood cell antibody are incubated with patient sample. If there is sufficient concentration and function of complement in the patient sample, the classical pathway is activated and hemolysis results.

CH$_{100}$ assay: A diffusion assay used to assess the function of the classical pathway of complement. This test is based on the principle of mixing sensitized sheep red blood cells with agar and placing serum in wells. As diffusion occurs, complement in the serum hemolyzes the cells, producing a measurable clear zone that is proportional in size to the complement activity.

Chancre: A firm, eroded, painless papule with raised margins found in the early stages of syphilis that usually progresses to a clean-based, nonbleeding, painless ulcer.

Chemotactic factor: A substance that directs the migration of cells into an area.

Chemotaxis: The directed movement of cells in response to a concentration gradient of a stimulus.

Chessboard titration: Used in indirect immunofluorescence, a serial dilution of conjugated antiserum is reacted with a serial dilution of positive control serum to determine the optimal dilution of conjugated antiserum.

Chiasmata: The crossover of genetic information from one chromosome to the sister chromosome.

Chimeras: The exchange of tissue between fraternal twins during fetal life so that each twin is exposed to the other's tissue antigens during development and tolerates the antigens as "self."

Chronic granulomatous disease: An immune deficiency in which defective neutrophils do not generate the respiratory burst necessary for intracellular killing of microorganisms.

Chronic lymphocytic leukemia (CLL): Most often, a B-cell malignancy characterized by the clonal expression of B cells which are present in the peripheral blood and the bone marrow; malignant B cells are morphologically similar to small resting lymphocytes.

Clonal deletion: One proposed mechanism of immune tolerance in which an immature B cell exposed to a low concentration of antigen arrests its maturation so that it cannot respond to subsequent antigen exposure.

Clone: A population of genetically identical cells derived from a single parent cell.

Cluster of differentiation (CD): Leukocyte glycoproteins that are identified by a monoclonal antibody clone; official nomenclature approved by international consensus.

Cold agglutinins: Autoantibodies of the IgM class that agglutinate human erythrocytes at temperatures less that 37°C and that may be found following *Mycoplasma pneumoniae* infection and other diseases.

Common acute lymphoblastic leukemia antigen (CALLA): A 100 kDa glycoprotein (CD10) that serves as a useful marker, since it is present in 75% of non-T, non-B acute lymphocytic leukemia and 40% of lymphoblastic lymphoma.

Common variable immunodeficiency: Immunodeficiency characterized by decreased serum immunogobulins, recurrent infections, and occuring in adults with a previously healthy immune system.

Competitive immunoassay: An assay in which labeled and unlabeled ligand compete for a limited number of binding sites on the binding reagent.

Complement: A humoral mechanism of the nonspecific immune response consisting of at least 14 proteins that proceed in a cascading sequence of activation, which results in cell lysis; organized into two pathways: classical and alternative.

Complement fixation: A serologic technique in which the test system and indicator system compete for the binding of complement. If complement binds to the specific test antigen-antibody complex, complement will be unavailable to react with the visible indicator system of sensitized sheep red blood cells.

Concanavalin A (Con A): A mitogen derived from the jack bean and used to stimulate T-cell mitosis.

Congenital rubella syndrome: During pregnancy, maternal infection with the rubella virus may result in the virus crossing the placenta and infecting the fetus; detrimental effects of rubella syndrome include congenital heart disease, cataracts, and neurosensory deafness.

Congenital syphilis: The transfer of *Treponema pallidum* across the placenta, which can result in late abortion, stillbirth, neonatal disease, or latent infection; transferral of the organisms can occur at any stage of syphilis.

Conjugate: In immunoassays, either labeled antibody or labeled antigen.

Constant domain: A portion of immunoglobulin peptide which is a sequence of approximately 110 amino acids that show little amino acid substitution and are therefore consistent within an immunoglobulin class or light chain type.

Convalescent phase: In infectious disease, the recovery.

Countercurrent immunoelectrophoresis: A gel precipitation reaction in which one column of wells contains antibody and a second column of wells contains the antigen. When placed in an electrical field, each migrates toward the other until precipitation occurs at the zone of equivalence. It is commonly used to detect autoantibodies, microbial antigens, and antibodies to infectious agents.

CREST: A mild form of scleroderma manifested by *c*alcinosis, *R*aynaud's phenomenon, *e*sophageal dysmotility, *s*clerodactyly, and *t*elangiectases.

Cromolyn (disodium cromoglycate): A therapeutic drug that protects asthmatic patients and others by stabilizing the lysosomes and preventing the release of mediators from mast cells.

Crossreactivity: The ability of an antibody to react with antigens closely related to, but different

than, the antigen that induces the antibody production.

Cryoglobulins: Serum proteins that reversibly precipitate or gel between 0° and 4°C.

Crystal scintillation: Used to measure γ radioactivity, this technique detects the energy released during decay that excites a fluor that releases a photon of visible light.

Curie (Ci): The traditional unit of radioactivity; it equals 3.7×10^{10} Bq.

Cutaneous lymphoma: Also referred to as mycosis fungoides, this disease is characterized by malignant T lymphocytes in the skin; malignant T cells in the blood are called Sézary cells.

Cyclosporin: An immunosupressive drug used in transplantation that inhibits interleukin-2 production and secretion.

Cytokines: Protein molecules secreted by leukocytes that transmit messages to regulate cell growth, differentiation, and activity.

Cytotoxicity: Cell destruction; cytotoxicity techniques are commonly used to detect HLA antigens in transplantation.

Cytotoxic T cells (T_c): A subpopulation of T lymphocytes that destroys cells by direct cell-to-cell interaction without the presence of antibody.

Cytotropic: Having an affinity for a cell; IgE is cytotropic for basophils and mast cells.

Dane particle: A complete hepatitis B virion.

Davidsohn differential: A hemagglutination test in which the characteristics of the heterophile antibody are defined by their adsorbtion by guinea pig and beef cell antigens. The heterophile antibodies associated with infectious mononucleosis are adsorbed by beef erythrocytes but not by guinea pig antigen.

Decay: Related to radionuclides, the nuclear emission of particles or photons from an unstable nucleus; disintegration.

Delayed hypersensitivity (cell-mediated immune reaction): Type IV hypersensitivity mediated by lymphokines released from sensitized T lymphocytes.

Denaturation: The loss of natural conformation of a protein or DNA strands.

Density gradient centrifugation: The most common procedure for the separation of mononuclear cells in which diluted blood is added to a tube containing a density gradient preparation and centrifuged. Four layers can be identified from top to bottom of the tube: plasma, mononuclear cells, density gradient, and finally red cells and granulocytes.

Diapedesis: The emigration of cells through a blood vessel wall to enter the adjacent tissue.

DiGeorge syndrome (thymic hypoplasia): An immunodeficiency disease characterized by the failure of parathyroid and thymus glands to develop during fetal life; decreased or absent T lymphocytes and hypocalcemic tetany become apparent shortly after birth.

Direct agglutination: An agglutination reaction in which the antigen is found naturally on the surface of cells (such as red blood cells or bacteria).

Direct anti–human globulin test: An agglutination procedure to detect in vivo sensitized red blood cells using anti–human globulin reagent.

Direct immunofluorescence: An immunofluorescence technique in which an antibody labeled with a fluorochrome reacts with a tissue, cell, or microbial test antigen; also known as direct fluorescent antibody test.

Disseminated intravascular coagulation: A secondary pathophysiologic state in which coagulation proteins and platelets are consumed in the microcirculation causing bleeding tendencies; the activated coagulation enzymes also catabolize C3 resulting in decreased serum concentration of C3.

Double diffusion: Also known as the Ouchterlony technique; both antigen and antibody diffuse in gel and may react.

Electrophoresis: A procedure to separate molecules in a electrical field based on differences in migration related to the net charge.

Electrostatic force: The attraction of a positively charged portion of a molecule for a negatively charged portion of a molecule.

ELISA: Enzyme-linked immunosorbent assay; one form of enzyme immunoassay which requires a solid phase and enzyme-labeled reagent antibody.

Elution: The separation of antibody from antigen.

Endodermal: Pertaining to the inner layer of a tissue.

Endpoint nephelometry: Maximal light scatter is measured and is related to the concentration of antigen present.

Enumeration: Number or count.

Enzyme immunoassay: A ligand assay in which the label is an enzyme and the binding reagent is an antibody.

Eosinophil chemotactic factor of anaphylaxis (ECF-A): A preformed mediator released during mast cell degranulation that attracts eosinophils to the site of activated mast cells.

Eosinophilia: An increased number of eosinophils in the peripheral blood, usually associated with allergic reactions or parasitic infections.

Epi-illumination fluorescence microscope: A fluorescence microscope in which excitation light travels from the light source through the excitation filter and is reflected by the dichroic mirror at a 45° angle to the specimen. Light emitted from the specimen travels through the objective, dichroic mirror, and barrier filter before it is viewed.

Epitope (antigenic determinant): The portion of the immunogen molecule that can bind with antibody.

Epstein-Barr virus: A double-stranded enveloped virus belonging to the herpesvirus group capable of transforming B lymphocytes, which then become self-perpetuating.

Equivalence: The relative concentration of antibody and antigen that produces maximal antigen-antibody complex formation.

F(ab')$_2$: The fragment of an immunoglobulin molecule generated by pepsin cleavage consisting of the two antigen combining sites joined by disulfide bonds.

Fab: The fragment of an immunoglobulin molecule generated by papain cleavage that binds to one antigen.

Fc: The fragment of immunoglobulin molecule generated by papain cleavage that cannot bind to the antigen. The Fc portion of rabbit IgG crystallizes; hence, this is the crystallizable fragment.

Febrile agglutinins: Antibodies produced in response to bacterial infections in which fever is a prominent feature.

Ficoll-Hypaque solution: A density gradient that allows separation of peripheral blood cells.

Flare: In type I hypersensitivity, the red edge of a wheal.

Flocculation: The loose lattice formed when soluble antibody reacts with a colloidal suspension of a lipid antigen; for example, as seen in a reactive pattern in the rapid plasma reagin test.

Flow cytometry: The method in which a large number of cells pass through an aperture, where they are exposed to light or electric current to generate a signal that is measured. Cell surface markers, cell size, and cell volume are detected by this technique.

Fluid phase diffusion: One of the earliest precipitation reactions to detect unknown antigen or antibody, in which soluble antigen is layered on top of soluble antibody in a capillary tube and each diffuses toward the other until antibody-antigen complex and precipitate at the interface.

Fluorescence: A form of luminescence in which a molecule absorbs light energy of one wavelength and emits light energy of a longer wavelength in less than 10^{-4} seconds.

Fluorescence microscopy: Modified darkfield microscopy that uses special components to separate excitation wavelengths of light from emission wavelengths of light.

Fluorescent treponemal antibody absorption test (FTA-ABS): An indirect fluorescent antibody test that uses dried Nichols strain *Treponema pallidum* as the antigen. Absorbed patient serum is added to the antigen and fluorescein isothiocyanate labeled anti–human gammaglobulin is added to visualize the patient antibody.

Fluorochrome: An organic compound that fluoresces when exposed to short wavelengths of light and that is used as a label in fluorescence immunoassays and immunofluorescence.

Forbidden-clone theory: A theory of autoimmunity that states that during fetal development those lymphocyte clones that are capable of reacting to self are eliminated.

Forward angle: In nephelometry, detection of light scatter at less than 90° from the transmitted light.

Fulminant: Occurring with great rapidity.

γ emission: A portion of the electromagnetic radiation spectrum that consists of very short wavelengths originating from an unstable nucleus.

Gamma globulin: A heterogenous mixture of proteins which migrate to the gamma region under standard conditions for serum protein electrophoresis; most IgG and some IgM and IgA molecules are found in this region, however, other serum proteins can be found in this region.

Gammaglobulin: A biologic preparation of antibodies administered to provide humoral protection.

γ heavy chain disease: A heavy chain disease characterized by fever, recurrent infection, lymphadenopathy, and progressive proliferation of plasma cells.

Gel: In immunologic procedures, agarose.

Goodpasture's syndrome: An autoantibody directed against the alveolar and glomerular basement membranes that induces a type II cytotoxic reaction that leads to complement activation, inflammation, localized damage, and loss of pulmonary and renal function.

Graft-versus-host disease (GVHD): The clinical and pathologic sequelae that occur when immunocompetent T cells in the graft recognize and attack antigens of the immunoincompetent host.

Granulocyte macrophage colony stimulating factor (GM-CSF): A lymphokine that induces the growth of hematopoietic cells that are committed to become granulocytes or monocytes.

Granuloma: A general term for a cellular reaction in which there is a mononuclear cell infiltrate in tissue.

Granulomatous hypersensitivity: Type IV hypersensitivity in which persistent antigen stimulates a mononuclear cell infiltrate.

Graves' disease: An autoimmune disease of the thyroid in which an autoantibody to the thyrotropin receptor (thyroid stimulating hormone receptor) stimulates the thyroid independent of the normal feedback control.

Gummas: Lesions commonly seen in tertiary syphilis that are believed to be the result of delayed hypersensitivity; lesions may occur in the skin, bones, mucosa, and muscles.

Hairy cell leukemia (leukemic reticuloendotheliosis): A disease characterized by infiltration of irregular "hairy" B lymphocytes with cytoplasmic projections into the bone marrow and spleen but without peripheral lymphadenopathy.

Half-life: The time needed for 50% of a radionuclide to decay and to become more stable; also 50% of a protein to be catabolized.

Haplotype: Closely linked loci on a single chromosome that are inherited as a unit.

Hapten: A low molecular weight substance that is antigenic (can bind to an immune product) but not immunogenic (cannot stimulate an immune response).

Haptoglobin: An acute-phase protein that binds irreversibly to free hemoglobin, thus forming a complex that is rapidly cleared by the mononuclear phagocyte system.

Hashimoto's thyroiditis: An autoimmune thyroid disease characterized by a chronic lymphocytic infiltrate.

Heavy chain: One peptide of the immunoglobulin molecule consisting of three or four constant domains and one variable domain.

Heavy chain disease: Rare lymphoproliferative disorders characterized by the presence of fragments of free heavy chains without light chains.

Helper T cells (T$_H$): A subpopulation of circulating T lymphocytes that function to help other antigen-specific T or B cells to proliferate and differentiate into functional effector cells.

Hemagglutination: A serologic technique in which antigen-antibody interaction results in the clumping of red blood cells.

Hemagglutination inhibition: A serologic technique in which virus particles neutralize antibody and prevent antibody from clumping red blood cells.

Hemolysin (amboceptor): Sheep red blood cell antibody that causes hemolysis of sheep red cells in the presence of complement.

Hemolytic disease of the newborn (HDNB): This disease is caused by maternal–fetal red cell incompatibility. Most commonly, an RhD-negative mother becomes sensitized to the D antigen present on fetal red blood cells; the maternal antibody crosses the placenta and increases the destruction of fetal red blood cells.

Hepatomegaly: Enlargement of the liver.

Heterodimer: A protein which is composed of the two different peptide chains.

Heterogeneous immunoassay: A test procedure that requires the separation of the free label from the bound label before quantitation.

Heterologous: Xenogeneic; in immunologic reactions, when antibody combines with an antigen that did not induce its production.

Heterophile antibody: An antibody that is produced in response to one antigen and that reacts with a second, genetically unrelated antigen.

Heterozygous: Having a different allele at the locus on each of the paired chromosomes.

Histamine: A bioactive amine and preformed mediator released from mast cells during allergic responses that is responsible for the immediate effects of bronchoconstriction, increased mucous production, pruritus, increased vasopermeability, and vasodilation.

Histocompatibility: Related to the degree of sameness between two tissues; if the donor and recipient are sufficiently different, one tissue may react against the other.

Histiocytes: Macrophages that are fixed in various tissues and that are actively involved in phagocytosis.

HIV: See human immunodeficiency virus.

Hive: Wheal and flare reaction in type I hypersensitivity; welt.

HLA: Human leukocyte antigen; the products of the major histocompatibility complex that are present on a cell surface.

Hodgkin's disease: A lymphoma characterized by binucleated Reed-Sternberg cells.

Homogenous immunoassay: A test method that does not require a separation step prior to quantitating the label because the bound label selectively separates from the free label or its activity is different when free.

Homologous: Allogeneic; in immunologic reactions, when antibody combines with the antigen which induced its production.

Homology: The degree of sameness; usually used to compare the similarity between genomes (such as HIV-1 and HIV-2) or amino acid sequences (such as IgG1 and IgG2).

Homozygous: Having the same allele at a single locus on both chromosomes.

Human immunodeficiency virus (HIV): The etiologic agent of AIDS.

Humoral immunity: A form of adaptive immunity in which B lymphocytes and plasma cells produce specific antibodies that recognize and react to a challenge.

Hyaluronidase: An enzyme produced by group A β-hemolytic streptococci.

Hybridize: The association of a probe with homologous base pairs.

Hybridoma: The fusion of a B cell with a myeloma cell line that results in a new immortal daughter cell.

Hydrogen bonding: The attraction of two negatively charged atoms for the positively charged hydrogen ion to create a weak bond.

Hydrophobic force: The attraction between nonpolar groups in an aqueous environment.

Hyperemia: An increased flow of blood into the affected area following injury.

Hypergammaglobulinemia: Increased concentration of immunoglobulins in the blood.

Hypersensitive pneumonitis (extrinsic allergic alveolitis): A type III hypersensitivity reaction in which inhaled antigens combine with pre-existing antibodies to initiate inflammation.

Hypersensitivity: An exaggerated immune response that causes tissue damage to the host.

Icteric: Pertaining to jaundice.

Identity: In gel precipitation reactions, a smooth continuous line formed when one antigen, identical to the second antigen, reacts with antiserum.

Idiotopes: Antigenic determinants within the variable region of an immunoglobulin molecule.

Idiotype: Antigenic variation within the variable domain of an immunoglobulin molecule.

Idiotype network: The interaction between one product of the immune system (such as an antibody) and another product of the immune system (such as a second antibody); the result is the regulation of the production of immune molecules.

IgA: The class of antibody defined by the alpha chain; serum and secretory forms exist.

IgD: The class of antibody defined by the delta chain; the most abundant immunoglobulin on the surface of mature B cells.

IgE: The class of antibody defined by the epsilon chain; also known as reaginic antibody; homocytotropic for mast cells and basophils.

IgG: The class of antibody defined by the gamma chain; the most abundant immunoglobulin in serum.

IgM: The class of antibody defined by the mu chain; the largest immunoglobulin in size.

IgG index: The comparison of the ratio between cerebrospinal fluid and serum IgG compared to cerebrospinal fluid and serum albumin. An index greater that 0.7 suggests IgG production in the central nervous system.

Immediate hypersensitivity: An exaggerated immune reaction within minutes following exposure to the antigen or allergen.

Immune adherence: The covalent bonding between the cleaved form of C3 (C3b) as part of an immune complex and cell surfaces that promotes their removal by the reticuloendothelial system.

Immune complex: An antigen-antibody complex; pathologic immune complexes may be deposited in tissue and cause an inflammatory response.

Immune complex disorder: The pathophysiology associated with clinical features secondary to immune complex formation and deposition.

Immune status: The measurement of specific antibody to determine whether an individual is resistant or susceptible to an infection.

Immune surveillance theory: The immune response of normal individuals that regularly eliminates malignant or potentially malignant cells, thereby preventing tumor growth.

Immunoelectrophoresis (IEP): An immunologic method in gel in which a mixture of proteins is separated by electrophoresis. Antiserum is placed in troughs and diffuses toward the separated proteins until precipitin arcs appear in the zone of equivalence. Used to characterize monoclonal proteins in serum or urine.

Immunofixation electrophoresis: An immunologic method in gel in which a mixture of proteins is separated by electrophoresis. Antiserum is applied to the gel and proteins are fixed (precipitated). Used to characterize monoclonal proteins in serum and urine.

Immunogen: A substance that causes a detectable immune response.

Immunogenicity: The property of an antigen to produce an immune response.

Immunoglobulin: Antibody.

Immunoglobulin class: Isotype.

Immunoglobulin subclass: Minor variation in the constant region of an immunoglobulin class that results in variation in physical and biologic function.

Immunologic deficiency theory: A theory of autoimmunity that states that a defect in immune regulation is responsible for autoimmunity.

Immunology: The study of the mechanisms that protect an individual from injury.

Immunometric assay: An immunoassay in which the amount of antigen in the test sample is directly proportional to the measured bound labeled antibody; sandwich assay.

Immunonephelometry: Nephelometry in which the suspended particles are antigen-antibody complexes.

Immunosuppression: Reduced activity of T and B lymphocytes and macrophages, including decreased antibody and cytokine production.

Immunotherapy: Therapy to manipulate the immune system against disease and malignancy.

Incubation: In infectious desease, the time between exposure to the organism and the appearance of signs and symptoms.

Indirect anti–human globulin test: An agglutination procedure to detect in vitro antibody-antigen reactions using anti–human globulin reagent. It is commonly used to detect red cell compatibility.

Indirect immunofluorescence: An immunofluorescence technique used to detect circulating patient antibody after it reacts with a source of known antigen. The bound patient antibody is detected by its reaction with fluorochrome-labeled antibody; also known as indirect fluorescent antibody test.

Inducer cells: A T-cell subset that directs the specific immune response against T-dependent antigens.

Infection: A state in which microorganisms establish and multiply within a host.

Inflammation: The physiologic processes evoked in response to tissue injury that provide protective mechanisms to destroy, dilute or isolate the injured site.

Innate immunity: Immunity that is present from birth in all individuals and that is activated in the same manner each time the individual is exposed to a challenge.

Innocent bystander cells: Cells in the vicinity of an immune event, most often activated complement, that may be destroyed even though the immune event is directed against different cells.

Interferon: A group of chemical mediators with antiviral, immunomodulatory and antiproliferative effects.

Interleukin-1 (IL-1): A soluble mediator produced primarily by macrophages that promotes IL-2 and IL-2R production by T cells.

Interleukin-2 (IL-2): A lymphokine produced and secreted by antigen-sensitized helper T lymphocytes that promotes growth of other activated T cells and induces interferon production.

Interleukin-3 (IL-3): A lymphokine that stimulates proliferation of early progenitor cells in the bone marrow.

Interleukin-4 (IL-4): Also known as B-cell growth factor 1, this lymphokine stimulates proliferation of antigen-activated B cells and induces differentiation of proliferating B cells into antibody-secreting plasma cells.

Interleukin-6 (IL-6): Also known as B cell growth factor 2, this cytokine B promotes cell differentiation into plasma cells.

Isograft: Tissue transplanted between genetically identical individuals.

Isohemagglutinin: Nonimmune IgM antibodies of the ABO blood group.

Isotype: Antigenic variation of heavy and light chains found in all healthy members of a species as defined by differences between the constant domains of the peptide.

J chain: A glycoprotein with a molecular weight of 15 kDa believed to initiate polymerization of IgM and secretory IgA.

Jaundice: The symptom characterized by a yellow coloration of the skin and sclera; it is associated with hyperbilirubinemia and may be seen in hepatitis.

Junctional diversity: During gene rearrangement in a B cell, changes that result from imprecision when gene pieces are recombined; this results in antibody with different specificity.

Kinin activation: The interaction of C2a with plasmin to produce polypeptides that promote smooth muscle contraction, mucous gland secretion, vascular permeability, and pain.

Kupffer cells: The most active phagocytic cells of the reticuloendothelial system which line the sinusoids of the liver.

Latency: The stage of acquired or congenital syphilis characterized by the absence of signs and symptoms, yet nontreponemal and treponemal antibody tests are positive.

Leukemia: Malignant proliferation of white blood cells originating in the bone marrow with a peripheral blood phase.

Leukotriene: A class of mediators synthesized from arachidonic acid in the 5-lipooxygenase pathway in mast cells; LTC_4, LTD_4 and LTE_4 constrict bronchial smooth muscle, stimulate mucus production and secretion, and cause erythema and wheal formation.

Ligand: A molecule that combines with specific complementary configurations of the binding reagents (such as receptors, proteins, or antibody).

Light chain: The peptide of the immunoglobulin molecule consisting of approximately 220 amino acids with one variable domain and one constant domain.

Linkage disequilibrium: The difference between the observed frequency of the 2 alleles occuring at two linked loci and the expected frequency of the 2 alleles occurring together due to random segregation.

Luminescence: The property of a molecule to emit a photon of light as it reverts to the stable ground state.

Lymph node: An encapsulated collection of lymphocytes and antigen-presenting cells that is a site of antigen interaction, lymphocyte recirculation, and lymphocyte proliferation.

Lymphadenopathy: Enlarged lymph nodes.

Lymphocyte phenotyping: Identification of cell surface or cytoplasmic markers that enable the class (T or B lymphocyte) or subclass or lymphocyte (helper T cell or suppressor T cell) to be quantitated.

Lymphocytosis: An increased number of lymphocytes in peripheral blood.

Lymphokine-activated killer cells (LAK): Cells that respond to IL-2, share many cell surface antigens with NK cells and can lyse target cells.

Lymphoma: Malignant tumor of cells from the lymph node.

Lymphoplasmapheresis: A method to remove lymphocytes and immunoglobulin from the blood.

Lymphoproliferative diseases: The clonal expansion of the cells of the immune system that undergo malignant transformation at a particular maturational or activation stage.

Lysozyme: An enzyme found in secretions that disrupts the cell wall of bacteria, thus killing the organism.

Major histocompatibility complex (MHC): A group of closely linked genes that produces peptides present on cell surfaces and humoral peptides that are important in transplantation, immune regulation, and immune responsiveness.

M antigens: Proteins in the cell wall of group A streptococci that determine the serotype and allow the bacterium to adhere to the host cell.

Maturational arrest: The phenomenon that results in the accumulation of malignant lymphocytes with a similar degree of maturation.

M component: A monoclonal immunoglobulin that commonly appears as a spike when seen on serum protein electrophoresis.

Mediator cells: Cells that participate in immunologic reactions by releasing biochemical substances.

Megaloblastic anemia: Decreased red blood cell function due to dysynchronous maturation of the nucleus and cytoplasm that results in mature blood cells that are larger than normal.

Mesodermal: Pertaining to the middle layer of a tissue between the endoderm and the ectoderm.

MHC Class I antigen: A dimer present on nucleated cell surfaces that is composed of β_2 microglobulin noncovalently bound to the major histocompatability complex product, a single glycoprotein chain composed of 338 amino acids with a molecular weight of 44,000 d.

MHC Class II antigen: A heterodimer major histocompatibility product composed of two glycoprotein chains, an α and a β chain, which are not covalently bound to each other but are located next to each other on the cell membrane.

MHC restriction: The phenomenon that occurs when a lymphocyte population is activated only when the antigen is presented with the appropriate MHC Class molecule.

Mitogenic factor: A substance produced by thymic macrophages that induces T-cell development.

Mitogens: Substances that induce cell division. For T and/or B cells these substances serve as the stimulus in lymphocyte transformation assays.

Mixed lymphocytes culture (MLC): A laboratory technique in which lymphocytes are transformed when exposed to genetically dissimilar lymphocytes; commonly used to detect MHC Class II molecules.

Monoclonal antibody: The transformation of a single clone of B cells to produce one class of immunoglobulin with one specificity.

Mononuclear phagocyte system: Mononuclear phagocytes located primarily in the reticular connective tissue framework of the spleen, liver, and lymphoid tissue; also called the reticuloendothelial system.

μ heavy chain disease: A rare heavy chain disease that mimics chronic lymphocytic leukemia because vacuolated lymphocytoid plasma cells frequently appear in the peripheral blood.

Multiple myeloma: A malignant growth of a single clone of plasma cell that results in a excess of homogeneous immunoglobulin.

Mycoplasma: A genus of organism lacking a cell wall; the species *Mycoplasma pneumoniae* is the etiologic agent in most cases of atypical pneumonia and can cause upper respiratory tract infections.

Mycosis fungoides: Cutaneous T cell lymphoma.

Nasopharyngeal carcinoma: A rare form of squamous cell carcinoma associated with Epstein-Barr virus infection.

Natural killer cells (NK): A group of lymphocytes that contain cytoplasmic granules and are capable of destroying virus-infected, neoplastic, or allogeneic cells without previous sensitization.

Neoantigens: New antigens expressed by tumor cells.

Neoplasm: An abnormal growth of tissue.

Nephelometric endpoint: Maximal or peak light scatter due to immune complex formation.

Nephelometric inhibition immunoassay: A nephelometric assay in which haptens form soluble complexes with hapten antiserum and prevents detectable complexes from forming between haptens bound to carrier proteins and hapten antiserum.

Nephelometry: A direct measurement of light scattered by particles suspended in solution.

Nephritic factor: An autoantibody of the IgG class which binds to alternative pathway C3 convertase preventing the normal decay of alternative pathway C3 convertase, which results in uncontrolled C3 activation.

Nezelof's syndrome: A cellular immune deficiency syndrome that is marked by T-cell dysfunction and abnormal immunoglobulin synthesis.

Nitroblue tetrazolium (NBT) test: A laboratory test used to measure the respiratory burst of neutrophils.

Non-competitive immunoassays: An assay in which labeled reagent antibody binds proportionally to the concentration of antigen; also called immunometric assays or sandwich assays.

Non-Hodgkin's lymphoma: A heterogenous group of lymphoid neoplasms that originate from lymph node cells and that lack Reed-Sternberg cells.

Non-icteric: Lacking jaundice.

Non-identity: In gel precipitation reactions, a crossed precipitin line formed when two different antigens react with antiserum.

Non-immune precipitation: In ligand assays, precipitation of protein and protein-bound ligand by altering its solubility without using antibody.

Non-specific staining: A nonimmunologic interaction of the conjugated antibody with an antigen; it may be due to the presence of free fluorochrome, interference from serum protein other than immunoglobulin, or mishandled specimens.

Nucleocapsid: A virion without a capsule.

Null cells: Peripheral blood mononucluear cells which do not express typical B or T cell markers.

Oligoclonal banding: Using high resolution gel electrophoresis of cerebrospinal fluid, the appearance of several discrete bands in the gamma region.

Oncology: The study and treatment of tumors or neoplasms.

Opsonins: Substances that enhance phagocytosis by increasing the rate and quality of uptake of a particle.

Opsonization: The process of coating an antigen with antibody or complement to provide more effective phagocytosis.

Partial identity: In gel precipitation reactions, a single precipitin line with a spur formed when one antigen shares common elements with the second, and both antigens react with the antiserum.

Passive agglutination (indirect): An agglutination reaction in which an inert carrier particle is coated with a specific antigen.

Passive hemagglutination: An agglutination reaction in which red blood cells serve as the particle and are coated with the antigen.

Passive immunity: The transient protection acquired when preformed immune products, such as antibodies, sensitized lymphocytes, and lymphokines, are administered to an individual.

Pathogenicity: The ability to cause disease.

Paul Bunnel test: A screening test to detect heterophile antibodies by reacting dilutions of heat-inactivated patient serum with a standard concentration of sheep erythrocytes and observing agglutination.

Phagocytosis: In the non-specific immune response, the process of engulfment and uptake of particles from the environment by polymorphonuclear neutrophils and macrophages.

Pharyngitis: Inflammation of the throat, often associated with pain.

Phosphorescence: A type of luminescence in which the length of time between excitation and emission of light is long (greater than 10^{-4} s).

Phytohemagglutinin (PHA): A mitogen derived from a kidney bean plant that transforms predominantly T cells.

Platelet-activating factor: A phosphorylcholine derivative that is chemotactic for neutrophils and can aggregate platelets.

Pluripotent stem cell: A precursor cell that can differentiate into many different cell types; cells of the immune system originate from primordial cells in the embryonic yolk sac and later in the bone marrow.

Pokeweed mitogen (PWM): A mitogen that stimulates predominantly B cells in a T-dependent process.

Polyclonal antibody: The increased production of different classes of immunoglobulins due to the transformation of many clones of B cells.

Polyethylene glycol: Commonly used in nephelometric assays to promote antigen-antibody complex formation.

Polymerase chain reaction (PCR): a technique to amplify a target sequence of DNA using primers.

Polymorphism: Allelic variation at a single gene locus.

Postcapillary high endothelial venule: Specialized endothelial cells of postcapillary venules in the lymph node to which T and B cells adhere and which allow lymphocytes to leave the blood stream and enter the interstitial fluid of the lymph node.

Postzone: Relative antigen excess compared to the antibody concentration that results in diminished or absent detected antigen-antibody complex.

Precipitation reaction: The formation of an insoluble complex composed of soluble antigen and soluble antibody.

Precipitins: Antibody that results in precipitation reactions.

Primary amyloidosis: A rare disorder characterized by the accumulation of a complex, extracellular, proteinaceous substance dominated by a fibrillar component.

Primary lymphoid tissue: The site of lymphocyte maturation; includes the bone marrow and thymus in the adult.

Primary syphilis: The first stage of *Treponema pallidum* infection characterized by the appearance of a chancre.

Primed: Immune cells that have been previously exposed to an antigen.

Probe: A small segment of DNA or RNA that can recognize a complementary strand.

Prodromal phase: In infectious disease, the time when non-specific symptoms appear and which occurs between the incubation phase and the acute phase.

Properdin (P): A protein of the alternative complement pathway that stabilizes the C3bBb complex to prolong the activity of C3 and C5 convertase.

Prostaglandin D2: An arachidonic acid derivative produced in mast cells that is responsible for the prolonged wheal and flare reaction in immediate hypersensitivity.

Prozone: Relative antibody excess compared to the antigen concentration that results in diminished or absent detectable antigen-antibody complex.

Pruritis: Itching.

Purified protein derivative (PPD): Antigenic material derived from a filtrate of *Mycobacterium tuberculosis* culture used in the skin test to determine exposure to *M. tuberculosis*.

Radial immunodiffusion (RID): Gel precipitation reaction in which monospecific antiserum is incorporated into the gel and soluble antigen is placed in the wells. Antigen diffuses in all directions, combines with the antibody, and forms a precipitin ring surrounding the well.

Radioallergosorbent test (RAST): A classic method to measure allergen-specific IgE in serum using a radiolabeled detector molecule.

Radioimmunosorbent test (RIST): A classic method to measure total IgE in serum using a radiolabeled detector molecule.

Radioisotope: An atom with an unstable nucleus that spontaneously emits radiation as it decays to a stable nucleus.

Radionuclide: Isomers that emit radioactivity and have a measurable life span; can be used in labeled immunoassays.

Rapid plasma reagin card test (RPR): A rapid macroscopic flocculation test performed on a disposable cardboard slide that uses the VDRL antigen plus charcoal particles added to allow macroscopic visualization of the flocculation.

Rate nephelometry: Multiple measurements during the formation of antigen-antibody complexes; the rate or speed with which the complexes form is related to the concentration of antigen present.

Raynaud's phenomenon: Ischemia in the extremities sometimes when exposed to cold temperatures.

Recombination: The exchange of genetic information between one chromosome and the homologous chromosome during meiosis.

Reagin: In syphilis serology, the antibody detected in nontreponemal testing.

Reagin screen test (RST): A macroscopic flocculation test based on the use of modified VDRL antigen with added Sudan black B for visualization of flocculation. The test can be read qualitatively and quantitatively for the screening and diagnosis of syphilis.

Reaginic antibody: Immunoglobulin E.

Reannealing: The reassociation of two denatured DNA strands.

Relative risk: The chance that an individual who expresses an HLA antigen that is associated with a disease will develop the disease compared to an individual who develops the disease but lacks the HLA antigen.

Restriction endonucleases: Enzymes which digest DNA or RNA at specific nucleotide sequences.

Reticuloendothelial system (RES): Mononuclear phagocytes located primarily in the reticular connective tissue framework of the spleen, liver, and lymphoid tissue.

Retrogenetic antigens (oncofetal antigens): Antigens that are normally expressed by fetal tissue and that can be expressed in transformed adult tissue.

Retrovirus: An RNA virus that contains reverse transcriptase, which enables the virus to make DNA from viral RNA.

Reverse passive agglutination: A passive agglutination reaction in which the carrier particle is coated with antibody.

Reverse transcriptase: An enzyme which converts RNA into DNA.

Rheumatic fever (RF): Following untreated streptococcal pharyngitis, this immune-mediated acute inflammatory disease is characterized by carditis, chorea, and erythema marginatum.

Rheumatoid factor (RF): An antibody directed against the Fc portion of an IgG molecule; only those of the IgM class are serologically detectable.

Rocky Mountain spotted fever (tick-borne typhus): A febrile disease marked by skin rash, fever, headache, and myalgia; caused by *Rickettsiae rickettsii*.

Rosette: In immunology, when three or more sheep red blood cells surround and bind to the surface of a lymphocyte; nonimmune rosettes identify T lymphocytes and sheep red blood cells coated with antibody or complement identify predominantly B lymphocytes.

Rubella (German measles): A mild contagious illness caused by the rubella virus and characterized by an erythematous maculopapular rash occurring primarily in children 5–14 years old and in young adults.

Sandwich assay: An immunoassay in which the binding reagent (usually antibody) is immobilized to an inert surface; unlabeled antigen binds to the immobilized antibody and is quantitated after labeled antigen is added; noncompetitive immunoassay.

Secondary immune response: The cellular and humoral events of the specific immune response that occur when antigen is repeatedly encountered; this immune response is greater, faster, and wider than the primary immune response due to immunologic memory.

Secondary lymphoid tissue: The sites which provide antigen and lymphocyte interaction; includes mucosal-associated lymphoid tissue, lymph nodes, bone marrow and spleen.

Secondary syphilis: The disseminated stage of *Treponema pallidum* infection that is marked by skin rashes, low-grade fever, malaise, and the presence of large numbers of treponemas throughout the body; all serologic tests are positive during this stage of the disease.

Secretory component (SC): A glycoprotein associated with secretory IgA and secretory IgM which is believed to add resistance to proteolytic enzyme digestion.

Sensitization: In serologic reactions, the binding of an antigen with antibody; in immune physiology, previous exposure to a antigen.

Sequela: A disease caused by a previous disease.

Sequestered antigen theory: A theory of autoimmunity that states that some self-antigens are hidden from cells of the immune system.

Seroconversion: The detection of specific antibody in the serum of an individual in whom this antibody was previously undetectable.

Seropositive: The presence of antibody in serum demonstrated by serologic testing.

Serum sickness: An immune complex disorder frequently found in patients who have received heterologous serum during immunotherapy and produced antibodies to the serum proteins.

Severe combined immunodeficiency (SCID): The most severe of the immunodeficiencies, characterized by the decrease or absence of both T and B lymphocytes.

Sézary cells: Malignant T cells from mycosis fungoides that are present in the peripheral blood.

Slow-reacting substances of anaphylaxis (SRS-A): Allergic metabolites of arachadonic acid (leukotrienes B_4, C_4, and D_4) that sustain smooth muscle contraction, vasodilation, and increased vasopermeability.

Specificity: The ability of an antibody to distinguish between two antigens.

Specific staining: Fluorescence that results from an immunologic reaction between the conjugated antibody and the antigen.

Splenomegaly: Enlargement of the spleen.

Staphylococcal protein A (SpA): A cell wall protein that interacts with the Fc receptor on B cells and is mitogenic for B cells.

Stasis: The complete cessation of blood flow during severe injury.

Stoke's shift: In fluorescence, the difference in nanometers between the excitation and emission wavelengths.

Streptococcus pygenes: Group A, gram-positive, β-hemolytic bacteria that cause oropharyngitis, pyoderma, scarlet fever, and rheumatic fever.

Streptozyme: A rapid, passive hemagglutination slide test to detect antibodies to any of the 5 streptococcal extracellular enzymes produced by group A β-hemolytic streptococci; patient serum and sheep erythrocytes coated with streptococcal enzymes are mixed together and observed for agglutination.

Sucrose density gradient ultracentrifugation: A technique used to separate IgM antibodies physically from IgG antibodies; the antibody-rich fraction can then be tested for the presence of a specific antibody.

Surface immunoglobulin (sIg): The unique surface marker on B cells that is synthesized by the B cell, is expressed on its surface, and serves as the antigen receptor.

Surrogate testing: One test performed to indirectly indicate a response to an antigen.

Swiss-type agammaglobulinemia: An autosomal recessive immunodeficiency that occurs in infants and is characterized by nonfunctional T and B cells.

Syngeneic: Members of the same species that are genetically identical.

Systemic lupus erythematosus (SLE): A chronic inflammatory, multisystem, autoimmune disease characterized by periods of remission and exacerbation.

TCR: T-cell receptor; a complex which is able to recognize antigen, to recognize MHC molecules, and is associated with CD3.

T-dependent antigens: Antigens that require helper T cells to generate an antibody response.

T- independent antigens: Substances capable of activating B cells without help from T cells.

Terminal deoxynucleotidyl transferase (TdT): An enzyme needed for DNA replication found predominantly in immature T cells.

Tertiary syphilis (gummatous syphilis): A slow, progressive, inflammatory disease that can produce clinical illness 2 to 40 years after initial infection and that results in neurologic and cardiovascular damage.

Theophylline: A methylxanthine that relaxes bronchial smooth muscle.

Thymocyte: Lymphoid cells of the thymus that mature and differentiate into T lymphocytes before being released into the peripheral circulation.

Thymoma: An epithelial cell tumor of the thymus.

Thymosin: A thymic hormone that promotes T-cell differentiation.

Thymus: Derived from the embryonic pharyngeal pouches, this organ provides a microenvironment in which T cells mature.

Titer: The relative concentration of antibody; in serologic testing to detect antibody, it is the reciprocal of the last serum dilution to demonstrate the presence of antibody.

Tolerance: Immunologic unresponsiveness to an antigen.

Tracer: Labeled antigen or hapten used in immunoassays, especially radioimmunoassays.

Transformation: Lymphocyte proliferation in response to a stimulus that become immunoblasts with increased cell size, nuclear size, and DNA content; the ability of lymphocytes to respond is useful to assess and monitor congenital defects, immunosuppressive therapy, and lymphokine production; in tumors, a process whereby a normal cell grows uncontrollably.

Transmitted light microscope: A fluorescence microscope in which light travels from the light source through the excitation filter, darkfield condenser, specimen, and barrier filter before it is viewed.

Treponema pallidum: An aerobic bacterium belonging to the order Spirochaetales that causes syphilis.

Treponema pallidum immobilization test (TPI): A confirmatory test for syphilis based on measuring the ability of antibody and complement to immobilize a suspension of organisms.

Tritiated thymidine: Tritium (a radioactive form of hydrogen) is incorporated into the purine base, thymidine.

Tumor: Swelling; neoplasm.

Tumor necrosis factor: Specific cytokines which promote cell death.

Turbidimetry: The measurement of light transmitted through a suspension of particles.

Unheated serum reagin test (USR): A nontreponemal, microscopic flocculation screening test that uses the choline chloride-EDTA modified VDRL antigen. Primarily used to monitor the efficacy of syphilis treatment.

Van der Waals force: A weak attractive force between the electron cloud of one atom and the nucleus of another atom.

Vaccination: The planned exposure to an infectious agent or its antigens to develop immunity against the infectious agent.

Vasculitis: A group of syndromes that have common clinicopathologic features associated with an inflammatory reaction in vessel walls.

Variable domain: A portion of the immunoglobulin peptide which is a sequence of approximately 110 amino acids and that shows amino acid variability and thus contribute to the antigen combining site of the immunoglobulin.

Venereal disease research laboratory slide test (VDRL): A standard nontreponemal screening test based on the principle of microscopic examination of patient heat-treated serum (source of reagin antibodies) for its ability to flocculate with VDRL antigen which contains 0.03% cardiolipin, 0.9% cholesterol, and 0.21% lecithin.

Viral cytopathic effect: Pathologic changes in cells resulting from viral infection.

Viral hemagglutination: A natural phenomenon that occurs when virus agglutinates red blood cells by binding to receptors on the surface of red blood cells.

Virion: A virus particle.

Virulence: The degree of pathogenicity.

Waldenström's macroglobulinemia: A rare disorder characterized by an uncontrolled proliferation of a single clone of plasma cells that synthesize homogenous IgM.

Weil-Felix test: An assay to detect rickettsial antibodies by observing agglutination with certain strains of *Proteus vulgaris*.

Western blot: The technique in which serum antibody will react with an antigen that is separated by polyacrylamide gel electrophoresis; a labeled reagent detects the serum antibody.

Wheal: Smooth, slightly elevated skin lesion with an irregular edge that is often pruritic and associated with type I hypersensitivity.

Wiskott-Aldrich syndrome: An X-linked recessive disorder that involves multiple immune defects, the presence of eczema, thrombocytopenic purpura, increased susceptibility to infection, and increased IgA and IgE levels.

Xenogeneic: Denoting members of different species with a different genetic background.

Xenograft: Tissue transplant from a donor of one species to a recipient of a different species.

Zidovudine (3'azido-3'deoxythymidine): Used to treat HIV infection, this purine analog inhibits reverse transcriptase, thus preventing viral RNA from being converted to DNA.

Index

NOTE: A *t* following a page number indicates tabular material, an *f* following a page number indicates an illustration, and a *g* following a page number indicates a glossary entry.

ENGINEERING
GRAPHICS

Books by the Authors

Basic Technical Drawing, rev. ed., by H. C. Spencer and J. T. Dygdon (Macmillan Publishing Company, 1980)

Basic Technical Drawing Problems by H. C. Spencer and J. T. Dygdon (Macmillan Publishing Company, 1972)

Descriptive Geometry, 8th ed., by E. G. Paré, R. O. Loving, I. L. Hill, and R. C. Paré (Macmillan Publishing Company, 1991)

Descriptive Geometry Worksheets with Computer Graphics, Series A, 8th ed., by E. G. Paré, R. O. Loving, I. L. Hill, and R. C. Paré (Macmillan Publishing Company, 1991)

Descriptive Geometry Worksheets with Computer Graphics, Series B, 8th ed., by E. G. Paré, R. O. Loving, I. L. Hill, and R. C. Paré (Macmillan Publishing Company, 1991)

Engineering Graphics, 5th ed., by F. E. Giesecke, A. Mitchell, H. C. Spencer, I. L. Hill, R. O. Loving, J. T. Dygdon, and J. E. Novak (Macmillan Publishing Company, 1993)

Engineering Graphics Problems, Series 1, 5th ed., by H. C. Spencer, I. L. Hill, R. O. Loving, J. T. Dygdon, and J. E. Novak (Macmillan Publishing Company, 1993)

Principles of Engineering Graphics by F. E. Giesecke, A. Mitchell, H. C. Spencer, I. L. Hill, R. O. Loving, and J. T. Dygdon (Macmillan Publishing Company, 1990)

Principles of Engineering Graphics Problems by H. C. Spencer, I. L. Hill, R. O. Loving, and J. T. Dygdon (Macmillan Publishing Company, 1990)

Principles of Technical Drawing by F. E. Giesecke, A. Mitchell, H. C. Spencer, I. L. Hill, J. T. Dygdon, and J. E. Novak (Macmillan Publishing Company, 1992)

Technical Drawing, 9th ed., by F. E. Giesecke, A. Mitchell, H. C. Spencer, I. L. Hill, J. T. Dygdon, and J. E. Novak (Macmillan Publishing Company, 1991)

Technical Drawing Problems, Series 1, 9th ed., by F. E. Giesecke, A. Mitchell, H. C. Spencer, I. L. Hill, J. T. Dygdon, and J. E. Novak (Macmillan Publishing Company, 1991)

Technical Drawing Problems, Series 2, 9th ed., by H. C. Spencer, I. L. Hill, J. T. Dygdon, and J. E. Novak (Macmillan Publishing Company, 1991)

Technical Drawing Problems, Series 3, 9th ed., by H. C. Spencer, I. L. Hill, J. T. Dygdon, and J. E. Novak (Macmillan Publishing Company, 1991)